Current Clinical Dental Terminology

*A glossary of accepted terms in
all disciplines of dentistry*

SECOND EDITION

Current Clinical
Dental Terminology

*A glossary of accepted terms in
all disciplines of dentistry*

Compiled and edited by

CARL O. BOUCHER
D.D.S., F.A.D.P., F.A.C.P., F.A.C.D.

Professor of Graduate Prosthodontics, The Ohio State University
College of Dentistry, Columbus, Ohio; Member of the Graduate Faculty
of the College of Dentistry; formerly Chairman of the Prosthodontic Division,
The Ohio State University, Columbus, Ohio; Editor, The Journal of Prosthetic Dentistry;
Editor, Glossary of Prosthodontic Terms; formerly Editor, Ohio Dental
Journal; Diplomate, American Board of Prosthodontics; Member,
Subcommittee on Terminology, International Organization for
Standardization/TC 106 for Dentistry

With forty-six contributors and collaborators

THE C. V. MOSBY COMPANY
Saint Louis 1974

SECOND EDITION

Copyright © 1974 by The C. V. Mosby Company

All rights reserved. No part of this book may be reproduced in any manner without written permission of the publisher.

Previous edition copyrighted 1963

Printed in the United States of America

Distributed in Great Britain by Henry Kimpton, London

Library of Congress Cataloging in Publication Data

Boucher, Carl O   ed.
        Current clinical dental terminology.

        1. Dentistry—Terminology.   I.   Title.
[DNLM: 1. Dictionaries, Dental.   WU 13 B753c   1973]
RK28.B68   1973   617.6′003   73-4651
ISBN 0-8016-0719-1

CB/CB/B   9   8   7   6   5   4   3   2   1

CONTRIBUTORS
AND COLLABORATORS

ANESTHESIOLOGY

Contributor

C. RICHARD BENNETT
D.D.S., Ph.D.

Associate Professor and Head of the Department of Anesthesiology, University of Pittsburgh School of Dental Medicine, Pittsburgh, Pa.; Assistant Professor, Department of Anesthesiology, University of Pittsburgh School of Medicine, Pittsburgh, Pa.; Associate Professor of Physiology and Pharmacology, University of Pittsburgh School of Dental Medicine, Pittsburgh, Pa.; Associate Professor, Graduate Faculty, University of Pittsburgh School of Dental Medicine, Pittsburgh, Pa.; Chief of Dental Services, Presbyterian-University Hospital, Pittsburgh, Pa.; Staff Anesthesiologist, Presbyterian-University Hospital, Pittsburgh, Pa.; Consultant, Children's Hospital, Magee Women's Hospital, Montefiore Hospital, Eye and Ear Hospital, Oakland Veterans Administration Hospital, Leech Farm Veterans Administration Hospital, Pittsburgh, Pa.; Consultant (Pharmacology), Council on Dental Therapeutics of the American Dental Association; Member, American Society of Oral Surgeons, Council on Hospitals.

CLEFT PALATE

Contributor

M. MAZAHERI
M.Sc., M.D.D., D.D.S.

Director, Clinical Services, Lancaster Cleft Palate Clinic, Lancaster, Pa.; Dental Surgeon, Lancaster General Hospital, Lancaster, Pa.; Lecturer, University of Pennsylvania, College of Dental Medicine, Philadelphia; Clinical Assistant Professor of Surgery, Pennsylvania State University College of Medicine, Hershey, Pa.

Collaborator

ROBERT T. MILLARD
B.S., M.A.

Director of Speech and Hearing Department, Lancaster Cleft Palate Clinic, Lancaster, Pa.; Hospital Staff and Consultant Position, Speech and Hearing Diagnostician, Research Institute, St. Joseph's Hospital, Lancaster, Pa.; Consultant for Speech and Hearing Disorders, Milton Hershey Schools, Hershey, Pa.

COMPLETE PROSTHODONTICS

Contributor

CARL O. BOUCHER
D.D.S., F.A.D.P., F.A.C.P., F.A.C.D.

Professor of Graduate Prosthodontics, The Ohio State University College of Dentistry, Columbus, Ohio; Member of the Graduate Faculty of the College of Dentistry; formerly Chairman of the Prosthodontic Division, The Ohio State University, Columbus, Ohio; Editor, The Journal of Prosthetic Dentistry; Editor, Glossary of Prosthodontic Terms; formerly Editor, Ohio Dental Journal; Diplomate, American Board of Prosthodontics; Member, Subcommittee on Terminology, International Organization for Standardization/TC 106 for Dentistry.

DENTAL JURISPRUDENCE

Contributor

HARVEY SARNER
B.S., LL.B.

Graduate of University of Minnesota School of Law; Instructor in Dental Jurisprudence, Indiana University School of Dentistry; private practice of law in Chicago.

DENTAL MATERIALS

Contributor

RALPH W. PHILLIPS
M.S., D.Sc.

Assistant Dean for Research and Research Professor of Dental Materials, Indiana University School of Dentistry, Indianapolis, Ind.

Collaborators

MARJORIE L. SWARTZ
M.S.

Professor of Dental Materials, Indiana University School of Dentistry, Indianapolis, Ind.

RICHARD D. NORMAN
D.D.S., M.S.

Professor of Dental Materials, Indiana University School of Dentistry, Indianapolis, Ind.

ENDODONTICS

Contributor

DUDLEY H. GLICK
B.S., D.D.S.

Clinical Professor, Department of Graduate Endodontics, University of Southern California, Los Angeles; Consultant, Endodontic Section, Veterans Administration Hospital, Long Beach, Calif.

Collaborators

ALFRED L. FRANK
D.D.S.

Clinical Professor, Department of Graduate Endodontics, University of Southern California, Los Angeles; Consultant, Endodontic Section, Veterans Administration Hospital, Long Beach, Calif.

JAMES H. S. SIMON
A.B., D.D.S.

Chief, Endodontic Section, Veterans Administration Hospital, Long Beach, Calif.; Clinical Assistant Professor of Endodontics, University of Southern California, Los Angeles, Calif.

FIXED PARTIAL PROSTHODONTICS

Co-contributors

SAMUEL E. GUYER
D.D.S.

Professor of Fixed Prosthodontics and Chairman, Department of Fixed Prosthodontics, Washington University School of Dental Medicine, St. Louis, Mo.; Diplomate and Member, American Board of Prosthodontics.

STANLEY D. TYLMAN
A.B., M.S., D.D.S.

Professor Emeritus, Crown and Bridge Prosthodontics, University of Illinois College of Dentistry, Chicago, Ill.

Collaborators

JOHN D. ADAMS
B.S., D.D.S.

Professor and Chairman, Department of Crown and Bridge, West Virginia University School of Dentistry, Morgantown, W. Va.

E. C. BROOKS
D.D.S.

Visiting Clinical Professor, Fixed Prosthodontics, Washington University School of Dental Medicine, St. Louis, Mo.

BOLESLAW MAZUR
B.S., M.S., D.D.S.

Professor of Fixed Prosthodontics, Loyola University School of Dentistry, Maywood, Ill.

GNATHOLOGY

Contributor

HARVEY STALLARD
Ph.B., Ph.D., D.D.S., Sc.D.

Ecologist and Orthodontist and an Associate and Colleague of B. B. McCollum and Charles E. Stuart in their studies of jaw motions and jaw relations and their methods of recording them.

Collaborator

CHARLES EDWARD STUART
D.D.S.

MAXILLOFACIAL PROSTHETICS

Contributor

WILLIAM R. LANEY
B.S., D.M.D., M.S.

Associate Professor of Dentistry, Mayo Medical School, and Consultant, Section of Prosthodontics, Department of Dentistry, Mayo Clinic and Mayo Foundation, Rochester, Minn.; Diplomate and Secretary-Treasurer, American Board of Prosthodontics.

OPERATIVE DENTISTRY

Contributor

GERALD D. STIBBS
B.S., D.M.D.

Professor of Restorative Dentistry and Special Assistant to the Dean, University of Washington School of Dentistry, Seattle, Wash.; formerly Chairman, Departments of Operative Dentistry and of Fixed Partial Dentures, and Director of Dental Operatory, University of Washington School of Dentistry, Seattle, Wash.

Collaborators

A. IAN HAMILTON
M.A., Ph.D., D.D.S.

Professor of Restorative Dentistry, University of Washington School of Dentistry, Seattle, Wash.

WILLIAM W. HOWARD
B.S., D.M.D.

Clinical Associate, University of Oregon Dental School, Portland, Ore.

ORAL DIAGNOSIS

Contributor

DONALD A. KERR
A.B., D.D.S., M.S.

Professor and Chairman, Department of Oral Pathology, University of Michigan School of Dentistry, Ann Arbor, Mich.; Professor of Pathology (for Dentistry), University of Michigan Medical School, Ann Arbor, Mich.; Staff Member, Department of Dentistry, University of Michigan Medical School, Ann Arbor, Mich.

Collaborator

RICHARD M. COURTNEY
D.D.S., M.S.

Associate Professor, Department of Oral Pathology, University of Michigan School of Dentistry, Ann Arbor, Mich.; Assistant Professor (for Dentistry), University of Michigan Medical School, Ann Arbor, Mich.

ORAL IMPLANTOLOGY

Contributor

A. NORMAN CRANIN
D.D.S.

Director, Dental and Oral Surgery, The Brookdale Hospital Medical Center, Brooklyn, N. Y.; Associate Clinical Professor of Dentistry, Mt. Sinai School of Medicine of the City University of New York; Clinical Professor of Oral Surgery, Brookdale Dental Center, New York University College of Dentistry, New York, N. Y.; Diplomate, American Board of Oral Medicine and New York Board of Oral Surgery; Associate Editor, The Journal of Prosthetic Dentistry.

Collaborator

LORD CECIL RHODES
D.D.S.

Director, Rhodes Dental Hospital, Norfolk, Va.; Member, American Academy of Implant Dentistry.

ORAL MEDICINE

Contributor

MAJOR M. ASH, Jr.
B.S., M.S., D.D.S.

Professor of Dentistry, University of Michigan School of Dentistry, Ann Arbor, Mich.

ORAL PATHOLOGY

Contributor

JOSEPH L. BERNIER
D.D.S., M.S., F.I.C.O., F.D.S., R.C.S.(Eng.)

Major General, U. S. Army (Ret'd); former Chief, Army Dental Corps; Professor and Chairman, Department of Oral Pathology, Georgetown University School of Dentistry, Washington, D. C.

ORAL PHYSIOLOGY

Co-contributors

DOUGLAS A. ATWOOD
M.D., D.M.D.

Chairman, Department of Prosthetic Dentistry, Harvard School of Dental Medicine, Boston, Mass.; Assistant Dean for Developments and Director of Clinics, Harvard School of Dental Medicine, Boston, Mass.; Junior Associate in Surgery (Dentistry), Peter Bent Brigham Hospital, Boston, Mass.; Director, Training Center for Clinical Scholars in Oral Biology, Harvard School of Dental Medicine, Boston, Mass.

SIDNEY I. SILVERMAN
B.S., D.D.S.

Professor and Chairman, Removable Prothodontics, Brookdale Dental Center, New York University College of Dentistry, New York, N. Y.; Diplomate, American Board of Prosthodontics; Consultant, Veterans Hospital, New York City; Attending Dental Surgeon, University Hospital, New York University.

ORAL RADIOLOGY

Contributor

LINCOLN R. MANSON-HING
D.M.D., M.S.

Professor and Chairman, Department of Dental Radiology, University of Alabama in Birmingham School of Dentistry, Birmingham, Ala.; Editor and Past President of the American Academy of Dental Radiology; Consultant to Veterans Administration Hospital, Birmingham, Ala.

Collaborator

DAVID F. GREER
B.S., D.M.D., M.S.

Associate Professor of Dentistry, Department of Dental Radiology, University of Alabama in Birmingham School of Dentistry, Birmingham, Ala.

ORAL SURGERY

Contributor

MORGAN L. ALLISON
D.D.S.

Reagents Professor, Chairman of Continuing Education, and Chairman, Section on Anesthesiology, The Ohio State University College of Dentistry, Columbus, Ohio; Director, Clinical Division of Dentistry, The University Hospitals, The Ohio State University, Columbus, Ohio; Associate Professor of Physiology, The Ohio State University College of Medicine; Diplomate, American Board of Oral Surgery.

Collaborators

CHARLES C. ALLING
M.Sc., D.D.S.

Colonel, U. S. Army (Ret'd); Professor and Chairman of Oral Surgery, University of Alabama in Birmingham School of Dentistry, Birmingham, Ala.; Chief, Section of Oral Surgery, University Hospital, University of Alabama, Birmingham, Ala.

†LEONARD MONHEIM
B.S., M.S., D.D.S.

ORTHODONTICS

Contributor

EARL E. SHEPARD
D.D.S.

Clinical Professor of Orthodontics, Washington University School of Dental Medicine, St. Louis, Mo.

Collaborators

WILLIAM ALLEN
M.S., D.D.S.

Professor of Orthodontics, Washington University School of Dental Medicine, St. Louis, Mo.

FRED FABRIC
Ph.D, M.S., D.D.S.

Formerly Assistant Professor of Orthodontics, Washington University School of Dental Medicine, St. Louis, Mo.

PEDODONTICS

Contributor

RALPH E. McDONALD
D.D.S., M.S.

Professor of Pedodontics and Dean, Indiana University School of Dentistry, Indianapolis, Ind.

PERIODONTICS

Contributor

HENRY M. GOLDMAN
D.M.D.

Dean, Boston University School of Graduate Dentistry; Professor of Stomatology, School of Graduate Dentistry; Professor and Chairman, Department of Stomatology, Boston University School of Medicine, Boston, Mass.

PHARMACOLOGY

Contributor

J. ROY DOTY
Ph.D.

Formerly Secretary, Council on Dental Therapeutics of the American Dental Association.

PRACTICE MANAGEMENT

Contributor

†JAMES B. BUSH
D.D.S., M.S.

REMOVABLE PARTIAL PROSTHODONTICS

Contributor

DAVIS HENDERSON
D.D.S.

Professor and Chairman, Division of Removable Partial Prosthodontics, University of Florida College of Dentistry, Gainesville, Fla.; Diplomate and Member, American Board of Prosthodontics.

Collaborators

CHESTER K. PERRY
D.D.S., M.Sc.

Professor of Denture Prosthetics, University of Detroit School of Dentistry, Detroit, Mich.; Diplomate and Member, American Board of Prosthodontics.

OLIVER C. APPLEGATE
D.D.S., D.D.Sc.

Professor Emeritus and formerly Director of Partial Denture Prosthetics, School of Dentistry, and W. K. Kellogg Foundation Institute of Graduate and Postgraduate Dentistry, University of Michigan, Ann Arbor, Mich.

APPENDIX

Contributor

DUNCAN McCONNELL
Ph.D.

Professor of Dentistry (Research), The Ohio State University College of Dentistry, Columbus, Ohio; Professor of Geology and Mineralogy, The Ohio State University, Columbus, Ohio.

†Deceased.

†Deceased.

To my wife

whose patience, tolerance,
help, understanding, and encouragement
made this book possible

FOREWORD

This glossary is an important step toward efficient communication in dentistry. By its very nature it emphasizes that language is a precision tool that must be used with understanding and skill. Moreover, it brings into sharp focus a problem that teachers of science writing have stressed for some time—the need for uniform terminology. If too many terms are used for the same thing or too many meanings used for the same term, the original purpose of technical words is lost, for technical language can be justified only if it is more accurate or more efficient than lay language.

The extensiveness of this glossary should not cause concern. It is not an indication that dentistry has become so complex that dental writing must be difficult. On the contrary, a knowledge of the correct use of scientific dental terms will make writing easier and will result in a better understanding of that which is written. The dental writer should also keep in mind that only a fraction of the words he uses are technical. A study just completed under a National Institutes of Health grant shows that 710 dental and scientific words account for 80 percent of the professional terms used in dental journals.

The writer who wants to get his message across as quickly and as effectively as possible will welcome the glossary as a new tool that will add the power of precision to his professional language. But he will never forget that effective writing demands far more than the ability to use technical terms. He must have something worthwhile to say and he must possess a broad knowledge of language.

†George J. Kienzle, B.A.
Formerly Professor and Director,
The Ohio State University
School of Journalism,
Columbus, Ohio

†Deceased.

x

PREFACE

This glossary of clinical dental terminology contains the tools of communication currently used in twenty-three areas of dental practice. It also includes an appendix with basic information of interest to dentists and dental students. The forty-six contributors and collaborators are leaders in their respective fields, and they represent all geographic sections of the United States. By using words that convey the precise message they want to express, they have been effective in communicating their concepts and techniques to dentists throughout the world. This glossary supplies the words they use and the meanings of the words so that there can be no misunderstanding.

Over 10,000 terms and definitions have been supplied and more than one definition for some of the terms have been suggested. Since each discipline in dentistry seems to have its own language, terms have been found to have different meanings in the different areas of dental practice, leading to confusion in the literature and misunderstanding among dentists, dental teachers, and researchers. This glossary gives the various meanings assigned to the same terms by different specialties. The special area of practice in which each definition is used is indicated in parentheses at the end of the definition.

The objective of this glossary is to provide a means for better understanding of the broad range of interest in dentistry and better communication between practitioners and between teachers and their students.

The number of terms having different meanings has been reduced in this second edition of the glossary. As this revision was developed, an effort was made to combine definitions or to select preferred definitions that would satisfy the requirements of all concerned. The result has been a reduction in the number of definitions in relation to the number of terms, which is a step toward more effective communication and better understanding of the principles, concepts, and practices of dentistry. The fact that the definitions of some terms (as included in the first edition) have been combined indicates that the differences in the concepts of the various areas of dental practice are not as great as some have believed. As long as one word has a meaning for the speaker, writer, or teacher different from the meaning it has for the listener, reader, or student, there will be misunderstanding of the message that is intended. This glossary can help in the selection of the spoken or written word and in the effective reception of the intended idea by the student. Constant practice by all who use the tools of dental communication will develop the habit of using the right word to express an idea in the best possible manner. This glossary is intended to be helpful to dental teachers, students, essayists, clinicians, practitioners, hygienists, assistants, laboratory technicians, and manufacturers, as well as operators of dental prepayment plans. It can smooth the road to understanding among all who have a part in providing dental health care.

The terms used in two additional areas of dental practice have been included in this second edition of the glossary. Gnathology and maxillofacial prosthetics use a number of terms that are not commonly employed by other disciplines in dentistry. Definitions of some terms are uniquely related to their philosophies or techniques. Their inclusion should help in understanding gnathology and maxillofacial prosthetics.

The main section of the glossary contains alphabetically arranged definitions of terms as they are understood and used in each area of clinical dental practice. Many of the definitions have been simplified as a result of critical analysis of those in the first edition. The many contributors and their collaborators have made outstanding contributions to this important step toward better understanding; they have my sincere appreciation. The appendix includes conversion tables for weights and measures, which are especially valuable at this time because of the ongoing change to the metric system throughout the world.

The efforts of all the contributors and collaborators were essential to this revision of the glossary. They have my thanks and sincere appreciation for a job well done.

One of the problems of dental students, hygiene students, and assistants has been to learn how to pronounce the words used by the dental profession that are new to them. Guidance in this direction is provided in this edition. I am grateful to my wife for supplying the diacritical marks that indicate the correct pronunciation of the often complicated words.

I wish to acknowledge the assistance of those persons who have assisted in preparation of the revised material for this book. My thanks go again to my wife, who prepared a card for every term and definition and arranged them in alphabetical order; later she read proof of the typed manuscript in its final form.

Also, I wish to gratefully acknowledge the assistance of the persons who did the typing: Penny George, Susan McClain, and Colleen Ringle.

Carl O. Boucher

ACKNOWLEDGMENTS

Grateful acknowledgment is made to the authors and publishers of the following publications used as reference sources by the various contributors and collaborators:

Adopted terminology, American Academy of Pedodontics, 1961.

Adriani, J.: The pharmacology of anesthetic drugs, ed. 4, Springfield, Ill., 1960, Charles C Thomas, Publisher.

Aita, J. A.: Congenital facial anomalies with neurologic defects, Springfield, Ill., 1969, Charles C Thomas, Publisher.

Allen, E. V., and Barker, H.: Peripheral vascular diseases, Philadelphia, 1962, W. B. Saunders Co.

American Academy of Maxillofacial Prosthetics, Workshop on Nomenclature, 1971 Annual Meeting.

American Academy of Oral Roentgenology: Glossary of terms used in dental radiology, 1964.

American Public Health Association: Services for children with cleft lip and cleft palate, New York, 1955; copyright by American Public Health Association, Inc.

Anderson, G. M.: Practical orthodontics, ed. 9, St. Louis, 1960, The C. V. Mosby Co.

Anderson, W. A. D., editor: Pathology, ed. 6, St. Louis, 1971, The C. V. Mosby Co.

Angle, E. H.: Angle system of regulation and retention of the teeth, and treatment of fractures of the maxillae, ed. 7, Philadelphia, 1902, S. S. White Dental Manufacturing Co.

Annotated glossary of terms used in endodontics, C. G. Maurice, Chairman, Nomenclature Committee, American Association of Endodontists, Oral Surgery, Oral Medicine and Oral Pathology, St. Louis, 1968, The C. V. Mosby Co.

Archer, W. H.: Oral surgery; a step-by-step atlas of operative techniques, ed. 3, Philadelphia, 1961, W. B. Saunders Co.

Ash, Major M.: A handbook of differential oral diagnosis, St. Louis, 1961, The C. V. Mosby Co.

Bard, P.: Medical physiology, ed. 10, St. Louis, 1956, The C. V. Mosby Co.

Bassett, R. W., Ingraham, R., and Koser, J. R.: An atlas of gold restorations, Los Angeles, 1964, University of Southern California.

Beckman, H.: Pharmacology—the nature, action and use of drugs, ed. 2, Philadelphia, 1961, W. B. Saunders Co.

Behrman, S. J.: The implantation of magnets in the jaw to aid denture retention, J. Prosthet. Dent. 10:807-841, 1960.

Bennett, C. R.: Monheim's general anesthesia in dental practice, ed. 4, St. Louis, 1974, The C. V. Mosby Co.

Bennett, C. R.: Monheim's local anesthesia and pain control in dental practice, ed. 5, St. Louis, 1974, The C. V. Mosby Co.

Bernier, J. L.: Management of oral disease, ed. 2, St. Louis, 1959, The C. V. Mosby Co.

Berry, M. F., and Eisenson, J.: Speech disorders: principles and practices of therapy, New York, 1956, Appleton-Century-Crofts.

Bhaskar, S. N.: Synopsis of oral pathology, ed. 3, St. Louis, 1969, The C. V. Mosby Co.

Black, H. C.: Black's law dictionary, St. Paul, Minn., West Publishing Co.; by permission of West Publishing Co., copyright holder.

Blackwell, R. E.: G. V. Black's operative dentistry, ed. 9, South Milwaukee, 1955, Medico-Dental Publishing Co.

Blakiston's new Gould medical dictionary, ed. 2, New York, 1956, The Blakiston Division, McGraw-Hill Book Co.

Blass, J. L.: Motivating patients for more effective dental service, Philadelphia, 1958, J. B. Lippincott Co.

Bodine, R. L., Jr.: Implant dentures: prosthodontic-favorable, J. Prosthet. Dent. 10:1132-1142, 1960.

Boucher, C. O., editor: Swenson's complete dentures, ed. 6, St. Louis, 1970, The C. V. Mosby Co. (Seventh edition to be published in 1975.)

Bowen, W. B.: Applied anatomy and kinesiology, Philadelphia, 1934, Lea & Febiger.

Boyle, P. E.: Kronfeld's histopathology of the teeth and their surrounding structures, ed. 3, Philadelphia, 1949, Lea & Febiger.

Brauer, J. D., and others: Dentistry for children, ed. 3, New York, 1952, The Blakiston Division, McGraw-Hill Book Co.

Brodnitz, F. S.: Keep your voice healthy, New York, 1953, Harper & Brothers (Harper & Row, Publishers).

Burnett, G. W., and Scherp, H. W.: Oral microbiology and infectious disease, Baltimore, 1957, The Williams & Wilkins Co.

Carnahan, C. W.: The dentist and the law, St. Louis, 1955, The C. V. Mosby Co.

Chusid, J. G., and McDonald, J. J.: Correlative neuroanatomy and functional neurology, ed. 11, Los Altos, Calif., 1962, Lange Medical Publications.

Cohen, M. M.: Pediatric dentistry, ed. 2, St. Louis, 1961, The C. V. Mosby Co.

Colby, R. A., Kerr, D. A., and Robinson, H. B. G.: Color atlas of oral pathology, ed. 3, Philadelphia, 1971, J. B. Lippincott Co.

Collins, V. J.: Principles of anesthesiology, Philadelphia, 1966, Lea & Febiger.

Cooper, H. K.: Integration of services in the treatment of cleft lip and cleft palate, J. Am. Dent. Assoc. **47:**27-32, 1953.

Cooper, H. K.: Oral aspects of rehabilitation, J. Am. Coll. Dent. **27:**52-59, 1960.

Cooper, H. K., Long, R. E., Cooper, J. A., Mazaheri, M., and Millard, R. T.: Psychological, orthodontic, and prosthetic approaches in rehabilitation of the cleft palate patient, Dent. Clin. North Am. **4:**381-393, July, 1960.

Cranin, A. N.: Nomenclature, J. Implant Dent. **2:**41-44, 1956.

Cranin, A. N.: Some philosophic comments on the endosseous implant, Dent. Clin. North Am. **14:**173-184, 1970.

Cranin, A. N., and Dennison, T. A.: Blade and anchor construction technics, J. Am. Dent. Assoc. **83:**833-839, 1971.

Denton, G. B.: The vocabulary of dentistry and oral science, Chicago, 1958, American Dental Association.

Dobbs, E. C.: Pharmacology and oral therapeutics, ed. 12, St. Louis, 1961, The C. V. Mosby Co.

Dorland's illustrated medical dictionary, ed. 24, Philadelphia, 1965, W. B. Saunders Co.

Etter, E.: Glossary of words and phrases used in radiology and nuclear medicine, Springfield, Ill., 1960, Charles C Thomas, Publisher.

Fairbanks, G.: Voice and articulation drill book, New York, 1940, Harper & Brothers (Harper & Row, Publishers).

Finn, S. B., Volker, J. F., and Cheraskin, E.: Clinical pedodontics, Philadelphia, 1957, W. B. Saunders Co.

Fischer, B.: Orthodontics, ed. 2, Philadelphia, 1957, W. B. Saunders Co.

Gabel, A. B.: American textbook of operative dentistry, ed. 9, Philadelphia, 1954, Lea & Febiger.

Gellhorn, E.: Physiological foundations of neurology and psychiatry, Minneapolis, 1953, University of Minnesota Press; copyright 1953 by the University of Minnesota.

Gilmore, H. W., and Lund, M. R.: Operative dentistry, ed. 2, St. Louis, 1973, The C. V. Mosby Co.

Glasser, O.: Medical physics, Chicago, 1944, Year Book Medical Publishers, Inc.

Goldberg, N. L., and Gershhoff, A.: The implant lower denture, Dent. Dig. **55:**490, 1949.

Goldman, H. M., and Cohen, D. W.: Periodontal therapy, ed. 4, St. Louis, 1968, The C. V. Mosby Co.

Goldman, H. M., and Cohen, D. W.: An introduction to periodontia, ed. 4, St. Louis, 1969, The C. V. Mosby Co.

Goldman, H. M., Schluger, S., Cohen, D. W., Chaikin, B., and Fox, L.: An introduction to periodontia, ed. 3, St. Louis, 1966, The C. V. Mosby Co.

Goldman, H. M., Schluger, S., Fox, L., and Cohen, D. W.: Periodontal therapy, ed. 2, St. Louis, 1960, The C. V. Mosby Co.

Goodman, L. S., and Gilman, A.: The pharmacological basis of therapeutics, ed. 2, New York, 1955, The Macmillan Co.

Goodman, L. S., and Gilman, A.: The pharmacological basis of therapeutics, ed. 4, New York, 1970, The Macmillan Co.

Gorlin, R. J., editor: Summary of the Workshop on Ulcerative and Bullous Disorders of the Orofacial Region, J. Dent. Res. **50:**795-815, 1971.

Gorlin, R. J., and Goldman, H. M.: Thoma's oral pathology, ed. 6, St. Louis, 1970, The C. V. Mosby Co.

Gorlin, R. J., and Pindborg, J. J.: Syndromes of the head and neck, New York, 1964, Mc-Graw-Hill Book Co.

Goth, A.: Medical pharmacology—principles and concepts, ed. 7, St. Louis, 1974, The C. V. Mosby Co.

Graber, T. M.: Orthodontics, principles and practice, Philadelphia, 1961, W. B. Saunders Co.

Grant, D. A., Stern, I. B., and Everett, F. G.: Orban's periodontics, ed. 4, St. Louis, 1972, The C. V. Mosby Co.

Gray, G. W., and Wise, C. M.: Bases of speech, ed. 3, New York, 1958, Harper & Brothers (Harper & Row, Publishers).

Gregory, W. K.: Evolution emerging, vol. 1, New York, 1957, The Macmillan Co.

Grossman, L. I.: Endodontic practice, ed. 7, Philadelphia, 1970, Lea & Febiger.

Gruebbel, A. O., consulting editor: Symposium on Practice Administration, Dent. Clin. North Am. 5:March, 1961.

Guide to dental materials and devices, ed. 6, Chicago, 1972-1973, American Dental Association.

Harris, T. A. B.: Mode of action of anesthetics, Baltimore, 1951, The Williams & Wilkins Co.

Healey, H. J.: Endodontics, St. Louis, 1960, The C. V. Mosby Co.

Henderson, D., and Steffel, V. L.: McCracken's partial denture construction, ed. 3, St. Louis, 1969, The C. V. Mosby Co.

Hine, M. K., editor: Review of dentistry, ed. 5, St. Louis, 1970, The C. V. Mosby Co.

Hollinshead, W. H.: Functional anatomy of the limbs and back, Philadelphia, 1952, W. B. Saunders Co.

Howard, W. W.: An atlas of operative dentistry, St. Louis, 1968, The C. V. Mosby Co.

Ingle, J. I.: Endodontics, Philadelphia, 1965, Lea & Febiger.

Ingraham, R., Koser, J. R., and Quint, H.: An atlas of gold foil and rubber dam, Buena Park, Calif., 1961, Uni-Tro College Procedures Press.

Jermyn, A. C.: Peri-implantoclasia—cause and treatment, J. Implant Dent. 5:25-49, 1958.

Johnston, J. F., Phillips, R. W., and Dykema, R.: Modern practice in crown and bridge prosthodontics, Philadelphia, 1960, W. B. Saunders Co.

Kantner, C. E., and West, R.: Phonetics, New York, 1941, Harper & Brothers (Harper & Row, Publishers), pp. 39-54.

Kazanjian, V. H., and Converse, J. M.: The surgical treatment of facial injuries, ed. 2, Baltimore, 1959, The Williams & Wilkins Co.

Kerr, D. A., Ash, M. M., Jr., and Millard, H. D.: Oral diagnosis, ed. 3, St. Louis, 1970, The C. V. Mosby Co.

Kilpatrick, H. C.: High speed and ultraspeed in dentistry, Philadelphia, 1959, W. B. Saunders Co.

Kruger, G. O., editor: Textbook of oral surgery, ed. 4, St. Louis, 1974, The C. V. Mosby Co.

Langley, L. L., and Cheraskin, E.: The physiological foundation of dental practice, St. Louis, 1956, The C. V. Mosby Co.

Levy, I. R.: Textbook for dental assistants, ed. 2, Philadelphia, 1942, Lea & Febiger.

Loechler, P. S., and Mueller, M. W.: Successful implant dentures, North-west Dent. 31:134-139, 1952.

Longacre, J. J., editor: Craniofacial anomalies, Philadelphia, 1968, J. B. Lippincott Co.

Mann, W. R., and Easlick, K. A.: Practice administration for the dentist, St. Louis, 1955, The C. V. Mosby Co.

McCall, J. O.: Practical dental assisting, Brooklyn, 1948, Dental Items of Interest Publishing Co., Inc.

McCoy, J. D., and Shepard, E. E.: Applied orthodontics, ed. 7, Philadelphia, 1956, Lea & Febiger.

McDonald, R. E.: Dentistry for the child and adolescent, ed. 2, St. Louis, 1974, The C. V. Mosby Co.

McGehee, W. H. O., True, H. A., and Inskipp, E. F.: A textbook of operative dentistry, ed. 4, New York, 1956, The Blakiston Division, McGraw-Hill Book Co.

Metals handbook, Metals Park, Ohio, 1961, American Society for Metals.

Mitchell, D. F., Standish, S. M., and Fast, T. B.: Oral diagnosis/oral medicine, Philadelphia, 1971, Lea & Febiger.

Morrey, L. W., and Nelsen, R. J.: Dental science handbook, Washington, D. C., 1970, U. S. Department of Health, Education, and Welfare.

Morrison, G. A.: In the dentist's office, Philadelphia, 1959, J. B. Lippincott Co.

Moyers, R. E.: Handbook of orthodontics, Chicago, 1958, Year Book Medical Publishers, Inc.

Nagle, R. J., and Sears, V. H.: Dental prosthetics, St. Louis, 1959, The C. V. Mosby Co.

National Bureau of Standards Handbook 59, Permissible dose from external sources of ionizing radiation, Washington, D. C., 1954, U. S. Government Printing Office.

Nomenclature Committee, The Academy of Denture Prosthetics: Glossary of prosthodontic terms, ed. 3, St. Louis, 1968, The C. V. Mosby Co.

Nomenclature Committee, American Association for Cleft Palate Rehabilitation: Proposed morphological classification of congenital cleft lip and cleft palate, Cleft Palate Bull. **10:** 11-16, 1960.

Oral surgery glossary, Committee on Hospital Oral Surgery Service, 1971, American Society of Oral Surgeons.

Orban, B.: Oral histology and embryology, ed. 2, St. Louis, 1949, The C. V. Mosby Co.

Orban, B., and Wentz, F. M.: Atlas of clinical pathology of the oral mucous membrane, St. Louis, 1960, The C. V. Mosby Co.

Orten, J. M., and Neuhaus, O. W.: Biochemistry, ed. 8, St. Louis, 1970, The C. V. Mosby Co.

Peyton, F. A., and Craig, R. G.: Restorative dental materials, ed. 4, St. Louis, 1971, The C. V. Mosby Co.

Phillips, R. W.: Skinner's science of dental materials, ed. 7, Philadelphia, 1973, W. B. Saunders Co.

Poppel, M. H., editor: Radiopaque diagnosis agents, Ann. N. Y. Acad. Sci. **78:**705, 1959.

Prinz, H.: Dental materia medica and therapeutics, ed. 5, St. Louis, 1922, The C. V. Mosby Co.

Robbins, S. L.: Textbook of pathology, Philadelphia, 1962, W. B. Saunders Co.

Romer, A. S.: The vertebrate body, Philadelphia, 1962, W. B. Saunders Co.

Ruch, T. C., and Fulton, J. F., editors: Medical physiology and biophysics, Philadelphia, 1960, W. B. Saunders Co.

Salzmann, J. A.: Principles of orthodontics, ed. 3, Philadelphia, 1950, W. B. Saunders Co.

Salzmann, J. A.: Orthodontics: principles and prevention, vol. I, Philadelphia, 1957, J. B. Lippincott Co.

Salzmann, J. A.: Orthodontics: practice and techniques, vol. II, Philadelphia, 1957, J. B. Lippincott Co.

Sarnat, B. G.: The temporomandibular joint, Springfield, Ill., 1951, Charles C Thomas, Publisher.

Sassouni, V., with the collaboration of Forrest, E. J.: Orthodontics in dental practice, St. Louis, 1971, The C. V. Mosby Co.

Schroeter, C.: Dentition of man, Seattle, 1966, University of Washington Press.

Schwartz, J. R.: Inlays and abutments, Brooklyn, 1952, Dental Items of Interest Publishing Company, Inc.

Schwarzrock, L. H., and Schwarzrock, S. P.: Effective dental assisting, ed. 2, Dubuque, Iowa, 1959, William C. Brown Co.

Seltzer, S.: Endodontology, New York, 1971, The Blakiston Division, McGraw-Hill Book Co.

Selye, H.: Stress of life, New York, 1956, McGraw-Hill Book Co.

Shafer, W. G., Hine, M. K., and Levy, B. M.: A textbook of oral pathology, Philadelphia, 1958, W. B. Saunders Co.

Sharry, J. J.: Complete denture prosthodontics, ed. 2, New York, 1968, McGraw-Hill Book Co.

Shepard, E. E.: Technique and treatment with the twin-wire appliance, St. Louis, 1961, The C. V. Mosby Co.

Sherrington, C. S.: The integrative action of the nervous system, ed. 2, New Haven, Conn., 1947, Yale University Press.

Sicher, H., and DuBrul, E. L.: Oral anatomy, ed. 5, St. Louis, 1970, The C. V. Mosby Co.

Silverman, S. I.: Oral physiology, St. Louis, 1961, The C. V. Mosby Co.

Silverman, S. I., and Tobis, J. S.: Nutrition and dental care in a physical medicine and rehabilitation program, Arch. Phys. Med. **39:** 555-559, 1958.

Slobody, L. B.: Survey of clinical pediatrics, New York, 1959, The Blakiston Division, McGraw-Hill Book Co.

Sodeman, W. A.: Pathologic physiology, ed. 2, Philadelphia, 1957, W. B. Saunders Co.

Sommer, R. F., Ostrander, F. D., and Crowley,

M. C.: Clinical endodontics, ed. 3, Philadelphia, 1966, W. B. Saunders Co.

Souder, W. H., and Paffenbarger, G. C.: Physical properties of dental materials, National Bureau of Standards Circular No. C433, Washington, D. C., 1942, U. S. Government Printing Office.

Stedman's medical dictionary, ed. 22, Baltimore, 1972, The Williams & Wilkins Co.

Stibbs, G. D.: Textbook of operative dentistry, St. Louis, 1967, The C. V. Mosby Co.

Stibbs, G. D.: Cavity preparations, Seattle, 1969, The University of Washington Press.

Stinaff, R. K.: Dental practice administration, ed. 3, St. Louis, 1968, The C. V. Mosby Co.

Storch, C. B.: Fundamentals of clinical fluoroscopy, New York, 1951, Grune & Stratton, Inc.

Taber, C. W.: Cyclopedic medical dictionary, ed. 8, Philadelphia, 1958, F. A. Davis Co.

Tarpley, B. W.: Technique and treatment with the labiolingual appliance, St. Louis, 1961, The C. V. Mosby Co.

The American college dictionary, New York, 1962, Random House, Inc.; by permission of Random House, Inc.

Terkla, L. G., and Laney, W. R.: Partial dentures, ed. 3, St. Louis, 1963, The C. V. Mosby Co.

Thoma, K. H.: Oral surgery, ed. 5, St. Louis, 1969, The C. V. Mosby Co.

Thoma, K. H., and Robinson, H. B. B.: Oral and dental diagnosis, ed. 5, Philadelphia, 1960, W. B. Saunders Co.

Thurow, R. C.: Edgewise orthodontics, ed. 3, St. Louis, 1973, The C. V. Mosby Co.

Tiecke, R. W., Stuteville, O. H., and Calandra, J. C.: Pathological physiology of oral disease, St. Louis, 1959, The C. V. Mosby Co.

Tocchine, J. J.: Restorative dentistry, New York, 1967, The Blakiston Division, McGraw-Hill Book Co.

Travis, L., and others: Handbook of speech pathology, New York, 1957, Appleton-Century-Crofts.

Tylman, S. D.: Theory and practice of crown and fixed partial prosthodontics (bridge), ed. 6, St. Louis, 1970, The C. V. Mosby Co.

Van Riper, C., and Irwin, J. V.: Voice and articulation, Englewood Cliffs, N. J., 1958, Prentice-Hall, Inc.

Webster's third new international dictionary of the English language (unabridged), Springfield, Mass., 1961, G. & C. Merriam Co.

Weinmann, J. P., and Sicher, H.: Bone and bones, St. Louis, 1955, The C. V. Mosby Co.

West, R., Ansberry, M., and Carr, A.: The rehabilitation of speech, New York, 1957, Harper & Brothers (Harper & Row, Publishers).

Wheeler, R. C.: A textbook of dental anatomy and physiology, ed. 4, Philadelphia, 1965, W. B. Saunders Co.

Wuehrmann, A. H.: Radiation protection and dentistry, St. Louis, 1960, The C. V. Mosby Co.

Wuehrmann, A. H., and Manson-Hing, L. R.: Dental radiology, ed. 2, St. Louis, 1969, The C. V. Mosby Co.

CONTENTS

Pronunciation guide

ā	as in	wait
ă	as in	bat
ah	as in	ma
ē	as in	me
ĕ	as in	met
e	as in	her
ī	as in	my
ĭ	as in	bit
ō	as in	boat
ŏ	as in	hot
o	as in	or
oo	as in	loose
ū	as in	due
ŭ or uh	as in	but
ul	as in	full

Current Clinical Dental Terminology

A glossary of accepted terms in
all disciplines of dentistry

❧ A ❧

Å Abbreviation for Ångström unit.

a nativitate (nă-tĭv′ĭ-tāt) A condition existing at birth or from infancy; denotes that a disability is congenital. (D. Juris.)

A point (see **point, A**)

aa (ana) Greek term meaning of each. (Oral Med.; Pharmacol.)

ab antecedente A notice given previously or a condition existing earlier. (D. Juris.)

abacterial (ā-băk-tē′rē-ăl) Nonbacterial; free from bacteria. (Anesth.)

abandonment Discontinuance of treatment, with or without cause. (D. Juris.)

abatement (ah-bāt′mĕnt) Decrease in severity of pain or symptoms. (Anesth.)

Abbé-Estlander operation (ăb-ā′ ĕst′lănd-er) (see **operation, Abbé-Estlander**)

abduce (ăb-doos′) To draw away; abduct. (Anesth.)

abduct (ăb-dŭkt′) To draw away from the median line or from a neighboring part or limb. (Anesth.)

abduction (ăb-dŭk′shŭn) The process of moving away from each other, as the two vocal bands; opposite of adduction. (Oral Physiol.)

aberrant (ăb-ĕr′ănt) Deviation from the usual or normal course, location, or action. (Oral Surg.)

abnormal frenum attachment (see **attachment, abnormal frenum**)

abrade (ah-brād′) To wear away by friction.

abrasion (ah-brā′zhŭn) Grinding or wearing away of tooth substance by mastication, incorrect brushing methods, bruxism, or similar causes. (Fixed Part. Prosth.; Remov. Part. Prosth.)

— An area from which the normal surface tissue (enamel, cementum, dentin) has been removed from a tooth by an abrasive or by an abrading action. (Oper. Dent.)

— Rubbing or scraping of a surface. The mechanical wearing away of the teeth by forces other than those of mastication. (Oral Diag.)

— Normal or abnormal loss of tooth structure due to friction caused by physiologic or pathologic forces interacting between the tooth and an abrasive substance or object or between the tooth and another tooth or teeth. (Oral Path.)

— A wound produced by the rubbing or scraping off of the covering surface. (Oral Surg.)

— Abnormal wear of tooth and/or soft tissues produced by abrasive dentifrices, faulty toothbrushing, buccolingual movement of the teeth (on contact areas of teeth), or habit patterns such as bruxism and clenching. (Periodont.)

dentifrice a. Wearing away of the cementum and dentin of an exposed root by an abrasive-containing dentifrice. (Oral Diag.)

denture a. Grinding or wearing away of any denture part by improper finishing, mastication, incorrect brushing methods, bruxism, or similar causes. (Remov. Prosth.)

gingival a. (see **gingiva, abrasion**)

abrasive (ah-brā′sĭv) A substance that will wear away a material by friction. Used in dentistry for cutting and polishing; e.g., stones and disks for cutting and pumice and metal oxides for polishing. (Remov. Part. Prosth.; D. Mat.; Oper. Dent.)

a. disk (see **disk, abrasive**)

a. point, rotary (see **point, abrasive, rotary**)

a. strip (see **strip, abrasive**)

abscess (ăb′sĕs) A circumscribed localized collection of pus in tissue. (Endodont.; Oral Diag.)

— A localized collection of pus in a cavity formed by the disintegration of tissue and surrounded by a limiting "membrane." (Oper. Dent.; Oral. Path.) (see also **pyogenic**)

alveolar a. (periapical a.) An abscess occurring in the apical region of an alveolus as a sequela of pulp death. May be acute or chronic. (Oper. Dent.)

dentoalveolar a. An acute inflammation of the periapical tissues characterized by a localized accumulation of pus. (Oral Diag.)

periapical a. An abscess occurring at the apical region of a tooth due to the death of the pulp of that tooth. (Oral Path.)

periodontal a. A localized area of acute or chronic inflammation found in the gingival corium, infrabony pockets, or periodontal membrane. Polymorphonuclear leukocytes are the inflammatory cells principally seen in the acute type, whereas round cells, plasma cells, and lymphocytes predominate in the chronic type. Chronic abscesses may be encapsulated, whereas acute periodontal abscesses present a diffuse inflammatory reaction. (Periodont.)

pulpal a. An abscess occurring within pulpal tissue. (Endodont.)

absence of teeth, congenital (see **anodontia**)

1

absorb (ăb-sorb′) To suck up, as through pores. (Anesth.)

absorbefacient (ăb-sor″bah-fā′shĕnt) Causing or that which causes absorption. (Anesth.)

absorbent (ăb-sorb′ĕnt) A substance that causes absorption of diseased tissue; taking up by suction. (Anesth.; Pharmacol.)

absorption (ăb-sorp′shŭn) The passage of a substance into the interior of another by solution or penetration. (Anesth.)

— Taking up of fluids or other substances by the skin, mucous surfaces, absorbent vessels, or dental materials. (Comp. Prosth.; Remov. Part. Prosth.)

— The process by which radiation imparts some or all of its energy to any material through which it passes. (Oral Radiol.)

   a. coefficient The ratio of the linear rate of change of intensity of roentgen rays in a given homogeneous material to the intensity at a given point within the same mass. (Anesth.)

abstraction (ăb-străk′shŭn) Term used to indicate teeth or other maxillary and mandibular structures that are inferior to (below) their normal position; away from the occlusal plane. (Orthodont.)

abutment (ah-bŭt′mĕnt) The terminal tooth or root that retains or supports a prosthesis. It is united to the prosthesis proper by means of the retainer. (Fixed Part. Prosth.)

— A tooth or tooth root used for the support, retention, and stabilization of a fixed or removable prosthesis. (Remov. Part. Prosth.)

   auxiliary a. (awg-zĭl′yă-rē) A tooth other than the tooth that supports the primary direct retainer; serves to support a unit of a removable partial denture. (Remov. Part. Prosth.)

   a. groove (see **groove, abutment**)

   intermediate a. A natural tooth without other natural teeth in proximal contact; used as a support in addition to two primary abutments. (Fixed Part. Prosth.; Remov. Part. Prosth.)

   isolated a. A tooth standing alone, with an edentulous area both anterior and posterior to it. (Remov. Part. Prosth.)

   a. locater A thin resin base made on a diagnostic cast into which holes have been cut to predetermine locations of the cuspids and molars on a subperiosteal implant. (Oral Implant.)

   multiple a. The unit resulting from the fixed splinting of natural teeth; used as an abutment. (Remov. Part. Prosth.)

   primary a. A tooth used for the direct support, retention, and stabilization of a removable partial denture. (Remov. Part. Prosth.)

   a. splint (see **splint, abutment**)

a.c. (ante cibum) Latin phrase meaning before eating. (Oral Med.; Pharmacol.)

acanthesthesia (ah-kăn″thĕs-thē′zē-ah) Sensation of a prick; a form of paresthesia. (Anesth.)

acanthion (ah-kan′thē-on) The tip of the anterior nasal spine. (Orthodont.)

acanthosis (ăk-ăn-thō′sĭs) Hyperplasia of the prickle cell layer of the epithelium. (Oral Diag.)

— An increase in the number of cells in the prickle cell layer of stratified squamous epithelium, leading to thickening of the entire epithelial layer and a broadening and fusing of rete pegs. (Oral Path.)

acapnia (ah-căp′nē-ah) A condition characterized by diminished carbon dioxide in the blood. (Anesth.)

acarbia (ah-kar′bē-ah) A condition in which the blood bicarbonate is lowered. (Anesth.)

acatalasemia (ā″kăt-ah-lā-sē′mē-ah) An apparent congenital lack of the enzyme catalase in blood and other tissues, in many cases leading to a progressive necrosis of the oral tissues (Takahara's disease). (Oral Med.)

accelerator (ăk-sĕl′ĕr-ā″tor) A catalytic agent used to hasten a chemical reaction; e.g., NaCl or K_2SO_4 added to plaster of paris and water to hasten setting. (Comp. Prosth.; Remov. Part. Prosth.)

— A substance that hastens a chemical reaction; not necessarily a catalyst, since accelerators sometimes enter into the reaction. (D. Mat.)

   platelet thrombin a. (see **factor, platelet 2**)

   prothrombin conversion a. I (**factor V, labile factor, plasma a. globulin, proaccelerin, serum a. globulin**) Considered by some to be a factor in serum and plasma that catalyzes the conversion of inactive prothrombin to an active form. (Oral Med.)

   prothrombin conversion a. II (**cothromboplastin, extrinsic thromboplastin, factor VII, serum prothrombin conversion a. [SPCA], stable factor**) Considered by some to be one of the factors in the blood that accelerate the conversion of active prothrombin to thrombin by thromboplastin. Vitamin K deficiency reduces the activity of this factor. (Oral Med.)

   serum a. (see **factor V**)

accelerin (see **factor V**)

acceptance The act of a person to whom something is offered or tendered by another whereby he receives that which is offered with the intention of retaining it, such intention being evidenced by a contract, either expressly or by conduct. (D. Juris.)

absolute a. An express and positive agreement to pay a bill according to its text. (D. Juris.)

conditional a. An agreement to pay a bill on the fulfillment of a condition. (D. Juris.)

implied a. An acceptance interpreted by law from the acts or conduct of the patient. (D. Juris.)

access (ăk'sĕs) The convenience form required to afford sufficient space for an adequate visual field and for the proper use of instruments for cavity preparation and insertion of a restorative material. (Oper. Dent.)

a. cavity The opening required to effect entrance to the pulp chamber to allow for adequate cleaning, shaping, and filling of the root canal system. (Endodont.)

accessory canal (ăk-sĕs'ō-rē) (see **canal, accessory root**)

accident An unforeseen event, occurring without intent of the person whose act causes it; an unexpected or unusual occurrence; the result of an unknown cause or the unprecedented consequence of a known cause; a casualty. (D. Juris.)

cerebrovascular a. (CVA) Apoplexy resulting from hemorrhage into the brain or occlusion of the cerebral vessels due to embolism or thrombosis. (Oral Med.)

unavoidable a. An accident not occasioned, either remotely or directly, by the want of such care or skill as the law holds every person bound to exercise. (D. Juris.)

account A statement in writing of obligations and credits or of acknowledgments and disbursements; a list of items of debts and credits with their respective dates. (D. Juris.)

a. book A book in which are entered the financial transactions of a business or profession. Such books may be admitted in evidence. (D. Juris.)

open a. A straightforward arrangement between the dentist and the patient for the handling of financial payments due the dentist and owed by the patient. (Pract. Man.)

accretions (ah-krē'shŭns) Accumulation of foreign material such as mucinous plaque, materia alba, and supragingival and subgingival calculus on teeth. (Oral Diag.; Periodont.)

A.C.E. mixture Abbreviation for a mixture of alcohol, chloroform, and ether. (Anesth.)

acenesthesia (ah-sē-nĕs-thē'zē-ah) Absence of a

feeling of well-being, present in such disorders as hypochondriasis and neurasthenia. (Anesth.)

acentric relation (ā-sĕn'trĭk) (see **relation, jaw, eccentric**)

acescence (ah-sĕs'ĕns) Slight acidity. (Anesth.)

acetate (ăs'ĕ-tāt) Any salt of acetic acid. (Anesth.)

acetone (ăs'ĕ-tōn) Dimethylketone; normally present in urine in small quantities but found in increased amounts in diabetes. (Oral Diag.)

acetylcholine (ăs''ĕ-tĭl-kō'lēn) An ester of choline that acts as the neurohumoral agent at each of the autonomic ganglia, parasympathetic postganglionic fibers, and somatic motor fibers. (Anesth.)

— An ester of choline actively involved as a chemical mediator at the neuromuscular junction, at autonomic ganglia, and between parasympathetic nerve endings and visceral effectors. (Oral Physiol.)

ACh Abbreviation for acetylcholine. (Anesth.)

achlorhydria (ah-klor-hī'drē-ah) Absence of free hydrochloric acid in the stomach even under conditions of histamine stimulation. (Oral Med.)

achondroplasia (ah-kŏn-drō-plā'zē-ah) **(chondrodystrophia fetalis)** A dominant hereditary disease characterized by defective formation of endochondral bone, producing short limbs, a head with a large cranial vault, and an underdeveloped cranial base; the torso is normal. (Oral Diag.)

— A heredofamilial disease characterized principally by a failure of normal endochondral bone formation, although membranous bones are also affected. It results in dwarfism and malocclusion, and prognathism may occur. (Oral Med.)

— A hereditary disturbance of endochondral bone formation that is transmitted as a mendelian dominant factor. Resultant retardation or aplasia of endochondral growth creates dwarfism, retrusion of the maxilla, and relative mandibular prognathism. (Oral Path.)

— A hereditary cartilage disorder that begins in prenatal life and results in a nonendocrine dwarfism. (Pedodont.)

achromatopsia (ah-krō-mah-tōp'sē-ah) Total color blindness.

acid (ăs'ĭd) A chemical substance that, in an aqueous solution, undergoes dissociation with the formation of hydrogen ions; pH ranges from 0 to 6.9. (Anesth.)

acetic a. The acid of vinegar, sometimes used as a solvent for the removal of calculus from a removable dental prosthesis. (Remov. Part. Prosth.) (see also **solvent**)

ascorbic a. (see **vitamin C**)

carbolic a. (see **phenol**)

cevitamic a. (see **vitamin C**)

folic a. (see **vitamin B$_c$**)

hydroxypropionic a. (see **acid, lactic**)

lactic a. (hydroxypropionic a.) A monobasic acid, $C_3H_6O_3$, formed as an end product in the intermediary metabolism of carbohydrates. The accumulation of lactic acid in the tissues is in part responsible for the lowering of pH during inflammatory states; e.g., it is believed that the drop in pH will hasten bone resorption in periodontitis because the minerals in the bone are stable within the matrix only at the normal tissue pH of 7.4. (Periodont.)

nicotinic a. (niacin, P.-P. factor, pyridine 3-carboxylic a., vitamin P.-P.) One of the vitamins of the B complex group and its vitamer, niacinamide, specific for the treatment of pellagra. Niacinamide functions as a constituent of coenzyme I (DPN) and coenzyme II (TPN). Nicotinic acid is found in lean meats, liver, yeast, milk, and leafy green vegetables. (Oral Med.)

— An acid, $C_5H_4N(COOH)$, that forms part of the B complex group of vitamins. It is present and necessary in the body as a cofactor in intermediary carbohydrate metabolism. It is a constituent of certain coenzymes that function in oxidative-reductive metabolic systems. With niacinamide, it is a pellagra-preventive factor. (Periodont.)

orthophosphoric a. (see **acid, phosphoric**)

pantothenic a. One of the B complex vitamins whose importance in human nutrition has not been established. It is a constituent of coenzyme A and as such is presumed to be involved in adrenocortical function. (Oral Med.; Pharmacol.)

— A vitamin of the B complex, widely distributed in food and tissues and important for normal development in certain animals such as chicks and rats. Deficiency in rats produces retrograde changes in alveolar and supporting bone. (Periodont.)

phosphoric a. (H$_3$PO$_4$, orthophosphoric a.) The principal ingredient of silicate and zinc phosphate cement liquids. (D. Mat.)

pteroylglutamic a. (see **vitamin B$_c$**)

a. salt A salt containing one or more replaceable hydrogen ions. (Anesth.)

strong a. An acid that is completely ionized in aqueous solution. (Anesth.)

acidemia (ăs″ĭ-dē′mē-ah) Decreased pH of the blood, irrespective of changes in the blood bicarbonate. (Anesth.)

acidifier (ah-sĭd′ĭ-fī-er) A chemical ingredient (acetic acid) that maintains the required acidity of the fixer and stop-bath solutions. (Oral Radiol.)

acidophilic (as″ĭ-dō-fĭl′ĭk) Having an affinity for acid. (Anesth.)

acidosis (ăs″ĭ-dō′sĭs) Clinical term used to indicate acidemia or lowered blood bicarbonate with a tendency toward acidemia. (Anesth.)

— Disturbance of acid-base and water balance characterized by an excess of acid or inadequate base; e.g., metabolic acidosis of diabetes mellitus or respiratory acidosis due to respiratory depressants. (Oral Med.)

— Disturbance of acid-base balance characterized by an excess of acid or inadequate base. Causes include ingestion of acid, reduced elimination of carbon dioxide through the lungs, increased formation of acids as in diabetes, and loss of base by kidneys or through the intestinal tract. (Oral Physiol.)

compensated a. A condition in which the blood bicarbonate is usually lower than normal but in which the compensatory mechanisms have kept the pH within normal range. (Anesth.)

respiratory a. Acidemia produced by hypoventilation; results in an increase in plasma carbonic acid and plasma bicarbonate. (Anesth.)

uncompensated a. Acidemia usually accompanied by lowered blood bicarbonate, such as occurs after the ingestion of hydrochloric acid or in terminal nephritis. (In uncompensated carbon dioxide acidosis the bicarbonate may be normal.) (Anesth.)

acquaintance form (see **form, acquaintance**)

acquired centric relation (sĕn′trĭk) (see **relation, centric; relation, jaw, eccentric**)

acroanesthesia (ăk″rō-ăn-ĕs-thē′zē-ah) Anesthesia of the extremities. (Anesth.)

acrocephalia (ăk-rō-sĕ-fā′lē-ah) A deformity of the head characterized by an upward and forward bulge of the frontal bones and a flat occiput. (Oral Diag.)

acrodynia (ăk-rō-dĭn′ĭ-ah) **(erythredema polyneuropathy, Feer's syndrome, pink disease, Swift's syndrome, Selter's disease)** A disease of children in which manifestations occur with the eruption of the primary teeth. Syndrome includes raw-beef hands and feet, superficial sensory loss, photophobia, tachycardia, muscular hypotonia, changes in temperament, stomatitis, periodontitis, and premature loss of teeth.

Etiology has been related to mercury and deficiency of vitamin B₆ and essential fatty acids. (Oral Med.) (see also **erythredema polyneuropathy**)

acroesthesia (ăk-rō-ĕs-thē'zē-ah) Increased sensitivity; pain in the extremities. (Anesth.)

acromegaly (ăk-rō-mĕg'ah-lē) **(Marie's disease)** Enlargement of bones and soft parts of hands, feet, and face associated with hyperfunction of pituitary gland due to eosinophilic adenoma in adults. (Oral Diag.)

— A chronic type of endocrinopathy in the adult caused by an increased elaboration of growth hormone due to granulated cell hyperfunction usually associated with an adenoma or, rarely, with eosinophilic hyperfunction or carcinoma of the pituitary gland. It is characterized by enlargement of the feet, hands, tongue, and mandible, separation of the teeth, disturbances of sexual organs, and often diabetes mellitus. (Oral Med.)

acrosclerosis (ăk-rō-sklĕ-rō'sĭs) A special form of scleroderma that affects the extremities, head, and face and is associated with Raynaud's phenomenon. There may be marked thickening of the periodontal membrane. (Oral Med.)

— A connective tissue disease, involving the fingers, face, and upper part of the thorax, that combines the features of Raynaud's disease and scleroderma. Periodontal features include widening of the periodontal membrane space revealed on radiographic examination, with microscopic evidence of derangement of the alveolar group of periodontal fibers. (Periodont.)

acrylic, *adj.* (ah-krĭl'ĭk) Frequently improperly used as a noun. Should be used to modify nouns; e.g., acrylic resin, acrylic resin denture, and acrylic resin tooth. (see **resin, acrylic; denture, acrylic resin; tooth, acrylic resin**) (Comp. Prosth.; Remov. Part. Prosth.)

a. resin (see **resin, acrylic**)

ACTH (adrenocorticotropic hormone, adrenocorticotropin, adrenotropic hormone, corticotropic hormone, corticotropin) The adenohypophyseal hormone that stimulates the adrenal cortex to secrete cortical hormones. (Oral Med.)

— Adrenocorticotropic hormone, produced by basophilic cells of the anterior lobe of the pituitary gland, which exerts a reciprocal regulating influence on the production of corticosteroids by the adrenal cortex. (Oral Med.; Periodont.)

— The adrenocorticotropic hormone secreted by the anterior lobe of the pituitary gland. The effects of ACTH are nonspecific and secondary to other, more fundamental actions of this hormone. In hypophysectomized rats, ACTH is antagonistic to the growth hormone of the anterior pituitary gland. Since ACTH leads to the suppression of the formation of bone without interfering with the normal rate of resorption, it causes atrophy of the bones. (Oral Physiol.)

actinic cheilitis (ăk-tĭn'ĭk) (see **cheilitis, actinic**)

actinomycetes (ăk"tĭ-nō-mī-sē'tēz) Filamentous microorganisms that have been implicated in the formation of dental calculus and serve as a mode of attachment of dental calculus to the tooth surface. They have also been found in pathologic lesions of the alveolar processes (actinomycosis). (Periodont.)

actinomycosis (ăk"tĭ-nō-mī-kō'sĭs) **(lumpy jaw, streptothricosis)** An infection caused by an aerobic fungus, *Actinomyces bovis,* a normal inhabitant of the mouth that may cause lesions of the jaws. It is found clinically in cervicofacial, abdominal, and thoracic forms. The most common cervicofacial form originates in the mouth after trauma, such as a dental extraction. A firm, hard swelling develops, usually over the angle of the jaw. The swelling becomes fluctuant and suppurative and spreads to the face, producing chronic draining sinuses. Colonies of organisms may appear in the suppuration as "sulfur granules." (Oral Med.)

— A systemic mycotic infection caused by *Actinomyces bovis, Nocardia asteroides,* and *Actinomyces israelii.* The cervicofacial form is most common. A granulomatous lesion of soft tissue or bone containing characteristic colonies of microorganisms results. (Oral Path.)

action, neuromuscular An activity initiated and controlled by the coordinated action of muscles and nerves; e.g., the movements of the mandible during mastication, speech, etc. (Periodont.)

action potential The electrical potential developed in a muscle or nerve during activity. (Oral Physiol.)

activate (ăk'tĭ-vāt) To adjust an appliance so that it will exert effective force on the teeth and jaws. (Orthodont.)

activated resin (see **resin, autopolymerizing**)

activator (ăk'tĭ-vā-tor) An alkali, sodium carbonate, which is a component of the developing solution that softens and swells the gelatin of the film emulsion and provides the necessary alkaline medium for the developing agents to react with the sensitized silver halide crystals. (Oral Radiol.)

— A myofunctional appliance (Andresen, Monobloc, Oral Screen, Bimler). A removable type of orthodontic appliance that acts as a passive transmitter of force which is produced by the function of the activated muscles and applied to the teeth and alveolar processes in contact with it. (Orthodont.)

platelet a. (see **factor, platelet 3**)

prothrombin a., direct (see **prothrombinase**)

prothrombin a., extrinsic (see **prothrombinase**)

active Pertaining to the condition of an orthodontic appliance that has been adjusted to apply effective force to the teeth or jaws. (Orthodont.)

   a. reciprocation (see **reciprocation, active**)

activity, platelet thromboplastic (see **factor, platelet 2**)

acuity (ah-kū′ĭ-tē) Sharpness; clearness; keenness.

   auditory a. The sensitivity of the auditory apparatus; sharpness of hearing. It relates to the ability to hear a given tone with respect to the degree of intensity required to produce a sensation that is just perceptible; i.e., the lower the intensity required, the greater the acuity. (Oral Physiol.)

   visual a. Sharpness, acuteness, or clearness of vision. Visual acuity may be defective because of optical or neurologic dysfunction. Finger-counting and finger-movement tests can be given by the dentist in light, dark, and bright illumination. The patient is asked to identify objects at near and distant positions. When he has difficulty in determining form and contour of common objects, his judgment is not adequate in regard to decisions concerning the mold of the tooth, arch form, and facial contours in dental treatment. (Oral Physiol.)

acute (ah-kūt′) Having a short and relatively severe course; opposite of chronic. (Oral Diag.)

— A traumatic, pathologic, or physiologic phenomenon or process that is sudden and severe in onset. (Oral Surg.)

   a. phase reactions A phrase that refers to abnormalities in the blood associated with acute and chronic inflammatory and necrotic processes and detected by a variety of tests, including erythrocyte sedimentation rate, C-reactive protein, serum hexosamine, serum mucoprotein, and serum nonglucosamine polysaccharides. (Oral Med.)

adamantinoblastoma (ăd-ah-măn″tĭ-nō-blăs-tō′-mah) (see **ameloblastoma**)

adamantinoma (ăd-ah-măn″tĭ-nō′mah) (see **ameloblastoma**)

Adams-Stokes disease (see **disease, Adams-Stokes**)

Adams-Stokes syndrome (see **disease, Adams-Stokes**)

adaptation (ăd′ăp-tā′shun) Close approximation of restorative material to cavity walls; accurate adjustment of a matrix band or a shell to a tooth and/or to the contour of gingival tissues. (Oper. Dent.)

— A condition in reflex activity marked by a decline in the frequency of impulses when sensory stimuli are repeated several times. There are variations in adaptation of different sense organs: e.g., muscle spindles adapt slowly, making them suitable for serving long, sustained postural reflexes. Adaptation is not the same as fatigue. (Oral Physiol.)

— Alteration that an organ or organism undergoes to accommodate to its environment. (Oral Surg.)

adapter, band An instrument utilized as an aid in fitting an orthodontic band to a tooth. (Orthodont.)

addict, *n.* (ăd′ĭkt) One who has developed addiction to a drug. One who depends on a sedative, narcotic, or stimulant drug to the extent that his health, social behavior, and, in some cases, his life are endangered if the drug is withdrawn suddenly. (Anesth.; Oral Med.; Pharmacol.)

—, *v.* (ah-dĭkt′) To form a habit of using a drug. (Anesth.)

—, *v.* (ah-dĭkt′) To develop addiction. (Pharmacol.)

addiction Although there is no universally accepted definition, generally considered a condition involving two factors: (1) a compulsive behavior pattern and (2) an altered physiologic state that requires continued use of the drug to prevent withdrawal symptoms. (Pharmacol.)

addictive Pertaining to a drug whose repeated use may produce addiction. Present federal regulations place greater emphasis on the broader designation of potential for abuse. (Pharmacol.)

Addis' test (see **test, Addis'**)

Addison-Biermer anemia (ad′ĭ-sŭn bēr′mer) (see **anemia, pernicious**)

Addison's disease (see **disease, Addison's**)

additive An ingredient present in a food, drug, or cosmetic preparation in addition to the basic or essential constituents; e.g., alumina is a polishing additive in a dentifrice. (Pharmacol.)

adduct (ah-dŭkt′) To draw toward the center or midline. (Anesth.)

adduction (ah-dŭk′shŭn) The process of bringing toward each other, as two vocal bands; the opposite of abduction. (Oral Physiol.)

adenalgia (ăd-ĕ-năl′jē-ah) Pain in a gland, due usually to inflammation (adenitis). (Oral Surg.)

adenitis (ăd″ĕ-nī′tĭs) Inflammation of glandular tissue, usually manifested by pain (adenalgia). (Oral Surg.)

adenoameloblastoma (ăd″ĕ-nō-ah-mĕl″ō-blăs-tō′-mah) An epithelial neoplasm with a basic structure resembling enamel organs and glandular (adenomatous) tissue. It is generally benign. (Oral Diag.)

— An epithelial odontogenic tumor in which the ameloblastic epithelium forms numerous duct-like structures. It may be encapsulated. (Oral Path.)

adenocarcinoma (ăd″ĕ-nō-kar-sĭ-nō′mah) A malignant epithelial neoplasm with a basic structure of glandular (acinar) pattern, suggesting derivation from glandular tissue. (Oral Diag.; Oral Path.)

    acinar cell a. A malignant tumor whose cells appear as glandular tissue. (Oral Path.)

adenoma (ăd″ĕ-nō′mah) A benign epithelial neoplasm or tumor with a basic glandular (acinar) structure, suggesting derivation from glandular tissue. (Oral Diag.; Oral Path.)

    acidophilic a. (see **oncocytoma**)

    oxyphilic a. (see **oncocytoma**)

adenomatosis oris (ăd″ĕ-nō-mah-tō′sĭs) An enlargement of the mucous glands of the lip without secretion or inflammation. (Oral Diag.)

adenopathy (ăd″ĕ-nŏp′ah-thē) An enlargement or increase in size of glandular organs or tissues due usually to disease processes. (Oral Surg.)

adequacy, velopharyngeal A functional closure of the velum to the postpharyngeal wall that restricts air and sound from entering the nasopharyngeal and nasal cavities. (Cleft Palate)

ADH (see **hormone, antidiuretic**)

adhesion (ăd-hē′zhŭn) The physical attraction of unlike molecules for one another. (Comp. Prosth.)

— The molecular attraction existing between the surfaces of bodies in contact. (Comp. Prosth.; Remov. Part. Prosth.)

— Ability of a material to stick to itself or another material. A true adhesion is the result of chemical bonding. (D. Mat.)

— The abnormal joining of tissues to each other, occurring after repair of an injury. Adhesion tissue usually consists of fibrous connective tissue. (Oral Surg.)

    sublabial a. Abnormal union of the sublabial mucosa of the upper lip to the alveolar process; usually present in a unilateral or bilateral cleft of the lip. (Cleft Palate)

adhesive An intermediate material that causes two materials to stick together; a luting agent. (D. Mat.)

    a. foil (see **foil, adhesive**)

adjunct (ăj′ŭngkt) A drug or other substance that serves a supplemental purpose in therapy. (Oral Med.)

adjusting occlusion Altering, by increasing or decreasing, the occlusal contact of a restoration so that it will be in balanced or functional occlusion with the opposing contacting teeth. (Oper. Dent.)

adjustment (ah-jŭst′mĕnt) Modification of a denture or of the teeth on a denture after a denture has been fabricated and inserted in the mouth. (Comp. Prosth.; Remov. Part. Prosth.)

— In cellular and tissue structures, a change in the physiologic condition, creating needs that the tissues must satisfy in order to re-create the conditions of equilibrium or homeostasis by exchanging metabolites, eliminating wastes, and absorbing oxygen and nutritional elements. This pattern is the process of adjustment or adaptation. It is as valid for cellular function and organ system function as it is for total behavioral function, including social adjustment. Thus both physiologic and psychologic adjustments are made in an attempt to retain equilibrium and to have degrees of adjustment ranging from maximum to minimum. (Oral Physiol.)

    occlusal a. Modification of the occluding surfaces of opposing teeth to develop harmonious relationships between the teeth themselves, the neuromuscular mechanism, the temporomandibular joints, and the structures supporting the teeth. (Comp. Prosth.; Fixed Part. Prosth.; Remov. Part. Prosth.)

    — Judicious or selective grinding of tooth surfaces used as a therapeutic procedure directed toward establishment of periodontal health by producing acceptable patterns of tooth form, tooth position, tooth integration, and jaw position. Used in the treatment of occlusal traumatism. The reshaping of the outer surfaces of teeth in order to create patterns of tooth form and tooth contact that will be physiologically and biologically acceptable to the supporting tissues of the teeth, the masticatory musculature, and the integrated components of the temporomandibular joints. (Periodont.)

adjuvant (ăj'oo-vănt) In a prescription, an auxiliary active ingredient that supports the action of the basic drug. (Pharmacol.) (see also **basis**)

administration, sublingual Placing of a drug under the tongue to dissolve and to be absorbed through the mucous membrane. (Oral Med.; Pharmacol.)

admission Voluntary concession or admission that a fact or allegation is true. (D. Juris.)

adnexa (ăd-nĕk'sah) Conjoined anatomic parts. Tissues adjacent to or contained within a nearby space. (Oral Implant.)

adrenal corticoid (see **corticoid, adrenal**)

adrenal crisis (see **crisis, adrenal**)

Adrenalin (ah-drĕn'ah-lĭn) A proprietary preparation of epinephrine. (see **epinephrine**) (Anesth.; Oral Physiol.; Pharmacol.)

adrenaline British name for epinephrine. (Oral Med.; Pharmacol.)

adrenergic (ăd-rĕn-ĕr'jĭk) Transmitted by norepinephrine or activated by norepinephrine or the other sympathomimetic agents. (Anesth.; Oral Med.; Pharmacol.)

— Term applied to those nerve fibers that liberate epinephrine or norepinephrine at a synapse when a nerve impulse passes; a drug that mimics the action of adrenergic nerves. (Anesth.)

  a. blocking agent (see **agent, adrenergic blocking**)

  a. fibers (see **fibers, adrenergic**)

  a. receptors (see **receptors, adrenergic**)

adrenic (ăd-rĕ'nĭk) Pertaining to the adrenal gland. (Anesth.)

adrenocortical insufficiency (ah-drĕ"nō-kor'tĭ-kăl) (see **hypoadrenocorticalism**)

adrenocorticotropin (ah-drĕ"nō-kor"tĭ-kō-trō'pin) (see **ACTH**)

adrenolytic (ah-drĕ"nō-lĭt'ĭk) Capable of impeding the action of epinephrine or levarterenol (norepinephrine) or both (sympatholytic). (Anesth.; Oral Med.; Pharmacol.)

  a. agent (see **agent, adrenergic blocking**)

adrenotropic (ăd-rĕ'nō-trŏp'ik) Having a special affinity for the adrenal gland. (Anesth.)

adsorbent (ăd-sorb'ĕnt) A solid substance, usually chemically inert, that attracts and holds other substances, especially liquids, vapors, or

dissolved solids, to its surface. Effective adsorbents have a large specific surface area. (Oral Med.)

adsorption (ăd-sorp'shŭn) A process believed to be physical in nature in which molecules of a gas or liquid condense on or adhere to the surface of another substance. (Anesth.)

  root a. (see **resorption, root**)

ADT Abbreviation for *Accepted Dental Therapeutics,* a journal published by the Council on Dental Therapeutics of the American Dental Association.

adumbration (ăd"ŭm-brā'shŭn) A geometric lack of sharpness; an inherent property of a finite focal spot that causes the production of a penumbra. (Oral Radiol.)

advancement The surgical detachment of a soft tissue or bony structure, followed by its reattachment or relocation. (Oral Surg.)

advances Monies paid before the proper time of payment. (D. Juris.)

aeration (ā-er-ā'shŭn) The arteriolization of the venous blood in the lungs; ventilation. (Anesth.)

— The passage of air or gases into a liquid, e.g., the passage of oxygen from pulmonary alveoli into the blood. (Oral Physiol.)

aerodontalgia (ā"er-ō-dŏn-tăl'jē-ah) Pulpal pain with decreased barometric pressure. Latent symptoms of pulpitis may be triggered by high-altitude flying or confinement in a decompression chamber, but the symptoms may be confused with those of aerosinusitis. (Oper. Dent.; Oral Med.)

aeroembolism (ā"er-ō-ĕm'bō-lĭzm) (**air embolism**) An obstruction of a blood vessel that is caused by the entrance of air into the bloodstream. (Anesth.)

aerosinusitis (ā"er-ō-sī"nŭ-sī'tĭs) Painful symptoms related to the maxillary sinus due to a change in barometric pressure (compression or recompression). Symptoms of odontalgia may be consistent with those of aerodontalgia. (Oral Med.)

aerosol (ā'er-ō-sŏl) A colloid in which gas is the dispersion medium; used as a wetting agent. The word is commonly used as a synonym for dioctyl sodium sulfosuccinate. (Oper. Dent.)

— A substance dispensed, usually from a special container, in the form of a foam or mist. (Oral Med.)

aesthetics (see **esthetics**)

affect (af'ekt) A freudian term for the feeling of pleasantness or unpleasantness produced by a stimulus; also the emotional complex influencing a mental state; the feeling experienced in connection with an emotion. (Oral Physiol.)

afferent (ăf'er-ĕnt) Conveying from a periphery to a center. (Anesth.)

a. impulse An impulse that arises in the periphery and is carried into the central nervous system. An afferent nerve conducts the impulse from the site of origin to the central nervous system. (Anesth.)

affiliation (ah-fĭl-ē-ā'shŭn) The incorporation or formation of a partnership by two or more dentists for the purpose of practicing the profession of dentistry. (Pract. Man.)

afflux (ăf'lŭks) The rush of blood to a part. (Anesth.)

affricative (ah-frĭk'ah-tĭv) A fricative speech sound initiated by a plosive. (Cleft Palate)

aftercondensation (see **postcondensation**)

afterperception (af″ter-per-sĕp'shŭn) (see **postperception**)

aftersensation (see **postsensation**)

A:G ratio (see **ratio, A:G**)

agar (ah'găr) A polysaccharide derived from seaweed; the basic constituent of a reversible hydrocolloid. (D. Mat.) (see also **hydrocolloid, reversible**)

a. hydrocolloid A reversible hydrocolloid made from agar-agar. (Remov. Part. Prosth.)

agar-agar type (ah'găr-ah'găr) (see **hydrocolloid, reversible**)

age hardening (see **hardening, age**)

agenesis (ā-jĕn'ĕ-sĭs) Defective development or congenital absence of parts. (Oral Diag.; Oral Path.)

— Inhibition of bone growth, which may result in congenital cleft palate, osteogenesis imperfecta, multiple exostosis, or achondroplasia; may be associated with conditions such as prenatal stress. (Oral Physiol.)

agent A person who acts for, or in the place of, another, by authority from him. (D. Juris.)

anesthetic a. A drug that produces local or general loss of sensation. (Anesth.)

anti-inflammatory a. A drug that reduces inflammation perhaps through reduction of the capillary permeability, which is increased by inflammatory processes. (Oral Surg.; Pharmacol.)

bleaching a. An agent used in the modification or removal of discoloration; generally used on pulpless teeth. (Endodont.)

blocking a. An agent that occupies or usurps the receptor site normally occupied by a drug or a biochemical intermediary, e.g., acetylcholine or epinephrine. (Oral Med.; Pharmacol.)

adrenergic b. a. A drug that blocks the action of the neurohormones norepinephrine and/or epinephrine or of adrenergic drugs at sympathetic neuroeffectors. (Anesth.)

— A drug that selectively inhibits certain responses of adrenergic neuroeffectors to norepinephrine and other sympathomimetic agents. (Oral Med.; Pharmacol.)

adrenolytic b. a. An uncertain term sometimes used in reference to adrenergic blocking agents. (Anesth.; Oral Med.; Pharmacol.)

cholinergic b. a. A drug that inhibits the action of acetylcholine or cholinergic drugs at the postganglionic cholinergic neuroeffectors. An anticholinergic agent. (Anesth.)

ganglionic b. a. A drug that prevents passage of nerve impulses at the synapses between preganglionic and postganglionic neurons. (Anesth.)

myoneural b. a. A drug that prevents transmission of nerve impulses at the junction of the nerve and the muscle. (Anesth.)

chemotherapeutic a. A chemical of either natural or synthetic origin used for its specific action against disease, generally against infection. (Oral Med.; Pharmacol.)

oxidizing a. An agent that provides oxygen in reacting with another substance or, in the broader and more definitive chemical sense, a chemical capable of accepting electrons and thereby decreasing the negative charge on an atom of the substance being oxidized. (Oral Med.; Pharmacol.)

polishing a. An abrasive that produces a smooth, lustrous finish. (D. Mat.)

wetting a. Any agent that will reduce the surface tension of water. Generally used in investing wax patterns. (D. Mat.)

agglutinin (ah-gloo'tĭ-nĭn) An antibody that agglutinates red blood cells or renders them agglutinable. (Oral Med.)

aglossia (ah-glos'ē-ah) A developmental anomaly in which a portion or all of the tongue is absent. (Oral Path.)

— Congenital absence of the tongue. (Oral Diag.)

agnathia (ăg-nā'thē-ah) Absence of the lower jaw. (Orthodont.)

agnosia (ăg-nō'zē-ah) A loss of ability to recognize common objects, i.e., to understand the significance of sensory stimuli (e.g., tactile, auditory, or visual) due to brain damage. (Oral Physiol.)

agonist (ăg'ō-nĭst) An organ, a gland, a muscle,

or a nerve center that is so connected physiologically with another that the two function simultaneously in forwarding a given process; e.g., two muscles that pull on the same skeletal member and receive a nervous excitation at the same time. The opposite of antagonist. (Oral Physiol.)

agony Severe pain or extreme suffering; the death struggle. (Anesth.)

agranulocytopenia (ah-grăn″ū-lō-sī-tō-pē′nē-ah) (see **agranulocytosis**)

agranulocytosis (ah-grăn″ū-lō-sī-tō′sĭs) Decrease in the number of granulocytes in peripheral blood due to bone marrow depression by drugs and chemicals or replacement by a neoplasm. Manifest orally by necrotizing ulcerations. (Anesth.)
— A marked reduction in the formation of white blood cells, commonly accompanied by severe oral lesions and sometimes noma. (Oral Diag.)
— An extreme degree of agranulocytopenia in which virtually all granulocytes are absent from the circulating blood. A reduction of both the neutrophils and eosinophils below the normal level, as contrasted with neutropenia, in which the reduction is predominantly in neutrophils. (Oral Med.)
— A disease characterized by a marked reduction in the number of granulocytes in the peripheral blood and accompanied, in severe cases, by necrotizing ulcerations of the oral mucosa. (Oral Path.)
— A comparatively rare, grave condition in which there is an almost complete absence of polymorphonuclear leukocytes in the peripheral blood. Oral lesions are ulceronecrotic, involving the gingivae, tongue, buccal mucosa, or lips. Regional lymphadenopathy and lymphadenitis are prevalent. (Periodont.)

agreement The coming together in accord of two minds on a given proposition; a concord of understanding and intention with respect to the effect on their relative rights and duties. (D. Juris.)

AHF Antihemophilic factor. (see also **factor VIII**)

aid Assistance; support.
    a. in medicinal periodontal therapy Those pharmaceuticals employed in or necessary for the performance of periodontal therapy, including preoperative and postoperative sedatives and analgesics; topical, locally injected, and general anesthetics; postoperative dressings; antiseptics and antibiotics; desensitizing agents for hypersensitive teeth; and mouthwashes, dentifrices, and disclosing solutions. (Periodont.) (see also **therapy, periodontal**)
    a. in physiotherapy Agent used by the patient to cleanse the teeth and oral tissues and provide pseudofunctional stimulation of the gingival tissues to maintain periodontal health (an essential phase of periodontal therapy). Such aids include toothbrushes and dentifrices, balsa wood interdental stimulators, dental floss, interdental rubber and plastic tips, hydrotherapeutic mouth rinses, disclosing solutions, and gum brushes or finger cots (terry cloth) for gum massage. (Periodont.)

speech a. Therapy, a restoration, an appliance, or an electronic device used to improve speech. (Comp. Prosth.; Remov. Part. Prosth.)
    prosthetic s. a. A restoration used to close a congenital or acquired cleft or other opening in the hard palate, the soft palate, or both, or to replace lost or missing tissue necessary for the production of good speech. (Cleft Palate; Comp. Prosth.; Remov. Part. Prosth.)
        p. s. a., pharyngeal section Posterior section of the prosthetic speech aid; it lies in the nasopharyngeal region so as to block the escape of air through the nose. (Cleft Palate)
        p. s. a., temporary A prosthetic speech aid requiring periodic adjustment or renewal due to the growth and development of the maxillae and surrounding structures. (Cleft Palate)
        p. s. a., velar section Middle portion of the prosthetic speech aid, covering the cleft of the soft palate or hard palate. (Cleft Palate)

visual a. Any model, drawing, or photograph used to help the patient understand proposed treatment. (Pract. Man.)

air The invisible and odorless gaseous mixture that makes up the earth's atmosphere.
    a. chamber (see **chamber, relief**)
    complemental a. (see **volume, inspiratory reserve**)
    functional residual a. (see **capacity, functional residual**)
    minimal a. The volume of air in the air sacs themselves (part of the residual air). (Anesth.)
    reserve a. (see **volume, expiratory reserve**)
    residual a. (see **volume, residual**)
    supplemental a. (see **volume, expiratory reserve**)
    a. syringe (see **syringe, air**)

tidal a. (see volume, tidal)
a. turbine handpiece (see handpiece, air turbine)
airbrasive technique (see technique, airbrasive)
airway A clear passageway for air into and out of the lungs. A device for securing unobstructed respiration during general anesthesia or in states of unconsciousness. (Anesth.)
ala (ā'lah) A winglike process; e.g., the ala of the nose is the cutaneous-covered cartilaginous structure on the lateral aspect of the external naris. (Oral Surg.)
alarm reaction (see reaction, alarm; syndrome, general adaptation)
Albers-Schönberg disease (ăl'berz shān'berg) (see osteopetrosis)
Albright's syndrome (see syndrome, Albright's)
albumin (ăl-bū'mĭn) A protein that is a constituent of nearly all tissues. (Oral Diag.)
albuminuria (ăl-bū"mĭ-nū'rē-ah) (hyperproteinuria, proteinuria, proteuria) An increase in urinary albumin seen characteristically in nephritis, fever, toxemia of pregnancy, or any severe infection. (Oral Diag.)
— The presence of clinically detectable amounts of protein in the urine (usually less than 100 mg/24 hr may be found normally by special methods). The usual protein is albumin, although globulins, Bence Jones protein, and fibrinogen may be present and may exceed albumin. The condition may be due to prerenal or renal disease or to inflammation of the urinary tract. (Oral Med.)
alcohol A transparent liquid that is colorless, mobile, and volatile. Alcohols are organic compounds formed from hydrocarbons by the substitution of hydroxyl radicals for the same number of hydrogen atoms.
absolute a. Alcohol containing no more than 1% H_2O. (Anesth.)
sugar a. The product that results when the aldehyde and ketone groups of a sugar are converted to hydroxyl groups. (Oral Med.)
aldosterone (ăl-dŏs'ter-ōn) (electrocortin) An adrenal corticosteroid hormone that acts primarily to accelerate the exchange of potassium for sodium in the renal tubules and other cells. It is a potent mineralocorticoid but also has some regulatory effect on carbohydrate metabolism. (Oral Med.)
aldosteronism, primary (ăl-dŏs'ter-ōn-ĭzm) A hyperadrenal syndrome caused by abnormal elaboration of aldosterone and characterized by excessive loss of potassium and resultant muscle weakness. The symptoms are suggestive of tetany. The condition is often associated with an adenoma or cortical hyperplasia of the adrenal glands. (Oral Med.)

alganesthesia (ăl-găn"es-thē'zē-ah) Absence of a normal sense of pain. (Anesth.)
algesia (ăl-jē'zē-ah) Sensitivity to pain; hyperesthesia; a sense of pain. (Anesth.; Oral Surg.)
algesic (ăl-jē'sĭk) Painful. (Anesth.)
algesimetry (ăl-jē-sĭm'ē-trē) The measurement of response to painful stimuli. (Oral Med.)
— The determination of the effect of various therapeutic measures on the response to painful stimuli. (Oral Med.)
algetic (ăl-jĕt'ĭk) Painful. (Anesth.)
alginate (ăl'jĭ-nāt) A salt of alginic acid, e.g., sodium alginate, which, when mixed with water in accurate proportions, forms an irreversible hydrocolloid gel used for making impressions. (Comp. Prosth.; Oper. Dent.; Periodont.; Remov. Part. Prosth.)
— A salt of alginic acid extracted from marine kelp; used as the main ingredient in tinfoil substitutes for prosthetic dentistry and as the main constituent of irreversible hydrocolloid impression materials. (D. Mat.) (see also hydrocolloid, irreversible)
align (ah-līn') To move the teeth into their proper positions so as to conform to the line of occlusion. (Orthodont.)
alignment (ah-līn'mĕnt) Arrangement of the teeth in the alveolar process in the form of two parabolic curves. (Orthodont.)
tooth a. Arrangement of the teeth in relationship to their supporting bone (alveolar process), the adjacent teeth, and the opposing dentition. (Periodont.)
a. wire (see wire, alignment)
alkali (ăl'kah-lī) A strong water-soluble base. A chemical substance that, in aqueous solution, undergoes dissociation, resulting in the formation of hydroxyl (OH) ions. (Anesth.)
alkaline (ăl'kah-līn) Having the reductions of an alkali. A pH of 7.1 to 14 designates an alkaline solution. (Anesth.)
a. diet (see diet, alkaline)
a. reserve (see reserve, alkaline)
alkaloid (ăl'kah-loyd) Any one of the many nitrogen-containing organic bases derived from plants. The alkaloids are bitter and physiologically active. A number of the alkaloids are useful therapeutic agents. (Oral Med.; Pharmacol.)
synthetic a. A synthetically prepared compound having the chemical characteristics of the alkaloids. (Oral Med.; Pharmacol.)
alkalosis (ăl-kah-lō'sĭs) Chemical term used to indicate alkalemia or increased blood bicarbo-

nate with a tendency toward alkalemia. (Anesth.)

— Disturbance of acid-base balance and water balance, characterized by an excess of alkali or a deficiency of acids. Causes include ingestion of base, excessive loss of carbon dioxide due to hyperventilation, and loss of strong acids, as in protracted vomiting or intubation. (Oral Med.; Oral Physiol.)

compensated a. A condition in which the blood bicarbonate is usually higher than normal but in which the compensatory mechanisms have kept the pH within normal range. (Anesth.) (see also **alkalosis, uncompensated**)

respiratory a. Alkalemia produced by hypoventilation; as a result of hypoventilation the plasma carbonic acid decreases, and there is an excretion of bicarbonate in the urine to restore the carbonic acid:sodium bicarbonate ratio and prevent a change in pH. Plasma bicarbonate is therefore decreased in respiratory alkalosis but raised in metabolic alkalosis. (Anesth.)

uncompensated a. Alkalemia usually accompanied by an increased blood bicarbonate; occurs after the ingestion of sodium bicarbonate or after vomiting, with resultant loss of hydrochloric acid. (In compensated carbon dioxide alkalosis, the bicarbonate may be normal.) (Anesth.) (see also **alkalosis, compensated**)

allele (ah-lēl′) **(allelomorph)** One or more genes occupying the same location in a chromosome but differing because of a mutational change of one of them. (Oral Med.)

allelomorph (ah-lē′lō-morf) (see **allele**)

allergen (ăl′er-jĕn) Purified protein substance used to test a patient's sensitivity to food, pollen, etc. (Anesth.)

— A substance capable of producing an allergic response. Common allergens are pollens, dust, drugs, and foods. (Oral Med.)

allergy (ăl′er-jē) An antigen-antibody reaction resulting in a condition of unusual or exaggerated specific susceptibility to a substance that is harmless in similar amounts for the majority of members of the same species. (Anesth.)

— A hypersensitivity reaction of the body to an allergen; an antigen-antibody reaction manifested in several forms—e.g., anaphylaxis, asthma, hay fever, urticaria, angioedema, dermatitis, and stomatitis. (Oral Med.)

— A hypersensitivity of the organism to a specific protein; may manifest itself in one of the following system complexes: asthma and other disturbances of the respiratory tract, eczema and other forms of dermatitis, migraine headaches, and obscure pains in smooth muscles. (Oral Physiol.)

— An altered antigen-antibody reaction. An allergic reaction in the oral cavity may be manifest in the form of edema, erythema, vesiculation, and ulceration of the soft tissues. Microscopic sections reveal an excessive number of eosinophils in the subepithelial infiltrate. (Periodont.)

"spontaneous" clinical a. (see **atopy**)

allochiria (ăl-ō-kī′rē-ah) Tactile sensation experienced at the side opposite its origin. (Anesth.)

alloplast (ăl′ō-plăst) Transplant (implant) consisting of material originating from a nonliving source that is surgically inserted to replace missing tissue. (Oral Implant.; M.F.P.)

alloplastic (ăl′ō-plăs′tĭk) Nonbiologic (metal, ceramic, plastic) material. (Oral Implant.)

alloplasty (ăl′ō-plăs″tē) Plastic surgical procedure in which use is made of material not from the human body. (Oral Implant.)

alloxan (ah-lok′săn) A substance, mesoxalylurea, capable of producing experimental diabetes by destroying the islet cells of the pancreas. The resultant periodontal lesions include a nonspecific osteoporosis, without notable effects on the periodontal membrane, cementum, and gingivae. (Periodont.)

alloy (ăl′oy) Metals that are mutually soluble in a liquid state. (D. Mat.)

— The product of the fusion of two or more metals. (Oper. Dent.)

amalgam a. The alloy, or product of the fusion of several metals, usually supplied as filings, that is mixed with mercury to produce dental amalgam. (Oper. Dent.)

dental a. a. (see **amalgam**)

chrome-cobalt a. (see **alloy, cobalt-chromium**)

cobalt-chromium a. (chrome-cobalt a.) Base metal alloys available commercially as Stellites. Used in dentistry for metallic denture bases and partial dentures. (D. Mat.)

dental gold a. An alloy in which the principal ingredient is gold. (Oper. Dent.)

eutectic a. An alloy made of metals that are insoluble in the solid state; the alloy with the lowest melting point is the eutectic. (D. Mat.)

— Any combination of metals the melting point of which is lower than that of any of the individual metals of which it consists. One in which the components are mutually soluble in the solid state. It has a nonhomogeneous grain structure and is therefore likely to be brittle and to be subject to tarnishing and corrosion. (Oper. Dent.)

nickel-chromium a. A stainless steel. (D. Mat.)

silver a. (Objectionable as synonym for dental amalgam) An alloy in which the principal ingredient is silver. (Oper. Dent.)

alopecia (ăl-ō-pē′shē-ah) Normal or abnormal deficiency of hair. Baldness. (Oral Path.)

alphabet, international phonetic A set of internationally agreed-on alphabetical symbols, one for each sound; supplements the existing alphabet to fill out needed representation of sounds. (Cleft Palate)

alpha-estradiol (ăl″fah-ĕs-trah-dī′ŏl) An estrogenic steroid, prepared by dehydrogenation of estrone, which is one of the factors responsible for the maintenance of epithelial integrity of the oral tissues. A deficiency results in epithelial desquamation. (Periodont.)

alpha-hemihydrate (ăl″fah-hĕm-ē-hī′drāt) A physical form of the hemihydrate of calcium sulfate, $(CaSO_4)_2 \cdot H_2O$; dental artificial stone. (D. Mat.)

alpha-tocopherol (ăl″fah-tō-kŏf′er-ŏl) (see **vitamin E**)

alternative plan A compromise plan of treatment deviating from the ideal plan in scope and financial investment. (Pract. Man.)

alumina (ah-lū′mĭ-nah) Aluminum oxide, an abrasive sometimes used as a polishing agent. (D. Mat.)

Aluwax (ăl′ū-wăx) A commercially prepared wax wafer that contains aluminum; used as a template for the examination of occlusion and in occlusal adjustment. (Periodont.)

alveolalgia (ăl″vē-ō-lahl′jē-ah) (see **socket, dry**)

alveolar (ăl-vē′ō-lahr) Pertaining to an alveolus. (Oper. Dent.)

— Pertaining to a dental alveolus or to the bony processes of the maxillae or mandible that contain the teeth. Also pertains to a saclike or annular cell arrangement, e.g., glandular or pulmonary alveoli. (Oral Surg.)

a. crest (see **crest, alveolar**)

a. process (see **process, alveolar**)

a. ridge (see **ridge, alveolar**)

alveolectomy (ăl″vē-ō-lĕk′tō-mē) Excision of a portion of the alveolar process to aid in the removal of teeth, the restoration of the normal contour after the removal of teeth, and the preparation of the mouth for dentures. (Oral Surg.)

alveololingual sulcus (see **sulcus, alveololingual**)

alveolus (ăl-vē′ō-lŭs) An air sac of the lungs

formed by terminal dilations of the bronchioles. (Anesth.)

— The socket in the bone in which a tooth is attached by means of the periodontal ligament. (Comp. Prosth.; Orthodont.; Remov. Part. Prosth.)

— The cavity in the bony alveolar process of the mandible or maxillae in which the root of a tooth is held by the periodontal ligament. (Oper. Dent.; Oral Surg.)

amalgam (ah-mal′găm) **(dental a. alloy)** An alloy, one of the constituents of which is mercury. (D. Mat.; Oper. Dent.)

a. carrier (see **carrier, amalgam**)

a. carver (see **carver, amalgam**)

a. condenser (see **condenser, amalgam**)

copper a. An alloy composed principally of copper and mercury. (D. Mat.) (see also **amalgam**)

— An amalgam of copper and mercury, supplied in pellets or ingots that are heated and then triturated to a plastic mix. (Oper. Dent.)

dental a. An amalgam used for dental restorations and dies. (Oper. Dent.)

a. matrix (see **matrix, amalgam**)

a. plugger (see **condenser, amalgam**)

a. scrap (see **scrap, amalgam**)

silver a. A dental amalgam, the chief constituent of which is silver. A.D.A. composition specifications: silver, 65% minimum; tin, 25% minimum; copper, 6% maximum; zinc, 2% maximum. (Oper. Dent.)

spheroiding of a. A phenomenon occurring in plastic amalgam that has been condensed with excessive mercury content, in which it withdraws from angles and margins on removal of the condensing force and assumes a rounded or spheroidal appearance. It occurs in the plastic mass, not after hardening. (Oper. Dent.)

a. squeeze cloth A piece of linen used to hold plastic amalgam from which excess mercury is to be squeezed. (Oper. Dent.)

amalgamation (ah-măl″gah-mā′shŭn) Formation of an alloy by mixing mercury with another metal or other metals. (D. Mat.; Oper. Dent.) (see also **trituration**)

amalgamator (ah-măl′gah-mā-tor) A machine designed for mixing amalgam mechanically. (D. Mat.)

— A mechanical device used to triturate the ingredients of dental amalgam into a plastic mass. (Oper. Dent.)

ameloblastic fibroma (see **fibroma, ameloblastic**)

ameloblastic sarcoma (see **sarcoma, ameloblastic**)

ameloblastoma (ah-měl″ō-blăs-tō′mah) **(adamantinoblastoma, adamantinoma)** An epithelial neoplasm with a basic structure resembling the enamel organ and suggesting derivation from ameloblastic cells. It is usually benign. (Oral Diag.)

— An epithelial odontogenic tumor characterized by nests of cells composed of a single peripheral layer of cells resembling ameloblasts that enclose a central group of cells resembling stellate reticulum. (Oral Path.)

    acanthomatous a. An epithelial odontogenic tumor that differs from the simple ameloblastoma in that the central cells within the cell nests are squamous and may be keratinized rather than stellate. The peripheries of the cell nests are composed of ameloblastic cells. (Oral Path.) (see also **ameloblastoma**)

amelogenesis imperfecta (ah-měl″ō-jěn′ě-sĭs) A severe hypoplasia or agenesis of enamel that is inherited as a dominant characteristic. (Oral Diag.)

— A hereditary disturbance of the ectodermal component of the tooth germ resulting in agenesis, aplasia, hypoplasia, or hypocalcification of enamel. (Oral Path.)

amenorrhea (ah-měn-or-rē′ah) Absence or abnormal cessation of the menstrual cycle. (Oral Diag.)

ammeter (ăm′mē-ter) A contraction of amperemeter. An apparatus that measures the amperage of an electric current. (Oral Radiol.)

ammonia thiosulfate (ah-mō′nē-ah thī-ō-sŭl′fāt) An ingredient of the fixing solution that acts as a solvent for silver halides. A liquid concentrate that has a fixing power about three times that of solutions containing sodium thiosulfate (a powder). (Oral Radiol.)

ammoniacal silver nitrate (see **silver nitrate, ammoniacal**)

amnesia (ăm-nē′zē-ah) Lack or loss of memory, especially the inability to remember past experiences. (Anesth.)

amnesiac (ăm-nē′zē-ăk) A person affected by amnesia. (Anesth.)

amnesic (ăm-nē′zĭk) (see **sedative**)

amnestic (ăm-něs′tĭk) Amnesic; causing amnesia. (Anesth.)

amorphous (ah-mor′fŭs) A substance having no specific space lattice, the molecules being distributed at random. (D. Mat.)

ampere (ăm′pēr) (Amp) Practical unit of quantity of electric current, equal to a flow of 1 coulomb per second or the flow of 6.25×10^{18} electrons per second. The current produced by 1 volt acting through a resistance of 1 ohm. (Oral Radiol.)

amperemeter (ăm′pēr-mēt″er) (see **ammeter**)

amputation neuroma (see **neuroma, traumatic**)

amputation, pulp (see **pulpotomy**)

amputation, root (see **apicoectomy**)

amyloidosis (ăm″ĭ-loi-dō′sĭs) The formation and deposition of a white, insoluble protein in tissue, e.g., in oral tissues, especially the tongue. (Oral Diag.)

— Localized or generalized deposits of amyloid in the tissues of the body. Methods for determining its presence are the Congo red test, gingival biopsy, and biopsy of a parenchymal organ. (Oral Med.)

— A condition in which amyloid, a glycoprotein, is deposited intercellularly in tissues and organs. Four types of amyloidosis are recognized, two of which, primary amyloidosis and amyloid tumor, frequently produce nodules in the tongue and gingiva. (Oral Path.)

    primary a. Amyloidosis occurring without a known predisposing cause. Amyloid deposits are found in the tongue, lips, skeletal muscles, and other mesodermal structures. The disease may be manifested by polyneuropathy, purpura, hepatosplenomegaly, heart failure, and the nephrotic syndrome. (Oral Med.)

    secondary a. Amyloidosis occurring secondary to chronic diseases such as tuberculosis, leprosy, rheumatoid arthritis, multiple myeloma, and prolonged bacterial infections. Amyloid deposits are found in parenchymal organs. The disease is usually manifested by proteinuria and hepatosplenomegaly. (Oral Med.)

amyotonia (ah-mi″o-tō′nē-ah) Abnormal flaccidity or flabbiness of a muscle or group of muscles. (Oral Psysiol.)

anabolism (ah-năb′ō-lĭzm) The constructive process by which substances are converted from simple to complex forms by living cells; constructive metabolism. (Periodont.)

    energy a. The storage of energy in living tissues (one phase of metabolism, the other being catabolism). (Oral Physiol.)

    substance a. Constructive metabolism, the change of matter from a lower to a higher state of organization, especially into organized tissues. (Oral Physiol.)

anacatharsis (an-ah-kah-thar′sĭs) Vomiting. (Anesth.)

anaerobes (ăn-ā′er-ōbs) Microorganisms that can exist and grow only in the partial or complete absence of molecular oxygen. (Periodont.)

analeptic (ăn-ah-lěp′tĭk) An agent that acts to overcome depression of the central nervous system. (Anesth.)

— A strong central nervous system stimulant that is used to restore consciousness, especially from a drug-induced coma. (Oral Med.; Pharmacol.)

analgesia (ăn″al-jē′zē-ah) Loss of all pain sensation without the loss of consciousness as a result of the administration of a drug. (Anesth.)

— Insensibility to pain without loss of consciousness; induced by an anesthetizing agent, the administration of which may be controlled by the operator or by the patient. (Oper. Dent.)

— A state in which painful stimuli are not perceived or interpreted as pain. (Oral Med.; Pharmacol.)

— Lack of awareness of pain stimuli; usually induced by a drug, although trauma or a disease process may produce a general or regional analgesia. (Oral Surg.)

— Absence of sensibility to pain; induced by orally administered drugs (e.g., acetylsalicylic acid or codeine sulfate), topically applied anesthetic agents (e.g., lidocaine ointment), locally injected and inhalation anesthetics, suitably selected music and sounds (audio-analgesia), hypnosis, etc. (Periodont.)

infiltration a. The arrest of the sensory responses of nerve endings at the surgical site by injections of an anesthetic at that site. (Oral Surg.)

regional a. Reversible loss of pain sensation over an area of the body by blocking the afferent conduction of its innervation with a local anesthetic agent. (Anesth.)

analgesic (ăn-al-jē′sĭk) **(analgetic)** The property of a drug that enables it to raise the pain threshold. (Anesth.)

— A drug that obtunds the perception of pain without causing unconsciousness. (Oral Med.; Pharmacol.)

— An analgesic may be classified in one of two groups: an analgesic that blocks the sensory neural pathways of pain (e.g., procaine and its derivatives) or an analgesic that acts directly on the thalamus to raise the pain threshold and to lower reflex stimulation. (Oral Physiol.)

analgetic (ăn-al-jĕt′ĭk) (see **analgesic**)

analgia (ăn-al′jē-ah) Absence of pain. (Anesth.)

analog computer (see **computer, analog**)

analysis (ah-năl′ĭ-sĭs) Separation into component parts.

bite a. (see **analysis, occlusal**)

cephalometric a. (sĕf″ah-lō-mĕ′trĭk) Evaluation of the growth pattern or morphology based on cephalometric tracings. (Orthodont.)

dietary a. Evaluation of a diet on the basis of caloric intake; protein, fat, and carbo-

hydrate proportions; acid-alkali balance; roughage; and minerals and vitamins in order to determine any imbalance or deficiency that could be a causative factor in the production of disease. (Periodont.)

occlusal a. A study of the relations of the occlusal surfaces of opposing teeth. Examination and evaluation of the occlusion of the teeth. (Comp. Prosth.; Fixed Part. Prosth.; Remov. Part. Prosth.)

functional o. a. Examination of the occlusion and disclusion in gnathographically mounted casts and noting on prepared charts the ills of the tooth closures in relation to centric relation, deflective malocclusion both in lateral and centric attempts, the kind of malocclusion, the vertical and horizontal overlaps, and all the minutiae of importance. (Gnathol.)

radiochemical a. Determination of the absolute disintegration rate of a radionuclide in a mixture based on the counting rate of a sample that has been separated and purified, in measured yield, by appropriate chemical procedures. (Oral Radiol.)

analyzing rod (see **rod, analyzing**)

anamnesis (ăn-ăm-nē′sĭs) Past history of disease or injury based on the patient's memory or recall at the time of dental and/or medical interview and examination. (Oral Med.)

anaphylactic (an″ah-fĭ-lăk′tĭk) Pertaining to decreasing, rather than increasing, immunity. (Anesth.)

a. hypersensitivity (Arthus' reaction) A local tissue response that is the result of an Ah-AB caused by repeated intradermal injections with one antigen, resulting in inflammation and necrosis. (Periodont.)

anaphylactoid (ăn″ah fĭ-lăk′toid) Resembling anaphylaxis; pertaining to a reaction, the symptoms of which resemble those of the anaphylactic produced by the injection of serum and other nonspecific proteins. (Anesth.)

a. reaction (see **reaction, anaphylactoid**)

anaphylaxis (ăn″ah-fĭ-lăk′sĭs) A violent allergic reaction characterized by sudden collapse, shock, or respiratory and circulatory failure after injection of an allergen. (Oral Med.)

anaplasia (ăn″ah-plā′zē-ah) A regressive change in cells toward a more primitive or embryonic cell type. Anaplasia is a prominent criterion of malignancy in tumors. (Oral Path.)

anasarca (dropsy) (ăn″ah-sar′kah) Generalized edema. (Oral Med.)

anatomic (ăn-ah-tŏm′ĭk) Pertaining to the anatomy of a structure. (Comp. Prosth.)

a. crown (see **crown, anatomic**)

a. dead space The actual capacity of the respiratory passages that extend from the nostrils to and including the terminal bronchioles. (Anesth.)

a. form (see **form, anatomic**)

a. height of contour (see **contour, height of**)

a. impression (see **impression, anatomic**)

a. landmark (see **landmark**)

a. teeth (see **tooth, anatomic**)

anatomy (ah-năt′ō-mē) The science of the form, structure, and parts of animal organisms.

dental a. The science of the structure of the teeth and the relationship of their parts. The study involves macroscopic and microscopic components. (Periodont.)

radiographic a. The images on a radiographic film of the combined anatomic structures through which the roentgen rays (x rays) have passed. (Oral Radiol.)

anchorage The principle employed in tooth movement whereby the teeth used to move other teeth will move unless sufficient resistance is present to prevent movement. (Orthodont.)

cervical a. The anchorage extending from an appliance (neck strap) fitted around the neck. (Orthodont.)

compound a. The resistance obtained from two or more teeth. (Orthodont.)

extramaxillary a. (extraoral a.) Anchorage secured outside the mouth. (Orthodont.)

extraoral a. (see **anchorage, extramaxillary**)

intermaxillary a. (see **anchorage, maxillomandibular**)

intramaxillary a. Anchorage secured within the same arch. (Orthodont.)

intraoral a. A resistance obtained from inside the oral cavity. (Orthodont.)

maxillomandibular a. Anchorage secured from one dental arch to the other. (Orthodont.)

occipital a. The form of anchorage in which the resistance is borne by the top and back of the head and force is transmitted to the teeth by means of a headgear and heavy elastics connected to attachments on the teeth. (Orthodont.)

reciprocal a. Mutual resistance of one tooth against another by means of which both are moved. (Orthodont.)

simple a. Resistance obtained from a larger tooth or one more favorably situated. (Orthodont.)

stationary a. Application of force so that if the anchor tooth moves at all, it must move bodily. (Orthodont.)

Andresen appliance (see **activator**)

androgen (ăn′drō-jĕn) Any substance that possesses masculinizing qualities, such as testosterone. (Oral Physiol.)

anemia (ah-nē′mē-ah) A quantitative or qualitative hemoglobin deficiency of the blood: a decrease may occur either in the number of red blood cells or in the amount of hemoglobin they contain. (Oral Diag.)

— Term indicating that the concentration of hemoglobin or the number of red blood cells is below the accepted normal value with respect to age and sex. In true anemia the total concentration of hemoglobin or the total number of erythrocytes is below normal irrespective of concentration values. Symptoms, which may or may not be evident, include weakness, pallor, anorexia, and those related to the cause of the anemia. (Oral Med.)

— A condition in which the circulating erythrocytes are deficient in number or in total hemoglobin content per unit volume of blood. (Oral Path.)

— A decrease in blood volume caused by a decrease in erythrocytes resulting from hemorrhages, increased erythrocyte destruction, or decreased erythrocyte production. The latter may result from toxins and exposure to radium and x rays and occurs in a large group of blood dyscrasias. (Oral Physiol.)

Addison-Biermer a. (see **anemia, pernicious**)

aplastic a. Anemia characterized by a decrease in all marrow elements, including platelets, red blood cells, and granulocytes. (Oral Med.)

Biermer's a. (see **anemia, pernicious**)

Cooley's a. (see **thalassemia major**)

displacement a. (see **anemia, myelophthisic**)

erythroblastic a. (see **thalassemia major**)

hemolytic a. Anemia characterized by an increased rate of destruction of red blood cells, reticulocytosis, hyperbilirubinemia and/or increased urinary and fecal urobilinogen, and, generally, splenic enlargement. Hereditary hemolytic anemias include congenital hemolytic jaundice, sickle cell anemia, oval cell anemia, and thalassemia. Acquired hemolytic anemias include paroxysmal nocturnal hemoglobinuria and those due to immune mechanisms (erythroblastosis fetalis), transfusions of incompatible blood, infections, drugs, and poisons. Autoimmune hemolytic anemias are acquired hemolytic anemias associated with antibody-like substances that may not be true autoantibodies or even antibodies; they may be primary (idiopathic), or they may be secondary to lymphoma, lymphatic leukemia, disseminated lupus erythematosus, or sensitization to drugs and pollens. (Oral Med.)

hemorrhagic a. Deficiency in red blood cells and/or hemoglobin due to excessive bleeding. (Oral Diag.)

hyperchromic a. Anemia in which the erythrocytes are larger than normal in size, so that the content, but not the concentration, of hemoglobin is increased. (Oral Med.)

hypochromic a. Anemia caused by impaired hemoglobin synthesis due to a deficiency of iron or pyridoxine and to chronic lead poisoning. (Oral Med.)

microcytic h. a. Anemia in which the mean corpuscular volume (MCV), the mean corpuscular hemoglobin content (MCH), and the mean corpuscular hemoglobin concentration (MCHC) are all low, e.g., iron-deficiency anemia, hereditary leptocytosis, hemoglobin C anemia, and anemias due to pyridoxine deficiency and chronic lead poisoning. (Oral Med.)

iron-deficiency a. Deficiency in hemoglobin resulting from an inadequate intake or utilization of iron. (Oral Diag.)

— Anemia due to a deficiency of iron, characterized by hypochromic microcytic erythrocytes and a normoblastic reaction of the bone marrow. Iron deficiency may be due to an increased demand during growth or repeated pregnancies, to chronic or recurrent hemorrhage (e.g., menstrual abnormalities, hemorrhoids, or peptic ulcer), to a low intake of iron, or to impaired absorption, as in chronic diarrhea. (Oral Med.)

macrocytic-normochromic a. Anemia related to a failure of nucleoprotein synthesis caused by a deficiency of vitamin B_{12}, folic acid, or related substances. (Oral Med.)

Mediterranean a. (see **thalassemia major**)

megaloblastic a. Anemia characterized by hyperplastic bone marrow changes and maturation arrest due to a dietary deficiency, impaired absorption, impaired storage and modification, or impaired utilization of one or more hematopoietic factors. Included are pernicious anemia, nutritional macrocytic anemias associated with gastrointestinal disturbances, anemias associated with impaired liver function (e.g., macrocytic anemia of pregnancy), hypothyroidism, leukemia, and achrestic anemia. (Oral Med.)

myelophthisic a. (displacement a.) Anemia due to displacement or crowding out of erythropoietic cells of the bone marrow by foreign tissue, as in leukemia, metastatic carcinoma,

lymphoblastoma, multiple myeloma, osteoradionecrosis, and xanthomatosis. (Oral Med.)

normocytic-normochromic a. Anemia associated with disturbances of red cell formation and related to endocrine deficiencies, chronic inflammation, and carcinomatosis. (Oral Med.)

nutritional macrocytic a. Macrocytic-normochromic anemia occurring as a result of a deficiency of substances necessary for deoxyribonucleic acid synthesis; e.g., vitamin B_{12} and folic acid deficiency may be due to a lack of intrinsic factors, sprue, regional enteritis, etc. Folic acid deficiency may occur in chronic alcoholism, as a result of a diet deficient in meats and vegetables, and in diseases causing intestinal malabsorption. (Oral Med.)

oval cell a. (see **elliptocytosis**)

pernicious a. (Addison-Biermer a.) A reduction in red blood cells caused by a deficiency in vitamin B_{12} usually due to a lack of the intrinsic factor in the gastric secretion. A painful smooth tongue is usually associated with pernicious anemia. (Oral Diag.)

— A macrocytic-normochromic (megaloblastic) anemia associated with achlorhydria and a lack of a gastric intrinsic factor necessary for the binding and absorption of vitamin B_{12}, which is an erythrocyte-maturing factor. In addition to hematologic findings, atrophic glossitis and gastrointestinal and nervous disorders occur. (Oral Med.)

— A macrocytic hyperchromic anemia caused by the failure of the stomach to produce intrinsic factor, causing an inability to absorb vitamin B_{12}, which is needed for the maturation of erythrocytes. (Oral Path.)

— A disease of hematogenesis; a macrocytic and hyperchromic anemia resulting from a lack of essential factors in gastric secretion. Vitamin B_{12} provides specific therapy for the disease. Generalized lesions include achlorhydria, spinal cord degeneration, and gastrointestinal disturbances, and the oral mucosa is pale and atrophic. (Periodont.)

physiologic a. Anemia characterized by lowered blood values due to an increase in plasma volume that occurs most markedly during the sixth and seventh months of pregnancy. (Oral Med.)

sickle cell a. (drepanocythemia, sicklemia) A hereditary type of anemia confined to Negroes and characterized by the appearance of sickle-shaped cells in the blood. (Oral Diag.)

— A hereditary hemolytic anemia in which the presence of an abnormal hemoglobin (hemoglobin S) results in distorted sickle-shaped erythrocytes. Manifestations include episodic crises of muscle, joint, and abdominal pain; neurologic symptoms; and leg ulcers. It occurs almost exclusively in the Negro race. (Oral Med.) (see also **trait, sickle cell**)

— A hereditary familial hemolytic disease characterized by the capacity of the erythrocytes to assume a sickle shape. (Oral Path.)

spherocytic a. (see **jaundice, congenital hemolytic**)

anergy (ăn′er-jē) In terms of hypersensitivity, an inability to react to specific antigens; i.e., lack of reaction to intradermally injected antigens in measles, Hodgkin's sarcoma, and overwhelming tuberculosis. (Oral Med.)

anesthesia (ăn″ĕs-thē′zē-ah) Loss of feeling or sensation, especially loss of tactile sensibility, with or without loss of consciousness. (Anesth.; Oper. Dent.)

— Entire or partial loss or absence of feeling or sensation; produced by drugs or disease. (D Juris.)

basal a. A state of narcosis, induced prior to the administration of a general anesthetic, that permits the production of states of surgical anesthesia with greatly reduced amounts of general anesthetic agents. (Anesth.)

block a. Anesthesia induced by injecting the drug close to the nerve trunk, at some distance from the operative field. Generally used for operative procedures on maxillary molars and mandibular teeth, except the incisors. (Oper. Dent.) (see also **anesthesia, infiltration**)

endobronchial a. Anesthesia induced by introducing a single catheter into one bronchus or a double-lumen catheter into both main bronchi so that the lungs no longer communicate with each other. An anesthetic is then conducted into one or both of the bronchi as desired. (Anesth.)

general a. An irregular, reversible depression of the cells of the higher centers of the central nervous system that makes the patient unconscious and insensible to pain. (Anesth.)

glove a. Anesthesia with a distribution corresponding to that part of the skin which is covered by a glove. (Anesth.)

infiltration a. Anesthesia induced by injecting the anesthetic solution directly into or around the tissues that are to be anesthetized; used for operative procedures on the maxillary bicuspid, anterior teeth, and mandibular incisors. (Oper. Dent.) (see also **anesthesia, block**)

intranasal a. Topical anesthesia of the nasal membranes produced by direct applications of anesthetic agents. (Oral Surg.)

intraosseous a. Regional or local anesthesia produced by injection; anesthesia produced by the injection of an anesthetic agent into the cancellous portion of a bone. (Oral Surg.)

intrapulpal a. The injection of a local anesthetic directly into pulpal tissue under pressure. (Endodont.)

local a. (**regional a.**) Loss of pain sensation over a specific area of the anatomy without loss of consciousness. (Anesth.; Oper. Dent.)

regional a. Term used for local anesthesia. (Anesth.) (see also **anesthesia, local**)

topical a. A form of local anesthesia whereby free nerve endings in accessible structures are rendered incapable of stimulation by applying a suitable solution directly to the surface of the area. (Anesth.; Oper. Dent.)

anesthesiologist (ăn″ĕs-thē″zē-ŏl′ō-jĭst) A specialist in anesthesiology. (Anesth.)

anesthetic (ăn″ĕs-thĕt′ĭk) A drug that produces loss of feeling or sensation either generally or locally. (Oper. Dent.)

— A pharmaceutical preparation utilized to produce loss of feeling or sensation; applied topically, injected locally, administered by inhalation, or introduced parenterally. (Periodont.)

a. agent (see **agent, anesthetic**)

local a. A drug that has few, if any, irritating effects, when injected into the tissues, and, when absorbed into a nerve, will temporarily interrupt its property of conduction. (Anesth.)

— A drug, injected by either the block or the infiltration method, that produces local insensibility to pain. (Oper. Dent.)

topical a. A drug applied to the surface of tissues that produces local insensibility to pain. Used prior to the insertion of a hypodermic needle to prevent pain; also used to prevent pain associated with scaling or with the retracting of gingival tissues. (Oper. Dent.)

anesthetist (ah-nĕs′thĕ-tĭst) A person who administers anesthetics. (Anesth.)

anesthetize (ah-nĕs′thĕ-tīz) To place under anesthesia. (Anesth.)

aneurysm (ăn′ū-rĭzm) A localized dilation of an

artery in which one or more layers of the vessel walls are distended. (Oral Surg.)

arteriovenous a. (see **shunt, arteriovenous**)

angiitis, visceral (ăn″jē-i′tĭs) (see **disease, collagen**)

angina (ăn-jī′nah) A spasmodic, choking pain. Term is sometimes applied to the disease producing the pain, e.g., Ludwig's angina. Obviously, to call necrotizing ulcerative gingivitis "Vincent's angina" is incorrect. (Oral Med.)

— Attacks of choking, cramplike pain or pain due to "sore throat." (Oral Med.)

agranulocytic a. (see **agranulocytosis**)

Ludwig's a. A severe phlegmonous infection in the floor of the mouth and in the neck. The entire neck is boardlike in hardness, the tongue is elevated, and breathing is difficult. (Oral Diag.; Oral. Med.)

— A cellulitis involving the submaxillary, sublingual, and submental spaces and characterized clinically by a firm swelling of the floor of the mouth, with elevation of the tongue. (Oral Path.)

— A life-endangering, bilateral inflammation of the sublingual, submaxillary, and lateral pharyngeal spaces. A phlegmon. (Oral Surg.)

monocytic a. "Sore throat" associated with infectious mononucleosis. (Oral Med.)

a. pectoris Frequently a symptom of cardiovascular diseases; characterized by a severe, viselike pain behind the sternum that sometimes radiates to the arms, neck, or mandible. It may also consist of a sense of constriction or pressure of the chest. It is brought on by exertion or excitement and is relieved by rest. (Oral Med.)

Vincent's a. Incorrect term for involvement of the pharynx by the spread of acute necrotizing ulceromembranous gingivitis. (Oral Med.)

— Involvement of the throat, i.e., the pharynx and tonsillar areas, by a necrotizing and ulcerative inflammatory disease, associated with the presence of fusospirochetal organisms and apparently precipitated by stress and disturbed emotional states; lesions similar to necrotizing ulcerative gingivitis and stomatitis. (Periodont.)

angioedema (ăn″jē-ō-ĕ-de′mah) (see **edema, angioneurotic**)

angioma (ăn″jē-ō′mah) A benign tumor of vascular nature. (Oral Diag.) (see also **hemangioma; lymphangioma**)

— A benign lesion of either blood or lymph vessel origin. May represent congenital hamartoma or benign neoplasm. (Oral Path.) (see also **hamartoma; hemangioma; lymphangioma**)

angioneurotic edema (ăn″jē-ō-nū-raht′ĭk) (see **edema, angioneurotic**)

angle Degree of divergence of two or more lines or planes that meet each other; the space between such lines. (Oper. Dent.)

Bennett a. The angle formed by the sagittal plane and the path of the advancing condyle during lateral mandibular movement, as viewed in the horizontal plane. (Comp. Prosth.)

— An angle between the protrusive path of a point in the condyle and the path of this point when "orbiting" (curving) about the opposite condyle. (Gnathol.)

a. board A device used to facilitate the establishment of reproducible angular relationships between a patient's head, the x-ray beam, and the x-ray film. (Oral Radiol.)

cavosurface a. The angle in a prepared cavity, formed by the junction of the wall of the cavity with the surface of the tooth. The bevel of this angle is always reckoned from the plane of the enamel wall. (Oper. Dent.)

cranial base a. The angle formed by a line representing the floor of the anterior cranial fossa intersecting a line representing the axis of the clivus of the base of the skull. (Orthodont.)

cusp a. The angle made by the slopes of a cusp with the plane that passes through the tip of the cusp and is perpendicular to a line bisecting the cusp; measured mesiodistally or buccolingually. One half of the included angle between the buccal and lingual or mesial and distal cusp inclines. (Comp. Prosth.)

— The angle made by the slopes of a cusp with a perpendicular line bisecting the cusp; measured mesiodistally or buccolingually. (Remov. Part. Prosth.)

facial a. An anthropometric expression of the degree of protrusion of the lower face, assessed by measuring the inclination of the facial plane relative to a horizontal reference plane. (Orthodont.)

a. former One of a series of paired, hoe-shaped cutting instruments having the cutting edge at an angle other than a right angle in relation to the axis of the blade; used to form or accentuate angles, establish bevels, etc. in cavity preparation. Designed by C. E. Woodbury. (Oper. Dent.)

bayonet a. f. Hoe-shaped, paired cutting instrument; binangled with the blade parallel with the axis of the shaft; the cutting edge is not perpendicular to the axis of the blade. Used to accentuate angles in an "invisible" Class 3 cavity. (Oper. Dent.)

Frankfort-mandibular incisor a. (F.M.I.A.) Procumbency of the mandibular incisor to the Frankfort horizontal plane. (Orthodont.)

incisal a. (ĭn-sī′zăl ăng-ŭl) The degree of slope between the axis-orbital plane and the palatal discluding skidway of the upper incisor. (Gnathol.)

　i. guidance a. The angle formed with the occlusal plane by drawing a line in the sagittal plane between the incisal edges of the maxillary and mandibular central incisors when the teeth are in centric occlusion. (Comp. Prosth.; Remov. Part. Prosth.)

　i. guide a. The inclination of the incisal guide on the articulator. (Comp. Prosth.)

　　lateral i. g. a. The inclination of the incisal guide in the frontal plane. (Comp. Prosth.)

　　protrusive i. g. a. The inclination of the incisal guide in the sagittal plane. (Comp. Prosth.)

line a. An angle formed by the junction of two walls along a line; designated by combining the names of the walls forming the angle. (Oper. Dent.)

a. of mandible The gonial angle. The relation existing between the body of the mandible and the ramus of the mandible. (Orthodont.)

occlusal rest a. The angle formed by the occlusal rest with the upright minor connector. (Remov. Part. Prosth.)

point a. An angle formed by the junction of three walls at a common point; designated by combining the names of the walls forming the angle. (Oper. Dent.)

rest a. (see **angle, occlusal rest**)

symphyseal a. The angle of the chin, which may be protruding, straight, or receding, according to type. (Orthodont.)

Angle's classification, modified A classification of the different forms of malocclusion set up by Edward Hartley Angle, American orthodontist (1855-1930). (Orthodont.)

Class I The normal anteroposterior relationship of the lower jaw to the upper jaw. The mesiobuccal cusp of the maxillary first permanent molar occludes in the buccal groove of the mandibular first permanent molar; **Special Class I**—mutilated.

Type I All teeth in linguoversion.

Type II Narrow arches; labioversion of the maxillary anterior teeth and linguoversion of the mandibular lower anterior teeth.

Type III Linguoversion of the maxillary anterior teeth; bunched; lack of development in the proximal region.

Class II The posterior relationship of the lower jaw to the upper jaw. The mesiobuccal cusp of the maxillary first permanent molar occludes mesial to the buccal groove of the mandibular first permanent molar.

Division 1 Labioversion of the maxillary teeth.

Subdivision Signifies a unilateral condition.

Division 2 Linguoversion of the maxillary central incisor teeth.

Subdivision Signifies a unilateral condition.

Class III The anterior relationship of the lower jaw to the upper jaw; may have a subdivision. The mesiobuccal cusp of the maxillary first permanent molar occludes distal to the buccal groove of the mandibular first permanent molar.

Type I The alignment generally good but the arch relationship abnormal.

Type II Good alignment of the maxillary anterior teeth but linguoversion of the mandibular anterior teeth.

Type III The upper arch underdeveloped; the maxillary anterior teeth in linguoversion; the mandibular alignment good.

Subdivision A unilateral condition.

Ångström unit (see **unit, Ångström**)

angular cheilosis (see **cheilosis, angular**)

angulation (ăng″gū-lā′shŭn) The direction of the primary beam of radiation in relation to object and film. (Oral Radiol.)

horizontal a. The angle measured within the occlusal plane at which the central ray of the x-ray beam is projected relative to a reference in the vertical or sagittal plane. (Oral Radiol.)

vertical a. The angle measured within the vertical plane at which the central ray of the x-ray beam is projected relative to a reference in the horizontal or occlusal plane. (Oral Radiol.)

anguli, palatal (ăng′gū-lī) The lingual lobes of the upper anterior teeth with marked mesiodistal convexities; appear as a girdle on the cervical third of the palatal surfaces of the teeth. (Periodont.)

anhidrosis (ăn″hĭ-drō′sĭs) An abnormal deficiency in the production of sweat; may be associated with anodontia in ectodermal dysplasia. (Oral Diag.)

anhidrotic ectodermal dysplasia (see **hypohidrotic ectodermal dysplasia**) (Oral Med.)

anhydremia (ăn-hī-drē′mē-ah) A decrease in blood volume due to a decrease in the serum component of blood; occurs in shock or in any condition in which blood fluid is passed into the tissue and results in hemoconcentration. (Oral Physiol.)

anion (an′ī-ŏn) A negatively charged ion. (Oral Radiol.)

anionic detergent (ăn″ī-ahn′ĭk) (see **detergent, anionic**)

anisocytosis (ăn-ī″-sō-sī-tō′sĭs) Inequality in cell size, especially of red blood cells. (Oral Diag.)

anisognathous (ăn″ī-sŏg′nah-thŭs) Maxillary and mandibular dental arches or jaws are of different sizes. (Comp. Prosth.; Oral Diag.; Orthodont.; Remov. Part. Prosth.)

ankyloglossia (ăng″kĭ-lō-glahs′ē-ah) Tonguetie. (Oral Diag.)

— Fusion of the tongue with the floor of the mouth; the condition may be partial or complete. (Oral Path.)

ankylosis (ăng″kĭ-lō′sĭs) Abnormal fixation and immobility of a joint, including the gomphosis type of joint, that fixes the teeth to the jaw. The ankylosis may be fibrous or bony. (Oral Diag.)

— Fixation of a joint by a fibrous or bony union of the bones and joint components. (Oral Med.)

— Hypomobility in a joint due to pathologic proliferation of fibrous connective tissue or bone. (Oral Path.)

— Restriction of movement by the development of adhesions or ossification in the joint between two bones, at least one of which normally serves as a lever. (Oral Physiol.)

— Complete or partial loss of motion of a part normally movable. (Oral Surg.)

— Abnormal immobility and consolidation of a joint; consolidation of the alveolar bone and cementum of the teeth. (Orthodont.)

a. of active eruption A pathologic process that has stopped the eruptive movement of a tooth. (Periodont.)

false a. Inability to open the mouth due to trismus rather than to disease of the joint. (Oral Diag.)

fibrous a. Fixation of a joint by fibrous tissue; slight motion may be possible. (Oral Diag.)

a. of tooth (see **tooth, ankylosed**)

anlage (ăn′lah-gĕh) The first cells in the embryo that form any distinct part or organ of the body. (Oral Surg.)

anneal (ah-nēl′) (**homogenizing heat treatment, softening heat treatment**) The softening of a metal by controlled heating and cooling. The process makes a metal more easily contoured to a definite form—more easily adapted, bent, or swaged—and less brittle. (Comp. Prosth.; Remov. Part. Prosth.)

— Heat treatment of metals to relieve strain hardening through atomic diffusion in the solid state; solution of homogenizing heat treatment. Technically the term refers to a heating and cooling operation; however, it commonly connotes the softening of a metal. (D. Mat.; Oper. Dent.)

a. foil A process of subjecting noncohesive foil to heat to volatilize a protective gaseous coating on its surface, thus leaving the surface clean, making it cohesive, and restoring its property of cold welding. Present evidence does not indicate that the foil is actually annealed or softened by this procedure. (Oper. Dent.)

a. glass A process of regulated heating and subsequent cooling to remove strain hardening or work hardening of glass. (Oper. Dent.)

a. metal A process of regulated heating and subsequent cooling to remove strain hardening or work hardening of metal. (Oper. Dent.)

announcement A communication (usually printed) that states office policies or practice limitations to the public and the profession. (Pract. Man.)

anochromasia (ăn″ō-krō-mā′sē-ah) Variation in the staining quality of cells, particularly of degenerating red blood cells. (Oral. Diag.)

anociassociation (ah-nō″sē-ah-sō-sē-ā′shŭn) The blocking of neuroses, fear, pain, and harmful influences or associations to prevent shock. (Anesth.)

anode (ăn′ōd) The positive terminal of a roentgen ray (x-ray) tube; a tungsten block embedded in a copper stem and set at an angle of either 20° or 45° to the cathode. The anode emits roentgen rays (x rays) from the point of impact of the electronic stream from the cathode. (Oral Radiol.)

rotating a. An anode that rotates during x-ray production to present a constantly different focal spot to the electron stream and to permit use of small focal spots or higher tube voltages without overheating the tube. (Oral Radiol.)

anode-film distance (see **distance, target-film**)

anodontia (ăn-ō-dŏn′shē-ah) (**aplasia of dentition**) Failure of teeth to form; may be partial or complete. (Oral Diag; Orthodont.)

— Congenital absence of teeth; may be partial or total and may affect the permanent dentition or both the deciduous and the permanent dentitions. (Oral Path.)

    partial a. Absence of parts of the dentition resulting from arrested tooth development. (Pedodont.)

    total a. Complete absence of teeth resulting from arrested tooth development. (Pedodont.)

anodyne (ăn′ō-dīn) An agent or drug that relieves pain; milder than analgesia. (Anesth.; Oper. Dent.)

anomaly (ah-nŏm′ah-lē) A developmental disturbance of minor degree, e.g., gemination. (Oral Diag.)

— An aberration or deviation from normal anatomic growth, development, or function. (Orthodont.)

    dental a. An abnormality in which a tooth or teeth have deviated from the normal in form, function, or position. (Orthodont.)

    dentofacial a. Term indicating an oral or a dysgnathic anomaly. (Orthodont.)

    dysgnathic a. An anomaly that extends beyond the teeth and includes the maxillae, the mandible, or both. (Orthodont.)

    eugnathic a. An anomaly limited to the teeth and their immediate alveolar supports. (Orthodont.)

    gestant a. (see **odontoma**)

    maxillofacial a. Distortion of normal development of the face and jaws; a dysgnathic anomaly. (Orthodont.)

    oral a. An abnormal structure other than of the teeth. (Orthodont.)

anophaxia (ăn-ō-făx′ē-ah) A tendency for one eye to turn upward. (Anesth.)

anorexia (ăn-ō-rĕk′sē-ah) The partial or complete loss of appetite for food. (Oral Med.)

anoxemia (ăn-ahk-sē′mē-ah) A deficient aeration of the blood; a total lack of oxygen content in the blood. (Anesth.)

anoxia (ăn-ahk′sē-ah) A condition of total oxygen lack; term frequently misused as a symptom of hypoxia. (Anesth.)

— Oxygen deficiency. (Oral Physiol.)

anoxiate (ăn-ahk′sē-āt) To cause or produce anoxia. (Anesth.)

anoxic hypoxia (see **hypoxia, anoxic**)

antagonist A drug that counteracts, blocks, or abolishes the action of another drug. (Oral Med.; Pharmacol.; Oral Physiol.)

— A muscle that acts in opposition to the action of another muscle, e.g., flexor vs. extensor. (Oral Physiol.)

— A tooth in one jaw that occludes with a tooth in the other jaw. (Oral Physiol.)

    insulin a. Circulating hormonal and nonhormonal substances that stimulate glyconeogenesis; e.g., 11-oxysteroids and S hormones. (Oral Med.)

    loss of a. A situation in which a tooth loses its opponent in the opposite dental arch, resulting in loss of function and periodontal atrophy disease. (Periodont.)

    narcotic a. A narcotic drug that acts specifically to reverse depression of the central nervous system. (Anesth.)

antagonistic reflex (see **reflex, antagonistic**)

ante cibum (ăn″tē sī′bum) (see **a.c.**)

anterior Situated in front of; term used to denote the incisor and canine teeth or the forward region of the mouth. (Oper. Dent.; Orthodont.)

— The forward position. (Orthodont.)

    a. determinants of occlusion (see **occlusion, anterior determinants of cusp**)

    a. guide (see **guide, anterior**)

    a. nasal spine (see **spine, anterior nasal**)

    a. palatal bar (see **connector, anterior palatal major**)

    a. tooth arrangement (see **arrangement, tooth, anterior**)

anteroclusion Malocclusion of the teeth in which the mandibular teeth are in a position anterior to their normal position relative to the teeth in the maxillary arch. (Orthodont.)

anteversion The tipping or tilting of teeth or other maxillary and mandibular structures too far forward (anterior) from the normal or generally accepted standard. (Orthodont.)

anthelmintic (ăn″thĕl-mĭn′tĭk) A drug that acts against parasitic worms, especially intestinal worms. (Oral Med.; Pharmacol.)

anthrax (ăn′thraks) An infectious disease in herbivorous animals caused by a spore-forming bacillus. Primary lesions in human beings may be on the lips or cheeks. (Oral Diag.)

antibiotic (ăn-tĭ-bī-ŏt′ĭk) An organic substance produced by one of several microorganisms, especially certain molds, that is capable, in low concentration, of destroying or inhibiting the growth of certain other microorganisms. (Oral Med.; Pharmacol.)

    a. in hairy tongue (see **tongue, hairy**)

    oral reactions to a. Manifestations on the oral mucous membrane of reactions to antibiotics;

characterized by glossitis, angular cheilosis, and/or hairy tongue. Reactions may be due to imbalance of oral flora produced by the antibiotics or to hypersensitivity to the antibiotics. (Periodont.)

a. therapy (see **therapy, antibiotic**)

a. tongue (see **tongue, antibiotic**)

antibody (ăn′tĭ-bŏd-ē) A specific substance that is produced by an animal as a reaction to the presence of an antigen and that reacts specifically with an antigen in some observable way.

anticholinergic (ăn″tĭ-kō″lĭn-er′jĭk) **(parasympatholytic, cholinolytic)** A drug that acts to inhibit the effects of the neurohormone acetylcholine or to inhibit the cholinergic neuroeffects. A cholinergic blocking agent. (Anesth.; Oral Med.; Pharmacol.)

anticholinesterase (ăn″tĭ-kō″lĭn-es′ter-ās) A drug or chemical that inhibits or inactivates the enzyme cholinesterase, resulting in the actions produced by the accumulation of acetylcholine at cholinergic sites. (Anesth.; Oral Physiol.; Pharmacol.)

anticoagulant (ăn″tĭ-kō-ăg′ū-lănt) A drug that delays or prevents coagulation of blood. (Oral Med.; Pharmacol.)

anticonvulsive Relieving or preventing convulsion. (Anesth.)

antidote (ăn′tĭ-dōt) A substance that acts to antagonize the toxic effects of a drug, especially in overdose, or of a poison. (Anesth.; Oral Med.; Pharmacol.)

antiemetic (ăn″tē-ē-mĕt′ĭk) A drug used to prevent, stop, or relieve nausea and emesis (vomiting). (Anesth.; Oral Med.; Pharmacol.)

antiflux A material that prevents and confines the flow of solder, e.g., graphite. (D. Mat.)

antigen (ăn′tĭ-jĕn) A substance that incites the formation of antibodies when introduced into the blood or tissues. (Anesth.)

— A substance, usually a protein, that elicits the formation of antibodies which react with it when introduced parenterally into an individual or species to which it is foreign. (Oral Med.)

antihemophilic factor (an″tĭ-hē″mō-fĭl′ĭk) (see **factor VIII**)

antihistamine (ăn″tĭ-hĭs′tah-mĭn) A drug that counteracts the release of histamine, e.g., in allergic reactions; also has topical anesthetic and sedative effects as well as a drying effect on the nasal mucosa. (Oral Med.)

— A drug that antagonizes the effects of histamine in the body. (Oral Med.; Pharmacol.)

— A blocking drug; it prevents the access of histamine to its receptor site in the cell and thereby blocks the response of the effector cell to the antigen. (Oral Physiol.)

antihistaminic (ăn″tĭ-hĭs-tah-mĭn′ĭk) Referring to a drug that acts to prevent or antagonize the pharmacologic effects of histamine released in the tissues. (Anesth.)

antihypnotic (ăn″tĭ-hĭp-not′ĭk) Preventing or hindering sleep. (Anesth.)

antileptic (ăn″tĭ-lĕp′tĭk) Assisting, supporting, revulsive. (Anesth.)

anti-Monson curve (see **curve, reverse**)

antiphlogistic (ăn″tĭ-flō-jĭs′tĭk) Obsolete term for anti-inflammatory or antipyretic. (Oral Med.; Pharmacol.)

antipruritic (ăn″tĭ-proo-rĭt′ĭk) Relieving or preventing itching. (Oral Med.; Pharmacol.)

antipyretic (ăn″tĭ-pī-rĕt′ĭk) A drug that reduces fever primarily through action on the hypothalamus, thereby resulting in increased heat dissipation through augmented peripheral blood flow and sweating. (Oral Med.; Pharmacol.)

antisepsis (ăn″tĭ-sĕp′sĭs) The prevention of infection of a body surface, usually skin or oral mucosa, through the application of an antimicrobial agent. (Anesth.; Oral Surg.; Pharmacol.)

antiseptic (ăn″tĭ-sĕp′tĭk) An antimicrobial agent for application to a body surface, usually skin or oral mucosa, in an attempt to prevent or minimize infection at the area of application. (Anesth.; Oral Med.; Periodont.; Pharmacol.)

antisialagogue (ăn″tĭ-sī-ăl′ah-gawg) A drug that reduces, slows, or prevents the flow of saliva. (Anesth.; Oral Med.; Pharmacol.)

antisialic (ăn″tē-sī-ăl′ĭk) Checking or that which checks salivary secretions. (Anesth.)

antispasmodic (ăn″tĭ-spăz-mod′ĭk) **(antispastic)** A drug that relieves muscle spasms. (Anesth.)

antispastic (see **antispasmodic**)

antistreptolysin O (ăn″tĭ-strĕp-tol′ĭ-sĭn) An antibody against streptolysin O, a hemolysin produced by group A streptococci. A high titer is supporting evidence of rheumatic fever. (Oral Med.)

antithermic Reducing temperature. (Anesth.) (see also **antipyretic**)

antitussive (ăn″tĭ-tŭs′ĭv) A drug that relieves or prevents cough. (Oral Med.; Pharmacol.)

Antoni type tissue (see **tissue, Antoni types A and B**)

antrodynia (ăn″trō-dĭn′ē-ah) Pain in the maxillary antrum. (Oral Surg.)

antrostomy (ăn-trŏs′tō-mē) A surgical opening into an antrum, either through the medial wall into the nose or through the lateral wall into the oral cavity. (Oral Surg.)

antrum (ăn'trŭm) A maxillary sinus; the antrum of Highmore. A cavity in the maxilla, lined by ciliated columnar epithelium, the inferior border of which approximates the apices of the roots of the maxillary posterior teeth. (Periodont.)

a. of Highmore (see **sinus, maxillary**)

maxillary a. (see **sinus, maxillary**)

antuitrin S (ăn-tu'ĭ-trĭn) (see **hormone, pregnancy**)

ANUG A distinct, recurrent periodontal disease involving primarily the interdental papillae, which undergo necrosis and ulceration. (Periodont.)

anxiety Vague, unmotivated fear. (Oral Diag.)

— A complex emotional state, with fear or apprehension as its most prominent feature. Fear produced by past experiences or apprehension of future possibilities; may be centered around specific diseases or body organs. (Oral Med.)

— A condition of heightened and often disruptive tension accompanied by an ill-defined and distressing aura of impending harm or injury. Anxiety can disrupt physiologic functions through its effect on the autonomic nervous system. The patient may assume tense posture, show excessive vigilance, move the hands and feet restlessly, and speak with a strained, uneven voice. The pupils may be widely dilated, giving the appearance of unrestrained fright, and the hands and face may perspire excessively. In extremely acute forms of anxiety the patient may have generalized visceral reactions of respiratory, cardiac, vascular, and gastrointestinal dysfunction. The dentist must recognize the existence of anxiety, seek its etiology and relation to dental treatment, and determine how the patient's defenses against anxiety can be used to facilitate rather than inhibit treatment. (Oral Physiol.)

— A feeling of apprehension, uncertainty, and fear often associated with the genesis of harmful dental habits and with the occurrence of necrotizing ulcerative gingivitis. (Periodont.)

apathic (ah-păth'ĭk) Without sensation or feeling. (Anesth.)

apathism (ăp'ah-thĭzm) The state of being slow in responding to stimuli. (Anesth.)

apatite (ăp'ah-tīt) The inorganic mineral substance of teeth and bone. (see also **carbonate hydroxyapatite**)

APC (see **aspirin, phenacetin, caffeine**)

apertognathia (ah-per″tō-năth'ē-ah) "Open-bite" deformity. (Oral Surg.)

— An occlusion characterized by a vertical separation between the maxillary and mandibular

anterior teeth. Incorrectly called an "open bite." (Orthodont.)

Apert's syndrome (see **syndrome, Apert's**)

aperture An opening. (Anesth.)

apex The end of the root. (Endodont.)

a. blunderbuss An open or everted apex of a tooth, resembling the divergent form of the barrel of a blunderbuss rifle. (Endodont.)

apexification (ā-pĕk″sĭ-fĭ-kā'shŭn) The process of continued root development or apical closure of the root by hard tissue deposition. (Endodont.)

apexigraph (ā-pĕks'ĭ-grăf) A device for determining the position of the apex of a tooth root. (Endodont.)

aphagia (ah-fā'jē-ah) Inability to swallow. (Anesth.)

aphasia (ah-fā'zē-ah) Loss of power of expression through speech, writing, or signs, or of comprehending spoken or written language due to disease or injury of the brain centers (either sensory or motor or both). (Oral Physiol.)

aphtha (ăf'thah) (**aphthous stomatitis**) A small ulcer on the mucous membrane. (Oral Diag.)

—, pl. **-hae** Vesicles that undergo subsequent ulceration and are surrounded by a raised erythematous area. (Periodont.)

Bednar's a. (bĕd'narz) (**pterygoid ulcer**) An ulcer on the soft palate near the greater palatine foramen; seen in newborn infants. (Oral Path.)

Mikulicz' a. (mĭk'ū-lĭch) Recurrent ulceration of the oral mucosa, resembling herpes. (Oral Diag.) (see also **periadenitis mucosa necrotica recurrens**)

recurrent a. (see **stomatitis, herpetic; ulcer, aphthous, recurrent**)

recurrent scarring a. (see **periadenitis mucosa necrotica recurrens**)

aphthous stomatitis (ăf'thŭs) (see **aphtha; stomatitis, aphthous; stomatitis, herpetic**)

apical (ăp'ĭ-kal) Pertaining to the end portion of the root. (Endodont.)

a. base (see **base, apical**)

a. fiber (see **fiber, apical**)

apicectomy (ā″pĭ-sĕk'tō-mē) (see **apicoectomy**)

apicoectomy (ā″pĭ-kō-ĕk'tō-mē) (**apicectomy, apiectomy, root amputation, root resection**) Surgical removal of the apex or apical portion of a root. (Endodont.)

— Excision of the apical portion of a root in order to gain access to the periapical area to remove diseased tissues. (Oral Surg.)

apicostome (ā'pē-kō-stōm) An instrument for performing an apicostomy. (Endodont.)

apicostomy (ā-pē-kahs'tō-mē) The formation of

a surgical opening through the mucoperiosteum and the alveolar bone to the apical end of a tooth. (Endodont.)

apiectomy (ā″pē-ĕk′tō-mē) (see **apicoectomy**)

aplasia (ah-plā′zē-ah) Lack of origin or development, e.g., aplasia of dentition associated with ectodermal dysplasia. (Oral Diag.)

a. of dentition (see **anodontia**)

apnea (ăp′nē-ah) A temporary cessation of respiratory movements. (Anesth.)

apneumatic (ăp-nū-măt′ĭk) Free from air; used to describe something accomplished with the exclusion of air, e.g., an apneumatic operation. (Anesth.)

apoplexy (ăp′ō-plĕk″sē) A stroke caused by acute vascular lesions of the brain. (Oral Diag.)

apostematosa, cheilitis glandularis (see **cheilitis glandularis apostematosa**)

apothecaries' system (see **system, apothecaries'**)

apoxesis (ăp-ahk-sē′sĭs) (see **curettage, apical**)

apparatus (ăp″ah-rā′tŭs) Arrangement of a number of parts that act together to perform some special function.

attachment a. The tissues that invest and support the teeth for function: the cementum, the periodontal ligament, and the alveolar bone. (Periodont.)

masticating a. The structures involved in chewing, e.g., the teeth, the mandibular musculature, the mandible and its temporomandibular joints, the accessory mandibular and facial musculature, and the tongue, which are controlled by an exquisitely functioning neuromuscular mechanism. (Periodont.) (see also **system, stomatognathic**)

appellant (ah-pĕl′ănt) The party who, dissatisfied with the disposition of a case on the trial level, appeals to a higher court; one who appeals. (D. Juris.)

appliance (ah-plī′ăns) A device used to provide function or therapeutic effect, e.g., a dental prosthesis, a fixation splint, a removable occlusal overlay, or an obturator. (Comp. Prosth.; Remov. Part. Prosth.) (see also **restoration**)

acrylic resin and copper band a. A provisional device for splinting teeth. Copper bands are fitted accurately to the cervical portions of the teeth (which have been prepared for full coverage), over which either cold-curing or heat-processed tooth acrylic resin is applied and contoured so as to establish harmonious relationships with adjacent teeth or opposing dentition and to afford protection for the investing and supporting structures of the teeth encompassed within the splint. (Periodont.)

activator a. (see **activator**)

craniofacial a. A device used to immobilize and/or reduce mandibular or midfacial fractures. The attachment is either external, using wires or bars to headcaps or skeletal pins; or internal, using circumzygomatic wires, circummandibular wires, or wires passed through drill holes in the following: zygomatic process of the frontal bone, inferoanterior border of the zygomatic arch, infraorbital rim, anterior nasal spine, and inferior rim of the bony nares (piriform aperture). (Oral Surg.)

Crozat a. A removable orthodontic appliance constructed of wire. (Orthodont.)

edgewise a. An appliance using a rectangular labial arch wire ligated to brackets on bands cemented to individual teeth. (Orthodont.)

fixed a. (permanent a.) An appliance that is cemented to the teeth or attached by means of an adhesive material. (Orthodont.)

fracture a. (biphase pin fixation, external pin fixation, Stader splint) Any one of the various devices for extraoral reduction and fixation of fractures in which pins, clamps, or screws are placed in the fractured segments, the fractured parts aligned, and then the pins, clamps, or screws joined with metal bars or rigid plastic connectors, e.g., the Stader splint or Roger-Anderson pin fixation appliance. (Oral Surg.)

Hawley a. A removable device made to fit in the palate against the lingual surfaces of the teeth and used to retain the positions of teeth after they have been aligned by active orthodontic treatment. (Orthodont.)

hay rake a. A device used to limit abnormal excursions of the tongue. Consists of an upper acrylic resin palate secured by spring clasps, with a wire railing approximately 0.5 cm in height and 3 cm in length placed palatal to the upper incisors, giving the tongue a "stirrup" into which to thrust. In this manner, harmful effects of tongue thrusting are mitigated until the patient learns a new swallowing pattern. (Periodont.)

labiolingual a. An appliance utilizing the maxillary and mandibular first permanent molars as anchorage, with labial arches, 0.036 to 0.040 inch in diameter, introduced into horizontal buccal tubes attached to the anchor bands and lingual arches of the same diameter fitted into vertical or horizontal tubes fastened to the lingual side of the anchor bands. Various designs of wires of smaller diameter are fashioned into loops attached to both the labial and lingual arches to initiate different types of movement. (Orthodont.)

light round-wire a. An appliance utilizing small-gauge labial wires (0.016 inch or less) applied in a multibanded technique. This appliance was made particularly popular by P. R. Begg of Australia and utilizes expansion and contraction loops, as well as intermaxillary hooks, all formed into the main wire. A ribbon-arch type of bracket is used in producing tipping and bodily movements. (Orthodont.)

multibanded a. An appliance that incorporates bands other than the molar anchor bands. (Orthodont.)

obturator a. (see **obturator**)

orthodontic a. A mechanism for the application of force to the teeth and their supporting tissues to produce changes in their relationships and to control their growth and development. (Orthodont.)

— A device (fixed, removable, or a combination thereof) designed to move teeth into a more esthetic and functional (physiologic) alignment within the dental arch and in relationship to the opposing dentition. Orthodontic appliances may also be used to stabilize or immobilize teeth, reduce fractures of the maxillae or mandible, etc. (Periodont.)

removable o. a. An appliance so designed that it can be removed and replaced by the patient. (Orthodont.)

permanent a. (see **appliance, fixed**)

pin and tube a. A labial arch with vertical posts that insert into tubes attached to bands on the teeth. (Orthodont.)

prosthetic a. A complete or partial denture for children when groups of teeth are lost or are congenitally missing. Used to maintain space or masticatory function, or for esthetic reasons. (Pedodont.)

regulating a. An orthodontic appliance. (Orthodont.)

retaining a. (see **retainer**)

speech a. (see **aid, prosthetic speech**)

therapeutic a. A vehicle used to transport and retain some agent for therapeutic purposes, e.g., a radium carrier. (M.F.P.)

twin-wire a. An appliance utilizing fixed lingual arches and a labial arch consisting of two light round wires attached to brackets on the anterior teeth. (Orthodont.)

universal a. An appliance designed by Spencer R. Atkinson that includes bands for all the teeth in both arches. To each of the bands is attached a special bracket with two transverse slots for labial or buccal wires, the cervical slot opening buccally and the incisal or occlusal slot opening superiorly. The wires for the cervical bracket are 0.008 to 0.015 inch in diameter, whereas the occlusal bracket receives a flat wire measuring 0.010 to 0.015 × 0.028 inch. The wires are held in place by a single lock pin. A lingual arch with a 0.30-inch diameter fits into horizontal lingual molar sheaths. The round wire allows for mesiodistal and intrusive and extrusive movements, and the flat wire rotates and allows for buccolingual tooth movement. (Orthodont.)

applicator A device for applying medication; usually a slender rod of glass or wood, used with a pledget of cotton on the end. (Oper. Dent.)

appointment A mutually agreed-on time reserved for the patient to receive treatment. (Pract. Man.)

a. book A ledger or table of workdays divided into segments of time to enable the dentist to reserve specified lengths of time for patient treatment. (Pract. Man.)

a. card A small card given to the patient as a reminder of the time reserved for him. (Pract. Man.)

apposition (ăp-ō-sĭ'shŭn) The condition of being placed or fitted together; juxtaposition; coaptation. (Comp. Prosth.; Remov. Part. Prosth.)

approximal (approximating) Contiguous; adjacent; next to each other. (Oper. Dent.)

approximating (see **approximal**)

apraxia (ah-prăk'sē-ah) A loss of ability to execute a purposeful, goal-oriented, or skilled act due to selective damage to certain high-level brain centers, either sensory, motor, or both. (Oral Physiol.)

apron A piece of clothing worn in front of the body for protection.

a. band A labial incisal or gingival extension of an orthodontic band that aids in retention of the band and in proper positioning of the bracket. (Orthodont.)

lead a. An apron made of materials containing metallic lead or lead compounds for the purpose of reducing radiation hazards. (Oral Radiol.)

lingual a. (see **connector, linguoplate major**)

rubber dam a. A small strip of rubber dam, perforated to fit over an implant abutment that is used to inhibit introduction of cement into the peri-implant space. (Oral Implant.)

arc, reflex A system of nerves utilized in a reflex

or involuntary act, consisting primarily of an afferent nerve with sensory receptor, a nerve center, and an efferent nerve that stimulates the effector muscle or gland. (Oral Physiol.)

arch(es) A structure with a curved outline.

a. bar (see **bar, arch**)

basal a. (see **base, apical**)

dental a. The composite structure of the dentition and the alveolar ridge or the remains thereof after the loss of some or all of the natural teeth. (Comp. Prosth.; Fixed Part. Prosth.; Remov. Part. Prosth.)

> **d. a. contraction** (see **contraction**)
>
> **dentulous d. a.** A dental arch containing natural teeth.
>
> **edentulous d. a.** A dental arch from which all natural teeth are missing. The residual alveolar ridge. (Comp. Prosth.)
>
> > **partially e. d. a.** A dental arch from which one or more but not all teeth are missing. (Comp. Prosth.; Fixed Part. Prosth.; Remov. Part. Prosth.)

a. expansion (see **expansion**)

a. form (see **form, arch**)

high labial a. A labial arch wire adapted so as to lie gingival to the anterior tooth crowns; has auxiliary springs extending downward in contact with the teeth to be moved. (Orthodont.)

ovoid a. An arch that curves continuously from the molars on one side to the molars on the opposite side in such a way that two such arches placed back to back describe an oval. (Orthodont.)

palatine a. (glossopalatine a.) The pillars of the fauces; the two arches of mucous membrane enclosing the muscles at the sides of the passage from the mouth to the pharynx. (Oral Surg.)

passive lingual a. An orthodontic appliance effective in maintaining space and preserving arch length when bilateral primary molars are prematurely lost. (Pedodont.)

pharyngeal a. The branchial arches of the fetus. (Oral Surg.)

removable lingual a. An arch wire that is designed to fit the lingual surface of the teeth. It has two posts soldered on each end that fit snugly into the vertical tubes of the molar anchor bands. (Orthodont.)

stationary lingual a. An arch wire that is designed to fit the lingual surface of the teeth and is soldered to the anchor bands. (Orthodont.)

tapering a. A dental arch that converges from molars to central incisors to such an extent

that lines passing through the central grooves of the molars and premolars intersect within 1 inch anterior ot the central incisors. (Orthodont.)

trapezoidal a. An arch that has the same convergence as a tapering arch but to a lesser degree. The anterior teeth are somewhat squared to abruptly rounded from canine tip to canine tip. The canines act as corners of the arch. (Orthodont.)

U-shaped a. A dental arch in which there is little difference in diameter (width) between the first premolars and the last molars; the curve from canine to canine is abrupt, so that a dental arch in the shape of a capital U is formed. (Orthodont.)

a. width The width of a dental arch. The width, which varies in all diameters between the right and left opposites, is determined by direct measurement between the canines, between the first molars, and between the second bicuspids. These intercanine, interbicuspid, and intermolar distances can be cited as arch width. (Gnathol.)

a. wire (see **wire, arch**)

architecture, gingiva (see **gingiva, architecture**)

arcus senilis (ar′kŭs sē-nĭ′lĭs) An opaque grayish white ring at the periphery of the cornea occurring in elderly persons. (Oral Diag.)

area Region.

apical a. (see **base, apical**)

basal seat a. (denture-bearing a., denture-supporting a., stress-bearing a., stress-supporting a.) The portion of the oral structures that is available to support a denture; surfaces of oral structures that resist forces brought on them during function. (Comp. Prosth.; Remov. Part. Prosth.)

— The edentulous portion of a dental arch on which a fixed or removable prosthesis rests. (Periodont.)

contact a. (see **point, contact**)

denture-bearing a. (see **area, basal seat**)

denture-supporting a. (see **area, basal seat**)

impression a. The surface of the oral structures recorded in an impression. (Comp. Prosth.; Remov. Part. Prosth.)

pear-shaped a. (see **pad, retromolar**)

post dam a. (see **area, posterior palatal seal**)

posterior palatal seal a. The soft tissues along the junction of the hard and soft palates on which pressure, within the physiologic limits of the tissues, can be applied by a denture to aid in its retention. (Comp. Prosth.; Remov. Part. Prosth.)

postpalatal seal a. (see **area, posterior palatal seal**)

pressure a. An area of excessive displacement of soft tissue. An area in an impression where the tray shows through the impression material. (Comp. Prosth.; Remov. Part. Prosth.)

recipient a. That portion of the body on which a skin, bone, tooth, or other graft is placed. (Oral Surg.)

relief a. That portion of the surface of the mouth on which pressures are reduced or eliminated. (Comp. Prosth.; Remov. Part. Prosth.)

rest a. (rest seat) The prepared surface of a tooth or fixed restoration into which the rest fits, giving support to a removable partial denture. (Remov. Part. Prosth.)

rugae a. (rū'gī) **(rugae zone)** That portion of the hard palate in which rugae are found. (Comp. Prosth.; Remov. Part. Prosth.)

saddle a. (see **area, basal seat**)

stress-bearing a. (see **area, basal seat**)

stress-supporting a. (see **area, basal seat**)

supporting a. The areas of the maxillary and mandibular edentulous ridges that are considered best suited to carry the forces of mastication when the dentures are in function. (Comp. Prosth.) (see also **area, basal seat**)

— The surfaces of the residual ridges and/or teeth used for the support of a denture. (Remov. Part. Prosth.)

Argyll Robertson pupil (ar-gĭl') (see **pupil, Argyll Robertson**)

argyria (ar-jĭr'ē-ah) A bluish color of the skin or mucous membranes produced by the deposition of silver salts in collagen fibers after prolonged use of silver salts. (Oral Med.)

local a. Localized blue pigmentation of the oral mucosa from the deposition of silver amalgam in the submucosal connective tissue. (Oral Med.)

argyrosis (ar-jĭ-rō'sĭs) Pathologic bluish black pigmentation in a tissue due to the deposition of an insoluble albuminate of silver. (Oral Diag.; Oral Path.)

ariboflavinosis (ah-rī"bō-flā-vĭ-nō'sĭs) A nutritional disease due to a deficiency of riboflavin (vitamin B_2); characterized by angular cheilosis, seborrheic dermatitis, magenta tongue, and ocular disturbance. (Oral Med.)

Arkansas stone (ar'kan-saw) (see **stone, Arkansas**)

arm A definitely shaped extension or projection

of a removable partial denture framework. (Remov. Part. Prosth.)

reciprocal a. A clasp arm or other extension used on a removable partial denture to oppose any force arising from an opposing clasp arm on the same tooth. Reciprocation cannot be attained unless a similar arrangement is provided on the opposite side of the dental arch. (Remov. Part. Prosth.) (see also **arm, retention**)

retention a. An extension or projection that is part of a removable partial denture and is used to aid in the retention and stabilization of the restoration, e.g., a part of a direct retainer. (Remov. Part. Prosth.) (see also **arm, reciprocal**)

truss a. (see **connector, minor**)

upright a. (see **connector, minor**)

armamentarium (ar"mah-měn-tā'rē-ŭm) The equipment and materials of a practitioner or institution, including books, instruments, medicine, and surgical appliances. (Anesth.)

— A group of instruments, absorbent materials, chemicals, and other items necessary for the surgical or nonsurgical treatment of root canals. (Endodont.)

arrangement The pattern into which a group of things is organized.

financial a. An agreement between the dentist and patient on the method of handling the patient's account. (Pract. Man.)

tooth a. The placement of teeth on a denture or temporary base with definite objectives in mind. (Comp. Prosth.; Fixed Part. Prosth.; Remov. Part. Prosth.)

anterior t. a. The arrangement of anterior teeth to attain the desired esthetic or phonetic effects. (Comp. Prosth.; Fixed Part. Prosth.; Remov. Part. Prosth.)

arrest, cardiac Auriculoventricular dissociation, with ventricular standstill or severe ventricular bradycardia; ventricular fibrillation. (Oral Med.)

arrhythmia (ah-rĭth'mē-ah) Any variation from the normal rhythm of the heart. (Anesth.)

arrow point tracer (see **tracer, needle point**)

arterial innervation (see **innervation, arterial**)

arteriole (ar-tē'rē-ōl) A minute arterial branch proximal to a capillary. (Oral Physiol.)

arteriosclerosis (ar-tē"rē-ō-sklĕ-rō'sĭs) Nonspecific term that means hardening of the arteries. It may refer to atherosclerosis, hyperplastic arteriosclerosis, or Mönckeberg's sclerosis. (Oral Med.)

— Term applied to a group of diseases that affect the elasticity of the blood vessels. These degenerative processes generally affect only the tunica media and tunica intima. The disease that affects only the tunica intima is termed atherosclerosis. The latter is the common disease in which cholesterol is considered a principal etiologic agent. The effect of this disorder is to narrow the lumen of a blood vessel, causing rupture of the blood vessel or ischemia of an area of tissue the vessel supplies. (Oral Physiol.)

arteriosclerotic heart disease (ar-tē″rē-ō-sklĕ-rŏt′ĭk) (see **disease, heart, arteriosclerotic**)

arteriovenous shunt (ar-tē″rē-ō-vē′nŭs) (see **shunt, arteriovenous**)

arteritis, temporal (ar″ter-ī′tĭs) Inflammation of the temporal artery that produces a nodular, tortuous swelling of the temporal artery accompanied by burning, throbbing pain, initially in the teeth, temporomandibular joint, and eye, but ultimately localized over the artery. This disorder occurs primarily in patients over 55 years of age. (Oral Diag.)

artery A blood vessel through which the blood passes from the heart to the various structures of the body. There are three layers of tissue in every artery: the inner coat (tunica intima), composed of an inner endothelial lining, connective tissue, and an outer layer of elastic tissue (inner elastic membrane); the middle coat (tunica media), composed chiefly of muscle tissue; and the outer coat (tunica adventitia), composed chiefly of connective tissue. The structure of the three layers varies with the location, size, and purpose of the blood vessel. (Oral Physiol.)

large a. An elastic artery, having an abundant supply of elastic tissue and a great reduction of smooth muscle. The tunica intima is thick, and the endothelial cells are round or polygonal in shape. The tunica media is the thickest of the three layers. It contains few smooth muscle fibers, and its outer border has a special concentration of elastic fibers—the external elastic membrane. The tunica adventitia is relatively thin and ill defined, and is continuous with the loose connective tissue surrounding the vessel. (Oral Physiol.)

medium-sized a. Most of the arteries in the body; e.g., the facial, maxillary, radial, ulnar, and popliteal arteries. Thick muscular bands are found in the tunica media. Thin elastic fibers course circularly in the tunica media and run longitudinally in the tunica adventitia. The tunica adventitia is as thick as the tunica media, and its outer layer

gradually blends with the connective tissue that supports the artery and the surrounding structures. (Oral Physiol.)

arthralgia (ar-thrăl′jē-ah) Pain in a joint or joints. (Oral Med.)

arthritis (ar-thrī′tĭs) Any of a number of types of inflammation of a joint or joints. (Oral Diag.; Oral Med.)

allergic a. Arthralgia, swelling, and stiffness of joints·associated with food and drug allergies and serum sickness. (Oral Med.)

atrophic a. (see **arthritis, rheumatoid**)

bacterial a. (see **arthritis, infective**)

hypertrophic a. (see **osteoarthritis**)

infective a. (bacterial a.) Primary and secondary bacterial infections of the joints, e.g., by staphylococcus, gonococcus, streptococcus, or pneumococcus. (Oral Med.)

rheumatic a. (roo-măt′ik) An acute polyarticular and migratory arthritis of unknown cause but assumed to be related to group A streptococcal infection of the upper respiratory tract. (Oral Med.)

rheumatoid a. (roo′mah-toid) A chronic destructive inflammation of the joints of unknown origin, with associated constitutional manifestations. Chronic synovitis and regressive changes in the articular cartilage occur with pain, swelling, deformity, limitation of motion, and occasionally ankylosis of the joints. Variable systemic manifestations include weakness, loss of weight, anemia, leukopenia, splenomegaly, lymphadenopathy, and the formation of subcutaneous nodules. Small joints are principally affected. In most instances, onset is in the third or fourth decade of life. (Oral Med.)

— The most common form of chronic inflammatory disease of the joints. The etiology of widespread disease of connective tissue is not well known, but the cellular pathology is well understood. The principal clinical problem arises from the primary articular disorder and the tissue damage that results. Rheumatoid arthritis differs from osteoarthritis in that synovitis is the earliest pathologic change in the joint, whereas in osteoarthritis it is a late change. The sequence of pathologic alteration in rheumatoid arthritis is as follows: synovitis, pannus formation, fibrous ankylosis, and bony ankylosis. Rheumatoid arthritis occurs in the temporomandibular joint more frequently than does osteoarthritis. It is also one of a group of the collagen diseases that affects the connective tissue. These diseases, including scleroderma, rheumatic fever, periarteritis nodosa, lupus erythematosus, and some endocrine disorders, affect muscles, skin, and organs. (Oral Physiol.)

— A chronic disease of the joints, usually polyarticular and marked by inflammatory changes in the synovial membranes and articular structures and by atrophy and rarefaction of the bones. (Oral Surg.)

— A chronic joint disease, usually involving many articulations, presenting both inflammatory and degenerative lesions. A collagen disease of unknown etiology, capable of being controlled by the administration of ACTH or cortisone preparations. (Periodont.)

senile a. Arthritis occurring in patients of advanced age. (Comp. Prosth.)

specific infectious a. Arthritis caused by direct invasion and subsequent infection of joint structures by microorganisms from the bloodstream. Nearly all pathogenic bacteria have been isolated as etiologic agents. Fortunately, those organisms particularly responsible for purulent inflammation of the joints (staphylococcus, streptococcus, gonococcus, meningococcus, and pneumococcus) can now be controlled by antibiotics so that adequate therapy can prevent the severely crippling effects of infections caused by them. There is a group of nonpurulent inflammatory diseases that primarily affect the soft connective tissue of joints and the surrounding structures and that stabilize or activate joints and cause arthritis. (Oral Physiol.)

traumatic a. Acute or chronic inflammation of a joint as the result of acute or chronic injury. (Oral Med.; Oral Physiol.)

arthroplasty (ar′thrō-plăs″tē) Surgical correction of a joint abnormality. (Oral Surg.)

a. gap (see **gap arthroplasty**)

a. interposition (see **interposition arthroplasty**)

arthrostomy (ar-thrŏs′tō-mē) The surgical formation of an opening into a joint. (Oral Surg.)

articular cartilage (see **cartilage, articular**)

articulare Point of intersection of the dorsal contour of the mandibular condyle and the temporal bone. (Orthodont.)

articulate, *v.* (ar-tĭk′ū-lāt) To arrange or place. (Comp. Prosth.; Fixed Part. Prosth.; Remov. Part. Prosth.) (see also **arrangement, tooth**)

articulating paper Paper strips, coated with ink- or dye-containing wax, used for the marking or locating of occlusal interferences or deflec-

tive or interceptive occlusal contacts prior to making occlusal adjustment. (Comp. Prosth.; Periodont.)

articulation (ar-tĭk″ū-lā′shŭn) A joint. (Oral Physiol.) (see also **joint**)

— The state of being joined together by a joint or joints. (Cleft Palate; Comp. Prosth.; Remov. Part. Prosth.) (see also **arrangement, tooth**)

— Relationship of cusps of teeth during jaw movement. (Orthodont.)

anatomic a. A rigid or movable junction of bony part. (Comp. Prosth.; Remov. Part. Prosth.)

articulator a. The use of a device that incorporates artificial temporomandibular joints, permitting the orientation of casts in a manner duplicating or simulating various positions or movements of the mandible to assist in the arrangement of teeth. (Comp. Prosth.; Remov. Part. Prosth.)

balanced a. The simultaneous contacting of the upper and lower teeth as they glide over each other when the mandible is moved from centric relation to the various eccentric relations and back to centric relation again. (Comp. Prosth.) (see also **occlusion, balanced**)

dental a. The contact relationship of the upper and lower teeth when gliding into and away from centric occlusion. (Comp. Prosth.; Remov. Part. Prosth.)

mandibular a. (see **articulation, temporomandibular**)

speech a. The production of individual sounds in connected discourse; the movement and placement during speech of the organs that serve to interrupt or modify the voiced or unvoiced airstream into meaningful sounds; the speech function performed largely through the movements of the lower jaw, lips, tongue, and soft palate. (Cleft Palate; Comp. Prosth.; Remov. Part. Prosth.)

— The process by which the articulatory mechanism breaks up and modifies the laryngeal tones, creating new sounds within the oral cavity. The new sounds are essentially the consonants, which are defined as sounds accompanied by friction noises. A consonant is formed as the airstream passes opposing structures that are in partial or complete contact; e.g., the lips contact each other for "p" and "b," and the tongue touches the teeth and palate for "t" and "d." The articulatory mechanism involves the lips, teeth, palate, and tongue (the tongue is by far the most important articulatory structure). The final action of the articulatory apparatus is to join in a fluid sequence all the sounds that have been synthesized into symbols. Without articulatory capacity, the sounds produced by the speech mechanism would be only of variable pitch, volume, and quality, such as vowel sounds. (Oral Physiol.)

temporomandibular a. (temporomandibular joint, mandibular joint) The joint formed by the two mandibular condyles and the mandibular fossae, including the articulation of the condyloid processes of the mandible and the interarticular disks with the mandibular fossae of the temporal bone. (Comp. Prosth.; Remov. Part. Prosth.)

— A diarthrodial, ginglymus (sliding hinge) joint. It is paired, and the joints act alternately as axes of rotation for each other during lateral movements. Each joint limits the range of motion of the other. The sliding, or translational, action of the joint, coupled with both horizontal and vertical rotation, permits the mandible and its associated structures to move through a considerable space during function. (Oral Physiol.)

— The bilateral articulation between the glenoid or mandibular fossae of the temporal bones and the condyles (condyloid processes) of the mandible. The structures comprising the temporomandibular joint include the mandibular fossae of the temporal bone, the articular disks, the mandibular condyles, and the articular tubercles of the zygomatic process of the temporal bone. (Oral Surg.; Periodont.)

t. a., capsule The ligamentous covering of the temporomandibular joint. (Oral Surg.)

t. a., collagen disease Rheumatoid arthritis in which the joint may be so involved because of bone changes that the mandibular condyle is fused to the articular fossa in the base of the cranium. Fusion prevents mastication of food, and, as a result, the nutritional status of the patient degenerates rapidly since he is forced to live on a liquid diet. Inanition is a frequent concomitant of such fusion. If the osteoid changes do not result in fusion but only seriously limit the mobility of the condyle, the patient frequently resorts to a soft, high-carbohydrate, nondetergent diet, and obesity frequently ensues. (Oral Physiol.)

t. a., hormonal disturbances Hormonal disorders, which frequently affect growth patterns of the skeleton, involving the temporomandibular joint. The patient with acromegaly, for example, has a disproportionate growth of the mandibular in relation to the maxillae and the cranium. In the later stages of the disease, he is unable to close his mouth or to occlude his teeth because the enlarged coronoid process of the mandible cannot bypass the zygomatic process. This limitation of movement, coupled with muscle weakness, seriously affects the nutritional status of the patient. It also affects the esthetic appearance, which involves related emotional and psychologic problems. Other hormonal disorders have characteristic patterns and problems. (Oral Physiol.)

t. a., neuromuscular disorders Neuromuscular disorders involving the temporomandibular joint, in which the patient is unable to maintain appropriate patterns of mandibular closure consistent with good dental occlusion. The natural teeth degenerate rapidly and are frequently lost prematurely; when dentures are substituted, they cause the residual tissues to deteriorate rapidly. In addition to the chronic masticatory disability, the deglutitive mechanism functions poorly because of incoordinated lip and tongue action. Frequently, food is projected out of the mouth and wasted rather than ingested. This reduced ingestion coupled with higher energy and protein requirements of neurologically involved patients, frequently creates a state of chronic malnutrition. (Oral Physiol.)

t. a., neurosis (nū-rō'sĭs) A nervous disorder in which the patient with natural teeth frequently associates severe temporomandibular joint or facial pain with arthritis or some other chronic disease with which he is afflicted. This pain may be due to faulty dental occlusion. If such a patient has multiple disease problems, however, it is not uncommon for him to exhaust the services of numerous physicians and dentists before it is determined that the facial pain is due to faulty dental occlusion. (Oral Physiol.)

t. a., structure An integral portion of the stomatognathic system, permitting and partially controlling mandibular movement during mastication, speech, swallowing, etc. It is constituted, in relationship to its associated musculature, so as to allow hinge and translatory movements, or combinations thereof, of the mandible. (Periodont.)

articulator (ar-tĭk′ū-lā-tor) A mechanical device that represents the temporomandibular joints and jaw members to which maxillary and mandibular casts may be attached. (Comp. Prosth.; Fixed Part. Prosth.; Remov. Part. Prosth.)

    adjustable a. An articulator that may be adjusted to permit movement of the casts into recorded eccentric relationships. An articulator capable of adjustment to more than one eccentric position. (Comp. Prosth.; Remov. Part. Prosth.)

artifact (ar′tĭ-făkt) A blemish or image in the radiograph that is not preesnt in the roentgen image of the object; the result of faulty manufacture, manipulation, exposure, or processing of an x-ray film. (Oral Radiol.)

artificial respiration (see **respiration, artificial**)

artificial stone (see **stone, artificial**)

artifistulation (ar″tĭ-fĭst″ū-lā′shŭn) A procedure in which the alveolar plate of bone is surgically perforated to relieve pressure and ease pain caused by the accumulation of tissue exudate. (Endodont.)

aryepiglottic (ar″ē-ĕp″ĭ-glaht′ĭk) (see **arytenoepiglottic**)

arytenoepiglottic (ar″ē-tē″nō-ĕp″ĭ-glaht′ĭk) **(aryepiglottic)** Pertaining to the arytenoid cartilage and the epiglottis. (Anesth.)

arytenoid (ar-ē-tē-′noid) Resembling a ladle or pitcher mouth; relating to cartilage, gland, ligament, or muscle. (Anesth.; Oral Physiol.)

Aschheim-Zondek test (ăsh′hīm tsahn′dĕk) (see **test, pregnancy**)

ascites (ah-sī′tēz) An accumulation of serous fluid in the peritoneal cavity. (Oral Diag.)

ascorbic acid (see **vitamin C**)

asepsin (ah-sĕp′sĭn) An antiseptic analgesic; an antipyretic drug. (Anesth.)

asepsis (ah-sĕp′sĭs) Without infection; free of viable microorganisms. (Oral Surg.)

aseptic Not producing microorganisms or free from microorganisms. (Anesth.)

asialia (ah″sĭ-ā′lē-ah) (see **asialorrhea**)

asialorrhea (ah-sī″ah-lō-rē′ah) **(asialia)** A decrease in or lack of salivary flow. (Oral Med.) (see also **hyposalivation**)

asjike (ahs-jĭ′kē) (see **beriberi**)

aspect, buccal The facial surface of posterior teeth; the cheek side of a posterior tooth. (Periodont.)

asphalgesia (ăs-făl-jē′zē-ah) A burning sensation and convulsions sometimes experienced when touching certain articles during hypnosis. (Anesth.)

asphyxia (ăs-fĭk′sē-ah) A condition of suffocation due to restriction of oxygen intake plus interference with the elimination of carbon dioxide. (Anesth.)

aspirate, *n.* (ăs′pĭ-rāt) A phonetic unit whose identifying characteristic is the sound generated by the passage of air through a relatively open channel; the sound of "h"; a sound followed by or combined with the sound of "h." (Cleft Palate)

—, *v.* To draw out or take into by suction or to withdraw air. (Anesth.)

aspiration (ăs″pĭ-rā′shŭn) The act of breathing or drawing in; the removal of fluids or gases from a cavity by means of an aspirator. (Anesth.)

    a. biopsy (see **biopsy, aspiration**)

    a. pneumonia Pneumonia produced by aspiration of foreign material. (Oral Med.)

aspirator (ăs′pĭ-rā-tor) An apparatus used for removal of fluids or gases from a cavity. (Anesth.)

aspirin burn (see **burn, aspirin**)

aspirin, phenacetin, caffeine (APC, PAC) A pharmaceutical preparation used as an analgesic. (Periodont.)

assault A violent onset or attack. (D. Juris.)

    civil a. A technical assault; an unconsented touching of another. (D. Juris.)

    criminal a. An intentional and unlawful offer of injury of another by force. (D. Juris.)

    technical a. Placing of another in fear of receiving a bodily blow or contact to which he has not consented and which is not legally authorized; i.e., producing in another the apprehension of bodily harm. (D. Juris.)

assistant An agent or employee. (D. Juris.)

    dental a. An auxiliary to the dentist. (Pract. Man.) (see also **certified dental assistant**)

asthenia (as-thē′nē-ah) Loss of vitality or strength; a condition of debility; weakness. (Oral Med.)

asthenic (ăs-thĕn′ĭk) Term descriptive of an individual with a long, slender appearance who is thin and flat chested, with long limbs and a short trunk; comparable to the ectomorph in Sheldon's classification. (Oral Diag.; Oral Med.)

asthma (ăz′mah) Paroxysmal wheezing and difficulty in breathing resulting from bronchospasms frequently having an allergic basis and occasionally an emotional origin. (Oral Med.)

    cardiac a. Shortness of breath (paroxysmal dyspnea), sonorous rales, and expiratory wheezes that resemble bronchial asthma; related to cardiac failure. (Oral Med.)

astigmatism (ah-stĭg′mah-tĭzm) A defective curvature of the refractive surfaces of the eye, resulting in a condition in which a ray of light is not focused sharply in the retina but is spread over a more or less diffuse area. (Oral Physiol.)

astringent (ah-strĭn′jĕnt) Styptic; an agent that checks the secretions of mucous membranes and contracts and hardens tissues, limiting the secretions of glands. (Anesth.)

— A locally acting drug that tends to condense a tissue surface and reduce the permeability of cell membranes through the precipitation of proteins. (Oral Med.; Pharmacol.)

asymmetric (ā″sĭ-mĕ′trĭk) Unevenly arranged; out of balance; not the same on both sides; not a mirror image on both sides. (Orthodont.; Comp. Prosth.)

asynergy (ā-sĭn′er-jē) Lack of muscular coordination in special functions, e.g., hand-to-mouth movements for feeding. (Oral Physiol.)

asystole (ā-sĭs′tō-lē) Faulty contraction of the ventricles of the heart, resulting in incomplete or imperfect systole. (Anesth.)

ataractic (ăt-ah-răk′tĭk) **(ataraxic, tranquilizer)** One of a poorly defined group of drugs designed to produce ataraxia. The former concept, that their use involved no mental or motor impairment, is subject to question. (Anesth.; Oral Med.; Pharmacol.)

ataraxia (ăt″ah-răk′sē-ah) A state of complete serenity without impairment of mental or physical functions. (Oral Med.; Pharmacol.)

ataraxic (see **ataractic**)

ataxia (ah-tăk′sē-ah) Muscular incoordination characterized by irregular muscle activity. (Oral Diag.; Oral Physiol.)

locomotor a. (see **tabes dorsalis**)

atelectasis (ăt″ĕ-lĕk′tah-sĭs) The complete or partial collapse of a lung. (Anesth.)

atherosclerosis (ăth″er-ō-sklĕ-rō′sĭs) A degenerative disease principally affecting the aorta and its major branches, the coronary artery, and the larger cerebral arteries. The arterial changes include narrowing of the lumen of the vessels, weakening of the arterioles leading to rupture, an increased tendency toward development of atheromatous plaques, and thrombi. Atherosclerosis is a common cause of coronary thrombosis, congestive heart failure, aneurysms, hemorrhage, cerebral infarcts, and apoplexy. (Oral Med.)

athetosis (ăth″ĕ-tō′sĭs) A neuromuscular impairment in which voluntary control of movement is interfered with by extensive twisting and swaying spasms of the skeletal musculature; the spasms are especially conspicuous and disconcerting during emotional stress and on initiation of conscious voluntary acts. (Oral Physiol.)

athiaminosis (ah-thī″ah-mĭ-nō′sĭs) (see **beriberi**)

athletic (ăth-lĕt′ĭk) Pertaining to a bodily constitution characterized by a strong, muscular, robust appearance. (Oral Diag.)

atom (ăt′om) The smallest part of an element that is capable of entering into a chemical reaction. It consists of a positive nucleus and an extranuclear portion composed of electrons equal in number to the nuclear protons. (Anesth.; Oral Radiol.)

atomic (ah-tom′ĭk) Pertaining to the atom.

  a. energy (see **energy, atomic**)

  a. mass number (symbol A) The total number of nucleons (protons plus neutrons) of which an atom is composed. (Oral Radiol.)

  a. number (z) The number of electrons outside the nucleus of a neutral atom. It is also the number of protons in the nucleus. (Oral Radiol.)

  a. structure theory The theory that matter is composed of a vast number of particles, or atoms, bound together by a force of attraction. (Oral Radiol.)

  a. weight The weight of one atom of an element as compared to the weight of an atom of hydrogen. One atomic weight unit is equal to 1.660×10^{-24} grams. (Oral Radiol.)

atomizer (ăt′ŭ-mī-zer) An apparatus for changing a jet of liquid into a spray. (Anesth.)

atopy (ăt′ō-pē) **(atopic hypersensitivity, "spontaneous" clinical allergy)** A group of "allergic" disorders showing a marked familial distribution; although the susceptibility appears to be inherited, contact with the antigen must occur before hypersensitivity can develop. Disorders include asthma or hay fever due to pollens, gastrointestinal and skin reactions due to food, etc. (Oral Med.)

atresia (ah-trē′zē-ah) Absence or closure of a normal opening. (Oral Diag.)

— The congenital absence or occlusion of one or more ducts in an organ. (Oral Path.)

  aural a. Absence or closure of the auditory canal. (M.F.P.)

atrophy (ăt′rō-fē) A progressive acquired decrease in the size of a normally developed cell, tissue, or organ. It may be the result of a decrease in cell size, number of cells, or both. (Comp. Prosth.; Oral Diag.; Oral Path.)

adipose a. Atrophy due to a reduction in fatty tissue. (Comp. Prosth.)

alveolar a. A depletion of the size of the alveolar process of the jaws from disuse, overuse, or pathologic disturbance of the bone. (Comp. Prosth.; Remov. Part. Prosth.)

diffuse a. a. (see **periodontosis**)

bone a. Bone resorption both internally (in density) and externally (in form), e.g., of residual ridges. (Comp. Prosth.)

— A loss of bone substance or volume. Atrophy of bone ordinarily occurs without a corresponding change in the volume or external dimensions of bone, but the mass of bone tissue may be reduced as much as 75%. The internal architecture of the bone gradually becomes attenuated and finally disappears. Atrophied bone is brittle and of a more spongy consistency than normal bone. In cross section the cortex is thin and the periosteal surface is smooth and unchanged, but the intramedullary substance is composed of a yellow, fatty, cancellous bone tissue. Bone atrophy may be systemic, regional, or local. (Oral Physiol.)

a. of disuse A diminution of the number of principal fibers of the periodontal membrane due to functional disuse. The remaining periodontal fibers assume a plane of orientation more or less parallel to the long axis of the root—an afunctional fiber arrangement. In addition, the thickness of the periodontal membrane as observed radiographically and histologically is markedly reduced. (Periodont.)

— The regressive changes produced in the periodontium as a result of functional disuse of the teeth. Lesions include osteoporotic changes in supporting bone, an afunctional change in direction of periodontal fibers, and narrowing of the periodontal membrane space. (Periodont.; Remov. Part. Prosth.)

facial a. Failure of facial development. If it is bilateral, it may produce brachygnathia; unilateral types, although rare, are more common than the bilateral type. Causes include physical injury, neurovascular disease, and paralysis. (Oral Diag.)

muscular a. A wasting of muscle tissue, especially due to lack of use. (Comp. Prosth.)

— A loss of bulk and an increase in number and size of sarcolemmic nuclei in muscle. The striations of the fibers, however, are retained, and the fibers themselves are not all reduced to the same degree or to the same size. Those which were originally large probably require longer to atrophy, and some fibers actually hypertrophy when prolonged pathologic degenerative changes occur. There are numerous causes for simple atrophy of muscle, e.g., chronic malnutrition, immobilization, and denervation. The muscles of the face show lack of bulk associated with disuse when opposing teeth have been missing for many years. However, the marked degenerative changes associated with loss of dentoalveolar structures or systemic diseases do not occur as rapidly in the facial and masticatory muscles, since these muscles are never really in total disuse because they are used in speech, respiration, and deglutition. (Oral Physiol.)

periodontal a. The quantitative degenerative changes that occur in the attachment apparatus and supporting bone as a result of disease. (Periodont.)

— The atrophic, or degenerative, changes occurring in the attachment apparatus **and** supporting bone when a tooth loses its antagonist. Lesions include osteoporotic changes in the supporting bone, an afunctional change in the direction of periodontal fibers, and narrowing of the periodontal membrane space. (Oral Physiol.; Periodont.)

postmenopausal a. A thinning of the oral mucosa occurring after menopause. (Comp. Prosth.; Remov. Part. Prosth.)

pressure a. Tissue destruction and reduction in size as a consequence of prolonged or continued pressure on a local area or group of cells; acts by interfering with the vascular and lymphatic supply of the cells, thus preventing proper nutriment from reaching and being absorbed by the cells. Seen in occlusal traumatism. Interference with blood supply and local tissue metabolism results in a reduction in the size and number of viable cells. (Periodont.)

p. a. by epithelial attachment A theoretical type of atrophy. The theory, advanced to explain destruction of gingival fibers during gingival inflammation, states that gingival fiber degeneration is produced by pressure exerted by the proliferating pocket epithelium. It is now generally conceded that proteolytic substances produced in the tissues during inflammation are responsible for gingival fiber destruction; subsequently, the epithelium can proliferate apically. (Periodont.)

senile a. The normal atrophy or diminution of

all tissues due to advanced age. (Comp. Prosth.)

atropine (at'rō-pēn) An alkaloid that annuls parasympathetic effects and antagonizes the effects of pilocarpine. It acts directly on the effector cells, preventing the action but not the liberation of acetylcholine. It suppresses sweat and other glandular secretion. (Oral Physiol.)

attached gingiva (see **gingiva, attached**)

attachment A mechanical device for retention and stabilization of a dental prosthesis. Kinds of atttachments include frictional, internal, and slotted. (Remov. Part. Prosth.)

abnormal frenum a. (frē'nŭm) Aberrant insertions of labial, buccal, or lingual frenum capable of initiating, adversely modifying, or perpetuating periodontal disease by exerting retraction on the gingival margin, creating diastemata between teeth, limiting lip or tongue movements, etc. (Periodont.)

epithelial a. The continuation of the sulcal epithelium that is joined to the tooth structure and is located at the base of the sulcus, or pocket. (Periodont.)

migration of e. a. The apical progression of the epithelial attachment along the cementum of the tooth root, usually associated with inflammatory processes affecting the gingival tissues. Also the cervical movement of the epithelial attachment along the enamel during active tooth eruption. (Periodont.)

physiology of e. a. The processes by which epithelial attachment proliferates from enamel to cementum. The epithelial attachment is situated on the enamel surface during eruption of the teeth. Contrary to Gottlieb's theory, which states that with increasing age the epithelial attachment proliferates apically from the enamel until it is on the cementum and continues to do so throughout life, most recent investigators believe that the progress of the epithelial attachment onto the cementum is a result of pathologic influences. Thus stages II, III, and IV of Gottlieb's eruption stages are today considered to be pathologic in nature. (Periodont.)

gingival a. The attachment of the gingival tissues to the teeth, which serves to keep tissues adapted to tooth surface and to supplement the function of the attachment apparatus by holding the teeth in line. It also supplements the epithelial attachment by acting as a barrier to bacterial, mechanical, or chemical irritation. (Periodont.)

diseased g. a. The changes occurring in the gingival corium, the sulcal epithelium, and the outer epithelial covering of the gingivae as a result of a disease process. In the gingival pocket the inflammatory changes include ulceration of the sulcal epithelium, edema, hyperplasia, etc. (Periodont.)

intracoronal a. (precision a., slotted a.) A frictional retainer used in partial denture construction. It consists of a two-part mechanism: (1) the cryptlike unit built into the abutment crown or restoration and (2) an insert that extends and attaches to the prosthesis through a slot on the outside of the "crypt." (Remov. Part. Prosth.)

orthodontic a. A device, secured to the crown of a tooth, that serves as a means of attaching the arch wire to the tooth. (Orthodont.)

parallel a. A prefabricated device for attaching a denture base to an abutment tooth. Retention is provided by friction between the parallel walls of the two parts of the attachment. (Remov. Part. Prosth.)

precision a. (see **attachment, intracoronal**)

slotted a. (see **attachment, intracoronal**)

attack, heart (see **thrombosis, coronary**)

attenuation (ah-těn"ū-ā'shŭn) The process by which a beam of radiation is reduced in energy when passing through some material. (Oral Radiol.)

attraction The tendency of teeth or other maxillary or mandibular structures to become superior to (elevated above) their normal position. (Orthodont.)

attrition (ah-trish'ŭn) The normal loss of tooth substance due to friction caused by physiologic forces such as interaction between the tooth and an abrasive substance, generally food, or another tooth or teeth. (Oper. Dent.; Oral Diag.; Oral Path.)

attritional occlusion (see **occlusion, attritional**)

atypical (ā-tǐp'ē-kal) Pertaining to deviation from the basic or typical. (Oper. Dent.)

A.U. (see **unit, Ångström**)

audiogram (aw'dē-ō-grăm) A graphic summary of the measurements of hearing loss showing the number of decibels lost at each frequency tested. (Cleft Palate)

audiology (aw-dē-ahl'ō-jē) The study of the entire field of hearing, including the anatomy and function of the ear, the impairment of hearing, and the evaluation, the education or reeducation, and the treatment of persons with hearing loss. (Cleft Palate; Oral Physiol.)

audiometer (aw-dē-ahm'ě-ter) A device for the

testing of hearing; calibrated to register hearing loss in terms of decibels. (Cleft Palate)

augmentation (awg″mĕn-tā′shŭn) Assistance to respiration by the application of intermittent pressure on inspiration. (Anesth.)

— Increase of the size beyond the existing size, such as an implant placed over the mandibular or maxillary ridges. (Cleft Palate)

Aureomycin (aw″rē-ō-mī′sĭn) A proprietary brand of chlortetracycline.

auricle (aw′rĭ-kŭl) (1) Pinna, the external part of the ear. (2) Atrium, the chamber of the heart that receives the blood: on the right, from the general circulation, and on the left, from the pulmonary circulation. (Oral Physiol.)

auricular fibrillation (see **fibrillation, auricular**)

auricular tags Rudimentary appendages of auricular tissue occurring on the face along the line of union of the first branchial arch. (Oral Diag.)

auriculotemporal syndrome (see **syndrome, auriculotemporal**)

auscultation (aw″skul-tā′shŭn) The examination procedure of listening for sounds produced in a body cavity in order to detect or judge an abnormal condition, such as crepitus at a fracture site. (Anesth.; Oral Surg.)

autoclave (aw′tō-klāv) An apparatus for effecting sterilization by steam under pressure. (Anesth.)

autogenous bone graft (see **graft, autogenous bone**)

autograft (see **graft, autogenous**)

autoimmune disease (aw″tō-ĭ-mūn′) (see **disease, autoimmune**)

automatic condenser (see **condenser, mechanical**)

automatic mallet (see **condenser, mechanical**)

automatism (aw-tŏm′ah-tĭzm) A tendency to take extra or superfluous doses of a drug when under its influence. (Oral Med.; Pharmacol.)

autopolymer (aw-tō-pol′ĭ-mer) A cold-curing resin to which certain chemicals have been added to initiate and propagate polymerization; used for dental restorations, denture repair, and relining. (D. Mat.)

a. resin (see **resin, autopolymer**)

autopolymerization (aw″tō-pol″ĭ-mer-ĭ-zā′shŭn) **(cold-curing)** Polymerization without the use of external heat as a result of the addition of an activator and a catalyst. (Comp. Prosth.; Oper. Dent.; Remov. Part. Prosth.)

— The accomplishment of polymerization by chemical means without external application of heat or light. (D. Mat.)

autoprothrombin I (aw″tō-prō-thrŏm′bĭn) (see **factor VII**)

autoprothrombin II (aw″tō-prō-thrŏm′bĭn) (see **factor IX**)

autoradiography (aw″tō-rā-dē-ŏg′rah-fē) Photographic recording of radiation from radioactive material, obtained by placing the surface of the radioactive material in close proximity to a photographic emulsion. (Oral Radiol.)

autotransformer A transformer with a single winding, having a large number of connections, or taps. Used to deliver a precise voltage to the high-tension primary circuit. (Oral Radiol.)

autotransplant (see **graft, autogenous**)

auxiliary abutment (see **abutment, auxiliary**)

A.V. (AV) Abbreviation of atrioventricular or auriculoventricular. (Anesth.)

average life (mean life) The average of the individual lives of all the atoms of a particular radioactive substance; 1.443 times radioactive half-life. (Oral Radiol.)

avitaminosis (ā-vī″tah-mĭ-nō′sĭs) A disease or condition resulting from a deficiency of one or more vitamins in the diet (e.g., scurvy, which is due to ascorbic acid deficiency, and beriberi, which is due to thiamine deficiency). (Oral Diag.; Oral Med.; Oral Path.; Periodont.)

fat-soluble a. Any one of the diseases resulting from deficiency of the fat-soluble vitamins; i.e., vitamins A, D, and E. (Oral Med.)

avoirdupois system (see **system, avoirdupois**)

avulsed tooth (see **tooth, evulsed**)

avulsion (ah-vŭl′shŭn) (see **evulsion**)

nerve a. (see **evulsion, nerve**)

axial inclination (ăks′ē-ŭl) (see **inclination, axial**)

axial plane (see **plane, axial**)

axial wall plane (see **plane, axial wall**)

axiopulpal (ăk″sē-ō-pŭl′pŭl) Relating to the angle formed by the axial and pulpal walls of a prepared cavity. (Oper. Dent.)

axis (ăk′sĭs) A straight line around which a body may rotate. (Comp. Prosth.)

cephalometric a. (see **axis, Y**)

condylar a. An imaginary line through the two mandibular condyles around which the mandible may rotate during a part of the opening movement. (Comp. Prosth.)

condyle a. One of three axes of the jaw condyles: (1) the hinge axis, an intercondyle imaginary line across the face through both condyles; whenever either condyle is chosen to be a rotator, it will display (2) a vertical axis; and there is also (3) a sagittal axis. The hinge axis is a moving center for the opening and closing movements. The vertical axis is a center for the horizontal components of orbital movements. The sagittal axis is the center for the vertical components of orbital movements. (Gnathol.)

hinge a. (horizontal a.) An imaginary line between the mandibular condyles around which the mandible can rotate without translatory movement. (Fixed Part. Prosth.; Comp. Prosth.)

— The opening-closing axis of the hinge parts of the jaw joints. When this axis was first located and demonstrated instrumentally, onlookers supposed that it existed only in the hindmost stations of the condyles. It is a moving axis carried about by the sliding movements propelling the hinges. It can be located at the hindmost position because there all motions except the pure hinge movements can be excluded. In certain anthropoids it has been located in the anterior terminal position and found to check with the location obtained in the hindmost station. (Gnathol.)

h. a. determination Location of the hinge axis by fixing a face-bow rigidly to the lower teeth with a clutch made for the patient out of aluminum alloy or acrylic resin and cemented firmly to the teeth with plaster or zinc oxide–eugenol paste. The patient is trained to relax his jaw-protruding muscles and to exercise his jaw-retracting muscles so that only minimal chair guidance of the jaw may be needed. When the points of pure rotation are found, they are dotted with tattoo ink and then tattooed by using a tri-needle pen to insert the pigment beneath the outer skin without causing bleeding, pain, infection, or disfigurement. (Gnathol.) (see also **hinge-bow**)

h. a.–orbital plane A craniofacial plane determined by three tattooed points. Two are located one on each side of the face at the point of exit through the skin in front of the tragus of the imagined extended rearmost mandibular hinge axis. The third point is located on the right side of the nose at the level of the orbital rim just beneath the pupil when the patient is gazing directly forward. This plane corresponds to the anthropologic Frankfort plane and is joined with two

other projection planes used to describe the craniofacial relations of the gnathic organ. (Gnathol.)

horizontal a. (see **axis, hinge**)

long a. An imaginary line passing longitudinally through the center of a body. (Fixed Part. Prosth.; Oper. Dent.)

mandibular a. The most posterior simulated hinge axis of the mandible. (Comp. Prosth.)

opening a. An imaginary line around which the mandible may rotate during its opening and closing movements. (Comp. Prosth.)

orbital movements of a. Movements projected on the axis-orbital plane in gathering the input data for an articulator, which is an analog computer; the most extensive lateral and sagittal motions are recorded either on the axis-orbital plane or on more convenient planes parallel to it. The data recorded on the horizontal planes are the outward, forward, and backward thrust directions of the condyles and the lower cusps. (Gnathol.) (see also **computer, analog**)

a. of preparation The path taken by a restoration as it slides on or off the preparation. (Fixed Part. Prosth.)

sagittal a. The imaginary line around which the working condyle rotates in the frontal plane during lateral mandibular movement. The sagittal and vertical axes function concurrently. (Fixed Part. Prosth.)

a. shift Imprecise term used before the nine different directionalized laterotrusions were discovered and named. Often the axis of the mandible is treated as though it were an axle on an articulator. (Gnathol.)

vertical a. The imaginary line around which the working condyle rotates in the horizontal plane during lateral mandibular movement. The sagittal and vertical axes function concurrently. (Fixed Part. Prosth.)

Y a. (cephalometric a.) The angle of a line connecting the sella turcica and the gnathion, and related to a horizontal plane. An indicator of downward and forward growth of the mandible. (Orthodont.)

axon (ăk′son) An extension of a nerve cell body that conducts impulses away from the cell. Generally there is only one axon to a cell, and it may extend up to 3 feet in length. (Oral Physiol.)

❧ B ❧

B point (see **point, B**)

bacitracin (băs-ĭ-trā′sĭn) An antibiotic produced by a gram-positive, spore-forming organism of the *Bacillus licheniform* group; usually administered topically. (Periodont.)

back-action clasp (see **clasp, back-action**)

back pressure porosity (see **porosity, back pressure**)

backing A metal support that serves to attach a facing to a prosthesis. (Remov. Part. Prosth.)

bacteremia (băk-ter-ē′mē-ah) Presence of bacteria in the bloodstream. It may be transient, intermittent, or continuous. Transient bacteremia may result from dental procedures such as root planing or from tonsillectomy, or it may accompany the early phase of many infections. Continuous bacteremia is a feature of endocarditis. (Oral Med.; Periodont.)

— Presence of bacteria in the blood as might occur during root planing of the tooth of a rheumatic patient who has not been prophylactically premedicated with antibiotics. (Periodont.)

bacteria, presence of, in NUG Involvement of bacteria in ANUG, as evidenced by the response of acute signs and symptoms to the broad-spectrum antibiotics. Much speculation exists as to the specific causative agent or agents, some of which include fusospirochetes, *Bacteroides melaninogenicus, Borrelia vincentii,* and *B. buccalis.* (Periodont.) (see also **ANUG**)

bacteria, resident (oral) The microorganisms constant in the oral flora of an individual. (Periodont.)

bacterial culture (see **culture, bacterial**)

bacteriolytic action (băk-tē-rē-ō-lĭt′ĭk) Breaking down of bacteria by an enzyme or other agent, e.g., by antibacterial factors in saliva. (Oral Diag.)

Bacterium melaninogenicum (băk-tē′rē-ŭm mĕl″ah-nĭn-ō-jĕn′ē-cŭm) (see **Bacteroides melaninogenicus**)

Bacteroides (băk-tĕ-roi′dēz) A genus of Schizomycetes made up of rod-shaped, highly pleomorphic, gram-negative, nonspore-forming obligate anaerobic bacteria sometimes associated with periodontitis. (Periodont.)

B. melaninogenicus (Bacterium melaninogenicum) A small gram-negative diplobacillus found in the mouth and pharynx; an anaerobic organism sometimes associated with periodontitis. (Periodont.)

badge, film (see **film badge**)

bailment A delivery of goods to hold or on a contract, either expressed or implied, that the obligation shall be executed and the goods returned when use for which they were bailed shall have passed or be accomplished. (D. Juris.)

balance Term that has no value in prosthodontics unless it is combined with another word or phrase e.g., occlusal balance. (Comp. Prosth.; Remov. Part. Prosth.) (see also **occlusion**)

acid-base b. In metabolism, the balance of acid to base necessary to keep the blood pH normal (between 7.35 and 7.43). (Anesth.)

occlusal b. A condition in which there are simultaneous contacts of the occluding units on both sides of the opposing dental arches, and equilibrium of the various components of mastication. (Comp. Prosth.; Fixed Part. Prosth.; Orthodont.; Remov. Part. Prosth.; Periodont.)

balanced articulation (see **occlusion, balanced**)

balanced bite (see **occlusion, balanced**)

balanced occlusion (see **occlusion, balanced**)

balancing contact (see **contact, balancing**)

balancing contacts The contacts of teeth on the side opposite the bolus side. (Gnathol.)

balancing occlusal surfaces (see **surfaces, occlusal, balancing**)

balancing side The side opposite the working side of the dentition or denture; usually the side toward which the mandible is moved. (Comp. Prosth.) (see also **working side**)

— The balancing condyle is obsolete terminology for the orbiting condyle. In lateral chewing, the condyle on the bolus side is rotating about the vertical axis; hence the condyle on the opposite side becomes a satellite and for that reason is called the orbiting condyle to indicate that it must take a curved path about the inward- and outward-rotating condyle. (Gnathol.)

balloon, sinus A hollow rubber structure, expandable with either liquid or air, used to support depressed fractures of the walls of the maxillary sinus. Sometimes called a Shea-Anthony antral balloon. The balloon of a Foley catheter is frequently used for this purpose. (Oral Surg.)

balsam (bawl'sŭm) Any of many viscous, sticky, aromatic fluids derived from plants; consists of resins plus oils. (Oral Med.; Pharmacol.)

band A thin strip of metal closely encircling the crown of a tooth horizontally. (Orthodont.)

b. adapter (see **adapter, band**)

apron b. (see **apron band**)

orthodontic b. A strip of metal formed so as to encompass the crown of a tooth on a horizontal plane. When employed in tooth movement procedures, the banding permits bodily movement of the teeth. A succession of welded orthodontic bands, when applied to adjoining teeth with cementation, is useful for tooth stabilization (provisional splinting). (Orthodont.; Periodont.)

adjustable o. b. A band provided with an adjusting screw to permit alteration in size. (Orthodont.)

o. anchor b. A band applied to a tooth from which resistance is obtained for tooth movement. (Orthodont.)

o. clamp b. A band provided with a nut and screw, which hold the ends of the band in place. (Orthodont.)

seamless o. b. A continuous strip of metal in the form of a ring, usually precontoured to the shape of the tooth. (Orthodont.)

b. pusher An instrument used to adapt the metal band to the tooth. (Orthodont.)

b. remover An instrument used to remove bands from the teeth. (Orthodont.)

rubber b. (see **elastic**)

slip-b. A band formed when a metal is placed under a load and one grain tends to slip or slide on another. (D. Mat.)

striated b. One of the alternating lighter and darker bands occurring in some muscle fibers. The striated appearance of these muscle fibers is the result of optical effects on the muscle. The striated muscle is anisotropic; i.e., light does not travel through muscle in all directions with equal speed. Muscle has two refractive indices: a maximal index for light traveling through the long axis of a fiber, and a minimal index for light traveling through the plane of a cross section of a fiber. This double refraction, or birefringence, is caused by the two structural elements of muscle: the fine crystalline latticework and the coarse colloidal aggregates. (Oral Physiol.)

bandage A strip of material wrapped about or applied to any body part.

Barton's b. A figure-of-eight bandage passing below the mandible and around the cranial bone to give upward support to the mandible. (Oral Surg.)

thyroid b. A large bandage consisting principally of a towel applied around the neck so that it exerts moderate pressure to the anterolateral part of the neck. (Oral Surg.)

bank plan A financial arrangement made between the dentist, his patient, and a bank for financing dental accounts; the bank provides the capital for a rate of interest that enables the patient to pay his dental account over a longer period of time than would otherwise be possible—usually 12 to 18 months. (Pract. Man.)

bar A metal segment of greater length than width that serves to connect two or more parts of a removable partial denture. (Remov. Part. Prosth.) (see also **bar, connector**)

anterior palatal b. (see **connector, major, anterior palatal**)

arch b. Any one of several types of wires, bars, or splints conforming to the arch of the teeth and used for the treatment of fractures of the jaws and/or stabilization of injured teeth, e.g., Erich, Jelenko, Niro, Winter. (Oral Surg.)

buccal b. An orthodontic appliance auxiliary consisting of a rigid metal wire extending from the buccal side of the molar band anteriorly. (Orthodont.)

b. clasp (see **clasp, bar**)

connector b. A connector of greater thickness and reduced width as compared to a plate type of connector, which has greater width and is thinner. (Remov. Part. Prosth.)

fixable-removable cross arch b. (see **connector, cross arch bar splint**)

Gilson fixable-removable b. (see **connector, cross arch bar splint**)

Kennedy b. (see **connector, minor, secondary lingual bar**)

labial b. A major connector that is located labial (or buccal) to the dental arch and that joins bilateral parts of a mandibular removable partial denture. (Remov. Part. Prosth.)

lingual b. A major connector that is located lingual to the dental arch and that joins bilateral parts of a mandibular removable partial denture. (Remov. Part. Prosth.) (see also **connector, major, lingual bar**)

secondary l. b. (see **connector, minor, secondary lingual bar**)

palatal b. A major connector that crosses the palate and unites bilateral parts of a maxillary removable partial denture. (Remov.

Part. Prosth.) (see also **connector, major**)

posterior p. b. (see **connector, major, posterior palatal**)

Passavant's b. (see **pad, Passavant's**)

barbiturate (bar-bĭt'ū-rāt) A salt of barbituric acid. (Anesth.)

barium sulfate (bă'rē-ŭm) A white, finely ground, tasteless powder that is insoluble in water, solvents, and solutions of acids and alkalis; in radiography used as a contrast medium because of its opacity to roentgen rays and as a protective barrier in plaster walls. (Oral Radiol.)

Barlow's disease (see **scurvy, infantile**)

barrier, protective Material of a composition that will greatly absorb radiation; e.g., lead or concrete. There are primary and secondary protective barriers: the primary protective barrier is one that can be expected to absorb a great amount of radiation, such as the useful primary beam; the secondary barrier is one that can be expected to absorb small amounts of radiation, such as scattered radiation. (Oral Radiol.)

Barton's bandage (see **bandage, Barton's**)

basal bone (see **bone, basal**)

basal metabolic rate (bā'sal mĕt-ah-bahl'ĭk) (**BMR, basal metabolism**) The basal rate or energy exchange, determined by means of a clinical test of oxygen consumption in a subject who has had a good night's rest, has fasted for 12 to 14 hours, and has been physically, mentally, and emotionally at rest for 30 minutes. (Oral Physiol.)

— The rate at which metabolic processes take place under basal conditions; usually indicated as a percentage of the normal calorie production per surface area, the normal values ranging between ±20%. At present the main value of the BMR test is to assess the rate in patients taking thyroid hormone or an antithyroid drug. (Oral Med.)

— The heat production of a person at the lowest level of cell activity; the minimal amount of cell activity necessary for the continuous function of respiration, circulation, and secretion. (Anesth.)

basal metabolism (see **basal metabolic rate**)

basal seat The oral tissues and structures that support a denture. (Comp. Prosth.; Remov. Part. Prosth.)

b. s. area (see **area, basal seat**)

b. s. outline An outline on the mucous membrane or on a cast of the entire area that is to be covered by a denture. (Comp. Prosth.; Remov. Part. Prosth.)

basal surface (see **surface, basal**)

base A compound that yields hydroxyl ions in water solution and causes neutralization of acid to form a salt and water. It is capable of combining with a protein. A base turns red litmus paper blue and has a pH higher than 7. (Anesth.)

— A unit of a removable prosthesis that supports the supplied teeth and any intermediary material and, in turn, receives support from the tissues of the basal seat, which is the denture foundation. (Comp. Prosth.; Remov. Part. Prosth.)

acrylic resin b. A denture base made of an acrylic resin. (Comp. Prosth.; Remov. Part. Prosth.)

apical b. (basal arch) The portion of the jawbones that gives support to the teeth. (Orthodont.)

cement b. A layer of insulated, sometimes medicated dental cement placed in the deep portions of a cavity preparation to protect the pulp, reduce the bulk of the metallic restoration, or eliminate undercuts in a tapered preparation. (Oper. Dent.)

proximal c. b. A cement base placed in the deep area of the proximal surface of a cavity preparation. (Oper. Dent.)

denture b. The part of a denture that fits the oral mucosa of the basal seat, restores the normal contours of the soft tissues of the dentulous mouth, and supports the artificial teeth. (Comp. Prosth.; Remov. Part. Prosth.)

— The portion of a denture that overlies the soft tissue; usually fabricated of resin or combinations of resins and metal. (D. Mat.)

tinted d. b. A denture base that simulates the coloring and shading of natural oral tissues. (Comp. Prosth.; Remov. Part. Prosth.)

extension b. (free-end) A unit of a removable prosthesis that extends anteriorly or posteriorly, terminating without end support by a natural tooth. (Remov. Part. Prosth.)

film b. A thin, flexible, transparent sheet of cellulose acetate or similar material. (Oral Radiol.)

mandibular b. The body of the mandible, on which is situated the teeth and alveolar tissues. (Orthodont.)

b. material Any substance from which a denture base may be made, e.g., acrylic resin, vulcanite, polystyrene resin, and metal. (Comp. Prosth.; Remov. Part. Prosth.)

metal b. The metallic portion of a denture base forming a part or all of the basal surface of the denture. It serves as a base for the attachment of the plastic (resin) part of the denture and the teeth. (Comp. Prosth.)

— The basal surface of a denture constructed of metal (e.g., aluminum, gold, and cobalt-chromium), to which the teeth are attached. (Comp. Prosth.; Remov. Part. Prosth.)

plastic b. A denture base, baseplate, or record base made of a plastic material. (Comp. Prosth.; Remov. Part. Prosth.)

record b. (see **baseplate**)

shellac b. Certain resinous materials adapted to maxillary or mandibular casts to form baseplates. (Comp. Prosth.; Remov. Part. Prosth.)

sprue b. (see **crucible former**)

temporary b. (see **baseplate**)

tissue-supported b. A denture base that receives most or all of its support from structures other than natural teeth or facsimiles. (Remov. Part. Prosth.)

tooth-borne b. The denture base that restores an edentulous area and has abutment teeth at each end for support. The tissue that it covers is not used for support of the base. (Fixed Part. Prosth.; Remov. Part. Prosth.)

— A base that is entirely supported by the teeth bordering the edentulous area that it covers. (Remov. Part. Prosth.)

tooth-tissue–supported b. A base that has support from both the adjacent teeth and the edentulous area that it covers. (Remov. Part. Prosth.)

trial b. (see **baseplate**)

Basedow's disease (băs′ĕ-dōz) (see **goiter, exophthalmic**)

baseplate (record base, temporary base, trial base) A temporary form representing the base of a denture and used for making maxillomandibular (jaw) relation records, for arranging artificial teeth, or for trial placement in the mouth. (Comp. Prosth.; Remov. Part. Prosth.)

— Preformed shape fabricated of shellac, wax, or acrylic resin and used in denture construction. (D. Mat.)

stabilized b. A baseplate lined with a plastic or other material to improve its adaptation and stability. (Comp. Prosth.; Remov. Part. Prosth.)

b. wax (see **wax, baseplate**)

basic metabolic rate (see **basal metabolic rate**)

basion (bā′sē-ahn) The midline point at the anterior margin of the occipital foramen. (Orthodont.)

basis The principal active ingredient in a prescription. (Oral Med.; Pharmacol.)

basophil (bā′sō-fĭl) (see **leukocyte**)

basophilia (bā-sō-fĭl′ē-ah) (**basophilic granular degeneration, basophilic stippling**) An aggregate of blue-staining granules found in erythrocytes; seen in lead poisoning, leukemia, malaria, severe anemias, and certain toxemias. (Oral Med.)

basophilic line (bā-sō-fĭl′ĭk) (see **line, basophilic**)

Battle's sign (see **sign, Battle's**)

bayonet A binangled instrument, the nib or blade of which is generally parallel to the shaft; resembles a bayonet. (Oper. Dent.) (see also **angle former, bayonet; condenser, bayonet**)

beam A stream or approximately unidirectional emission of electromagnetic radiation or particles. (Oral Radiol.)

central b. The center of the beam of roentgen rays emitted from the tube. (Oral Radiol.)

useful b. The part of the primary radiation that passes through the aperture, cone, or other collimator. (Oral Radiol.)

beaver-tail retractor (see **retractor, beaver-tail**)

Bednar's aphtha (see **aphtha, Bednar's**)

beeswax A low-melting wax that is an ingredient of many dental waxes. (D. Mat.)

Behçet's syndrome (see **syndrome, Behçet's**)

Beilby's layer (see **layer, Beilby's**)

Bell method (see **method, Bell**)

Bell's palsy, sign, palsy test (see under appropriate noun)

Bence Jones protein (see **protein, Bence Jones**)

Benedict's test (see **test, Benedict's**)

benign (bē-nīn′) Term that signifies the inability of a neoplasm to metastasize when describing it. (Oral Path.)

Bennett angle, movement (see under appropriate noun)

benzoyl peroxide A chemical incorporated into the polymer of resins to aid in the initiation of polymerization. (D. Mat.)

beriberi (**asjike, athiaminosis, endemic multiple neuritis, endemic polyneuritis, hinchazon, inchacao, kakke, loempe, panneuritis endemica, perneiras**) A polyneuritis produced by deficiency of thiamine (vitamin B_1). (Oral Diag.)

— A nutritional disease due to a deficiency of thiamine. Classically it is characterized by multiple neuritis, muscular atrophy, weakness, cardiovascular changes, and progressive edema. (Oral Med.)

— A disease characterized by multiple neuritis, congestive heart failure, and generalized edema. Oral manifestations, which are not distinctive, consist of edema of the tongue, loss of the papillae and pain. The condition is due to a deficiency of thiamine (vitamin B_1). (Oral Path.)

— An avitaminosis produced by lack of thiamine in the diet. It is usually associated with fractional deficiency of the vitamin B complex factors. It produces a form of polyneuritis characterized by spasmodic rigidity of the lower limbs, muscular atrophy, paralysis, anemia, and muscular pains. (Periodont.)

beryllium window (ber-ĭl′ē-ŭm) Part of an x-ray tube made of beryllium through which the rays pass to the outside. (Oral Radiol.)

Besnier-Boeck-Schaumann disease (běz′nē-ā běk shaw′măn) (see **sarcoidosis**)

beta-hemihydrate (bā″tah-hěm-ē-hī′drāt) The physical state of hemihydrate of calcium sulfate–plaster of paris. (D. Mat.)

betatron (bā′tah-trahn) A machine that produces high-speed electrons through magnetic induction. (Oral Radiol.)

bevel An acute angle (under bevel) or an obtuse angle (standing bevel) made by one surface or line with another. A sloped edge or a surface having a slant at the edge. (Anesth.)

— The inclination that one line or surface makes with another when not at right angles; in cavity preparation, a cut that produces an angle of more than 90° with a cavity wall. (Oper. Dent.)

    cavosurface b. The incline or slant of the cavosurface angle of a prepared cavity wall in relation to the plane of the enamel wall. (Oper. Dent.)

    contra b. (reverse b.) A bevel located on the side of the blade opposite the customary side, usually on the one closest to the shaft or shank (or the one toward the lesser angle with the shaft). (Oper. Dent.)

    instrument b. The sloping keen edge of a cutting instrument. (Oper. Dent.)

    regular b. A bevel located on the customary side of a blade usually on the side most distal from the shank, or on that side which is at the more obtuse angle with the shaft. (Oper. Dent.)

    reverse b. (see **bevel, contra**)

B.H.N. (see **number, Brinell hardness; test, Brinell hardness**)

bicarbonate A salt resulting from the incomplete neutralization of carbonic acid, as from passing excess carbon dioxide into a base solution. (Anesth.)

bicuspid (bī-kŭs′pĭd) (see **premolar**)

bicuspidized molar (see **molar, bicuspidized**)

b.i.d. Abbreviation for *bis in die,* a Latin phrase meaning twice a day. (Oral Med.; Pharmacol.)

Biermer's anemia (bēr′merz) (see **anemia, pernicious**)

bifid tongue (bī′fĭd) (see **tongue, bifid**)

bifid uvula (see **uvula, bifid**)

bifurcation (bī-fer-kā′shŭn) The division into two parts or branches, as any two roots of a tooth. (Oper. Dent.)

    b. involvement (see **involvement, bifurcation**)

bilateral (bī-lăt′er-ŭl) Pertaining to both sides. (Orthodont.)

bilharziasis (bĭl″har-zī′ah-sĭs) (see **schistosomiasis**)

bilirubinemia (bĭl″ē-roo″bĭ-nē′mē-ah) Presence of bilirubin in the blood. It may be due to obstruction within or without the liver or to increased hemolysis. The total serum bilirubin in an adult is 0.2 to 0.7 mg/100 ml. (Oral Med.)

bilirubinuria (bĭl″ē-roo-bĭ-nū′rē-ah) Presence of bilirubin in the urine. More often refers to an excess of bilirubin in the urine due to excessive hemolysis. (Oral Med.)

billet (see **pluglet**)

billing The procedure of preparing a financial statement. (Pract. Man.)

bimaxillary (bī-măx′ĭl-ăr-ē) Pertaining to the right and left maxillae; sometimes incorrectly used to refer to the maxillae and mandible. (Comp. Prosth.)

— Pertaining to superior and inferior jaws. (Orthodont.)

    b. protrusion (see **protrusion, bimaxillary**)

Bimeter (bī′mē-těr) A gnathodynamometer with a central bearing point adjustable to varying heights. (Comp. Prosth.) (see also **gnathodynamometer**)

binangle (bĭn′ăngl) An instrument having two offsetting angles in its shank. The angles are such as to keep the cutting edge or the face of the nib within 3 mm of the axis of the shaft. (Oper. Dent.)

binder A substance usually sticky, that holds the solid particles in a mixture together, thus aiding in the preservation of the physical form of the mixture. (Oral Med.; Pharmacol.)

binding Reversible combination of various drugs with body constituents such as plasma proteins. (Oral Med.; Pharmacol.)

binocular loupe (see **loupe, binocular**)

biologic Pertaining to biology. (Remov. Part. Prosth.)

biology The science of life or living matter, in all its forms and phenomena. (Comp. Prosth.; Remov. Part. Prosth.)

biomechanics (bī″ō-mē-kăn′ĭks) (see **biophysics**)

biometrics (bī″ō-mĕt′rĭks) The science of the application of statistical methods to biologic facts. (Comp. Prosth.)

biophysics (bī″ō-fĭz-ĭks) **(biomechanics)** The science that deals with the forces that act on living cells of the living body, the relationship between the biologic behavior of living structures and the physical influences to which they are subjected, and the physics of vital processes. (Comp. Prosth.; Remov. Part. Prosth.)

dental b. The branch of biophysics that deals with the biologic behavior of oral structures as influenced by dental restorations. (Comp. Prosth.; Remov. Part. Prosth.)

biopsy (bī′ŏp-sē) The removal of a tissue specimen or other material from the living body and microscopic examination of it to aid in establishing a diagnosis. (Oral Diag.; Oral Path.; Oral Surg.; Periodont.)

aspiration b. (needle b.) The procedure of obtaining a biopsy specimen by aspiration through a needle; used for bone or deep soft tissue lesions. (Oral Path.; Oral Surg.)

excisional b. The removal of an entire lesion, usually including a significant margin of contiguous normal tissue, for microscopic examination and diagnosis. (Oral Path.; Oral Surg.)

exploratory b. Exploration combined with biopsy to determine method and degree of local extension, usually of bone or deep soft tissue lesions. (Oral Path.)

incisional b. The surgical removal of a selected mass of a lesion and, if possible, adjacent normal tissue for microscopic examination and diagnosis. (Oral Path.; Oral Surg.)

needle b. (see **biopsy, aspiration**)

punch b. Biopsy material obtained by use of a punch. (Oral Path.)

biotin (bī′ō-tĭn) (see **vitamin H**)

biotransformation Chemical and physical changes produced in drugs after they enter the body; e.g., hydrolysis and conjugation. (Oral Med.; Pharmacol.)

bird-face (see **brachygnathia; retrognathism**)

bis- Prefix meaning that two like or mirror-image moieties are joined together to form a chemical compound. (Oral Med.; Pharmacol.)

biscuit (associated with porcelain) The fired article before it is glazed. May be any stage after the fluxes have flowed enough to provide rigidity to the structure up to the stage where shrinkage is complete. Referred to as low, medium, or high biscuit, depending on the completeness of vitrification. (D. Mat.)

— (associated with ceramics) Firing bakes, or stages (referred to as low, medium, and high),

during the fusing of dental porcelain preceding the final, or glaze, bake. (Fixed Part. Prosth.)

bismuth poisoning (bĭz′mŭth) (see **bismuthosis**)

bismuthia (bĭz-mū′thē-ah) Discoloration of mucous membranes and skin from bismuth poisoning. (Oral Med.)

bismuthism (see **bismuthosis**)

bismuthosis (bĭz″mŭth-ō′sĭs) **(bismuth poisoning, bismuthism)** Acute or chronic bismuth intoxication due to the ingestion or injection of bismuth salts. Possible manifestations include abuminuria, exfoliative dermatitis, gastrointestinal disturbances and stomatitis. (Oral Med.) (see also **stomatitis, bismuth**)

— The pathologic tissue changes that occur as a result of therapeutic measures utilizing bismuth preparations; characterized by stomatitis, salivation, intestinal catarrh, nephritis, and the deposition of bismuth sulfide in the form of a dark blue line along the gingivae. (Periodont.)

bite The part of an artificial tooth on the lingual side between the shoulder and the incisal edge of the tooth. (Comp. Prosth.)

— An interocclusal record or relationship. The term bite should be reserved for a morsel of food, for the act of incision, and for use in connection with discussions of the amount of pressure developed in closing the jaws, etc. (Comp. Prosth.; Fixed Part. Prosth.; Remov. Part. Prosth.) (see also **denture space; distance, interarch; record, interocclusal; record, maxillomandibular**)

b. analysis (see **analysis, occlusal**)

balanced b. (see **occlusion, balanced**)

biscuit b. A maxillomandibular or interocclusal record made in soft wax. Usually in centric position. It is an obsolete type of record. (Comp. Prosth.; Remov. Part. Prosth.) (see also **record, maxillomandibular**)

b. block In intraoral radiography a film holder that the patient bites to provide stable retention of the film packet. (Oral Radiol.)

— Occlusion rim. (see also **rim, occlusion**)

close b. (see **distance, small interarch**)

closed b. An abnormal overbite. (Orthodont.)

— A decrease in the occlusal vertical dimension produced by factors such as tooth abrasion and loss or failure of eruption of supportive posterior teeth. (Periodont.) (see also **distance, reduced interarch**)

b. closing (see **dimension, vertical decrease**)

convenience b. (see **occlusion, acquired, eccentric**)

edge-to-edge b. An occlusion in which the incisal edge of maxillary incisors meets the incisal edge of mandibular incisors. (Orthodont.) (see also **occlusion, edge-to-edge**)

b. fork (see **fork, face-bow**)
b. guard (see **guard, bite**)
   b. g. splint (see **splint, acrylic resin bite-guard**)
locked b. (see **occlusion, locked**)
normal b. (see **occlusion, normal**)
open b. A condition in which the anterior mandibular teeth cannot be brought into the proper relation to the maxillary dentition due to a dislocation of the temporomandibular articulation, a mandibular fracture, a malunion of an old fracture, or a deformity of either the alveolar processes of the skeleton or the maxillae or mandible. (Oral Surg.)
— Failure of the occluding surfaces of some of the teeth to achieve contact when the jaws are brought into normal, full closure. (Orthodont.)
— A malformation in which the anterior teeth do not occlude in any mandibular position. (Periodont.)
b. opening (see **dimension, vertical, increasing occlusal**)
   b. o. bends Bends made in maxillary and mandibular light round wires mesial to the molar tubes. (Orthodont.)
b. plane (see **plane, bite**)
b. plate (see **plane, bite**)
b. raising (see **dimension, vertical, increasing occlusal**)
b. record (see **path, occlusal, registration**)
rest b. (see **position, rest, physiologic**)
b. rim (see **rim, occlusion**)
working b. (see **occlusion, working**)
biteplane (bīt′plān) Any removable appliance used to treat patients complaining of pains in the temporomandibular joints or the muscles near them. It is usually made of clear acrylic resin; it covers all the teeth and is sometimes kept in place by orthodontic wrought wire clasps. (Gnathol.)
bite-wing film (see **film, bite-wing**)
bite-wing radiograph (see **radiograph, bite-wing**)
biting, cheek (see **habit**)
biting, lip (see **habit**)
biting, nail (see **habit**)
biting pressure (see **pressure, occlusal**)
biting strength (see **strength, biting**)
blade (see **instrument parts**)
blanching, gingival (see **gingiva, blanching**)
Blandin and Nuhn's gland (see **gland, Blandin and Nuhn's**)
blastomatoid lesion (blăs-tō′mah-toid) Overzealous reactive process, which, because of tumescence, presents some features of neo-plasia. A specific tissue element, such as fibroblasts, endothelial cells, osteoblasts, osteoclastic giant cells, or nerves, predominates, in a specific lesion to form granuloma pyogenicum, giant cell reparative granuloma, traumatic fibroma, tori, or traumatic neuroma. (Oral Diag.)
— Reactive lesion having some of the characteristics of a neoplasm—granuloma pyogenicum, traumatic fibroma, fibroid epulis, and amputation neuroma. (Oral Med.)
Blastomyces braziliensis (blăs″tō-mī′sēz) A species of fungus causing South American blastomycosis; not found in the United States. (Oral Path.)
Blastomyces dermatitidis (blăs″tō-mī′sēz der″mah-tīt′ĭ-dĭs) A species of fungus causing North American blastomycosis. (Oral Path.)
blastomycosis (blăs″tō-mī-kō′sĭs) Infection due to the fungus *Blastomyces dermatitidis* (North American blastomycosis) or to *Blastomyces braziliensis* (South American blastomycosis); characterized by chronic suppurative lesions. The disseminated form is usually fatal. (Oral Path.)
South American b. A fungous infection that often begins when organisms enter the body through the oral mucosa, producing local ulcers or through an extraction site, producing papillary lesions. Dissemination leads to granulomatous lesion of the lymph nodes, gastrointestinal tract, liver and lungs, and to microabscesses of the skin. The causative agent is *Blastomyces braziliensis*. (Oral Path.)
bleaching The use of a chemical oxidizing agent (sometimes in combination with heat) to lighten pulpless tooth discolorations. (Endodont.) (see also **agent, bleaching**)
bleeding The flowing of blood.
   gingival b. (see **gingiva, bleeding**)
   occult b. Hemorrhage of such small proportions that the blood can be detected only by chemical test, the microscope, or the spectroscope. (Oral Surg.)
   b. points A series of puncture points made through the gingival tissue to delineate and mark the depth of the periodontal or gingival pockets; used as a guide for making the gingivectomy incision. (Periodont.)
blindness, color (**defective color vision**) Decreased ability to detect differences in color, necessitating objective testing of the patient's color vision prior to selection of a shade of artificial teeth, fillings, etc. (Oral Physiol.) (see also **achromatopsia**)
   blue-yellow c. b. Color disability in which

the spectrum is seen in reds and greens; a form of protanopia. (Oral Physiol.)

red-green c. b. The common form of color disability, in which the entire spectrum is constituted by yellows and blues; a form of protanopia. (Oral Physiol.)

Bloch-Sulzberger syndrome (see **syndrome, Bloch-Sulzberger**)

block A mental obstacle that prohibits a patient from having favorable responses to the dentist and his suggested treatment plans. (Pract. Man.)

field b. The reversible interruption of nerve conduction over terminal branches by infiltration of a suitable agent into the area. (Anesth.)

nerve b. The reversible interruption of conduction along a nerve trunk or its branches due to the absorption of a suitable agent. Also, regional anesthesia secured by extraneural or paraneural injection in close proximity to the nerve whose conductivity is to be cut off. (Anesth.)

blocking The process of obstructing or deadening, as a nerve. (Anesth.)

b. agent (see **agent, blocking**)

blockout (wax out) Elimination of undesirable undercut areas on a cast to be used in the fabrication of a removable denture. (Comp. Prosth.; Remov. Part. Prosth.)

blood The fluid circulating through the heart, arteries, capillaries, and veins; carries nutriment and oxygen to body tissues. (Oral Physiol.)

bad b. Lay term for syphilis. (Oral Med.)

b. calcium The level of calcium in the blood plasma; generally regulated by parathyroid gland activity in conjunction with the degree of calcium ingestion, absorption, utilization, and excretion. Normal value is 8.5 to 11.5 mg/100 ml of blood serum. (Periodont.)

b. cell count The ratio of red blood cells to white blood cells per cubic centimeter. (Anesth.)

— An estimation of the number and/or types of circulating blood cells, e.g., red blood cell (erythrocytic) counts, white blood cell counts, or differential counts. (Oral Diag.)

b. clot (see **clot, blood**)

color index of b. A figure gained by dividing the hemoglobin percentage by the red blood cell percentage. In most anemias the result is below 1, but in pernicious anemia it is characteristically above 1. (Oral Diag.)

b. disorders Hematologic dyscrasias that affect

the component cells and plasma elements of the blood. Generally divided into two broad groups: those in which there is an increase in bulk (e.g., plethora, hydremia, and polycythemia) and those in which there is a decrease in bulk (e.g., anhydremia, dehydration, and anemia). (Oral Physiol.)

b. groups The division of blood into types on the basis of the compatibility of the erythrocytes and serum of one individual with the erythrocytes and serum of another individual. The groups are immunologically and genetically distinct. (Oral Med.)

b. pressure (see **pressure, blood**)

b. sugar The concentration of sugar (chiefly glucose—"true blood sugar") in the blood. It is usually kept within a narrow range by an interplay of many factors: glycogenolysis, glyconeogenesis, intestinal absorption, insulin, insulin "antagonists," and other hormones. In the testing of total reducing substances, the normal range of concentration of fasting blood sugar is 80 to 120 mg/ml; in the testing of "true blood sugar," the normal range of concentration is 70 to 100 mg/ml. (Oral Med.)

b. urea nitrogen (BUN) Nitrogen in the form of urea in whole blood or serum. Its concentration is a gross measure of renal function. The upper limit of the normal range is 25 mg/100 ml. (Oral Med.)

volume index of b. The volume of red blood cells/total volume of blood times 100 = vol% of packed red blood cells (hematocrit index). A value greater than 1 indicates an abnormally large number or size of erythrocytes. (Oral Diag.)

blower, chip (see **syringe, air, hand**)

blowpipe A torch that employs gas-oxygen, oxygen, or acetylene to melt metal in dental casting or soldering procedures. (D. Mat.)

blue, methylene (mĕth'ĭ-lēn) A dye used to color bacteria for microscopic examination. (Oral Diag.)

— An aniline dye often used in 2% to 4% aqueous solution as an antiseptic, topical analgesic, and protective in the treatment of lesions of the oral mucous membranes and skin. (Periodont.)

blue nevus (see **nevus, blue**)

blunderbuss apex (see **apex, blunderbuss**)

BMR (see **basal metabolic rate**)

bodily movement (see **movement, bodily**)

body Any mass or collection of material.

Donovan b. An extracellular structure found

in macrophages in lesions of granuloma inguinale. (Oral Path.)

foreign b. Any object or material that is not normal for the area in which it is located. (Oral Surg.)

ketone b. The formation of excess acetoacetic acid, beta-hydroxybutyric acid, and acetone in the blood due to the excessive mobilization of fat. May be due to diabetes mellitus or decrease in carbohydrate intake. (Oral Med.)

Lipschütz b. Any one of the eosinophilic oval structures seen in the nuclei of cells found in herpes virus infections. (Oral Path.)

Schaumann b. (shaw'măn) A round to oval cytoplasmic inclusion composed of concentric deposits of an amorphous material. Seen in the giant cells of sarcoidosis, in beryllium lesions, and sometimes in other giant cells. (Oral Path.)

b. temperature (see **temperature, body**)

Verocay b. A component of Antoni type A tissue seen in neurilemoma. (Oral Path.) (see also **neurilemoma; tissue, Antoni type A**)

Boeck's disease (bĕks) (see **sarcoidosis**)

Boeck's sarcoid (bĕks) (see **sarcoidosis**)

Bogarad's syndrome (see **syndrome, auriculo-temporal**)

Bohn's nodules (see **nodules, Bohn's**)

Boley gauge (see **gauge, Boley**)

Bolton-nasion plane (see **plane, Bolton-nasion**)

Bolton plane (see **plane, Bolton-nasion**)

Bolton point, triangle (see under appropriate noun)

bolus (bō'lŭs) A mass of food ready to be swallowed or a mass passing through the intestines. (Periodont.)

bond The force that holds two or more units of matter together. (D. Mat.)

— The uniting or binding force between an orthodontic band or attachment and the enamel of the tooth. (Orthodont.)

primary or chemical b. A bond that requires some change in structure of matter. Primary bonds are ionic, covalent, or metallic. (D. Mat.)

secondary or physical b. (sometimes called van der Waals' forces) A bond that involves weak interatomic attractions such as variation in physical mass or location of electrical charge; e.g., molecular polarization—electrical dipoles and dispersion effects—and hydrogen bridges. (D. Mat.)

bone The material of the skeleton of most vertebrate animals; the tissue comprising bones. (Comp. Prosth.; Remov. Part. Prosth.)

— Any distinct piece of osseous framework or skelton of the body; structures formed of bone tissue. (Comp. Prosth.; Remov. Part. Prosth.)

— The tissue comprising bones; the material of which bones are made. (Oral Physiol.)

— Any discrete part of the bony skeleton, e.g., the mandible. (Oral Physiol.)

alveolar b. The specialized bone structure that contains the alveoli or sockets of the teeth and supports the teeth. (Comp. Prosth.; Orthodont.; Remov. Part. Prosth.)

— The compact bone that is deposited next to the periodontal ligament and is itself supported by supporting trabecular bone. (Periodont.)

a. b. metabolism The metabolic activity occurring within alveolar bone, which is generally slower than that occurring within metaphyseal bone but more rapid than that of diaphyseal bone. With metabolic equilibrium, catabolic processes normally occurring within bone are counterbalanced by anabolic activity. In situations in which catabolism exceeds anabolism, bone loss occurs; conversely, when anabolic processes exceed catabolic activity, excess bone is deposited. (Periodont.)

b. anabolism The building up of bone tissue, a process involving bone growth. (Periodont.)

b. apposition The continual deposition of bone occurring concurrently with bone resorption. Bone apposition involves the formation of an organic matrix by the osteoblasts, with subsequent mineralization by the deposition of calcium, phosphate, and carbonate on the organic mucopolysaccharide matrix (osteoid). (Periodont.)

b. architecture The structural pattern of the alveolar bone and its subjacent latticework of supporting bone. The alveolar bone is thin and compact adjacent to the periodontal membrane. The trabecular bone connects and reinforces the individual alveoli. The architecture of a bone is the result of functional stimuli to that bone, the stimuli varying as to type, intensity, and duration. (Periodont.)

basal b. That part of the mandible and maxillae from which the alveolar process develops. (Comp. Prosth.; Remov. Part. Prosth.)

— The mandibular and maxillary framework that is fixed and unchangeable and limits the extent to which teeth can be moved if the occlusion is to remain stable. (Orthodont.)

bundle b. The bone that forms the immediate bone attachment of the numerous bundles of collagen fibers of the periodontal ligament which have been incorporated into the bone. (Periodont.)

b. bur A drill designed to cut into bone. (Oral Implant.)

b., calcium content The amount of calcium stored in bone tissue. All or nearly all of the calcium in the blood is in solution in the plasma; the amount in the red blood cells is negligible. In normal man the concentration of calcium in the plasma is usually 9 to 11 mg/100 ml. It is in constant exchange with the calcium of the extracellular fluid and bones. The parathyroid gland maintains the constancy of the calcium concentration in the plasma. The bones serve as a reservoir of calcium and phosphate to provide for the other needs of the body and to supply minerals for deposition in the skeleton. (Oral Physiol.)

cancellous b. (spongiosa, spongy b., supporting b., trabecular b.) The bone that forms a trabecular network, surrounds marrow spaces that may contain either fatty or hematopoietic tissue, lies subjacent to the cortical bone, and makes up the main portion (bulk) of a bone. (Periodont.)

    c. b., atrophy of disuse Wasting of bone tissue occurring with loss of function of a part (e.g., a tooth). The supporting bone assumes an osteoporotic nature, and the marrow remains either fatty or hematopoietic. (Periodont.)

b. catabolism The tearing down of bone tissue, a process involving bone absorption or resorption. (Periodont.)

b. cell function (see **cell, function, bone**)

b. cell transformation (see **cell, transformation, bone**)

b. changes, mechanical factors Pressure and tension that play an important role in determining bone structure through influence on its cellular processes. Excessive, prolonged, and uncontrolled pressure and tension in orthodontic procedures can break down bone faster than bone deposition can take place. This results in mobile teeth in an unstable occlusion, which introduces trauma. Prosthetic appliances that place undue strain on abutment teeth or denture bases are causes of bone loss. This loss results in unfavorable leverage with the prosthetic appliances,

which, in turn, causes more bone loss. Poor vascularity is a concomitant of undue pressure and tension, and may inhibit repair and frequently may cause necrosis. (Oral Physiol.)

b. chips Small pieces of cancellous bone generally used to fill in bony defects and to precipitate recalcification. (Oral Surg.)

b. conduction (see **conduction, bone**)

compact b. Hard, dense bone comprising the outer cortical layer and consisting of an infinite variety of periosteal bone, endosteal bone and haversian systems. (Oral Physiol.)

b. crest The most coronal portion of alveolar bone often the area of the start of periodontal disease on inflammatory level as opposed to lesions of occlusal trauma, periodontosis, and systemic diseases that may involve the deeper region of the attachment apparatus. (Periodont.)

b. in deficiency diets Generally, in deficiency diets, bone resorption exceeds bone apposition in the trabecular bone. (Periodont.)

b. density The compactness of bone tissue. The demonstration of bone density by means of radiographs is directly dependent on the quantity of organic salts contained in the bone tissue. Thus a pathologic decrease in bone density appears in radiographs because of a disturbance of the organic salts or destruction of part of the bone. (Periodont.)

b. deposition Apposition or formation of new bone as a normal physiologic process in growth of the skeleton, as a repair process, or as a pathologic process (in conditions such as osteosarcoma and Paget's disease). Bone formation is initiated by the production of osteoid by the osteoblasts and later mineralized primarily with calcium salts, as the phosphate. (Periodont.)

b. development (see **bone, endochondral, formation; bone formation; bone, membrane, formation**)

b. disease Any disease that affects the osseous structures of the body; e.g., Paget's disease. (Periodont.)

effect of function on b. Changes that may occur in bone housing of teeth as a result of loss or increase of functioning of the oral structures. The bone housing of the tooth is dependent on the forces exerted on the tooth to maintain its structure. The passage of fluids of the periodontal membrane through the channels of the alveolar bone into the marrow spaces during function serves as a physiologic stimulus to bone formation. With loss of function, osteoporotic changes occur in supporting bone. With excessive function, osteoclastic action causes osteoporotic changes in supporting bone and resorption of bone lining the cribriform channels of the alveolar bone. The changes resulting from the increase in forces within physiologic limits are increased deposition of bone within the marrow spaces and thickening of the alveolar bone. (Periodont.)

effect of external radiation on b. Damage to bone resulting from external radiation. Bones of adults have a high degree of resistance to radiation, whereas the bones of children, particularly the growth processes of the long bones, are susceptible to injury. Such injury is not a hazard of ordinary diagnostic radiography, but overexposure may result from therapeutic radiation. Uninformed use of fluoroscopic equipment may also be responsible for injury. Damage to the bones of adults is most often seen after heavy and localized x-ray treatment or similar radiation from other external sources. Spontaneous fractures of the ribs, neck, femur and jaw have been reported under such circumstances. The lesion is responsible for necrosis. Serious marrow changes are always produced at dosage levels much lower than those approaching the threshold for damage to bone substance. Damage may be done to the vascular channels of both bone and bone marrow at somewhat higher doses than those needed to affect the hematopoietic function and the formed elements of the bone marrow. (Oral Physiol.)

endochondral b. (ĕn″dō-kŏn′dral) A bone that is developed in relation to antecedent cartilages (e.g., long bones, mandible). (Oral Physiol.) (see also **bone, membrane**)

e. b. formation Primarily a replacement of previously formed embryonic cartilage with an adult bony structure; a more complex bone formation than membrane bone. The actual replacement of cartilage by bone is only part of the process, however, because much of the bone is laid down directly external to the embryonic cartilage in the intramembranous pattern. The typical long bone cartilage tends to assume the definite form of the adult bone at an early stage, while it is still very small. The cartilage undergoes partial modification and degeneration near the middle of its length, and its cells begin

to multiply and arrange themselves in longitudinal columns. Blood vessels break into this central area beginning the destruction of cartilage. Osteoblasts enter with the blood vessels and lay down bone in place of destroyed cartilage. Ossification proceeds from the center of a bone toward each end. (Oral Physiol.) (see also **bone, membrane, formation**)

b. formation. The deposition of an organic mucopolysaccharide matrix (osteoid) which is subsequently mineralized with calcium salts. (Oral Physiol.) (see also **bone apposition; bone deposition**)

b. graft, autogenous (see **graft, autogenous bone**)

b. graft, donor site (see **donor site**)

b. graft, onlay (see **graft, onlay bone**)

b. graft, recipient site (see **recipient site**)

b. groove Osteotomy into or near the crest of the alveolar ridge for placement of an endosteal blade type of implant. (Oral Implant.)

b. g., canted An osteotomy sloped from the direct vertical, to avoid the mandibular canal or to keep the implant infrastructure within the medullary confines. (Oral Implant.)

gross appearance of b. Macroscopic appearance of bone tissue. Compact bone (usually surface bone) appears as a hard, compact mass in which openings of minute size are present. Spongy bone (generally present on the interior surface of bone) contains a framework or web of enough bony substance to preserve the shape and rigidity of the bony structure and a space that is occupied by vascular, fatty, and other tissues. Collectively, these latter tissues make up the bone marrow, which has the function of fat storage and blood cell formation. (Oral Physiol.)

b. healing The processes, which begin immediately after injury, of inflammation, then revascularization, and, finally, substitution of new bone that grows into an injured area from adjacent endosteum and periosteum. In membrane bones the process of healing consists of the proliferation and direct extension of new bone from the old. In long bones it involves the preliminary formation of a model of fibrous connective tissue and cartilage through which osteogenesis progresses into and across the fracture gap from each side. The fibrous connective tissue, cartilage, and bone are organized in the form of a complex structure termed callus. The interaction of cells and tissue resulting in the healing of a fracture is an example of the organization of diverse means to a common end. (Oral Physiol.)

internal reconstruction of b. The formation of bone on the tensional side of the periodontal ligament with concurrent resorption from the marrow space; contralaterally, resorption of alveolar bone with apposition from the endosteum in the marrow space. (Periodont.)

interproximal b. The bone that forms the septa between the teeth; consists primarily of a spongiosa of supporting bone covered by a layer of cortical bone. (Periodont.) (see also **septum, interdental**)

b. involvement Changes in the alveolar and/or supporting bone occurring as a sequel to, or accompanying, inflammatory or dystrophic disease; usually of a resorptive nature. (Periodont.)

b. lamella Bone having the appearance of layers of thin leaves or plates, produced by the lines that represent periods of inactivity of bone formation. These lamellae may be parallel to the surface of the bone or concentrically arranged around haversian canals. (Periodont.)

lamellar b. Bone that has an apparent lamellation produced by incremental lines parallel to the surface, with a relation to change in fibril direction. (Periodont.)

malar b. (zygomatic b.) A quadrangular bone on each side of the face that unites the frontal and the superior maxillary bones with the zygomatic process of the temporal bone. It forms the cheek prominence, a portion of the lateral wall and floor of the orbit, and parts of the temporal fossa and infratemporal fossa. (Periodont.)

marble b. (see **osteopetrosis**)

b. marrow The soft vascular tissue that fills bone cavities and cancellous bone spaces and consists primarily of fat cells, hematopoietic cells, and osteogenetic reticular cells. (Oral Physiol.)

b. matrix (see **matrix, structure of bone**)

membrane b. A bone developed within membrane but having no antecedent cartilage (e.g., parietal, frontal, bones of upper face). (Oral Physiol.) (see also **bone, endochondral**)

    m. b. formation The simpler of the two types of bone formation: membrane bone formation and endochondral bone formation.

The membrane bone forms directly from the mesenchyme. The bone develops first as a thin, flattened, irregular bony plate or membrane in the dermis. It gradually expands at its margins and becomes thickened by the deposition of successive layers of additional bone on the inner and outer surfaces. The membrane bones are restricted to the skull, jaws, and shoulder girdles. Bones of the skull and face that are composed of membrane bone are the parietal and frontal bones, all the bones of the upper part of the face, the squama of the temporal bone, the tympanic bone, the medial plate of the pterygoid process of the sphenoid bone, and the superior part of the occipital squama. (Oral Physiol.) (see also **bone, enchondral, formation**)

membranes of b. Membrane structures associated with the growth, development, and repair of bone: the periosteum, a connective tissue layer adjacent to bone surfaces; periodontal membrane, a modified periosteum associated with tooth structure; and endosteum, a thin layer of connective tissue lining the walls of the bone marrow spaces. (Oral Physiol.)

b. metabolism (see **metabolism, bone**)

microscopic appearance of b. Composition of bone tissue as viewed under a microscope. Microscopically, bone is composed of osteocytes embedded within lacunae in a calcified intercellular matrix. Extending from the lacunae are minute canals called canaliculi, which communicate with canaliculi of adjacent lacunae. Through this system of canals, nutrient material reaches the osteocytes and provides avenues for the removal of waste products of metabolism. Bone is deposited in incremental layers (lamellae) around haversian canals, the lamellae toward the surface of the bone being more or less parallel to it. (Periodont.)

b. mineral content, chemistry of The hardness of bone results from its mineral content in the organic matrix. The minerals (commonly designated as bone salts) and the organic matrix make up the interstitial substance of bone. The bone salts consist essentially of Ca^{++}, $PO_4 \equiv$, OH^-, carbon dioxide, and water, together with small amounts of other ions, especially Na^+, Mg^{++}, K^+, Cl^-, and F^-. The conditions for calcification of bone are based on systemic and local conditions. The systemic conditions include the supply and transport of the minerals necessary for calcification and the delivery of the minerals to the locus of calcification in the required concentration. The local conditions include several enzymatic and nonenzymatic interrelated factors. Thus bone tissue shares the internal environment with other tissues of the body and must respond to the total body activity for regulation of the fluid and electrolyte balance. (Oral Physiol.)

onlay b. (see **graft, onlay bone**)

perichondrial b. Bone that is deposited in concentric layers around the long shaft of the bone in a manner similar to the growth of endochondral bone. When a bone extends its length, it is necessary for the shaft to increase proportionately in diameter. Thus the perichondrial bone, more appropriately called the periosteal bone, is thickest in the middle part of the long bones. Periosteal bone continues to be deposited long after the inner shaft bone has been ossified. (Oral Physiol.)

b. pH The hydrogen ion concentration in bone tissue. The normal pH of bone tissue is 7.4. At this pH the minerals of bone are stable within the matrix. With the lowering of pH in inflammation, especially with the accumulation of lactic acid, bone resorption can occur. (Periodont.)

physical properties of b. Although bone is a living tissue composed of protein matrix on which have been deposited mineral salts of calcium, phosphorus, magnesium, and, to a lesser extent, sodium and potassium, its physical properties can be tested just as those of such inanimate objects as brick, wood, and steel. Compact bone has the following physical characteristics: specific gravity, 1.92 to 1.99; tensile strength, 13,000 to 17,000 lb/in²; compressive strength, 18,000 to 24,000 lb/in²; compressive strength parallel to the long axis, 7,150 lb/in²; compressive strength at right angles to the long axis, 16,800 lb/in². It is these physical characteristics that make bone particularly suitable for carrying out its functions of weight bearing, leverage, and protection of vulnerable viscera. The mandible and the maxillofacial bones collectively represent the characteristics of bone. The mandible particularly, with its hard, dense, cortical layer and its linear trabeculations, provides a bone that can both resist pressure and create the mechanical lever arm necessary for the generation and distribution of the masticatory forces. (Oral Physiol.)

b. plate (see **plate, bone**)

b. rarefaction A decreased density of bone, i.e., a decrease in the weight per unit of volume. Largely because radiographs do not distinguish clearly among conditions resulting in a decrease in the density of the shadows cast by bones, and because the nature of the condition is often obscure both clinically and at autopsy, the tendency is to use the terms atrophy, osteoporosis, and rarefaction interchangeably. (Oral Physiol.)

b. recession (see **recession, bone**)

resorption and repair of b. An adaptive physiologic mechanism occurring as long as the individual retains his natural dentition. (Periodont.) (see also **resorption of bone**)

resting lines in b. Lines created by alternating periods of bone formation and rest, giving a tierlike appearance to lamellar bone. (Periodont.)

reversal lines in b. Irregular lines containing concavities directed away from the bundle bone and serving as a histologic indication that resorption has taken place up to that line from the marrow side. (Periodont.)

b. seeker Any compound or ion that migrates preferentially into bone in the living organism. (Oral Radiol.)

b. sensibility (see **pallesthesia**)

b. sequestrum (see **sequestrum**)

sphenoid b. An irregular, wedge-shaped bone located at the base of the skull in front of the temporal bone and the basilar portion of the occipital bone. It is composed of a body that is more or less cuboidal in shape and hollowed out interiorly to form the sphenoidal air sinuses. Extending from the body laterally are two great wings and two small wings. Projecting below the body are two pterygoid processes. The lateral surfaces of the pterygoid processes give origin to the external ptergoid muscles, whereas the medial surfaces give origin to the internal pterygoid muscles. The sphenoid bone is important in dentistry because its processes and inferior surface provide places of origin of internal and external pterygoid muscles. (Periodont.)

spongy b. (see **bone, cancellous**)

b. strength Ability of bone to withstand stress and strain. In the fetal skeleton the internal architecture of bone is organized to withstand functional stress although the bones are still in a prefunctional state. The strength of a bone increases with the amount of strain to which it is subjected. The stimulating effect of the stress results in increased deposits of calcium in the bone shaft and especially at the ends of the bones. The spongy cancellous tissue within the bone is stimulated to grow along the lines of pressure resulting from the weight of the body. These cancelli are small supporting girders situated along the lines of stress. During growth, collagen fibers are embedded within the deposits of calcium, just as elastic iron wires are embedded in reinforced concrete. As a result of these strengthening features that are developed during growth, the bones of an adult can withstand great stress. (Oral Physiol.)

b. support The amount of alveolar and trabecular bone adjacent to a tooth than can provide attachment, investment, and support for the tooth; an important prognostic attribute during periodontal therapy. (Periodont.)

supporting b. (see **bone, cancellous**)

    s. b., atrophy of disuse (see **bone, cancellous, atrophy of disuse**)

b. surgery (see **surgery, osseous**)

thickened margin of b. Widening of the crest of the alveolus, primarily on the buccal and/or lingual aspects, varying from a thick ledge to a "beading" of the bone margin; results in a more or less bulbous contour of the gingival tissue overlying it. (Periodont.)

trabecular b. (see **bone, cancellous**)

undermining resorption of b. State in which the necrotic mass arising by excessive pressure is eliminated by resorption of the bone adjacent to the area of pressure necrosis. (Periodont.)

b. wax (see **wax, bone**)

woven b. So termed because of the character and pattern resulting from the interweaving of broad bands of bone. (Periodont.)

zygomatic b. (see **bone, malar**)

Bonwill-Hawley chart (see **chart, Hawley**)

Bonwill's triangle (see **triangle, Bonwill's**)

bony crater A concave resorptive defect in the alveolar crest, usually occurring interdentally, but occasionally interradicularly, and presenting two osseous walls (facial and lingual). (Periodont.)

bony crepitus (see **crepitus, bony**)

borax Often a principal ingredient in casting fluxes. Used in gypsum products as a retarder for the setting reaction and a strengthener for hydrocolloids. (D. Mat.)

border The circumferential margin or edge. (Comp. Prosth.)

    denture b. (denture edge, denture periphery) The limit, boundary, or circumferential margin of a denture base. The margin of the denture base at the junction of the polished surface with the impression (tissue) surface. The curved boundary surface of a denture base. (Comp. Prosth.; Remov. Part. Prosth.)

    mandibular b. (mandibular plane) Tangent to the lower border of the mandible. A line joining point gonion to point gnathion. (Orthodont.)

b. molding Shaping of an impression material by the manipulation or action of the tissues adjacent to the borders of an impression. (Comp. Prosth.)

b. movement (see **movement, border**)

b. seal The contact of the denture border with the underlying or adjacent tissues to prevent the passage of air or other substances. (Comp. Prosth.)

b. structures The oral structures that bound the borders of a denture. (Comp. Prosth.)

    b. s., movement The action of the muscles and other structures adjacent to the borders of a denture. (Remov. Part. Prosth.)

b. tissues, movement The action of the muscles and other structures adjacent to the borders of a denture. (Remov. Part. Prosth.)

boutons terminaux (see **end-feet**)

Bowen's disease (see **disease, Bowen's**)

box, light (see **illuminator**)

boxing The building up of vertical walls, usually in wax, around an impression to produce the desired size and form of the base of the cast and to preserve certain landmarks of the impression. (Comp. Prosth.)

— The procedure of enclosing an impression occlusal path record, etc. with a strip of wax, clay, or wet asbestos for the purpose of confining, shaping, and more effectively condensing the material of which the cast is to be made. (Remov. Part. Prosth.)

b. strip (see **strip, boxing**)

brachycephalic (brăk″ē-sĕ-făl′ĭk) Descriptive term applied to a broad, round head having a cephalic index of more than 80. (Orthodont.)

brachygnathia (brăk″ĭg-nā′thē-ah) **(bird-face, micrognathia)** Marked underdevelopment of the mandible. (Oral Diag.) (see also **retrognathism**)

bracing Resistance to the horizontal components of masticatory force. (Comp. Prosth.; Remov. Part. Prosth.)

bracket A small metal attachment fixed to a band that serves as a means of fastening the arch wire to the band. (Orthodont.)

bradycardia (brăd-ē-kar′dē-ah) Abnormal slowness of the heart as evidenced by a slowing of the pulse rate (under 50 beats/minute). Anesth.)

bradydiastole (brăd″ē-dī-ăs′tō-lē) Abnormal prolongation of the distole. (Anesth.)

bradypnea (brăd″ē-nē′ah) Abnormal slowness of breathing. (Anesth.)

bradythesia (brăd″ē-thē′zē-ah) Slowness or dullness of perception. (Anesth.)

brain, electrical activity of Electrical energy that can be observed as waves with electroencephalographic equipment. This equipment records electrical rhythms in the brain. These rhythms and patterns have been organized into a system that imputes values for the state of health. The system also imputes values for conditions in disease in which the patterns deviate from those pattern symbols that can be reproduced consistently in a state of health. Electrical evidence of brain activity of the cerebral cortex reveals that different potential patterns are produced by different states of mental activity, e.g., tension, mental work, and sleep. (Oral Physiol.)

brainstem The part of the brain, presumably the oldest part phylogenetically, in which are located centers for many simple but basically important reactions within the nervous system. The brainstem includes the primitive forebrain, the midbrain, and the hindbrain. The predominant structure in the hindbrain is the medulla oblongata; the dominant structures in the forebrain are the pituitary gland and the unpaired optical vesicles. Derived from the brainstem late in development are the cerebellum from the hindbrain, and the thalamus, the basal nuclei, and the cerebral cortex from the forebrain. The principal nuclei of the cranial nerves are the medulla oblongata and part of the midbrain. (Oral Physiol.)

branchial nerve (see **nerve, branchial**)

breach of contract (see **contract, breach of**)

breath Air inhaled and exhaled in respiration. (Anesth.)

　bad (offensive) b. (see **halitosis**)

breathing, mouth The process of inspiration and expiration of air primarily through the oral cavity. It is commonly seen in nasal conditions such as deviated septum, hypertrophied adenoids, and allergies, and may produce excessive drying of the oral mucosa with a tendency to gingival hyperplasia. (Periodont.)

bregma (brĕg′mah) The point at which sagittal and coronary sutures meet. (Orthodont.)

Bremsstrahlung radiation (see **radiation, Bremsstrahlung**)

Breuer's reflex (see **reflex, Hering-Breuer**)

bridge Colloquial expression for a fixed partial denture. (Fixed Part. Prosth.; Remov. Part. Prosth.) (see **denture, partial, fixed**)

　cantilever b. (see **denture, partial, fixed, cantilever**)

　fixed b. (see **denture, partial, fixed**)

　removable b. A colloquial expression for a removable partial denture. (see also **denture, partial, removable**)

　b. splint (see **splint, fixed partial denture**)

Brill-Symmers disease (see **lymphoma, giant follicular**)

Brinell hardness number (see **number, Brinell hardness**)

Brinell hardness test (see **test, Brinell hardness**)

brittle Friable; technically, a brittle material is one in which the proportional limit and ultimate strength are close together in value. (D. Mat.) (see also **ductility**)

broach An instrument with numerous protruding barbs from a metal shaft. It is generally used to engage the dental pulp for extirpation. (Endodont.)

　barbed b. An instrument used for removing the pulp or debris from the root canal. (Endodont.)

　b. holder An instrument similar to a pin vise used to hold a broach. (Endodont.)

　pathfinder b. (see **broach, smooth**)

　smooth b. (**pathfinder, pathfinder b.**) An instrument used for locating the orifice of a root canal and exploring the canal to determine the accessibility of the root end. (Endodont.)

Broders' classification (see **index, Broders'**)

Broders' index (see **index, Broders'**)

bromism (brō′mĭzm) The toxic state induced by excessive exposure to or ingestion of bromine or bromine-containing compounds. (Oral Med.; Pharmacol.)

bromopnea (brōm″ahp-nē′ah) (see **halitosis**)

bronchia (brŏng′kē-ah) Bronchial tubes smaller than bronchi and larger than bronchioles. (Anesth.)

bronchiarctia (brŏng″kē-ark′shē-ah) The stenosis of a bronchial tube. (Anesth.)

bronchiectasis (brŏng″kē-ĕk′tah-sĭs) A chronic disease characterized by dilation of the bronchi and bronchioles, clinically recognizable by fetid breath and paroxysmal coughing, with expectoration of mucopurulent matter; dilation of the bronchi, either local or general. (Anesth.)

— Permanent dilation of the bronchioles resulting in a chronic stasis of exudate in the lungs. (Oral Med.)

bronchiocele (brŏng′kē-ō-sēl″) A dilation or

swelling of a branch smaller than a bronchus. (Anesth.)

bronchiole (brŏng'kē-ōl) A terminal division of a bronchium. (Anesth.)

bronchium (brŏng'kē-ŭm) One of the subdivisions of a bronchus. (Anesth.)

bronchoconstriction (brŏng″kō-kahn-strĭk'shŭn) The reduction of the caliber of the bronchi. (Anesth.)

bronchodilation (brŏng″kō-dī-lā'shŭn) The dilation of a bronchus; the operation of dilating a stenosed bronchus. (Anesth.)

bronchodilator (brŏng″kō-dī-lā'tor) A drug that dilates, or expands, the size of the lumina of the air passages of the lungs by relaxing the muscular walls. (Anesth.)

— A drug that causes the bronchi to dilate. (Oral Med.; Pharmacol.)

bronchospasm (brŏng'kō-spăzm) A spasmodic contraction of the muscular coat of the bronchial tubes, such as occurs in asthma. (Anesth.)

bronchostenosis (brŏng″kō-stĕ-nō'sĭs) Stenosis of the bronchi; bronchiarctia. (Anesth.)

Brooke's tumor (see **epithelioma adenoides cysticum**)

brown pellicle (see **pellicle, brown**)

bruise In medical jurisprudence a contusion; an injury made on the flesh of a person by an instrument without destroying its continuity, i.e., without breaking the skin. (D. Juris.)

bruit (broot) Extracardiac blowing sound heard at times over peripheral vessels; generally denotes cardiovascular disease. (Oral Diag.)

brush, polishing An instrument consisting of natural, synthetic, or wire bristles, mounted on a mandrel or in a hub to fit on a lathe chuck; used to carry abrasive or polishing media to polish teeth, restorations, and prosthetic appliances. (Oper. Dent.)

  bristle p. b. A polishing brush with natural or synthetic bristles. (Oper. Dent.)

  wheel p. b. A polishing brush with bristles mounted like spokes of a wheel. (Oper. Dent.)

  wire p. b. A polishing brush with bristles of wire, usually steel or brass. (Oper. Dent.)

brushing (see **abrasion, denture**)

bruxism (brŭk'sĭzm) An involuntary clenching of the teeth associated with forceful lateral or protrusive jaw movements; results in rubbing, gritting, or grinding together of the teeth. (Comp. Prosth.; Oper. Dent.; Oral Surg.; Orthodont.; Pedodont.)

— The nonfunctional gnashing, grinding, or clenching of the teeth. (Remov. Part. Prosth.)

— Grinding of the teeth. A habit, usually associated with emotional stress, anxiety, fear, or fatigue, in which mandibular teeth are moved laterally or protrusively while contacting the maxillary teeth resulting in abnormal wear patterns on the teeth. It also results frequently in occlusal traumatism and, generally, if prolonged, in a decrease in the occlusal vertical dimension. (Periodont.)

— The involuntary gnashing, grinding, or clenching of teeth. It is usually unconscious, whether the individual is awake or asleep; often associated with fatigue, anxiety, emotional stress, or fear; and frequently triggered by occlusal irregularities, usually resulting in either abnormal wear patterns on the teeth, periodontal breakdown, or joint or neuromuscular problems. (Oral Physiol.)

  b., nocturnal occlusal wear An effect of bruxism that consists of a flattened, highly wearglazed facet and not including an overall wear pattern. (Periodont.)

bruxomania (brŭk″sō-mā'nē-ah) A neurotic condition resulting in bruxism; a psychogenic condition often related to that phase of bruxism which occurs unconsciously while the individual is awake, except during mastication. (Comp. Prosth.; Remov. Part. Prosth.)

BSP (see **test, bromsulphalein**)

bubo (bū'bō) A lymph node that is enlarged secondary to an infection. The process may lead to suppuration; seen in primary syphilis, chancroid, plague, malaria, and other infectious processes. (Oral Med.)

buccal (bŭk'ŭl) Pertaining to or adjacent to the cheek. (Comp. Prosth.; Oper. Dent.; Orthodont.; Remov. Part. Prosth.)

  b. aspect (see **aspect, buccal**)

  b. contour (see **contour, buccal**)

  b. flange (see **flange, buccal**)

  b. notch (see **notch, buccal**)

  b. shelf (see **shelf, buccal**)

  b. splint (see **splint, buccal**)

  b. surface (see **surface, buccal**)

  b. tube (see **tube, buccal**)

  b. vestibule (see **vestibule, buccal**)

buccoclusion (bŭk″ō-kloo'zhŭn) An occlusion in which the dental arch or group of teeth is buccal to the normal position. (Orthodont.)

buccolingual relationship (see **relationship, buccolingual**)

buccolingual stress (see **stress, buccolingual**)

buccoversion (bŭk″ō-ver'zhŭn) Any deviation from the normal line of occlusion toward the cheeks. (Orthodont.)

— The position of a tooth when it lies or is inclined buccal to the basal alveolar process or to the line of occlusion. (Periodont.)

buck knife (see **knife, buck**)

buckling The crowding of anterior teeth in the dental arch; the malalignment may be an etiologic factor in the genesis of periodontal disease. (Periodont.)

budget plan A method of financing dental accounts in which arrangements are made for the patient to pay a series of small amounts on his account, usually over a period of 12 to 18 months. (Pract. Man.)

buffer Any substance in a fluid that tends to lessen the change in hydrogen ion concentration, which otherwise would be produced by adding acids or alkalis. (Anesth.; Oral Med.; Pharmacol.)

bulb, speech (see **aid, speech, prosthetic, pharyngeal section**)

bulla (bŭl′ah) A large blister or vesicle filled with fluid. (Oral Diag.)

— A circumscribed, elevated lesion of the skin containing fluid and measuring over 5 mm in diameter. (Oral Path.)

BUN (see **blood urea nitrogen**)

Bunnell test (see **test, Paul-Bunnell**)

bur A rotary cutting instrument of steel or tungsten carbide; supplied with cutting heads of various shapes and two or more sharp-edged blades; used as a rotary grinder. (Oper. Dent.)

　carbide b. A bur made of tungsten carbide; used at high rotational speeds. (Oper. Dent.)

　crosscut b. A bur with blades slotted perpendicularly to the axis of the bur. (Oper. Dent.)

　end-cutting b. A bur that has cutting blades only on the end of its head. (Oper. Dent.)

　excavating b. A bur used to remove dentin and debris from a cavity. (Oper. Dent.)

　finishing b. A bur with numerous, fine-cutting blades placed close together; used to contour metallic restorations. (Oper. Dent.)

　intramucosal insert base-preparing b. (see **insert, intramucosal**)

　inverted cone b. A bur with a head shaped like a truncated cone, the larger diameter being at the terminal (distal) end. (Oper. Dent.)

　plug-finishing b. (see **bur, finishing**)

　round b. A bur with a sphere-shaped head. (Oper. Dent.)

　straight fissure b. A bur without crosscuts that has a cylindrically shaped head. (Oper. Dent.)

　tapered fissure b. A bur that has a long head

with sides that converge from the shank to a blunt end. (Oper. Dent.)

burden of proof in law of evidence. The necessity or duty of proving a fact or facts in contention on an issue between the parties in a course of action. (D. Juris.)

Burkitt's tumor (African lymphoma) A type of lymphosarcoma seen in African children. About half the patients have lesions in the jawbones. Recent evidence suggests a possible viral etiology. (Oral Diag.)

Burlew wheel A proprietary brand of abrasive-impregnated, knife-edged, rubber polishing wheel; used on a mandrel in the dental handpiece to smooth metallic restorations and tooth surfaces. (Oper. Dent.)

　high luster B. w. Burlew wheel in which jeweler's rouge or iron peroxide is used as the abrasive agent. (Oper. Dent.)

　midget B. w. (sulci B. w.) A miniature form of Burlew wheel. (Oper. Dent.)

　sulci B. w. (see **Burlew wheel, midget**)

burn A lesion caused by contact of heat, radiation, friction, chemicals, etc. with tissue. Thermal burns are classified as follows: *first degree,* manifested by erythema; *second degree,* manifested by formation of vesicles; *third degree,* manifested by necrosis of the mucosa or dermis; *fourth degree,* manifested by charring into the submucous or subcutaneous layers of the body. (Oral Surg.; Periodont.)

　aspirin b. An irregularly shaped, whitish area on the mucosa caused by the topical application of acetylsalicylic acid. (Periodont.)

burnisher An instrument with rounded edges used to burnish, polish, or work-harden metallic surfaces, contour matrices, and spin or stretch margins of cast restorations. (Oper. Dent.)

　ball b. A burnisher with a working point in the form of a ball. (Oper. Dent.)

　beaver-tail b. (see **burnisher, straight**)

　fishtail b. A burnisher that slightly resembles a fish's tail or a hammer in shape; one end of the blade is flattened and the other is ball shaped. The flat end is useful in everting the edges of a rubber dam around teeth. (Oper. Dent.)

　straight b. A burnisher that resembles a beaver's tail in shape; the broad, flat blade is smoothly continuous with the shank, meeting it in a slight curve; the edges and the point are smoothly rounded. (Oper. Dent.)

burnishing A process related to polishing and abrading; the metal is moved by mechanically distorting the normal space lattice. Commonly accomplished during the polishing of soft golds. (D. Mat.)

burnout Elimination by heat of an invested pattern from a set investment to prepare the mold to receive casting metal. (Oper. Dent.)

high heat b. The use of temperature over 1100° F to effect wax elimination. (Oper. Dent.)

inlay b. (wax b.) Elimination of wax from an invested inlay flask. (Oper. Dent.) (see also **wax elimination**)

radiographic b. Excessive penetration of the x-ray beam of an object or part of an object, producing a totally black overexposed area on the radiograph. (Oral Radiol.)

wax b. (see **burnout, inlay; wax elimination**)

business area The area adjacent to the reception room in which the receptionist conducts the business affairs of the office and directly through which patients must pass both to enter and leave the dental office. (Pract. Man.)

business hours (office hours) Those hours of the day during which professional, public, or other kinds of business are ordinarily conducted. (D. Juris.)

business office The room reserved for the dentist in which he conducts the business side of his dental practice. Used by many dentists for the consultation appointment; it can also serve as an area in which he can isolate himself for relaxation during brief periods of the day. (Pract. Man.)

butt To place directly against the tissues covering the residual alveolar ridge; to bring any two square-ended surfaces into contact, as a butt joint. (Comp. Prosth.; Fixed Part. Prosth.; Remov. Part. Prosth.)

button Term that refers to excess metal remaining from casting and sprue; located at the end of the sprue, opposite the casting. (D. Mat.)

implant b. (see **insert, intramucosal**)

buttonhole approach A method of surgical treatment of a periodontal abscess in which, after an incision is made in the fluctuant abscess, an additional attempt is made to curet the area adjoining the root and the fundus of the abscess through the destroyed portion of the alveolar plate or bone. (Periodont.)

C

cachexia (kah-kĕk'sē-ah) Weakness, loss of weight, atrophy, and emaciation caused by severe or chronic disease. (Oral Med.)
  hypophyseal c. (see **disease, Simmonds'**)
  hypopituitary c. (see **disease, Simmonds'**)
café-au-lait spots (see **spots, café-au-lait**)
caffeine, phenacetin, aspirin (kăf'ēn, fĕh-năs'ŭh-tin) (**PAC**) An analgesic compound. (see also **aspirin, phenacetin, caffeine**)
Caffey's disease (see **hyperostosis, infantile cortical**)
calcific metamorphosis (of dental pulp) A frequently observed reaction to trauma; characterized by partial or complete obliteration of the pulp chamber and canal. (Endodont.)
calcification, dystrophic Pathologic deposition of calcium salts in necrotic or degenerated tissues. (Oral Path.)
calcification, metastatic Pathologic deposition of calcium salts in previously undamaged tissues. This process is due to an excessively high level of blood calcium such as in hyperparathyroidism. (Oral Path.)
calcifying epithelial odontogenic tumor (Pindborg tumor) An uncommon tumor arising from odontogenic epithelium characterized by focal areas of calcification. It has the same age, sex, and site distribution as the ameloblastoma. (Oral Diag.)
calcination (kăl"sĭ-nā'shŭn) A process of removing water by heat; used in the manufacture of plaster and stone from gypsum. (D. Mat.)
calcinosis (kăl-sĭ-nō'sĭs) Deposition of calcium salts in various tissues due to hypercalcemia and tissue degeneration. (Oral Diag.)
— Presence of calcification in or under the skin. The condition may occur in a localized form (c. circumscripta) or in a generalized form (c. universalis). (Oral Path.)
calcium The element that is the basic component of teeth and bones. It is also found in all cells of the body. The normal level of calcium in the blood is 9 to 11.5 mg/100 ml. (Oral Diag.)
— A basic element, with an atomic weight of 40.07, found in nearly all organized tissues. Essential for mineralization of bone and teeth. A deficiency of calcium in the diet or in utilization may lead to rickets or osteoporosis. Overexcretion in hyperparathyroidism leads to osteoporotic manifestations. (Periodont.) (see also **factor IV**)
blood c. (see **blood calcium**)
c. fluoride A compound that is used as a flux in the manufacture of some silicate cements. (D. Mat.)
c. hydroxide A white powder that is mixed with water or other medium and used as a base material in cavity liners and for pulp capping. (D. Mat.)
c. phosphate An odorless, tasteless white powder, the various forms of which are sometimes used as abrasives in dentifrices. (D. Mat.)
c. salts Calcium present in salivary fluid as phosphates and carbonates. These salts are believed to form dental calculus on their precipitation from saliva. (Periodont.)
c. sulfate (see **alpha-hemihydrate; beta-hemihydrate; gypsum**)
c. tungstate A chemical substance used in crystal form to coat screens; the screens fluoresce when struck by roentgen rays. (Oral Radiol.)
calculus (calcareous deposit) Tartar, the hard mineral deposit on teeth. Bacteria of filamentous types appear to be important constituents of calculus. Deposits of calculus may also form in salivary gland ducts, in kidneys, etc. (Oral Diag.)
— A concretion composed of calcium phosphate, calcium carbonate, magnesium phosphate, and other elements within an organic matrix composed of desquamated epithelium, mucin, microorganisms, and other debris. (Oral Path.)
— The accretion formed on the teeth by precipitation of calcium and magnesium salts from the saliva in the form of phosphates and carbonates, with a dental plaque of organic material serving as a nidus for formation. Deposited on a mucopolysaccharide matrix; possesses apatite structure; contains desquamated cells, debris, and various members of the oral microbial flora, among which the filamentous organisms are often considered as essential for deposition and attachment of calculus to the teeth. (Periodont.)
dental c. A salivary deposit of calcium phosphate and carbonate with organic matter on the teeth or a dental prosthesis. (Remov. Part. Prosth.)

hard c. Dental calculus containing a high percentage of calcified material (e.g., calcium phosphate or calcium carbonate) with a relatively small amount of organic material. It is extremely dense, and considerable force is required to remove it with hand instruments. (Periodont.)

serumal c. Previously used term for calculus found below the gingival margin. (Periodont.)

subgingival c. Calculus deposited on the tooth structure and found apical to the gingival margin within the confines of the gingival cervix, gingival pocket, or periodontal pocket. Usually darker, more pigmented, and denser than supragingival calculus. (Periodont.)

supragingival c. Calculus deposited on the teeth occlusal or incisal to the gingival crest. (Periodont.)

calibrated probe (see **probe, calibrated**)

calibration of x-ray unit (see **unit, calibration, x-ray**)

caliper, axis-orbital A caliper used to capture and freeze needed data on facial relations until they can be put into an articulator that will receive them. It consists of (1) a hinge-bow, the arms of which have been made equal, set on the bow's base far enough apart to suit facial dimensions and joined so that the three members share the same plane; (2) a bite fork covered with compound; (3) an orbital indicator of the axis-orbital plane; (4) an upright rod to hold the orbital indicator in place; (5) a toggle to freeze the bow's base to the bite fork; and (6) a second toggle to attach and allow adjustments for the support of the indicator. *Syn:* hinge-bow transfer recorder. (Gnathol.)

Callahan's method (see **method, chloropercha**)

callus The tissue near and about the broken fragments of a bone that becomes involved in the repair of the fracture through various stages of exudate, fibrosis, and new bone formation. (Oral Physiol.)

Camper's line (see **line, Camper's**)

camphorated parachlorophenol, N.F. XI (par″ah-klō″rō-fē′nol) A mixture of not less than 33% or more than 37% of parachlorophenol, and not less than 63% or more than 67% of camphor; used to treat root canals. (Endodont.)

canal(s) Portion of the root that contains the pulp tissue and is bounded by dentin. (Endodont.)

accessory root c. A lateral branching of the main root canal, usually occurring in the apical third of the root. (Endodont.)

branching c. (see **canal, collateral pulp**)

collateral pulp c. (branching c.) A dental pulp canal branch that emerges from the root at a place other than the apex. (Endodont.)

interdental c. (nutrient c.) The nutrient channels that pass upward through the body of the mandible mainly betweeen the central and lateral incisors, and that may extend posteriorly as far as the bicuspid region. Seen as radiolucent lines on radiographs. (Periodont.)

mandibular c. A channel extending from the mandibular foramen on the medial surface of the ramus of the mandible to the mental foramen. It contains mandibular blood vessels (arteries and veins) and the intraosseous portion of the mandibular branch of the trigeminal nerve. (Periodont.)

nutrient c. (see **canal, interdental**)

pulp c. The space in the radicular portion of the tooth occupied by the pulp. (Endodont.)

— The root canal; the area that extends from the pulp chamber to the root apex and contains pulpal tissue, blood supply, lymphatic drainage, innervation to the tooth, etc. (Periodont.)

root c. The space in the anterior part of the root of a tooth that contains the pulp tissue. (Endodont.) (see also **canal, pulp**)

r. c., measurements A technique employing the use of radiographs for determining the length of the root canal. (Endodont.)

canaliculus (kăn-ah-lĭk′ū-lŭs) A minute channel that extends from or to the lacunae of bone and cementum and contains filamentous processes of the cells that occupy the lacunae; interconnects with canaliculi extending from neighboring lacunae. (Periodont.)

cancer A malignant neoplasm. Term is sometimes incorrectly used to include all neoplasms, benign or malignant. Carcinoma and sarcoma are more limiting terms. (Oral Diag.)

cancrum oris (kăng′krŭm aw′rĭs) (see **stomatitis, gangrenous**)

Candida albicans (kăn′dĭ-dah ăl′bĭ-kănz) A yeastlike fungus that is a normal inhabitant of the mouth and that causes thrush. Formerly called *Monilia albicans;* hence moniliasis is used as a synonym for thrush. (Oral Diag.)

— A budding, yeastlike fungus present in the normal flora of the mucous membrane of the female genital tract and respiratory and gastrointestinal (including the mouth) tracts. (Oral Med.)

— A yeastlike fungus, normally present in oral microorganismal flora, that is capable of assuming a pathogenic role in the production of oral and systemic moniliasis (thrush, monilial infection, etc.). (Periodont.)

candidiasis (kăn″dĭ-dĭ′ah-sĭs) Infection by *Candida albicans*. (Oral Med.) (see also **moniliasis; thrush**)

canine (kā′nĭn) **(cuspid)** One of the four pointed teeth in man, situated one on each side of each jaw, distal to the lateral incisor; forms the keystone of the arch. The term canine is increasingly preferred to cuspid. (Oper. Dent.)

c. fossa (see **fossa, canine**)

canker (kăng′ker) (see **herpes labialis**)

c. sore (see **sore, canker**)

cannula (kăn′ū-lah) A tube for insertion into the body; its caliber is usually occupied by a trocar during the act of insertion. (Anesth.)

cantilever bridge (see **denture, partial, fixed, cantilever**)

cantilever partial denture (see **denture, partial, fixed, cantilever**)

cantle A fragment, piece, portion. (Oper. Dent.)

capacity Legal qualification, competency, power, or fitness. (D. Juris.)

functional residual c. (normal c.) The volume of gas in the lungs at resting expiratory level. (Anesth.)

iron-binding c. A measure of the binding capacity of iron in the serum; helps to differentiate the causes of hypoferremia. This capacity tends to increase in iron deficiency and diminishes in chronic diseases and during infection. (Oral Med.)

normal c. (see **capacity, functional residual**)

total lung c. The volume of air in the lungs at the end of maximal inspiration. (Anesth.)

vital c. The maximal volume of air that can be expired after maximal inspiration. (Anesth.; Cleft Palate)

— The total lung capacity minus the residual volume of air. It represents the general state of respiratory conditioning of a patient in relation to the ventilating capacity. A healthy, well-conditioned patient with a high vital capacity has the capacity for an increased chest expansion, great depth of inspiration, and a reduced rate of respiration. Conversely, a poorly conditioned, sick, or disabled patient generally has a reduced vital capacity and thus cannot ventilate adequately to provide the oxygen required for any unusual muscular activity. (Oral Physiol.)

capillarity The phenomenon by which a film of fluid is drawn and held between two closely approximating surfaces. This is a special hazard in the wearing of a removable partial denture that makes contact with enamel surfaces of abutment teeth. (Remov. Part. Prosth.)

capillary(ies) The terminal vessels uniting the arterial with the venous systems of the body. Capillaries are organized into extensive branching reticular beds to provide a maximum surface for exchange of fluids, electrolytes, and metabolites between tissues and the vascular system. The capillary bed has the largest cross-section area of the entire vascular system. When all the capillaries are opened simultaneously, they draw off a sufficient volume of blood from the tissue to cause temporary cerebral anemia, which may result in syncope or shock. (Oral Physiol.)

— The minute vessels connecting the arterioles with the venules, forming an extensive network within the tissues. (Periodont.)

c. attraction The quality or state that, because of surface tension, causes elevation or depression of the surface of a liquid that is in contact with a solid. Considered to be one of the factors in retention of complete dentures. (Comp. Prosth.)

c. regulation The control of each capillary by means of its principal regulating mechanisms, which are under the influence of local conditions. The role of the nervous system is less significant in capillary activity than in activity of arterial vessels. Capillary circulation is essentially under the joint control of the chemical messengers, substances from distant sources in the blood, and from specific chemical products of tissue metabolism. (Oral Physiol.)

capitulum (kah-pĭt′ū-lŭm) A little head. Term is used by some European writers instead of head or condyle. (Comp. Prosth.)

c. mandibulae (see **process, condyloid**)

capping, pulp The covering of an exposed dental pulp with a material that protects it from external influences and that does not interfere with pulpal healing. (Endodont.)

— A technique and material used for covering an exposed, healthy pulp with an agent that will protect the pulp tissue and stimulate the formation of secondary dentin in an effort to maintain the health and vitality of the pulp of the tooth. (Oper. Dent.)

direct p. c. Application to the exposed pulp of a drug or material compatible with the vital pulp for the purpose of stimulating repair of the injured pulpal tissue. (Pedodont.)

indirect p. c. A procedure that stimulates formation of secondary dentin by means of a chemical (usually calcium hydroxide) placed over a layer of carious dentin remaining over the potentially exposed pulp. The drug is sealed in place by means of another, more durable material (amalgam or cement) for a period of time, after which the treatment and remaining carious material is removed. (Oper. Dent.; Pedodont.)

capsule, joint A fibrous sac or ligament that encloses a joint and limits its motion. It is lined with synovial membrane composed of specialized connective tissue that has a collagenous matrix richly supplied with blood vessels, lymphatics, and nerves. It contains few elastic fibers or characteristic connective tissue cells. (Oral Physiol.)

temporomandibular j. c. (see **articulation, temporomandibular, capsule**)

carat A standard of fineness of gold, 24 carats being taken as expressing absolute purity, and the proportion of gold to other metals in an alloy in a mixture represented as so many carats. (D. Juris.)

— Measurement of gold content of alloys, pure gold having 24 carats. (D. Mat.)

carbide bur (see **bur, carbide**)

carbohemia (kar″bō-hē′mē-ah) Imperfect oxidation of the blood. (Anesth.)

carbohemoglobin (kar″bō-hē″mō-glō′bĭn) Hemoglobin compounded with CO_2. (Anesth.)

carbohydrate tolerance (see **tolerance, carbohydrate**)

carbon dioxide absorber A device that removes carbon dioxide from a mixture of bases. (Anesth.)

carbon markings The markings made on the teeth when, with articulating paper interposed, the mandibular teeth are brought in contact with the maxillary teeth in the centric path of closure, or when the mandible is carried through its various excursive movements with mandibular and maxillary teeth in contact. A diagnostic procedure for the detection of occlusal interferences. (Periodont.)

carbonate hydroxyapatite (kăr′bon-āt hī-drok″sē-ăp′ah-tīt) Term indicating the composition and crystal structure of hard tissues.

carcinoma (kar-sĭ-nō′mah) A malignant epithelial neoplasm. (Oral Diag.; Oral Path.)

adenocystic c. (basaloid mixed tumor) A pseudoadenomatous basal cell carcinoma originating from salivary glands. It grows slowly but is malignant. (Oral Diag.)

—An adenocarcinoma, the cells of which resemble basal cells and form ductlike or cystlike structures. (Oral Path.)

basal cell c. (basal cell epithelioma, rodent ulcer, turban tumor) An epithelial neoplasm with a basic structure resembling the basal cells of the epidermis; develops from basal cells of the epidermis or from the outer cells of hair follicles or sebaceous glands. It is malignant, but metastasis is extremely rare. (Oral Diag.)

— An epithelial neoplasm the cells of which are a basal layer type that develop on exposed skin surfaces, particularly the middle third of the face. It rarely if ever metastasizes but is locally invasive. It does not arise from oral mucosa. (Oral Path.)

basosquamous c. Carcinoma that histologically exhibits both basal and squamous elements. It may occasionally be seen in the oral cavity; considered to have a greater tendency to metastasize than basal cell carcinoma. (Oral Path.)

epidermoid c. (squamous cell c.) A malignant epithelial neoplasm with cells resembling those of the epidermis. The term squamous cell carcinoma is used for intraoral lesions of this nature. (Oral Diag.)

— A malignant epithelial tumor of the salivary gland; characterized by mucus-producing cells and metaplastic squamous epithelium. (Oral Diag.; Oral Path.)

exophytic c. A malignant epithelial neoplasm with marked outward growth like a wart or papilloma. (Oral Diag.)

intraepithelial c. (see **disease, Bowen's**)

mucoepidermoid c. A malignant epithelial tumor of the salivary gland; characterized by acini with mucus-producing cells. (Oral Diag.)

c. in situ (see **disease, Bowen's**)

squamous cell c. (see **carcinoma, epidermoid**)

transitional cell c. A malignant tumor arising from a transitional type of stratified epithelium. (Oral Path.)

cardiac Relating to the heart.

c. arrest (see **arrest, cardiac**)

c. massage (see **massage, cardiac**)

c. output The volume of blood put out by the heart per minute; the product of the stroke volume and the heart rate per minute. Cardiac output adjusts itself to the needs of the body in accordance with environmental influences, e.g., physical work, emotional stress, food intake, body posture, and temperature changes. A flow of blood to and from the heart causes greater stretch of normal heart muscle, which automatically causes greater stroke volume. Control is partially autonomous and partially under the control of the central nervous system on a subconscious level. The normal muscle requires ten to fifteen times more blood during function than at rest. Cardiac output diminishes when the heart is diseased. (Oral Physiol.)

cardioinhibitory (kar″dē-ō-ĭn-hĭb′ĭ-tor-ē) Restraining or inhibiting the movements of the heart. (Anesth.)

cardiokinetic (kar″dē-ō-kĭ-nĕt′ĭk) Exciting the heart; a remedy that excites the heart. (Anesth.)

cardiopulmonary Pertaining to the heart and lungs. (Anesth.)

care As a legal term, the opposite of negligence. (D. Juris.)

  reasonable c. The degree of care that might be expected from the reasonable person under particular circumstances. (D. Juris.)

caries (kā′rē-ēz) A process of progressive destruction of the hard tissues of the teeth initiated by bacterially produced acids at the tooth surface. In general medicine this term refers to death and decay of bone. (Oral Diag.)

— An irreversible disease of the calcified portions of teeth; characterized by demoralization of inorganic components and destruction of organic components of the tooth. (Oral Path.; Pract. Man.)

  dental c. A localized, progressive, molecular disintegration of tooth structure. Term designates a disease and has no plural. (Oper. Dent.)

  — Dissolution and disintegration of the enamel and/or dentin of a tooth. (Oral Path.; Remov. Part. Prosth.)

  — Tooth decay; a disease of the calcified structures of the teeth, characterized by decalcification of the mineral components and dissolution of the organic matrix. (Periodont.)

  arrested d. c. State existing when the progress of the decay process has halted. (Oper. Dent.)

  healed d. c. (see **caries, dental, arrested**)

  incipient d. c. A decayed part of a tooth that does not need restoration at the time of examination. (Pract. Man.)

  prevention of d. c. Action taken to stop the development of dental caries, including giving attention to factors such as diet, oral hygiene, fluoridation, and sound

restorative dental procedures. (Oper. Dent.)

  proximal d. c. Decay occurring in the mesial or distal surface of a tooth. (Oper. Dent.)

  radiographic index of d. c. A system of indicating the relative depth or degree of penetration of the carious process into the tooth substance. (Oper. Dent.)

  rampant d. c. A suddenly appearing, widespread, rapidly burrowing type of caries, resulting in early involvement of the pulp and affecting those teeth regarded as immune to ordinary decay. (Pedodont.)

  recurrent d. c. Extension of the carious process beyond the margin of a restoration due to inadequate extension of the outline form of the cavity or to incomplete marginal sealing of the restoration in the cavity. (Oper. Dent.)

  d. c. removal Mechanical elimination of carious dentin and debris from a cavity preparation. (Oper. Dent.)

  residual d. c. (residual carious dentin) Decayed material left in a prepared cavity and over which a restoration is placed. (Oper. Dent.)

  roentgenographic index of d. c. (see **caries, dental, radiographic index of**)

  secondary d. c. Decalcification of enamel beginning at the dentinoenamel junction and caused by a rapid lateral spreading of decay from an original carious lesion. (Oper. Dent.)

  senile d. c. (senile decay) Caries noted particularly in old age when supporting tissues have receded; occurs in cementum, usually on proximal surfaces of the teeth. (Oper. Dent.)

carious (ka′rē-ŭs) Pertaining to caries or decay. (Oper. Dent.)

  c. dentin (see **dentin, carious**)

carnauba wax (see **wax, carnauba**)

Carnoy's solution (see **solution, Carnoy's**)

carotene (kăr′ō-tēn) An orange pigment found in carrots, leafy vegetables, and other foods that may be converted to vitamin A in the body. (Oral Diag.)

carotenemia (kăr″ō-tĕ-nē′mē-ah) Excess carotene in the blood, producing a pigmentation of the skin and mucous membranes that resembles jaundice. (Oral Diag.)

carotid (ka-rot′ĭd) Either one of the two main right and left arteries of the neck. (Anesth.)

carrier A person harboring a specific infectious agent without clinical evidence of disease and who serves as a potential source or reservoir of infection for others. May be a healthy carrier or a convalescent carrier. (Oral Med.)

amalgam c. An instrument used to carry plastic amalgam to the prepared cavity or mold into which it is to be inserted. (Oper. Dent.)

foil c. (see **foil passer**)

cartilage A derivative of connective tissue arising from the mesenchyme. Typical hyaline cartilage is a flexible, rather elastic material with a semitransparent, glasslike appearance. Its ground substance, or matrix, is a complex protein (chondromucoid) through which there is distributed a large network of connective tissue fibers. There are cartilage cells distributed throughout the matrix that are rounded and that do not have the branching characteristics of bone cells. The cells are isolated in the matrix they have secreted and normally have no blood vessels. Therefore nutrients and metabolites are exchanged with the circulation by passage through the ground substance (matrix). (Oral Path.)

— A type of connective tissue found in many forms, e.g., external ear, ala of the nose, and articular surfaces of some bones. (Oral Physiol.)

— A form of connective tissue containing cellular elements (chondrocytes) embedded within lacunae, which appear as cavities within the cartilage matrix. Forms the basis of endochondral bone formation and serves to relate articular surfaces of bone. (Periodont.)

articular c. A thin layer of hyaline cartilage located on the joint surfaces of some bones. Not usually found on articular surfaces of temporomandibular joints, which are covered with an avascular fibrous tissue. (Oral Physiol.)

cricoid c. The lowest cartilage of the larynx. (Anesth.)

caruncle, submaxillary The orifice of the sublingual (Wharton's) duct that opens into the mouth on a small papilla on either side of the lingual frenum. (Comp. Prosth.)

carver (carving instrument) An instrument used to shape a plastic material such as wax or amalgam. (Oper. Dent.)

amalgam c. An instrument used to shape plastic amalgam. (Oper. Dent.)

carving Shaping and forming with instruments. (Oper. Dent.)

case Term often incorrectly used instead of the appropriate noun, e.g., patient, flask, denture, or casting. "Case" is not synonymous with "patient" because the latter is the human being affected with the disease. Correct usage would

be with reference to a specific instance of disease or injury, e.g., a case of typhoid fever. (Comp. Prosth.; Remov. Part. Prosth.)

c. charting Recording of pocket depth and topography, orientation of the lesions in relation to roots, delineation of gingival features, a description of zones of attached gingiva and alveolar mucosa, aberrant frenum and muscle attachments, depth and character of vestibular trough, occlusal factors, faulty tooth contact relations, nature and location of inflammatory changes, etc. (Periodont.)

c. dismissal The technique of illustrating to the patient what has been accomplished, usually done during the last appointment of a series. (Pract. Man.)

c. history (see **history, case**)

c. presentation Explanation to the patient of his dental needs. (Pract. Man.)

c. summary Enumeration of all the services to be performed for an estimated amount of money. (Pract. Man.)

cassette (kah-sĕt´) A light-tight container in which x-ray films are placed for exposure to x radiation; usually backed with lead to eliminate the effect of backscattered radiation. (Oral Radiol.)

cardboard c. (cardboard filmholder) A cardboard envelope, of simple construction, suitable for use in making radiographs on "direct exposure" or "no-screen" types of x-ray films. (Oral Radiol.)

screen-type c. A cassette usually made of metal, with exposure side of low atomic number material such as Bakelite, aluminum, or magnesium and containing intensifying screens between which a "screen type" of film or films may be placed for exposure to x radiation. (Oral Radiol.)

cast, *n.* An object formed or poured into a matrix or impression, e.g., metal or plaster. (Comp. Prosth.; Remov. Part. Prosth.)

— A positive reproduction of the form of the tissues of the upper or lower jaw made in an impression and over which denture bases or other dental restorations may be fabricated. (Comp. Prosth.; Remov. Part. Prosth.; Orthodont.)

— A plaster or stone replica of the shape of the dentition and adjoining tissues. Used as a diagnostic aid. (Periodont.)

c. bar splint (see **splint, cast bar**)

dental c. A positive likeness of a part or parts of the oral cavity. (Comp. Prosth.; Remov. Part. Prosth.)

diagnostic c. A positive likeness of dental

structures for the purpose of study and treatment planning. (Comp. Prosth.; Remov. Part. Prosth.)

— The properly related replica, in dental plaster or stone, of the teeth, adjacent tissues, and oral structures; possesses distinct topographic attributes which are guides to diagnosis and treatment. (Periodont.)

gnathostatic c. A cast of the teeth trimmed so that the occlusal plane is in its normal position in the mouth when the cast is set on a plane surface. Such casts are used in the gnathostatic technique of orthodontic diagnosis. (Oral Diag.)

implant c. A positive reproduction of the exposed bony surfaces made in a surgical bone impression and on which an implant frame is designed and fabricated. (Oral Implant.)

　　diagnostic i. c. A cast made from a conventional mucosal impression on which the wax trial denture and surgical impression trays are made or selected. (Oral Implant.)

investment c. (see **cast, refractory**)

c., keying of The process of so forming the base (or capital) of a cast that it can be remounted accurately to permit the adjustment of occlusal relations of supplied teeth that may have been moved by the volume changes that occur during the fabrication of the resin base. Also referred to as the split-cast method of returning a cast to an articulator. (Remov. Part. Prosth.)

master c. An accurate replica of the prepared tooth surfaces, residual ridge areas, and/or other parts of the dental arch reproduced from an impression from which a prosthesis is to be fabricated. (Comp. Prosth.; Fixed Part. Prosth.)

　　corrected m. c. A dental cast that has been modified by the correction of the edentulous ridge areas as registered in a supplemental, correctable impression. (Remov. Part. Prosth.)

occlusion c. A replica of the occlusal surfaces of a dental arch against which a prosthesis is to be fitted. (Remov. Part. Prosth.)

preextraction c. A cast made before the extraction of teeth. (see **cast, diagnostic**)

preoperative c. (see **cast, diagnostic**)

record c. A positive replica of the dentition and adjoining structures, used as a reference for conditions existing at a given time. (Orthodont.)

refractory c. A cast made of materials that will withstand high temperatures without disintegrating and that, when used in partial denture casting techniques, has expansion to compensate for metal shrinkage. (Comp. Prosth.; Remov. Part. Prosth.)

study c. (see **cast, diagnostic**)

working c. An accurate reproduction of a master cast; used in preliminary fitting of a casting to avoid injury to the master cast. (Remov. Part. Prosth.)

—, *v.* To throw metal into an impression to form the casting. (D. Mat.)

—, *v.* To produce a casting in a mold. (Oper. Dent.)

casting, *n.* A metallic object formed in a mold. (Comp. Prosth.; D. Mat.; Remov. Part. Prosth.)

　　vacuum c. The casting of a metal in the presence of a vacuum. (Comp. Prosth.; Remov. Part. Prosth.) (see also **casting machine, vacuum**)

—, *v.* Forming a casting in a mold. (Comp. Prosth.; D. Mat.; Remov. Part. Prosth.)

casting flask (see **flask, refractory**)

casting machine A mechanical device used for throwing or forcing a molten metal into a refractory mold. (Comp. Prosth.; D. Mat.; Oper. Dent.; Remov. Part. Prosth.)

　　air pressure c. m. A casting machine that forces metal into the mold by compressed air. (D. Mat.)

　　centrifugal c. m. A casting machine that forces the metal into the mold by centrifugal force. (Comp. Prosth.; D. Mat.; Oper. Dent.; Remov. Part. Prosth.)

　　pressure c. m. A casting machine in which the principal casting force is air pressure. (Oper. Dent.)

　　vacuum c. m. A casting machine in which the metal is cast by evacuation of gases from the mold. Atmospheric pressure actually forces metal into mold. (D. Mat.; Oper. Dent.)

casting model (see **cast, refractory**)

casting ring (see **flask, refractory**)

casting temperature (see **temperature, casting**)

casting wax (see **wax, casting**)

Castle's intrinsic factor (see **factor, Castle's intrinsic**)

catabolism (kah-tăb′ō-lĭzm) The destructive process (opposite of the anabolic-metabolic processes) by which complex substances are converted into more simple compounds. A proper relation between anabolism and catabolism is essential for the maintenance of bodily homeostasis and dynamic equilibrium. (Periodont.)

c. of energy Dissipation of energy in living tissues as work or heat (one phase of metabolism, the other being anabolism). (Oral Physiol.)

c. of substance Destructive metabolism; the conversion of living tissues into a lower state of organization and ultimately into waste products. (Oral Physiol.)

catalase reaction (kăt′ah-lās) The response of bubbling in the presence of hydrogen peroxide given by blood exudates or transudates. (Oral Implant.)

catalysis (kah-tăl′ĭ-sĭs) The increase in rate of a chemical reaction, induced by a substance called a catalyst, which itself takes no part in the reaction and remains unchanged. (Anesth.)

catalyst A substance that induces an increased rate of a chemical reaction without itself entering into the reaction or being changed by the reaction. (Oral Physiol.)

catamenia (kăt″ah-mē′nē-ah) Menstruation. Frequently used to designate age at onset of menses. (Oral Diag.)

catatonia (kăt″ah-tŏ′nē-ah) A form of schizophrenia characterized by alternating stupor and excitement. A patient's arms often retain any position in which they are placed. (Oral Med.)

catgut Sheep's intestine prepared as a suture and used for ligating vessels and closing soft tissue wounds. (Oral Surg.)

cathode A negative electrode from which electrons are emitted and to which positive ions will be attracted. In x-ray tubes, the cathode usually consists of a helical tungsten filament behind which a molybdenum reflector cup is located to focus the electron emission toward the target of the anode. (Oral Radiol.)

cation (kăt′ĭ-ahn) A positively charged ion. (Oral Radiol.)

cationic detergent (see **detergent, cationic**)

cat-scratch disease (see **fever, cat-scratch**)

causalgia (kaw-zăl′jē-ah) A postextraction localized pain phenomenon usually characterized by a continuous burning sensation. (Endodont.)

— A severe pain caused by injury to a large peripheral nerve. (Oral Diag.) (see also **neuralgia**)

cause A ground of action; a suit or action in court; any legal process by which one undertakes to obtain his claim. (D. Juris.)

proximate c. (see **proximate cause**)

caustic, *adj.* Destructive of living tissue by chemical burning action. (Oral Med.; Pharmacol.)

cavity A carious lesion or hole in a tooth. A com-

mon but incorrect term used for a prepared cavity. When used without a modifier, the term cavity is understood to be referring to a carious cavity unless the context indicates a prepared cavity. (Oper. Dent.)

access c. (see **access cavity**)

axial surface c. A cavity occurring in a tooth surface where the general plane is parallel to the long axis of the tooth. (Oper. Dent.)

c. classification Any method of separating, arranging, or considering cavities or lesions of the teeth in groups, each group of which possesses similar qualities or characteristics. Carious lesions are classified according to the surfaces of a tooth on which they occur (labial, buccal, occlusal, etc.); type of surface (pit and fissure, or smooth surface); and numerical grouping (G. V. Black's classification). (Oper. Dent.)

artificial c. c. (G. V. Black)

Class 1 Cavities beginning in structural defects of the teeth, as in pits and fissures.

Class 2 Cavities in proximal surfaces of bicuspids and molars.

Class 3 Cavities in proximal surfaces of cuspids and incisors that do not involve removal and restoration of the incisal angle.

Class 4 Cavities in proximal surfaces of cuspids and incisors that require removal and restoration of the incisal angle.

Class 5 Cavities in the gingival third (not pit cavities) of the labial, buccal, or lingual surfaces of the teeth.

Class 6 (not included in Black's classification) Cavities on incisal edges and cusp tips of the teeth. (Oper. Dent.)

complex c. A cavity that involves more than one surface of a tooth. (Oper. Dent.)

DO c. A cavity on the distal and occlusal surfaces of a tooth. (Oper. Dent.)

c. floor The base-enclosing side of a prepared cavity. (Oper. Dent.) (see also **cavity, prepared**)

gingival c. (gingival third c.) A cavity occurring in the gingival third of the clinical crown of the tooth (G. V. Black's Class 5). (Oper. Dent.)

c. lining Material applied to the prepared cavity to seal the dentinal tubules for protection of the pulp. (D. Mat.)

— A coating or insulating layer applied to the deep surface of a prepared cavity before the restoration is inserted. (Oper. Dent.)

c. medication Drug used to clean or treat a cavity prior to inserting a dressing, base, or restoration. (Oper. Dent.)

MO c. A cavity on the mesial and occlusal surfaces of a tooth. (Oper. Dent.)

MOD c. A cavity on the mesial, occlusal, and distal surfaces of a tooth. (Oper. Dent.)

nasal c. (nasal fossa) Two irregular spaces that are situated on either side of the midline of the face, extend from the cranial base to the roof of the mouth, and are separated from each other by a thin vertical septum. In radiographs the nasal cavity appears over the roots of the upper incisors as a large, structureless, radiolucent area. (Periodont.)

pit and fissure c. A cavity that begins in minute faults in the enamel caused by imperfect closure of the enamel. (Oper. Dent.)

c. preparation The orderly operating procedure required to establish in a tooth the biomechanically acceptable form necessary to receive and retain a restoration. A constant requirement is provision for prevention of failure of the restoration through recurrence of decay or inadequate resistance to applied stresses. (Oper. Dent.)

prepared c. The form developed in a tooth to receive and retain a restoration. (Oper. Dent.)

　floor of p. c. The flat bottom or enclosing base wall of a prepared cavity; on an axial plane it is called the axial wall, and on the horizontal plane it is called the pulpal wall. (Oper. Dent.)

　p. c., impression A negative likeness of a tapered type of prepared cavity. Made of one of the impression materials, e.g., wax, compound, hydrocolloid, Thiokol, or silicone rubber base material. A die or positive reproduction of the cavity is made from it, and the cast or ceramic restoration is constructed on it. (Oper. Dent.)

proximal c. A cavity occurring on the mesial or distal surface of a tooth. (Oper. Dent.)

pulp c. The space in a tooth bounded by the dentin; contains the dental pulp. The part of the pulp cavity within the coronal portion of the tooth is the pulp chamber, and the part found within the root is the pulp canal, or root canal. (Oper. Dent.)

self-cleansing ability of the oral c. The architectural and functional attributes of the various oral structures, including movements of the tongue, cheeks, and lips; flow of saliva; physiologic gingival form; proper tooth contacts; proper tooth form, etc. (Periodont.)

simple c. A cavity that involves only one surface of a tooth. (Oper. Dent.)

smooth surface c. A cavity formed by decay beginning in surfaces of teeth that are without pits, fissures, or enamel faults. (Oper. Dent.)

c. toilet G. V. Black's final step in cavity preparation. Consists of freeing all surfaces and angles of debris; often includes medication and insulation procedures. Term is rather objectionable due to general connotation; débridement is frequently suggested as more euphemistic. (Oper. Dent.)

c. varnish (see **varnish, cavity**)

c. wall (see **wall, cavity**)

cavosurface angle (see **angle, cavosurface**)

cavosurface bevel (see **bevel, cavosurface**)

cell(s) The basic unit of vital tissue. One of a large variety of microscopic protoplasmic masses that make up organized tissues. Each cell has a cell membrane, protoplasm, a nucleus, and a variety of inclusion bodies. Each type of cell is a living unit, with its own metabolic requirements, functions, permeability, ability to differentiate into other cells, reproducibility, life expectancy, etc. (Oral Physiol.)

bone c., function Specific function of each type of bone cell: osteoblast, formation of bone; osteocyte, maintenance of bone as a living tissue; and osteoclast, destruction or resorption of bone. (Oral Physiol.)

bone c., transformation Alteration of bone cell from one type to another. Because bone cells that have common ancestors are closely interrelated, frequent transformations occur from one to another of the morphologically different forms during the period of active growth. These transformations occur most frequently in developing bone but can be demonstrated in adult bone under certain conditions. The most striking examples of these alterations can be observed during the healing of fractures and in hyperthyroidism following the administration of the thyroid hormone. (Oral Physiol.)

c., carbohydrate The simplest nutritional complex in structure; generally present in the form of sugar and glycogen. Carbohydrates are found in the bloodstream but are not part of the vital structure of the blood cell. Rather, they are inert bodies stored in the tissue cells as glycogen, which is readily released when glucose unites with oxygen to provide energy, water, and carbon dioxide. (Oral Physiol.)

c., chemical composition In addition to 80% to 95% water content in the cell, also a variety of salt ions of inorganic salts in solution—notably potassium, phosphorus, calcium, and sulfur, and trace elements of the metals iron, copper, zinc, manganese, and cobalt. In addition to these ions, there are various simple compounds in solution that are in the process of becoming either part of the chemical structure of the cell or the end products of the metabolic processes. Most important are the organic compounds, which are responsible for vital cellular structure and activity. (Oral Physiol.)

connective tissue c. The fibroblast, which for purposes of clarity is characterized by such terms as perivascular connective tissue cell, or young connective tissue cell. (Oral Physiol.)

defense c. A cell, mobilized within inflamed, irritated, or otherwise diseased tissue, that acts as a protective element to neutralize or wall off the foreign irritant. Defense cells include plasma cells, polymorphonuclear leukocytes, and the cells of the reticuloendothelial system. (Periodont.)

c. differentiation The development of the cells into the various basic cell units of tissue: the epithelial cell and the nerve cell, which arise from the ectodermal tissue layer of the embryo; and the blood, muscle, bone, cartilage, and other connective tissue cells, which arise from the mesodermal tissue of the embryo. The mature tissue cell has many intermediary, transitional forms that are sequential in their development from the primitive, less differentiated anlage cell forms. These intermediary forms are evident clinically in disease in the blood dyscrasias, tumors, and inflammation, and in health in the normal processes of growth, development, healing, and repair. (Oral Physiol.)

endosteal c. A reticular cell that is modified and identified by its location; the endosteum is a condensation of the stroma of the bone marrow. (Oral Physiol.)

c., energy consumption The use of energy by the cells to maintain their integrity, to perform some purposeful activity, e.g., muscle contraction or nerve conduction, and to reproduce themselves. These activities depend on the transfer of energy from the environment to the organism for cell consumption

by mechanical, biophysical, and biochemical processes. (Oral Physiol.)

c., energy storage Accumulation of energy resources in the body. The most obvious energy resources of the body are glycogen stores in muscle tissue and fat compounds in the tissue spaces. These energy sources are held in a reservoir in the body in the form of potential energy. Other energy agents necessary for the production of energy may be in continuous and sometimes critical supply, e.g., oxygen. The basic supplies of energy are ultimately dependent on a continuous and consistently adequate nutritional intake. Nutritional intake is dependent in part on masticatory function. (Oral Physiol.)

c., energy transfer and release of energy The diverse phenomena for the transfer and release of energy, which deal with many biophysical principles, e.g., those relating to osmotic pressure, gas diffusion, membrane permeability, acid-base electrolyte balance, enzyme activity, the biochemical aspects of hemodynamics, and carbohydrate, fat, and protein metabolism. (Oral Physiol.)

Gaucher's c. A large (up to 40 μm in diameter) reticuloendothelial cell that is round to oval and contains a small, eccentrically located nucleus in the abundant, finely granular cytoplasm. (Oral Path.)

germ c. A cell of an organism whose function it is to reproduce an entity similar to the organism from which the germ cell originated. Germ cells are characteristically haploid. (Oral Radiol.)

giant c. A large cell frequently having several nuclei. (Oral Path.)

c. homeostasis (see **homeostasis, cell**)

Langerhans' c. Star-shaped cells of unknown function that appear to be permanent residents of the epithelium. (Periodont.)

c. membrane differentiation Specialization of cell membrane for the performance of various specific functions. The cell membrane is the surface at which cells carry on specific functions, at which stimuli are received, at which metabolites are interchanged between the extracellular and intracellular environment, and at which one cell relates to another. Cells have proximal surfaces and distal surfaces and are arranged with a polarity, if they are epithelial cells associated with a lumen where secretory or digestive function is performed. Some cells have brushed borders for greater surface, others have cilia, and still others (e.g., nerve endings) have special receptor or motor end organs at the membrane surface. The morphologic differentiation of portions of the cell membrane is associated with specialization of function. (Oral Physiol.)

c. membrane permeability The interchange of materials between the cell and its environment, regulated by the cell membrane at the cell surface. There is considerable controversy over how the passage of electrolyte substance through the membrane is achieved. Some speculations suggest that electrolytes go into chemical union with the membrane, pass through it, and are released within the cell; go into chemical solution in a lipoid component of the membrane and are thus transported; or, by bombardment against the cell membrane, pass through interstices in the membrane. It is possible that all three methods are in constant activity. (Oral Physiol.)

mesenchymal c. An embryonic connective tissue cell with an outstanding capacity for proliferation. Capable of further differentiation into reticular cells or osteoblasts. When persisting in the adult organism, the cells are usually arranged in loose connective tissue along the small blood vessels or in reticular fibers. They are identified by their location and their capacity to differentiate into other cell types, such as smooth muscle cells in the formation of new arteries, phagocytes in inflammatory processes, and bone cells in the formation of new bone tissue. (Oral Physiol.)

c. metabolism (see **metabolism, cell**)

c., method of examination Observation of both living specimens and fixed and stained preparations of tissue with the light microscope (as in classic cytology), ultraviolet and infrared microscopy, electron microscopy, x-ray diffraction, autoradiography, phase contrast, fluorescence, and polarization microscopy. (Oral Physiol.)

muscle c., development Increase in size of each muscle cell, resulting in an increase in muscle bulk during growth and development. The total number of muscle cells is fixed at birth and does not increase through the years. (Oral Physiol.)

plasma c. A cell of disputed origin (lymphatic vs. undifferentiated mesenchymal cell) that is seen in chronic inflammation and certain disease states and tumors but not normally in the circulating blood. The cell is larger than a lymphocyte and has an eccentric nucleus with basophilic nuclear chromatin peripherally located like figures on a clock face. Currently, the cells are believed to produce and carry antibodies. (Oral Path.) —A cell that contains eccentrically located nuclei, resembles a lymphocyte, and is derived from differentiation of the mesenchymal cells of the tissue. It is prevalent in inflamed tissues, and its presence is almost invariably construed as denoting the existence of inflammation and antibody formation. (Periodont.)

c. regeneration The process by which cells reproduce themselves. Regenerative processes vary among the kinds of tissues. Epithelial cells are able to regenerate by means of mitotic division, and they generally reproduce the appropriate cell forms. Hence, in the healing process they flatten out to cover large denuded areas before regenerative division takes place. This temporary modification is only an intermediary stage when protection of the underlying structure is the principal regenerative drive. Bone has a high degree of repair and regenerative capacity; muscle has only a moderate degree of regenerative function that is limited to cell membrane and is generally replaced by connective tissue. Nerve cells have the poorest regenerative capacity and when injured cause the most serious functional disorders because they serve a regulatory and integrative function. (Oral Physiol.)

reticular c. A cell of reticular connective tissue, such as in the stroma of the bone marrow, where it retains both osteogenic and hematopoietic potencies; it is identified by its location, morphology, potency, and direct origin from mesenchymal cells. (Oral Physiol.)

Sternberg-Reed c. A giant tumor cell believed to be derived from reticular cells; it contains from one to many nuclei and is seen in Hodgkin's disease. (Oral Path.)

Tzank c. A degenerated epithelial cell caused by acantholysis and found especially in pemphigus. (Oral Path.)

c., water content The major constituent of protoplasm, representing 80% to 95% of the cell content. In general, it is observed that the water content is greatest in cells in which chemical metabolism is high. Embryonic cells have a higher water content and a higher metabolism than do corresponding cells in the mature adult. (Oral Physiol.)

cellulitis (sĕl-ū-lī′tĭs) Inflammation in cellular tissue; term is commonly applied to suppurative inflammation of the loose areolar tissue of the cheeks and neck. (Oral Diag.)

— A diffuse inflammatory process that spreads along fascial planes and through tissue spaces without gross suppuration. (Oral Path.; Oral Surg.)

Celluloid strip (see **strip, plastic**)

cellulose, oxidized (sĕl′ū-lōs) Cellulose, in the form of cotton, gauze, or paper, that has been more or less completely oxidized by nitrogen dioxide to polyanhydroglucuronic acids. (Oral Surg.)

cement A material that produces a mechanical interlocking effect on hardening. (Comp. Prosth.; Orthodont.)

dental c. Any one of the materials used in dentistry as luting agents, bases, and temporary restorations. (D. Mat.) (see also **cement, dental, acrylic resin; cement, dental, zinc oxide–eugenol; cement, silicate; cement, zinc phosphate**)

— Material used as a luting agent, a thermal insulation in cavity preparation, temporary restorations, or pulp capping. Usually supplied as a powder of varied color and as a liquid; its composition varies with the type and purpose. Ingredients are mixed to the degree of consistency desired. (Oper. Dent.)

— One of a variety of compounds used in dentistry in semifluid form to seal and retain a restoration in a fixed position within or on a tooth or on or about the face. (Remov. Part. Prosth.)

acrylic resin d. c. A dental cement, dispensed as a powder and a liquid, that is mixed as any other cement. The powder contains polymethyl methacrylate, a filler, a plasticizer, and a polymerization initiator. The liquid monomer is methyl methacrylate, with an inhibitor and an activator. (Oper. Dent.)

d. c. base An insulating layer of cement placed in the deeper portion of a prepared cavity to insulate the pulp. (Oper. Dent.)

copper d. c. Basically a zinc phosphate cement, with either cuprous oxide (Cu_2O) or cupric oxide (CuO) as an additive. (D. Mat.)

— A zinc phosphate cement to the powder of which has been added a copper oxide. (Oper. Dent.)

germicidal d. c. Usually a zinc phosphate cement to which has been added copper

or silver salts to render it bactericidal. (Oper. Dent.)

Kryptex d. c. (see **cement, silicophosphate**)

silicious d. c. (see **cement, silicate**)

zinc oxide–eugenol d. c. Least irritating of the cements. The powder is essentially zinc oxide with strengtheners and accelerators. The liquid is basically eugenol. It is used as a sedative cement base, a temporary luting medium, and an interim temporary restoration. (Oper. Dent.)

c. dressing Postoperative dressing applied after periodontal surgery and consisting of an admixture of zinc oxide, rosin, zinc stearate, tannic acid powder, asbestos fibers, mineral oil, eugenol, etc. Possesses analgesic hemostatic, and protective qualities. (Periodont.)

c. d., Kirkland (see **dressing, Kirkland cement**)

c. line (see **line, cement**)

polycarboxylate c. Dental cement used for cementation of cast restorations and orthodontic appliances, and as bases. Prepared by mixing a zinc oxide powder with a liquid of polycarboxylic acid. (D. Mat.)

sealer c. A compound used in filling a root canal; it is inserted in a plastic condition, solidifies after placement, and fills any irregularities in the surface of the canal. A solid cone of silver or gutta-percha is normally used with the sealer cement. (Endodont.)

silicate c. A relatively hard, translucent, restorative material used primarily in anterior teeth. It resembles dental porcelain in appearance and is sometimes referred to as synthetic porcelain. Prepared by mixing a liquid and a powder. The powder is an acid-soluble glass prepared by the fusion of CaO, SiO, Al_2O_3, and other ingredients with a fluoride flux. The liquid is a buffered phosphoric acid solution. (D. Mat.; Oper. Dent.)

silicophosphate c. (Kryptex c.) A combination zinc phosphate and silicate cement. Less translucent, less irritating, and less soluble than silicate and stronger than zinc phosphate cement. Sometimes used as a luting agent or as a temporary resoration in posterior teeth. (D. Mat.; Oper. Dent.)

zinc phosphate c. A material used for cementation of inlays, crowns, bridges, and orthodontic appliances; occasionally used as a temporary restoration. Prepared by mixing a powder and a liquid. The powders are composed primarily of zinc oxide and magnesium oxides. The principal constituents of the liquid are phosphoric acid, water, and buffer agents. (D. Mat.; Oper. Dent.)

cemental line (see **line, cemental**)

cemental repair (see **repair, cemental**)

cemental spicule (spĭk'ūl) (see **spicule, cemental**)

cemental spike (see **spicule, cemental**)

cemental tear A small portion of cementum forcibly separated, either partially or completely, from the underlying dentin of the root as a result of occlusal force; seen on the tension side in occlusal traumatism. (Periodont.)

cementation (sē-mĕn-tā'shŭn) Attachment of a restoration to natural teeth or attachment of parts by means of a cement. (Comp. Prosth.; Oper. Dent.)

— The process by which the band or bands are attached to the teeth by means of an adhesive material. (Orthodont.)

cementicle (sē-mĕn'tĭ-cul) A calcified body sometimes found in the periodontal ligament of older individuals. It is presumed that degenerated epithelial cells form the nidus for this calcification. (Oral Path.)

cementifying fibroma (see **fibroma, cementifying**)

cementing line (see **line, cemental**)

cementoblast (sē-mĕn'tō-blăst) The cell that forms the organic matrix of cementum. Derived from the inner aspect of the dental sac during the initial formation of cementum or from the mesenchymal cell of the periodontal membrane after completion of primary cementogenesis. The cementoblast, trapped within cellular cementum, becomes a cementocyte. (Periodont.)

cementoclasia (sē-mĕn"tō-klā'zē-ah) Destruction of cementum by cementoclasts. (Orthodont.)

cementocyte (sē-mĕn'tō-sīt) The cell, found within lacunae of cellular cementum, that possesses protoplasmic processes which course through the canaliculi of the cementum; derived from cementoblasts trapped within newly formed cementum. (Periodont.)

cementoenamel junction (see **junction, cementoenamel**)

cementoid The most recent layer covering the surface of cementum that is uncalcified. (Periodont.)

cementoma (sē-mĕn-tō'mah) (**traumatic osteoclasia**) A neoplasm formed of cementum. Although cementum, by definition, is attached to the tooth, the term cementoma is commonly applied to calcified, radiopaque peri-

apical masses (second stage) and to the noncalcified, radiolucent, periapical lesions (first stage) that precede them. (Oral Diag.)

— An odontogenic tumor associated with the apices of teeth. It may be present as a mass of fibrous connective tissue, as fibrous connective tissue with spicules of cementum, or as a calcified mass resembling cementum and having few cellular elements. (Oral Path.)

first-state c. (see **fibroma, periapical**)

cementopathia (sē"mĕn-tō-păth'ē-ah) The concept wherein necrotic, diseased cementum and lack of productivity of cementum are implicated in the causation of periodontitis and periodontosis. (Periodont.)

cementoproximal Pertaining to the proximal surface apical to the cementoenamel junction of the clinical crown of a tooth. (Oper. Dent.)

cementum (sē-mĕn'tŭm) A specialized, calcified connective tissue that covers the anatomic root of a tooth. (Oper. Dent.)

— The hard, calcified substance formed by the cementoblasts. It is arranged in lamellar form and covers the root dentin. Fibrillar, noncellular cementum covers the cervical portion of the root, with the cellular cementum covering primarily the apical one third of the root surface. May be primary, deposited by cementoblasts derived from the embryonal dental sac, or secondary, formed by cementoblasts derived from mesenchymal cells of the periodontal membrane. (Periodont.)

acellular c. The calcified bonelike structure formed by the cementoblasts. Principally covers the cervical portion of the tooth root but occasionally extends over almost all of the root except the apical portion. It contains embedded ends of collagen fibers of the gingival corium and periodontal membrane, but no cementocytes. (Periodont.)

attachment of calculus to c. A phenomenon in which cementum adheres to areas of cemental resorption and/or cemental irregularity. Calculus may invade spaces formerly occupied by periodontal fibers; processes of filamentous organisms of dental calculus may extend into the cemental surface; or the organic matrix of the calculus may attach itself to the secondary cuticle. (Periodont.)

cellular c. Portion of the calcified substance covering the root surfaces of the teeth. It is bonelike in nature and contains cementocytes embedded within lacunae, with protoplasmic processes of the cementocytes coursing through canaliculi that anastomose with canaliculi of adjacent lacunae. The lacunae are dispersed through a calcified matrix arranged in lamellar form. Cellular cementum is localized primarily at the apical portion of the root but may deposit over the acellular cementum or may serve to repair areas of cemental resorption. (Periodont.)

collagen fibrils of c. Fibrils that penetrate the cementum surface and are continuous with the periodontal fibers necessary for tooth support. (Periodont.)

lamellar c. Cementum in which layers of appositional cementum are arranged in a sheaflike pattern, the layers of cementum being more or less parallel to the cemental surface and demarcated by incremental lines that represent periods of inactivity of cementum formation. (Periodont.)

necrotic c. Nonvital cementum that is situated coronal to the bottom of the periodontal pocket. (Periodont.)

secondary c. Term used to imply all subsequent layers of cementum formed after the primary layer. It may be either cellular or acellular. (Periodont.)

center, rotation A point or line around which all other points in a body move. (Comp. Prosth.; Remov. Part. Prosth.)

central bearing Application of forces between the maxillae and mandible at a single point that is located as near as possible to the center of the supporting areas of the upper and lower jaws. The purpose is to distribute closing forces of the jaws evenly throughout the areas of the supporting structures during the registration and recording of maxillomandibular (jaw) relations and during the correction of occlusal errors. (Comp. Prosth.; Fixed Part. Prosth.)

c.-b. device A device that provides a central point of bearing or support between upper and lower occlusion rims. It consists of a contacting point that is attached to one occlusion rim and a plate that provides the surface on which the bearing point rests or moves. (Comp. Prosth.; Remov. Part. Prosth.)

c.-b. tracing d. A central-bearing device that is used for making a tracing and/or for support between occlusion rims. (Comp. Prosth.; Fixed Part. Prosth.)

c.-b. point (see **point, central-bearing**)

central occlusion (see **occlusion, centric**)

centric (sĕn'trĭk) (objectionable as a noun) An adjective that should be used in conjunction with a noun. (Comp. Prosth.) (see **position, centric; relation, centric; occlusion, centric; occlusion, centric relation**)

c. checkbite (see **record, interocclusal, centric; record, maxillomandibular, centric**)

c. occlusion (see **occlusion, centric**)

c. position (see **position, centric**)

c. relation (see **relation, centric**)

centrifugal force (sĕn-trĭf-ū-găl) (see **force, centrifugal**)

cephalogram (sĕf'ah-lō-grăm) A cephalometric radiograph. On tracings of these films anatomic points, planes, and angles are drawn that assist in the evaluation of the patient's facial growth and development. (Oral Surg.)

cephalometer (sĕf"ah-lom'ĕ-ter) A head holder used in obtaining a cephalometric radiograph; a precision instrument that makes it possible to accurately reposition the patient's head for serial radiographs. (Oral Diag.; Oral Radiol.; Orthodont.)

radiographic c. An apparatus for making orthodiagraphic radiographs of both the profile and frontal views of the face and cranium. (Orthodont.)

cephalometric analysis (see **analysis, cephalometric**)

cephalometric landmark (see **landmark, cephalometric**)

cephalometric skeletal analysis Assessment of the facial type of skeleton; the relationship of the parts to each other, to the skull, and to an estimated "normal." (Oral Surg.)

cephalometrics (sĕf-ah-lō-mĕt'rĭks) Scientific study of the measurements of the head. (Orthodont.)

radiographic c. Study of the radiographic measurements of the head. (Orthodont.)

cephalometry (sĕf-ah-lom'ĕ-trē) Measurement of the bony structure of the head using reproducible lateral and anteroposterior radiograms. (Oral Diag.)

cephalophore (sĕf'ah-lō-for) A cephalostat designed to take in-sequence-oriented facial photographs and gnathostatic models (B. Fischer). (Orthodont.)

cephalostat (sĕf'ah-lō-stăt) An orienting device for positioning a patient's head in a standardized manner for measurement purposes. (Orthodont.) (see also **cephalometer**)

— A head-positioning device that assures reproducibility of the relations between an x-ray beam, a patient's head, and an x-ray film in radiography. (Oral Radiol.)

ceramics The art of making dental restorations,

or parts of restorations, from fused porcelain. (Fixed Part. Prosth.)

orthoclase c. (see **feldspar**)

cerebellum (sĕr-ĕ-bĕl′ŭm) The lower (back) brain between the pons and medulla oblongata and below the posterior portion of the cerebrum. (Anesth.)

— A major division of the brain behind the cerebrum and above the pons and fourth ventricle, consisting of a median lobe, two lateral lobes, and major connections, through pairs of peduncles, to the cerebrum, the pons, and the medulla oblongata. The cerebellum is intimately connected with the auditory vestibular apparatus and the proprioceptive system of the body and hence is involved in maintenance of body equilibrium, orientation in space, and muscular coordination and tonus. (Oral Physiol.)

cerebral palsy (see **palsy, cerebral**)

cerebrum (sĕr′ĕ-brŭm) The largest part of the brain, consisting of two hemispheres, where sensory stimuli are received and where motor impulses originate. (Anesth.)

— The largest portion of the brain. Operating at the highest functional level and occupying the upper part of the cranium, the cerebrum consists of two hemispheres united at the bottom by commissures of large bundles of nerve fibers. As with all parts of the nervous system, each part of the cerebrum has highly specific functions (e.g., a specific outer cortical area controls voluntary chewing, whereas certain inner subcortical areas are involved in involuntary jaw posture). (Oral Physiol.)

certified dental assistant A person who has completed the educational, experience, and testing requirements of the Certification Board of the American Dental Assistant Association. Since 1966 the requirements have been changed to include education in training programs accredited by the Council on Dental Education of the American Dental Association. (Pract. Man.)

cervical (ser′vĭ-kal) Relating to the neck, or cervical line, of a tooth. (Oper. Dent.)

c. convergence (see **convergence, cervical**)

c. line (see **junction, cementoenamel**)

chalazion forceps (kah-lā′zē-ahn) (see **forceps, chalazion**)

chamber An enclosed area

  ionization c. An instrument for measuring the quantity of ionizing radiation, in terms of the charge of electricity associated with ions produced within a defined volume of air. (Oral Radiol.)

  air-equivalent i. c. A chamber in which the materials of the wall and electrodes produce ionization essentially similar to that in a free-air ionization chamber. (Oral Radiol.)

  air-wall i. c. An ionization chamber with walls of material of low atomic number, having the same effective atomic number as atmospheric air. (Oral Radiol.)

  extrapolation i. c. An ionization chamber with electrodes whose spacing can be adjusted and accurately determined to permit extrapolation of its reading to zero chamber volume. (Oral Radiol.)

  free-air i. c. An ionization chamber in which a delimited beam of radiation passes between the electrodes without striking them or other internal parts of the equipment. The electric field is maintained perpendicular to the electrodes in the collecting region; as a result the ionized volume can be accurately determined from the dimensions of the collecting electrode and the limiting diaphragm. This is the basic standard instrument for dosimetry within the range of 5 to 400 kv. (Oral Radiol.)

  monitor i. c. An ionization chamber used for checking the constancy of performance of the roentgen-ray apparatus. (Oral Radiol.)

  pocket i. c. A small, pocket-sized ionization chamber used for monitoring radiation exposure of personnel. Before use it is given a charge, and the amount of discharge is a measure of the quantity of radiation received. (Oral Radiol.)

  standard i. c. (see **chamber, ionization, free-air**)

  thimble i. c. A small cylindrical or spherical chamber, usually with walls of organic material. (Oral Radiol.)

  thin-wall i. c. An ionization chamber having walls so thin that nearly all secondary corpuscular rays reaching them from external materials can penetrate them easily. (Oral Radiol.)

  tissue-equivalent i. c. A chamber in which the walls, electrodes, and gas are so selected as to produce ionization essentially equivalent to the characteristics of the tissue under consideration. (Oral Radiol.)

pulp c. (pulp cavity) The space located in the coronal portion of the tooth and occupied by the pulp. (Endodont.)

relief c. A recess in the impression surface of

a denture, created to reduce or eliminate pressure from the corresponding area of the mouth. (Comp. Prosth.; Remov. Part. Prosth.)

suction c. (see **chamber, relief**)

chamfer (shăm′fer) A marginal finish either curved or formed by a plane at an obtuse angle to the external surface of a prepared tooth. (Fixed Part. Prosth.)

— In extracoronal cavity preparations, a marginal finish that produces a curve from an axial wall to the cavosurface. (Oper. Dent.)

chancre (shăng′ker) (**autochthonous ulcer**) The primary lesion of syphilis, located at the site of entrance of the spirochete into the body, that occurs about three weeks after contact; begins as a papule and develops into a clean-based shallow ulcer. Secondary infection may produce suppuration. Has the appearance of a buttonlike mass because of the contiguous induration and rolled border. Weeping characteristics are also present. (Oral Diag.; Oral Med.; Oral Path.; Periodont.)

c. of lip The primary lesion of syphilis that often presents as an ulcerated or crusted, indurated lesion with a brownish or copper-colored weeping base when locating on the lip. The lesion is teeming with *Treponema pallidum*. (Periodont.)

soft c. (see **chancroid**)

chancroid (shăng′kroid) (**soft chancre**) A venereal disease caused by *Haemophilus ducreyi*. It is characterized by a soft chancre that is a necrotic draining ulcer similar to a chancre but without characteristic induration. A regional bubo may occur. (Oral Med.)

channel A hole drilled into dentin or metal for the purpose of receiving a pin. (Oper Dent.)

vascular c. A blood or lymph vessel through which inflammatory infiltrate and periodontitis can proceed from a localized superficial area to involve the deeper structures of the periodontium. (Periodont.)

characteristics, sex Primary: those organs concerned with reproduction, such as the gonads and genitalia. Secondary: differences in voice range and timbre, muscularity, and distribution of hair and adipose tissue. (Oral Med.)

Charcot's joint (see **joint, Charcot's**)

Charles' law (see **law, Charles'**)

chart A sheet of paper, pasteboard, etc. that presents a graphic representation of a condition or state.

Bonwill-Hawley c. (see **chart, Hawley**)

dental c. A diagrammatic chart of the teeth on which the findings from the clinical and radiographic examinations are recorded. (Pract. Man.)

Hawley c. (**Bonwill-Hawley c.**) Graded outlines of dental arch sizes based on the mesiodistal diameters of the six anterior teeth. (Orthodont.)

health c. A series of questions designed to reveal important data concerning the patient's general health. (Pract. Man.)

history c. Forms and records for obtaining a thorough medical and oral history combined with a complete record of findings that enables one to gather and have on hand the necessary records to render total patient care. (Periodont.)

tooth c. Diagrammatic representation of the teeth, showing all surfaces and usually the roots, on which the dentist indicates restorations present, decayed surfaces, and sometimes periodontal conditions. (Pract. Man.)

Charters' method (see **method, Charters'**)

charting Tabulation of the progress of a disease; the compilation of a clinical record. (Anesth.)

Chayes' attachment (shāz) Thought to be the first internal precision attachment. (Remov. Part. Prosth.) (see also **attachment, intracoronal**)

Cheadle's disease (chē′dĕlz) (see **scurvy, infantile**)

checkbite (see **record, interocclusal**)

centric c. (see **record, interocclusal, centric; record, maxillomandibular, centric**)

eccentric c. (see **record, interocclusal, eccentric**)

lateral c. (see **record, interocclusal**)

protrusive c. (see **record, interocclusal, protrusive**)

cheek biting A circumstance in which the individual cheek tissues are interposed between the teeth of the upper and lower dentitions. Occurs because of such factors as habit, the medial collapse of the tissues of the cheek, or tooth loss. Often results in hyperkeratotic lesions and irritations of the buccal mucosa, as well as abnormal stress on the teeth. (Periodont.)

cheilion (kī′lē-ahn) The corner of the mouth. (Orthodont.)

cheilitis (kī-lī′tĭs) (**perlèche**) Inflammation of the lip. (Oral Diag.; Oral Path.)

actinic c. (**solar cheilitis**) A condition of the lips characterized by swelling and a white, leathery covering with red areas of erosion; the lower lip is affected more than the upper. Usually found in persons who spend much time outdoors or in those with sensitive skin. (Oral Diag.)

— Crusting, desquamation, ulceration, atrophy, and inflammation of the lips, more especially the lower lip, due to chronic exposure to the elements and actinic rays of sunlight. (Oral Med.)

cigarette paper c. Focal areas of inflammation of the lips caused by cigarette paper sticking to the surface and subsequent traumatic injury produced by efforts to remove it. (Oral Diag.)

c. glandularis apostematosa A chronic disease of the lips characterized by sticky, mucoid exudation from the labial glands. (Oral Diag.)

— Chronic diffuse nodular enlargement of the lower lip associated with purulent inflammatory hyperplasia of the mucous glands and ducts. Rare, unknown etiology. (Oral Med.)

solar c. (see **cheilitis, actinic**)

cheiloplasty (kī'lō-plăs"tē) Corrective surgery or restoration of the lips. (Oral Surg.)

cheilorraphy (kī-lor'ah-fē) Surgical repair of a congenital cleft lip. (Oral Surg.)

cheiloschisis (kī-los'kĭ-sĭs) (see **harelip**)

cheilosis (kī-lō'sĭs) A noninflammatory condition of the lip usually characterized by chapping and fissuring. (Oral Diag.)

— Eroded fissuring at the corners of the oral orifice, resulting from vitamin B complex deficiency, decreased vertical dimension, drooling at the corners of the mouth orifice, and/or monilial infection. (Periodont.)

angular c. Transverse fissuring at the angles of the mouth attributable to deficiencies of the B complex group of vitamins, loss of the vertical dimension, drooling of saliva, and superimposed monilial infection. (Periodont.)

cheilotomy (kī-lot'ō-mē) Incision into, or excision of, a part of the lip. (Oral Surg.)

chelation (kē-lā'shŭn) Chemical reaction of a metallic ion (e.g., calcium ion) with a suitable reactive compound (e.g., ethylenediamine tetraacetic acid) to form a compound in which the metal ion is tightly bound. (Oral Med.; Pharmacol.)

chemamnesia (kĕm-ăm-nē'zē-ah) Reversible amnesia produced by a chemical or drug. (Anesth.)

chemoreceptor (kē"mō-rē-sĕp'tor) A receptor adapted for excitation by chemical substances. Carotid body or aortic (supracardiac) bodies. (Anesth.)

— A specialized sensory end organ adapted for excitation by chemical substances (e.g., olfactory and gustatory receptors) or specialized sense organs of the carotid body that are sensitive to chemical changes in the bloodstream. (Oral Physiol.)

chemotherapeutic agent (see **agent, chemotherapeutic**)

cherubism (chĕr'ū-bĭzm) **(familial intraosseous swelling)** A fibro-osseous disease of the jaws of genetic nature. The swollen jaws and raised eyes give a cherubic appearance; multiple radiolucencies are evident on radiographic examination. (Oral Diag.)

— A familial form of fibrous dysplasia that is characterized by unilateral or, more often, bilateral swelling of the jaws in children. (Oral Path.) (see also **dysplasia, fibrous**)

chew-in technique The method by which the dentist records a patient's occlusal paths in the wax patterns to be used in making restorations. In making the grooves and ridges in the wax patterns directly, the dentist asks the patient to make right-and-left and fore-and-aft sliding occlusal strokes to generate the paths of the opposite prominences. The patient morphogenerates his occlusion by nonchewing but by wearing mandibular strokes. The most elaborate chew-in technique follows a procedure of creating bispherical occlusion; that is, the occlusion for the left teeth is on one sphere, and the occlusion for the right teeth is on another sphere. The restorations are made first for the lower arch rather arbitrarily by making the cusps suit the spheres and having the direction of the ridges and the grooves determined by artistic judgment rather than by dictates from condylar data. After the lower restorations are put in the teeth, the upper incisors are restored to become the front guiders of the lateral and the protrusive sliding movements. As soon as the anterior teeth are fit in form and health, the upper postcanine teeth are prepared and filled with inlay wax and the patient is asked to pattern the grooves and the ridges by the sliding movements. From these wax data the patterns are finished by hand, invested, cast, and refined, and then put on the upper teeth, tested, and equilibrated in the mouth. (Gnathol.) (see also **path, occlusal, registration**)

chewing The movements of the mandible during mastication; controlled by neuromuscular action and limited by the anatomic structure of the temporomandibular joints. (Periodont.)

c. cycle (see **cycle, chewing**)

c. force (see **force, chewing**)

Cheyne-Stokes reflex (see **respiration, Cheyne-Stokes**)

Cheyne-Stokes respiration (see **respiration, Cheyne-Stokes**)

chickenpox (see **varicella**)

child In the law of negligence and in the laws for the protection of children, a term used as the opposite of adult (generally under the age of puberty), without reference to parentage and distinction of sex. (D. Juris.)

chin cup (see **cup, chin**)

chip blower (see **syringe, air, hand**)

chisel An instrument modeled after the carpenter's chisel; intended for cutting or cleaving enamel. The cutting edge is beveled on one side only; the shank may be straight or angled. (Oper. Dent.)

  contra-angle c. (posterior c.) A chisel-shaped, binangled, paired cutting instrument whose blade meets the shank at an angle greater than 12°; single beveled; said to be reverse beveled when the bevel is on the mesial side of the blade. (Oper Dent.)

  periodontal c. The simplest form of scaler; used with a push stroke for scaling or splitting of calculus, especially on mandibular anterior teeth. (Periodont.)

  posterior c. (see **chisel, contra-angle**)

  Wedelstaedt c. A chisel with a blade that is continuous with the shank; has no constricting neck; curves rather than angles into the shank; is available in varying widths; and has a regular or a contra-angle bevel. (Oper. Dent.)

chloramine solution (see **solution**)

chloride shift (klō'rīd) (see **phenomenon, Hamburger's**)

chloroformism (klō'ro-form″izm) The habitual use of chloroform for its narcotic effect; the anesthetic effect of vapor of chloroform. (Anesth.)

chloroformization (klō″rō-form″ĭ-zā'shŭn) The administration of chloroform. (Anesth.)

chloropercha (klor″ō-per'chah) A solution obtained by mixing various amounts of chloroform with gutta-percha. (Endodont.)

  c. method (see **method, chloropercha**)

chlorophyllin (klor″ō-fĭl'ĭn) Any of a number of products resulting from the reaction of certain decomposition products of chlorophyll with copper and/or other metallic ions. (Oral Med.; Pharmacol.)

chlortetracycline (klor″tĕt-rah-sī'klēn) **(Aureomycin)** A broad-spectrum antibiotic possessing bacteriostatic properties of some value in the treatment of disease produced by large viruses (the psittacosis and lymphogranuloma inguinale groups). (Periodont.)

choice of path of placement (see **placement, choice of path of**)

cholagogue (kō'lah-gahg) A drug that stimulates emptying of the gallbladder and flow of bile. (Oral Med.; Pharmacol.)

choleretic (kō″ler-ĕt'ĭk) A drug that stimulates production of bile by the liver. (Oral Med.; Pharmacol.)

cholesterol (kō-lĕs'ter-ol) A fatlike substance found in arterial atheromas, gallstones, cysts, etc. Normally, 140 to 220 mg. are present in 100 ml. of blood. (Oral Diag.)

cholinergic (kō-lĭn-er'jĭk) **(parasympathomimetic)** Producing or simulating the effects of acetylcholine. (Oral Med.; Pharmacol.)

  c. blocking agent (see **agent, blocking, cholinergic**)

cholinesterase (kō-lĭn-ĕs'ter-ās) An esterase that hydrolyzes acetylcholine. It is an enzyme that is widely distributed throughout the muscles, glands, and nerves of the body and that converts the acetylcholine into choline and acetic acid. (Oral Physiol.)

cholinolytic (kō″lĭn-ō-lĭt'ĭk) (see **anticholinergic**)

chondrodystrophia fetalis (kŏn″drō-dĭs-trō'fē-ah fē-tăl'ĭs) (see **achondroplasia**)

chondroectodermal dysplasia (kŏn″drō-ĕk-tō-dĕrm'al dĭs-plā'zē-ah) **(Ellis–van Creveld syndrome)** A syndrome characterized by the following tetrad: (1) bilateral polydactyly, (2) chondrodysplasia of the long bones, resulting in acromelic dwarfism, (3) anomaly of the teeth, nails, hair, and maxillary and mandibular region anteriorly, and (4) heart malformation. (Cleft Palate; Oral Med.)

chondroma (kahn-drō'mah) A benign neoplasm composed of cartilage-like tissue. (Oral Diag.)

— A benign tumor of cartilage. However, many chondrosarcomas arise in preexisting chondromas. (Oral Path.)

chondromyxosarcoma (kahn″drō-mĭk″sō-sar-kō'mah) Chondrosarcoma that exhibits an appreciable amount of myxomatous degeneration. (Oral Path.) (see also **chondrosarcoma**)

chondrosarcoma (kahn″drō-sar-kō'mah) A malignant neoplasm composed of cartilage-like tissue. (Oral Diag.; Oral Path.)

chorea (kō-rē'ah) **(St. Vitus' dance)** A disorder of the central nervous system resulting in purposeless, involuntary athetoid (writhing) movements of the muscles of the face and extremities. It may be associated with or follow rheumatic fever (Sydenham's chorea), hysteria, senility, or infections, or it may be a hereditary disorder (Huntington's chorea). (Oral Med.)

Christian's disease (see **disease, Hand-Schüller-Christian**)

Christmas disease (see **hemophilia B**)

chromosome (krō′mō-sōm) One of a number of small, dark-staining, and more or less rod-shaped bodies situated in the nucleus of a cell. At the time of cell division chromosomes divide and distribute equally to the daughter cells. They contain genes arranged along their length. The number of chromosomes in the somatic cells of an individual is constant (diploid number), whereas just half this number (haploid number) appears in germ cells; the number of chromosomes or diploid numbers, etc. within a species is usually constant. (Oral Radiol.)

  aberration c. Any rearrangement of chromosome parts as a result of breakage and reunion of broken ends. (Oral Radiol.)

chronic Characterized by a long, slow course as opposed to acute. (Oral Diag.)

cicatrix (sĭk′ah-trĭks, sĭ-kā′trĭks) (**scar**) The result of healing by second intention; characterized microscopically by excessive collagenation of the granulation tissue. (Oral Path.)

— The end product of repair of a wound, usually dense fibrous connective tissue; a scar. (Oral Surg.)

cicatrization (sĭk″ah-trĭ-zā′shŭn) Conversion of granulation tissue into scar tissue. (Oral Surg.)

Cieszynski's rule of isometry (see **rule of isometry, Cieszynski's**)

cineradiography (sĭn″ĕ-rā-dē-og′rah-fē) The making of motion pictures by means of roentgen rays and image intensification. Studies are used for diagnosis and research purposes. Speech patterns can be studied during the process of phonation; the action of the tongue, jaws, and palate can be studied during mastication and deglutition. (Cleft Palate; Comp. Prosth.)

cingulum (sĭng′gū-lŭm) The portion of incisor teeth and cuspids, occurring on the lingual or palatal aspects, that forms a convex protuberance at the cervical one third of the anatomic crown. Represents the lingual or palatal developmental lobe of these teeth. (Oper. Dent.; Periodont.)

  c. modification Alteration of the lingual form of an anterior tooth to provide a definite seat for the support of a rest unit of a removable partial denture. (Remov. Part. Prosth.)

circulation Movement of blood through blood vessels.

  coronary c. Circulation of blood within heart muscle.

  disturbance of c. Disorders and traumatic occurrences associated with alteration in either structure or function of the blood or the vascular system. (Oral Physiol.)

  peripheral c. The passage of fluids, electrolytes, and metabolites through the walls of terminal vessels of the vascular tree into and out of the tissue spaces. (Oral Physiol.)

  pulmonary c. Circulation of venous blood from right ventricle of the heart, to the lungs, and back to left atrium of the heart.

  systemic c. Circulation of oxygenated blood from left ventricle of the heart to the various tissues of body, and of venous blood back to right atrium of the heart. (Oral Physiol.)

circulatory system System for circulation of blood, consisting of heart, arteries, arterioles, capillaries, venules, and veins. (Oral Physiol.)

circumferential wiring (see **wiring, circumferential**)

citrin (sĭt′rĭn) (see **factor, platelet 1**)

civil action In civil law, a personal action to compel payment or the doing of some other thing that is civil (differentiated from criminal action). (D. Juris.)

civil law A statutory law as opposed to common law, or judge-made law. The dental practice act is a civil law. (D. Juris.)

claim In a juridical sense, a demand of some type made by one person on another; a challenge made by a person concerning the ownership of a thing (or money). (D. Juris.)

clamp A device used to effect compression.

  cervical c. (see **clamp, gingival**)

  gingival c. (**cervical c.**) A clamp intended to retract gingival tissues. (Oper. Dent.)

    Ferrier 212 g. c. A purposely unbalanced gingival clamp for retracting gingival tissue from the field of operation. It must be stabilized to position with modeling compound. Developed by W. I. Ferrier. (Oper. Dent.)

    Hatch g. c. An adjustable gingival clamp. (Oper. Dent.)

  molar c. (see **band, orthodontic clamp**)

  rubber dam c. A device made of spring metal and used to hold a rubber dam so that it will not slip off the tooth. (Endodont.)

— An instrument used to aid in holding a rubber dam in place or to improve the operating field under a rubber dam. (Oper. Dent.)

cotton roll r. d. c. A rubber dam type of clamp with a buccal and lingual wing or flange to hold cotton rolls in position in the mouth. (Oper. Dent.)

root r. d. c. A clamp whose jaws are designed to fit on the root surfaces of a tooth; usually used for the retention of a rubber dam. (Oper. Dent.)

Clarke-Fournier glossitis (foor-nē-ā′) (see **glossitis, interstitial sclerous**)

Clark's rule (see **rule, Clark's**)

clasp A metal attachment of a removable appliance that is adapted about a tooth or in the embrasures of teeth. (Orthodont.)

— The portion of a removable partial prosthesis that rests on and encompasses the abutment teeth so as to retain the partial denture and stabilize both the denture and the abutment teeth. (Periodont.)

— An extracoronal direct retainer of a removable partial denture; the assembly usually consists of two arms joined by a body that may connect with a rest. At least one arm of a clasp must terminate in the cervical convergence area of the tooth encircled. (Remov. Part. Prosth.)

Adams c. A formed wire clasp, of modified arrowhead design, utilizing the buccal mesial and distal proximal undercuts of a tooth for retention. (Orthodont.)

c. arm, fatigue of A situation in which the retentive arm of a clasp metal has undergone flexure at the same point repeatedly, and fracture has resulted. Tapering the clasp arm tends to distribute the flexure and to reduce such tendency to fracture. (Remov. Part. Prosth.)

arrowhead c. A wire clasp, for retention of removable appliances, whose active elements are in the shape of an arrowhead and engage the mesial and distal proximal undercuts on the buccal aspect of adjacent teeth. (Orthodont.)

back-action c. A clasp that originates on one surface of a tooth and traverses the suprabulge area to another surface, where it is supported by an occlusal rest; it then continues to encircle the tooth on the third surface, where it terminates in the infrabulge area beyond the opposite angle of the tooth surface where it originated. (Remov. Part. Prosth.)

bar c. A clasp whose arms are bar-type extensions from major connectors or from within the denture base; the arms pass adjacent to the soft tissues and approach the point of contact on the tooth in a cervico-occlusal direction. (Remov. Part. Prosth.)

b. c. arm A clasp arm that originates from the denture base or from a major or minor connector. It consists of the arm that traverses but does not contact the gingival structures and a terminal end that approaches its contact with the tooth in a cervico-occlusal direction. (Remov. Part. Prosth.)

cast c. A clasp made of an alloy that has been cast into the desired form and that retains its crystalline structure. (Remov. Part. Prosth.)

circumferential c. A clasp that encircles more than 180° of a tooth, including opposite angles, and that usually contacts the tooth throughout the extent of the clasp, at least one terminal being in the infrabulge area (cervical convergence). (Remov. Part. Prosth.)

c. c. arm A clasp arm that has its origin in a minor connector and that follows the contour of the tooth approximately in a plane perpendicular to the path of placement of the removable partial denture. (Remov. Part. Prosth.)

reciprocal c. c. a. An arm of a clasp located in such a manner as to reciprocate any force arising from an opposing clasp arm on the same tooth. (Remov. Part. Prosth.)

retentive c. c. a. (retention terminal) A circumferential clasp arm that is flexible and that engages the infrabulge area at the terminal end of the arm. (Remov. Part. Prosth.)

stabilizing c. c. a. A circumferential clasp arm that is rigid and that contacts the tooth at or occlusal to the surveyed height of contour. (Remov. Part. Prosth.)

combination c. A clasp that employs a wrought wire retentive arm and a cast reciprocal or stabilizing arm. A clasp that employs a bar type of retentive arm and a cast reciprocal or stabilizing arm. (Remov. Part. Prosth.)

continuous c. A secondary lingual bar. (Remov. Part. Prosth.)

Crozat c. A metallic attachment of a removable appliance adapted to the embrasures. (Orthodont.)

c. design A penciled outline, drawn on a cast, that denotes the outline for a clasp. (Remov. Part. Prosth.)

embrasure c. (ĕm-brā′zhŭr) A clasp used

where no edentulous space exists. It passes through the embrasure, utilizing two occlusal rests, and clasps the two teeth with circumferential clasps that have a common body. (Remov. Part. Prosth.)

flexibility of c. The property of a clasp that enables it to be bent without breaking and to return to its original form. Factors that affect the flexibility of a retentive clasp arm are its length, diameter, cross-section form, and structure, and the alloy of which it is made. (Remov. Part. Prosth.)

c. flexure (see **flexure, clasp**)

formed c. (see **clasp, wrought**)

mesiodistal c. A type of clasp that embraces the distolingual and mesial surfaces of a tooth and takes its retention in either or both mesial and distal undercuts. (Remov. Part. Prosth.)

retentive c., flexibility of Ability of the retentive clasp to deform sufficiently to escape from a retentive undercut area without permanent deformation. (Remov. Part. Prosth.)

Roach c. (see **clasp, bar**)

stress-breaking action of c. Relief for the abutment teeth from all or part of the occlusal forces. Partially achieved by means of a clasp having a retentive arm of tapered, round wrought alloy to give comparative maximum flexibility in any direction. (Remov. Part. Prosth.)

wrought c. (formed c.) A clasp made of an alloy that has been drawn into various forms of wire, by which process the crystalline structure has been converted to one of a fibrous nature. (Remov. Part. Prosth.)

classification Systems of grouping partially edentulous situations based on various conditions, e.g., location of the edentulous space, location of remaining teeth, position of direct retainers, and ability of oral structures to support a partial denture. (Remov. Part. Prosth.)

Angle's c. (see **Angle's classification, modified**)

Broders' c. (see **index, Broders'**)

cavity c. (see **cavity, classification**)

c. of habits Compilation of habits that may cause periodontal disease. Habit neuroses include lip biting, cheek biting, biting of foreign objects, and abnormal tongue pressure against the teeth. Occupational habits include thread biting, musician's habits, holding nails in the mouth, etc. Miscellaneous habits include thumb sucking, pipe smoking, incorrect toothbrushing habits, cracking nuts

with the teeth, mouth breathing, etc. (Periodont.)

Kennedy c. (see **Kennedy classification**)

c. of motions (Remov. Part. Prosth.)

Class 1 Motions of the fingers only.

Class 2 Motions of the fingers and wrist.

Class 3 Motions of the fingers, wrist, and elbow.

Class 4 Motions of the fingers, wrist, elbow, and upper arm.

Class 5 Motions of the fingers, wrist, elbow, upper arm, and body.

c. of periodontal diseases Division of periodontal diseases into three classes: (1) inflammation—gingival abrasion, gingivitis, marginal periodontitis; (2) dystrophy—disuse atrophy, occlusal traumatism, periodontosis; and (3) combinations of inflammatory and dystrophic diseases—periodontosis and periodontitis, occlusal traumatism, and periodontitis. (Periodont.)

c. of pockets Division of pockets into two classes: (1) suprabony-gingival and periodontal and (2) infrabony, according to number of osseous walls—three osseous walls, two osseous walls, one osseous wall. (Periodont.)

cleansing, biomechanical The process of cleaning and shaping a root canal with endodontic instrumentation in conjunction with irrigating solutions. (Endodont.)

cleansing solution (see **solution, cleansing**)

clearance A condition in which moving bodies may pass without hindrance. (Comp. Prosth.)

— Removal from the blood by the kidneys (e.g., urea or insulin) or by the liver (e.g., certain dyes). (Oral Physiol.)

interocclusal c. The difference in the height of the face when the mandible is at rest and when the teeth are in occlusion. This is determined by measuring the amount of space between the upper and lower teeth when the mandible is in the position of physiologic rest. The difference between the rest vertical dimension and the occlusal vertical dimension of the face, as measured in the incisal area. (Orthodont.) (see also **distance, interocclusal**)

occlusal c. A condition in which the lower teeth may pass the upper teeth horizontally without contact or interference. (Comp. Prosth.)

cleat A fixed point of anchorage, usually in the form of a metal spur or loop embedded in the acrylic resin base of a Hawley retainer or soldered onto an arch wire, to which a rubber dam elastic or other device is attached during orthodontic tooth movement. (Periodont.)

cleft(s) A longitudinal fissure or opening. (Oral Diag.)

facial c. Fissures along the embryonal lines of junction of the maxillary and lateral nasal processes; usually extend obliquely from the nasal ala to the outer border of the eye. (Oral Diag.)

gingival c. A cleft of the marginal gingiva; may be caused by many etiologic factors, such as incorrect toothbrushing, a breakthrough to the surface of pocket formation, or faulty tooth positions, and may resemble V-shaped notches. (Periodont.)

occult c. (see **submucous cleft**)

operated c. (**postoperative c.**) A cleft that has been surgically repaired. (Cleft Palate)

c. palate prosthesis (see **prosthesis, cleft palate**)

postoperative c. (see **cleft, operated**)

Stillman's c. Small fissures extending apically from the midline of the gingival margin in teeth subjected to trauma. Although these clefts may be found in traumatism, they are not necessarily diagnostic of occlusal trauma. (Oral Diag.)

submucous c. (see **submucous cleft**)

unoperated c. A cleft of the palate that has not been surgically repaired. (Cleft Palate)

cleidocranial dysostosis (see **dysostosis, cleidocranial**)

clenching The forceful intermittent application of the mandibular teeth against the maxillary teeth, with both horizontal and vertical components to the action; usually associated with emotional tensions and conflicts and often exerting detrimental effects on the teeth and their attachment apparatus. (Periodont.)

cleoid (klē'oid) A carving instrument having a blade shaped like a pointed spade or claw, with cutting edges on both sides and the tip. (Oper. Dent.)

climate, occlusal The new occlusal environment produced by occlusal adjustment, orthodontic tooth movement, and/or a periodontal prosthesis; characterized by properly located and finished crown margins, improved tooth position, favorable crown:root ratios, physiologic form and function of all surfaces of the teeth, anatomic and physiologic integration of the teeth with mandibular functional movement, adequate chewing efficiency, acceptable esthetics, negative occlusal perception, etc. (Periodont.)

clinic, table A display or demonstration of a topic, limited in scope, for transmitting information to a small number of persons at a time. (Orthodont.)

clinical crown (see **crown, clinical**)

clinical crown:clinical root ratio (see **ratio, clinical crown:clinical root**)

clinical diagnosis (see **diagnosis, clinical**)

clinoidale (klīn-oid'al) The most superior point on the contour of the anterior clinoid. (Orthodont.)

clonus (klō'nŭs) Alternating muscular spasm and relaxation in rapid succession. (Oral Physiol.)

closed bite (see **bite, closed**)

closed panel A method of administering dental services to selected groups of people by selected groups of dentists, not providing freedom of choice for either group. (Pract. Man.)

closed procedure Insertion of an implant into its host site through the intact overlying soft tissue. (Oral Implant.)

closure The act or condition of being brought together or closed up.

adjustive arcs of c. Arcs of jaw closure found in deflective malocclusion caused by an intercusping of the teeth that does not coincide with a centrically related jaw closure. By their incline plane mechanisms the deflectors tend to compel a shift in the mandibular occlusal position as the closure forces act. Proprioceptive reflexes ease such a closure without the limp from the incline planes. Proprioceptive reflexes never fully compensate for such malocclusions, especially those with lateralized mandibular occlusal positions. (Gnathol.)

arcs of mandibular c. Circular or elliptic arcs created by closure of the mandible. All closures of the mandible are about the opening-closing axis. If this axis is kept from being translated, the arcs of empty closures are circular. If the axis is being retracted parallel to the axis-orbital plane just before any contacts of the empty teeth are made, the arcs could be elliptic. Centrically related jaw closures are often prevented by teeth that deflect the closure direction either to the fore or to the side. (Gnathol.)

centric path of c. The path traversed by the mandible during closure when its associated neuromuscular mechanism is in a balanced state of tonus; usually results in a hinge-like movement of the mandible during closure. (Periodont.)

skeletal arcs of c. Jaw closure directions obtained by having the patient gain relaxation of his gnathic musculature. A collector of the data as the input for an articulator wants border movements about a border axis position when the mandible is moved by relaxed muscles. The dentist trains his patient to help him locate condylar centricity by gently pumping the mandible while suggesting easiness in the closure. As he does this, he learns to identify the approach to a completely relaxed musculature by a feeling of firmness because the hinges have equally retreated as far as the ligaments will allow. The cooperation of the patient in the movements also indicates that he has no fears to signal to the lateral pterygoid muscles. He also has had his teeth separated long enough from occlusal contacts to let the muscles forget the former protrusive closures needed to settle into an eccentric mandibular occlusal position. (Gnathol.)

velopharyngeal c. Closure of nasal air escape by the knee-action elevation of the soft palate and contraction of the posterior pharyngeal wall. (Cleft Palate.)

voluntary arcs of c. A jaw closure direction made by a patient having distoclusion to improve his looks. The belief was that skeletal muscles could be wholly governed by the conscious "will," which could cause stimuli to descend from the cerebral cortex down nerve trunks to the fibers needing contraction to fulfill the wishes of the will. Purely voluntary arcs of closure would require training, and the adjustments practiced would not lead to any significant adaptations. (Gnathol.)

clot Coagulated blood, plasma, or fibrin. (Oral Surg.)

blood c. A coagulum formed of blood of a semisolidified nature. Generally a clot acts as a protective dressing for a healing wound. (Periodont.)

clubbing (pulmonary osteoarthropathy) Deforming enlargement of the terminal phalanges of the fingers. It is usually acquired and may be associated with certain cardiac and pulmonary diseases. (Oral Diag.)

clutch A device made for gripping the teeth in a dental arch; also one to which face-bows or tracing devices may be attached rigidly enough to behave in space relations during the movements as if they were jaw outgrowths. (Gnathol.)

coagulating current (see **current, coagulating**)

coagulation time (see **time, coagulation**)

coated tongue (see **tongue, coated**)

coating, enteric (ĕn-ter'ĭk) A tablet covering that resists the action of the fluids and enzymes in the stomach but dissolves readily in the upper intestine. (Oral Med.; Pharmacol.)

coating material A biologically acceptable, usually porous nonmetal, applied over the surface of a metallic implant, with the expectation that tissue ingrowth will occur in the pores. Often a carbon, polymer, or ceramic substance. (Oral Implant.)

cobalt-chromium alloy (see **alloy, cobalt-chromium**)

code A system of recording information by symbols so that only selected people will know the meaning. Used also to conserve space. (Pract. Man.)

c. of ethics A series of principles used as a guide in assisting a dentist to fulfill the moral obligations of professional dental practice. (Pract. Man.)

codeine (kō'dēn) A crystalline alkaloid, morphine methyl ether, that is used as an analgesic and antitussive. (Periodont.)

Coecal (kō'kăl) Proprietary brand of dental stone (Hydrocal). (Oper. Dent.)

coefficient, absorption (see **absorption coefficient**)

coefficient, phenol The ratio of potency of a given germicide to that of phenol under standard conditions. (Oral Med.; Pharmacol.)

coefficient of thermal expansion (see **expansion, thermal, coefficient**)

cofactor V (see **factor VII**)

cognition (kog-nĭsh'ŭn) The higher mental processes of understanding, reasoning, knowledge, intellectual capacity, etc. (Oral Physiol.)

cognitive (kog'nĭ-tĭv) Pertaining to the faculty of knowing, perceiving, or being aware; an expression of intellectual capacity. (Oral Physiol.)

cognovit note (kog-nō'vĭt) A note that confesses judgment and to which the maker has no available defense. (D. Juris.)

cohere To stick together, to unite, to form a solid mass. (Oper. Dent.)

cohesion Ability of a material to adhere to itself. (D. Mat.)

cohesive Capable of cohering or sticking together so as to form a mass. (Oper. Dent.)

cold, clinical applications of Clinical uses of cold to treat cold injury (e.g., frostbite), to relieve pain in burn injury, to relieve pain in severe and acute inflammation (pulpitis), to reduce both toxic absorption and pain in gangrene of pulp, and to relieve pain and swelling in contusions, abrasions, and sprains. (Oral Physiol.) (see also **heat and cold, applied**)

cold, contraindications to clinical use Conditions

in which the clinical use of cold is inadvisable: cold allergy, peripheral neuropathy, and atrophy of skin (radiation damages). (Oral Physiol.)

cold-curing resin (see **resin, autopolymerizing**)

cold, physiologic effects of In reference to application of cold to a local area, marked vasoconstriction followed by vasodilation and edema. In extreme exposure the effects include a significant drop in temperature on the surface and a lesser drop in deeper tissue layers, depending on the degree of cold and duration of application; decreased phagocytosis; a decrease in local metabolism; analgesia to varying degrees of anesthesia of the part exposed to cold. (Oral Physiol.)

cold sore (see **sore, canker; herpes labialis**)

cold welding (see **welding, cold**)

cold work Deformation of the space lattice of metals by mechanical manipulation at room temperature. The process alters certain properties, e.g., ductility. (D. Mat.)

— Permanent deformation or change in shape of a structure accomplished at normal temperatures. (Oper. Dent.)

collapse A state of extreme prostration and depression with failure of circulation; abnormal falling in of the walls of any part or organ; with reference to a lung, an airless or fatal state of all or part of the lung. (Anesth.)

collar The small part of the root of a tooth that is a part of an artificial tooth (denture). (Comp. Prosth.)

collimation (kol″ĭ-mā′shŭn) Decrease in size of beam spread by means of a metal plate, usually lead, containing an aperture. The plate is placed in the path of the primary roentgen ray beam. (Oral Radiol.) (see also **diaphragm**)

— Literally, making parallel. In radiology, used with reference to the elimination of the peripheral (more divergent) portion of a useful x-ray beam, by means of metal tubes, cones, or diaphragms interposed in the path of the beam. (Oral Radiol.)

collimator (kol′ĭ-mā-ter) A diaphragm or system of diaphragms made of an absorbing material and designed to define the dimensions and direction of a beam of radiation. (Oral Radiol.)

collision tumor (see **tumor, collision**)

colloid (kol′oid) A suspension of particles in a dispersion medium, the particles generally ranging in size from 1 to 100 mμ. Hydrocolloids and silicate cements are examples of dental colloids. (D. Mat.)

   c. milium (kol′oid mĭl′ē-ŭm) Colloid degener-

ation of the elastic and collagen connective tissue in the upper corium, appearing microscopically as hyalinized areas. (Oral Path.)

color blindness (see **blindness, color**)

color, temper The color produced by the thickening of the oxide coating on carbon steel as temperature is increased. Used as an indication of the degree of tempering. (D. Mat.)

coloring, extrinsic Coloring from without, as in the application of color to the external surface of a prosthesis. (M.F.P.)

coloring, intrinsic Coloring from within. The incorporation of pigment within the material of a prosthesis. (M.F.P.)

coma A state of unconsciousness from which the patient cannot be aroused, even by powerful stimulation. It is gradual in onset, prolonged, and not spontaneously reversible. (Oral Physiol.)

   diabetic c. Unconsciousness accompanying severe diabetic acidosis. It may develop from omission of insulin, surgical complications, and/or disregard of dietary restrictions. Premonitory symptoms include weakness, anorexia, dry skin and mouth, drowsiness, abdominal pain, and fruity breath odor. Late symptoms are coma, air hunger, low blood pressure, tachycardia, dehydration, soft and sunken eyeballs, glycosuria, hyperglycemia, and a high level of acetoacetic acid. (Oral Med.) (see also **shock, insulin**)

combination clasp (see **clasp, combination**)

commercial In the colloquial application to the field of dentistry: merchandising and selling techniques, as contrasted to honest, ethical conduct. (Pract. Man.)

comminution of food (see **food, comminution of**)

common law Judge-made law. For example, professional responsibility is generally a matter of common law. Although not found in the statute books, this law is binding. (D. Juris.)

communicable period The period of time when the infectious agent that causes a communicable disease may be transmitted to a susceptible host; e.g., in diseases that initially involve the mucous membrane (i.e., diphtheria and scarlet fever), the period of communicability is from the time of exposure to the disease until termination of the carrier state, if one develops. (Oral Med.)

communication Information given; the sharing of knowledge; conference; bargaining prior to making a contract. (D. Juris.)

— The technique of conveying thoughts or ideas between two people or groups of people. (Pract. Man.)

confidential c. (see **communication, privileged**)

privileged c. (**confidential c.**) A class of communication between persons who owe each other fidelity and secrecy because of a confidential or fiduciary relationship. The law will not permit communications of this type to be divulged in a court. Examples of confidential relationships are those of husband and wife, attorney and client, and physician and patient. In dentistry the law of privileged communication applies only in the State of New York. (D. Juris.)

compact To form by uniting or condensing particles by the application of pressure; e.g., the progressive insertion and welding of foil and the building up of plastic amalgam in a preparation. (Oper. Dent.)

compaction The act of compacting or the state of being compact. (Oper. Dent.)

compensating curve (see **curve, compensating**)

compensation The monetary reward for rendering a service; insurance providing financial return to employees in the event of an injury that occurs during the performance of their duties and that prohibits work. Compulsory in many states. (Pract. Man.)

unemployment c. Insurance covering the employee so that he may be compensated for loss of income due to unemployment. (Pract. Man.)

compensatory wear (see **wear, compensatory**)

competence A measure of the degree of a person's ability to cope with all aspects of his environment. (Pract. Man.)

competent Having legal capacity, ability, or authority. (D. Juris.)

complaint The most troublesome of symptoms disclosed by the patient. (Oral Diag.)

chief c. The symptom or reason for which the patient seeks treatment. The most troublesome symptom. (Oral Diag.; Pract. Man.)

complemental air (see **volume, inspiratory reserve**)

complete denture (see **denture, complete**)

complex A combination of a number of things; the sum or total of various things.

craniofacial c. The bones and surrounding soft structures of the cranium and face. (Orthodont.)

dentofacial c. Term referring to the dentition and surrounding structures. (Orthodont.)

component(s) A part or element.

c. A (see **factor II**)

c. of force (see **force, component of**)

c. of partial denture (see **denture, partial, components of**)

salivary c. (see **lysozyme**)

thromboplastic cellular c. (TCC) (see **factor, platelet, 3**)

composite odontoma (see **odontoma, composite**)

composite resin (see **resin, composite**)

composition, modeling (see **plastic, modeling**)

compound A combination of atoms held together in a well-defined pattern by chemical bonds. In pharmacy, a mixture of drugs. (Anesth.; Oral Med.; Pharmacol.)

— A thermoplastic substance used as a nonelastic impression material. (D. Mat.)

— A nonelastic molding or impression material that softens when heated and solidifies without chemical change when cooled; i.e., a thermoplastic material. It is a mixture of resins and oils with an inert filler and coloring and flavoring agents. Used to stabilize clamps and separators on the teeth and for making dental impressions. (Comp. Prosth.; Oper. Dent.)

c. A, B, E, F, S (see **corticoid, adrenal**)

c. cone A compound in the form of a cone or pyramid; used for impressions of individual preparations. (Oper. Dent.)

impression c. (**modeling c.**) A compound used to secure an imprint or negative likeness. (Oper. Dent.)

intermetallic c. A compound of two metals in which the metals are only partially soluble in one another; exhibits a homogeneous grain structure, but the atoms do not intermingle randomly in all proportions. (Oper. Dent.)

modeling c. (see **compound, impression; plastic, modeling**)

c. tracing stick A compound dispensed in stick form. (Oper. Dent.)

tray c. A compound similar to impression compound but with less flow and more viscosity when soft, and more rigidity when chilled. (Oper. Dent.)

compression Act of pressing together or forcing into less space. (Oper. Dent.)

c. molding (see **molding, compression**)

c. of tissue (see **tissue, displaceability**)

compressive strength (see **strength, compressive**)

compromise (kahm′prō-mīz″) Arrangement arrived at, in or out of court, for settling a disagreement on terms considered by the parties to be fair. (D. Juris.)

compulsion (kahm-pŭl′shŭn) An irresistible impulse to perform some act contrary to one's better judgment and will. Oral habits (bruxism, clenching, etc.) are frequently generated by the promptings of inner compulsions. (Periodont.)

computer, analog A computer that represents the

factors of occlusion in physiomechanical analogies, such as the distance between the condyles, the slopes of the eminences, the slant of the occlusal plane, the curvature of the cuspal curves, the arcing directions of the working and the idling grooves of the post-canine teeth, the horizontal cross-section curves of the fossae of the upper incisors, the overlap relations of the lips and teeth, and the amount of discrepancy from centric relation in closures. (Gnathol.)

conceal (kahn-sēl') To withhold from utterance or declaration. (D. Juris.)

concrescence (kahn-krĕs'ĕns) The union of two teeth after eruption by the fusion of their cementum surfaces. (Oral Diag.)

— Fusion of teeth after their roots have formed. The union is effected by cementum. (Oral Path.) (see also **fusion**)

condensation (kahn"dĕn-sā'shŭn) A mechanical process used in dentistry to achieve adaptation and to improve physical properties, e.g., removal of excess mercury from amalgam and the rendering of a dense gold-foil restoration. (D. Mat.)

— Commonly used term for the insertion and compression, or compaction, of dental amalgam into a prepared cavity and the building up of a gold-foil restoration by compaction of foil pellets. Compaction is a more accurate term than condensation. (Oper. Dent.) (see also **compaction**)

condenser (kahn-dĕn'ser) (formerly called plugger) An instrument or device used to compact or condense a restorative material into a prepared cavity. Its working end is called the nib or point; the end of the nib is termed the face. The face may be smooth or serrated. (Oper. Dent.)

amalgam c. (amalgam plugger) An instrument used to condense plastic amalgam. (Oper. Dent.)

automatic c. (see **condenser, mechanical**)

back-action c. A condenser with the shank bent into a U shape so that the condensing force is a pulling motion rather than the usual pushing force. (Oper. Dent.)

bayonet c. A condenser in which the offset of the nib and the approximately right-angled bends in the shank permit a better line of force for condensation of foil. There are many variations in angles, length, and diameter of the nib. (Oper. Dent.)

electromallet c. (McShirley's electromallet) An electromechanical device for compacting gold foil, designed by R. C. McShirley.

Condensing points are held in either a straight or a right-angled handpiece; frequency of blows may be varied from 200 to 3600 strokes/min.; the intensity of the blow is controlled electronically. (Oper. Dent.)

foil c. A condenser used to compact gold foil. (Oper. Dent.)

long-handled f. c. A hand condenser of varied design for compacting gold foil. (Oper. Dent.)

foot c. A foil condenser with the nib shaped like a foot. (Oper. Dent.)

hand c. An instrument that compacts material, the force being applied by the muscular effort of the operator with or without supplementary force from a mallet in the hand of the assistant. (Oper. Dent.)

Hollenback c. (see **condenser, pneumatic**)

mechanical c. (automatic mallet) A device to supply an automatically controlled blow for condensing restorative material. It may be spring-activated, pneumatic, or electronically controlled. (Oper. Dent.)

parallelogram c. A condenser, the face of which is shaped like a rectangle or a parallelogram. (Oper. Dent.)

pneumatic c. (Hollenback c.) A mechanical device developed by George M. Hollenback to supply a compacting or condensing force. The force is delivered by controlled pneumatic pressure. Blows are variable in intensity, with speed variable up to 360 strokes/min. It has a straight and a right-angled handpiece; each uses condenser points of selected design. (Oper. Dent.)

c. point (see **point, condenser**)

round c. A condenser, the face of which has a circular outline. (Oper. Dent.)

c., stepping The orderly movement of a condenser point over the surface of gold foil or amalgam during its placement and compaction. (Oper. Dent.)

condensing force (see **force, condensing**)

condensing osteitis (see **osteitis, condensing**)

condensor (spreader) An instrument used in filling a root canal to compress the filling material in a lateral direction. (Endodont.)

conduct, dishonorable Conduct that mars the character and lessens the reputation; conduct that is shameful, disgraceful, base. (D. Juris.)

conduction The transfer of sound waves, heat, nerve impulses, or electricity. (Anesth.)

air c. The normal process of conducting sound waves through the ear canal to the membrane of the eardrum. (Cleft Palate)

— The process of transmitting sound waves to

the cochlea by way of the outer and middle ear. In normal hearing, practically all sounds are transmitted in this way, except those of the hearer's own voice, which are transmitted partly by bone conduction. (Oral Physiol.)

bone c. The transmission of sound waves or vibrations to the cochlea by way of the bones of the cranium. (Cleft Palate; Oral Physiol.)

impulse c. Conduction of an impulse along the nerve fiber, which is accompanied by an alteration of the electrical potential of the fiber tissue. There is thought to be an exchange of electrolytes across the nerve fiber membrane that appears to be selectively permeable to the sodium and potassium ions.

conductivity Capacity for conduction; ability to convey. (Anesth.)

electrical c. Ability of a material to conduct electricity. Metals are usually good conductors and nonmetals are poor conductors. (D. Mat.)

thermal c. Ability of a material to transfer heat. It is of great importance in dentistry, where a low thermal conductivity is desirable in restorative material and a high thermal conductivity is desirable when soft tissue is covered. (D. Mat.)

condylar (kahn'dĭ-lar) Pertaining to the mandibular condyle. The use of this word is restricted to the mechanical counterpart of the the condyle on the articulator. (Comp. Prosth.)

c. axis (see **axis, condylar**)

c. guide (see **guide, condylar**)

    c. g. inclination (see **guide, condylar, inclination**)

condyle (kahn'dīl) The rounded surface at the articular end of a bone. The use of this word is restricted to the anatomic structure. (Comp. Prosth.; Fixed Part. Prosth.; Remov. Part. Prosth.)

c. head Redundant term, the word condyle meaning head. Proper usage would be mandibular head or mandibular condyle. (Comp. Prosth.; Remov. Part. Prosth.) (see also **condyle**)

mandibular c. The articular process of the mandible; the condyloid process of the mandible. (Comp. Prosth.; Fixed Part. Prosth.; Remov. Part. Prosth.)

neck of c. (see **process, condyloid, neck of**)

orbiting c. (see **orbiting condyle**)

c. path The path traveled by the mandibular condyle in the temporomandibular joint during the various mandibular movements.

(Comp. Prosth.; Fixed Part. Prosth.; Remov. Part. Prosth.)

    lateral c. p. The path of the condyle in the glenoid fossa when a lateral mandibular movement is made. (Comp. Prosth.)

    protrusive c. p. The path of the condyle when the mandible is moved forward from its centric position. (Comp. Prosth.)

c. rod (see **rod, condyle**)

rotating c. The condyle that is on the side of the bolus formation, or the one that is braced and placed and rotated while the bolus is being chewed. (Gnathol.)

condylectomy (kahn"dĭl-ĕk'tō-mē) Surgical removal of a condyle. (Oral Surg.)

condyloid process (see **process, condyloid**)

condylotomy (kahn"dĭ-lot'ō-mē) Surgical division through, without removal of, a condyle; or removal of a portion, usually the articular surface, of a condyle. (Oral Surg.)

cone A solid substance, usually gutta-percha or silver, having a tapered form similar in length and diameter to a root canal; used to fill the space once occupied by the pulp in the root of the tooth. (Endodont.)

— An accessory device on a dental x-ray machine, designed to indicate the direction of the central axis of its x-ray beam and to serve as a guide in establishing a desired source-to-film distance. Such "cones" may be conical or tubular in form; provision for beam collimation and/or added filtration is often incorporated into the construction of the "cone." (Oral Radiol.)

c. distance (see **distance, cone**)

long c. A tubular "cone" designed to establish an extended anode-to-skin distance, usually within a range of from 12 to 20 inches. (Oral Radiol.)

short c. A conical or tubular "cone" having as one of its functions the establishment of skin distance of up to 9 inches. (Oral Radiol.)

confidence The desired reaction of a patient to the personality, appearance, intelligence, and technical ability of the dentist. (Pract. Man.)

congenital Present at birth and usually developed in utero. (Oral Diag.)

congestion (see **hyperemia**)

conjugate, *v.* To unite.

—, *n.* The product of conjugation. (Oral Med.; Pharmacol.)

conjugation In biochemistry, the union of a drug or toxic substance with a normal constituent of the body, such as glucuronic acid, to form an inactive product that is then eliminated. (Anesth.; Pharmacol.)

connective tissue (see **tissue, connective**)

connector The part of a fixed partial denture that unites the retainer(s) and the pontic(s). It may be rigid, as in a soldered joint, or non-rigid, as in the tapered-key or stress-breaker joint. (Fixed Part. Prosth.; Remov. Part. Prosth.)

— The part of a partial denture that unites its components. (Fixed Part. Prosth.; Remov. Part. Prosth.)

c. bar (see **bar, connector**)

cross arch bar splint c. A removable cross arch connector used to stabilize weakened abutments that support a fixed prosthesis by attachment to teeth on the opposite side of the dental arch. It can be removed by the dentist but not by the patient. (Remov. Part. Prosth.)

major c. A metal plate or bar (e.g., lingual bar, linguoplate, palatal bar) used to join the units of one side of a removable partial denture to those located on the opposite side of the dental arch. (Remov. Part. Prosth.)

anterior palatal m. c. A major connector uniting bilateral units of a maxillary removable partial denture. It is a thin metal plate that is located in the anterior palatal region and that achieves rigidity by means of the form imparted by the rugae and by lying in two planes. (Remov. Part. Prosth.)

lingual bar m. c. A type of connector used to unite the right and left components of a mandibular removable partial denture, and occupying a position lingual to the alveolar ridge. (Remov. Part. Prosth.)

linguoplate m. c. A major connector formed by the extension of a metal plate from the superior border of the regular lingual bar, across gingivae, and onto the cingulum of each anterior tooth. (Remov. Part. Prosth.)

posterior palatal m. c. (posterior palatal bar) A major connector located in the posterior palatal region; used to assist in bilateral unification when the anterior palatal bar alone would lack rigidity. (Remov. Part. Prosth.)

minor c. The connecting link between the major connector or base of a removable partial denture and other units of the restoration, e.g., direct and indirect retainers, rests, and extensions from major connectors

to which denture bases are attached. (Remov. Part. Prosth.)

secondary lingual bar m. c. (Kennedy bar) Often called a continuous clasp, or Kennedy bar. It rests on the cingulum area of the lower anterior teeth and serves principally as an indirect retainer and/or stabilizer for weakened anterior lower teeth. (Remov. Part. Prosth.)

nonrigid c. A connector used where retainers and/or pontics are united by a joint permitting limited movement. It may be a precision or a nonprecision type of connector. (Fixed Part. Prosth.)

rigid c. A connector used where retainers and/or pontics are united by a soldered, cast, or welded joint (in metallic fixed restorations) or are fused (in ceramic restorations). (Fixed Part. Prosth.)

saddle c. (see **connector, major**)

subocclusal c. A nonrigid connector positioned gingival to the occlusal plane. (Fixed Part. Prosth.)

consciousness A state in which the individual is capable of rational response to questioning and has all protective reflexes intact, including the ability to maintain a patent airway. (Anesth.)

consent Concurrence of wills; permission. (D. Juris.)

express c. Consent directly given by voice or in writing. (D. Juris.)

implied c. Consent made evident by signs, actions, or facts, or by inaction or silence. (D. Juris.)

consideration Inducement to make a contract. The cause, motive, or price that influences a contracting party to enter into a contract. (D. Juris.)

consonant A conventional speech sound produced, with or without laryngeal vibration, by certain successive contractions of the articulatory muscles that modify, interrupt, or obstruct the expired airstream to the extent that its pressure is raised. (Cleft Palate)

semivowel c. ("l, t") Consonants that are vowellike both perceptually and physiologically. (Cleft Palate)

constitution General makeup of the body as determined by genetic, physiologic, and biochemical factors. It may be markedly influenced by environment. (Oral Diag.)

construction, single denture The making of one upper or lower denture as distinguished from a set of two complete dentures. (Comp. Prosth.; Remov. Part. Prosth.)

consultant A professional or nonprofessional person who, by virtue of his special knowledge of professional or nonprofessional aspects of a dental practice, is sought out for advice and training. (Pract. Man.)

consultation Joint deliberation by two or more dentists and/or physicians to determine the diagnosis, treatment, or prognosis for a particular patient. The consulting doctors may examine the patient together or separately. (Oral Diag.)

— A meeting between the dentist, the patient, and other interested persons for the purpose of discussing the patient's dental needs, proposing treatment, and making business arrangements. (Pract. Man.)

contact (see **point, contact**)

balancing c. The contact established between the upper and lower dentures at the side opposite the working side (anteroposteriorly or laterally) for the purpose of stabilizing the dentures. (Comp. Prosth.)

deflective occlusal c. (cuspal interference) A condition of tooth contacts that diverts the mandible from a normal path of closure to centric jaw relation or causes a denture to slide or rotate on its basal seat. (Comp. Prosth.; Fixed Part. Prosth.; Remov. Part. Prosth.) (see also **contact, interceptive occlusal**)

faulty c. Imperfections in the contact between adjacent teeth. Often leads to food impaction between the teeth, with subsequent initiation or perpetuation of periodontal lesions. (Periodont.)

initial c. The first meeting of opposing teeth on elevation of the mandible toward the maxillae. The initial occlusal contact of opposing teeth when the jaw is closed. (Comp. Prosth.; Fixed Part. Prosth.; Remov. Part. Prosth.)

— Normal or noninterfering contact and intercuspation of the mandibular and maxillary teeth, occurring as the mandible, during a normal median closing movement or during any of the peripheral closing movements, closes into its final occlusal position. (Orthodont.)

interceptive occlusal c. An initial contact of teeth that stops or deviates from the normal movement of the mandible. (Comp. Prosth.; Fixed Part. Prosth.; Orthodont.) (see also **contact, deflective occlusal**)

premature c. Contact occurring when some of the teeth are in interceptive occlusion, or when some teeth are striking too hard; unphysiologic contact of opposing teeth during median closure, preventing complete or undeflected closure of the mandible. (Orthodont.) (see also **contact, deflective occlusal; contact, interceptive occlusal**)

— Early interference of opposing tooth surfaces, seen in discrepancies between centric occlusion and centric relation or other excursions, high and faulty restorations, etc., which may produce lesions of occlusal traumatism on teeth and their attachment apparatus. (Periodont.)

weak c. Less than optimal contact between two teeth or restorations, permitting food impaction and impingement on interdental supporting tissues. (Oper. Dent.)

working c. A contact of the teeth made on the side of the dental arch toward which the mandible has been moved. (Comp. Prosth.; Remov. Part. Prosth.)

— An occlusal contact in which tooth surfaces are rubbed together in empty chewing. The chief work produced by such relations is the creation of facets and ultimately long centric and broad centric arenas of wear. (Gnathol.)

contaminated Made radioactive by the addition of minute quantities of radioactive material. (Oral Radiol.)

contamination, radioactive Deposition of radioactive material in any place where it is not desired, and particularly where its presence may be harmful or may constitute a radiation hazard. (Oral Radiol.)

contingent (kahn-tǐn′jĕnt) Dependent for effect on something that may or may not occur. (D. Juris.)

continuant A speech sound in which the speech organs are held relatively fixed during the period of production. (Cleft Palate)

continuous bar retainer (see **retainer, continuous bar**)

continuous clasp (see **retainer, continuous bar**)

continuous loop wiring (see **wiring, continuous loop**)

contour, *n.* The external shape, form, or surface configuration of an object. (Comp. Prosth.; Remov. Part. Prosth.)

buccal c. The shape of the buccal aspect of a posterior tooth. It normally presents an occlusocervical convexity, with its greatest prominence at the gingival third of the clinical buccal surface, thus affording protection for the margin of the gingivae. (Periodont.)

gingival c. The form of the denture base or other material around the interproximal and cervical surfaces of artificial teeth. (Comp. Prosth.; Remov. Part. Prosth.)

— A festooning of the gingiva with a slightly

raised but still knifelike edge, rounding off toward the attached gingiva. (Periodont.)

height of c. A line encircling a tooth to designate its greatest circumference; the line encircling a tooth in a more or less horizontal plane and passing through the surface points of greatest radius; the line encircling a tooth at its greatest bulge or diameter with respect to a selected path of insertion. (Oper. Dent.)

— The greatest convexity of an object viewed from a predetermined position. (Remov. Part. Prosth.)

    anatomic h. of c. A line encircling a tooth to designate its greatest convexity. (Remov. Part. Prosth.)

    surveyed h. of c. A line, scribed or marked on a cast, that designates the greatest convexity with respect to a selected path of denture placement and removal. (Remov. Part. Prosth.)

proximal c. The form of the mesial or distal surface of a tooth. (Oper. Dent.)

restoration c. Where surfaces of teeth have been destroyed because of disease processes or excessive wear, the restoration of a proper contour for maintenance of healthy gingival tissue. (Periodont.)

tooth c. A shape of a tooth that is essential to a healthy gingival unit because it enables the bolus of food to be deflected from gingival margins during mastication. (Periodont.)

—, *v.* To create the external shape or form of an object, as of a denture. (Comp. Prosth.; Remov. Part. Prosth.)

contouring, occlusal Correction, by grinding, of gross disharmonies of the occlusal tooth form (e.g., uneven marginal ridges, plunger cusps, extruded teeth, and malpositioned teeth) in order to establish a harmonious occlusion and to afford protection to the periodontium of the tooth. (Periodont.)

contouring pliers (see **pliers, contouring**)

contra-angle (kahn″trah-ăng′gl) More than one angle. An instrument with a moderately long blade or nib, having two or more offsetting angles of such degree that the end of the instrument is kept within 3 mm of the axis of the shaft; it may have two angles (binangle) or three angles (triple angle). (Oper. Dent.)

contract An agreement, made after sufficient consideration, between two or more competent persons to do or not to do some legal thing. (D. Juris.)

breach of c. Violation or nonfulfillment of a contract or duty. (D. Juris)

express c. A contract that is an actual agreement between the parties, with the terms declared at the time of making, being stated in explicit language either orally or in writing. (D. Juris.)

implied c. A contract not evidenced by explicit agreement of the parties but inferred by the law from the acts and circumstances surrounding the transactions. (D. Juris.)

contraction Shortening, shrinkage, or reduction in length or size. (Oper. Dent.)

— A condition in which teeth or other maxillary and mandibular structures (such as the dental arch) are nearer than normal to the median plane. (Orthodont.)

metal c. Shrinkage associated with the congealing of a metal from its molten state to a solid after having been cast. (Remov. Part. Prosth.) (see also **expansion, thermal**)

muscle c. Development of tension in a muscle in response to a nerve stimulus. (Comp. Prosth.; Remov. Part. Prosth.)

— Muscle activity involving a change in length and/or tension. (Oral Physiol.)

    m. c., changes in striation bands Alterations in bands of striated muscle during contraction. Striated muscle is composed of a darker A band and a lighter I band. Both of these alternating bands develop tension during contraction but not to the same degree. In isometric contraction (clenched teeth), the sarcomere muscle unit remains unchanged in length, whereas the A band (the darker band) actually shortens and the I band (the lighter band) lengthens. When a muscle is passively stretched (as when the mandible is opened by gravity), the A band lengthens relatively more than the I band, and during isotonic contraction practically all the shortening is in the A segment. It is thus concluded that the contractile properties are not the same throughout the sarcomere—the unit of contractility. It is suggested that the darker A band has a greater concentration of contractile substance than the I band and that, in addition to contractile elemens, the I band contains elastic noncontractile elements that constitute a series of elastic components throughout the fibril. Thus there is, throughout a fiber, an arrangement of dark, contractile components alternating with lighter, elastic components. (Oral Physiol.)

    m. c., chemical factors in The chemical constituents and action involved in the contraction of muscle fibers. Muscle is a structure whose working units are built up largely from two proteins, actin and myosin, which appear to be organized into separate filaments running longitudinally through the muscle fibers. Neither type of filament runs continuously along the length of the fiber, although the effect is that of a continuous structure. The filaments are organized into a succession of groupings of one type of fiber. Each group is arranged in a regular palisade to overlap the next group of fibers, which are similarly arranged in palisades. This gives a banded appearance to the fiber. The thicker filaments contain myosin and are restricted to the A bands, where they give rise to a higher density and birefringence. The thinner filaments contain actin and extend to either side of the Z band, which is at the center of the I band. When the muscle contracts or is stretched, the two groups of filaments slide past each other like the alternating units of a sliding gate. The controlled sliding motion is presumably brought about through the mediation of oblique cross links between the filaments. These cross links are the structural expression of the biochemical interaction between actin and myosin. The chemical substance that initiates the interaction between these fibrils is adenosine triphosphate (ATP). The final effect of the interaction between adenosine triphosphate, myosin, and actin is to enable the two types of filaments to crawl past each other to create the shortened state of the muscle. (Oral Physiol.)

concentric m. c. Unresisted ordinary shortening of muscle. (Oral Physiol.)

eccentric m. c. Increase in muscle tonus during lengthening of the muscle. Eccentric contraction occurs when muscles are used to oppose movement but not to stop it—e.g., the action of the biceps in lowering the forearm gradually and in a controlled manner. Eccentric contractions are called isotonic because the muscle changes length. (Oral Physiol.)

isometric m. c. Increase in muscular tension without a change in muscle length, as in clenching the teeth. (Comp. Prosth.; Remov. Part. Prosth.)

isotonic m. c. Increase in muscular tension during movement without resistance (either lengthening or shortening), as in

free opening and closing of the jaws. (Comp. Prosth.; Remov. Part. Prosth.)

postural m. c. Maintenance of muscular tension (usually isometric muscular contraction) sufficient to maintain posture. (Comp. Prosth.; Remov. Part. Prosth.)

smooth m. c., mechanism of The mechanisms that regulate the functions of smooth muscle fibers. These regulatory mechanisms vary and are affected principally by two methods: (1) The parasympathetic and sympathetic nerve fiber endings of the autonomic nervous system form a reticulum around the muscle cells before entering them. The action of these fibers is antagonistic; they act directly on the muscle cell—not on each other. Examples of the structures principally under the control of the autonomic nerve mechanism are the blood vessels and the pilomotor fibers. (2) The selection response to rhythmic activity associated with the automaticity of a viscus or other organ is dependent on local or hormonal factors. An example of this mechanism is the function of the uterus under the control of the estrogenic hormone. (Oral Physiol.)

static m. c. Contraction in which opposing muscles contract against each other and prevent movement. This fixation action of a muscle in a static contraction is termed isometric since the muscle develops tension without changing its length. (Oral Physiol.)

contractor, independent One who has such control of the work contracted to be done that he is not subject to the direction of his employer regarding the manner or means of its performance. (D. Juris.)

contracture A permanent shortening (contraction) of a muscle. (Comp. Prosth.)

contraindication (kahn″trah-ĭn″dĭ-kā′shŭn) Any symptom or circumstance indicating the inappropriateness of a form of treatment otherwise advisable. (Anesth.)

contrast, radiographic (radiographic image) The differences in photographic or film density produced on a radiograph by structural composition of the object radiographed or by varying amounts of radiation. (Oral Radiol.)

r. c., long-scale An increased number of grays between the blacks and whites on a radiograph. Higher kilovoltages increase the scale of contrast. (Oral Radiol.)

r. c., short-scale A minimum number of grays

between the blacks and whites on a radiograph. Lower kilovoltages decrease the scale of contrast. (Oral Radiol.)

contributory negligence (see **negligence, contributory**)

control, stress Any method utilized to diminish or remove the stress load generated by occlusal contact, whether the contact is functional in origin or the result of a habit cycle. (Remov. Part. Prosth.)

contusion (kahn-tū′zhŭn) A bruise that is usually produced by an impact from a blunt object and that does not cause a break in the skin. (Oral Diag.; Oral Surg.)

convenience form (see **form, convenience**)

convenience relationship of teeth (see **relation, jaw, convenience; relation, jaw, eccentric; occlusion, convenience**)

convergence, cervical The angle formed between the cervicoaxial inclination of a tooth surface on the one side and a diagnostic stylus of a dental cast surveyor in contact with the tooth at its height of contour. (Remov. Part. Prosth.)

converter, rotary A motor generator set or unit which, when operated by one type of current, produces another; e.g., the conversion of alternating to direct current. (Oral Radiol.)

convertin (see **thromboplastin, extrinsic**)

coolant (koo′lănt) Air or liquid directed onto a tooth, tissue, or restoration to neutralize the heating effect of a rotary instrument. (Oper. Dent.)

Cooley's anemia (see **thalassemia major**)

Cooley's trait (see **thalassemia minor**)

Coolidge filament transformer, tube (see under appropriate noun)

coordination Harmonious functioning, e.g., of muscles. (Comp. Prosth.; Remov. Part. Prosth.)

cope The upper half of a flask in the casting art; hence also the upper, or cavity, side of a denture flask. (Comp. Prosth.)

coping (thimble) A thin metal covering or cap over a prepared tooth. Another restoration or part of a restoration may be fitted over the coping. May serve as a retainer or a base for the construction of a crown. (Comp. Prosth.; Fixed Part. Prosth.; Remov. Part. Prosth.)

paralleling c. A casting placed over an implant abutment to make it parallel to other natural or implant abutments. (Oral Implant.)

transfer c. A covering or cap, made of metal, acrylic resin, or other material, and used to position a die in an impression. (Comp.

Prosth.; Fixed Part. Prosth.; Remov. Part. Prosth.)

copolymer (kō-pahl′ĭ-mer) Polymerization of two or more monomers that have slightly different chemical formulas. Used in dentistry to impart certain desirable physical properties, e.g., flow. (D. Mat.)

copolymerization (kō-pahl-ĭ-mer-ĭ-zā′shŭn) Formation of a copolymer. (D. Mat.)

copper band appliance (see **appliance, acrylic resin and copper band**)

coproporphyrinuria (kahp″rō-por″fĭ-rĭ-nū′rē-ah) Presence of an abnormal concentration of coproporphyrin in the urine. Normal values range from 70 to 250 μg/day. An increased amount of coproporphyrin III occurs in the urine in clinical lead poisoning, exposure to lead without clinically apparent symptoms, infections, malignant disease, and alcoholic cirrhosis, after ingestion of small amounts of ethanol, or normally in some individuals. (Oral Med.)

cord(s) A long organ or body that is rounded.

spinal c. The central nervous system cord contained in the vertebral column. The spinal cord is essential to the regulation and administration of various motor, sensory, and autonomic nerve activities of the body. Through its pathways it conducts impulses from the extremities, trunk, and neck to and from the higher centers and to consciousness. It thus provides for simple reflexes, has control over visceral activities, and participates in the conscious activities of the body. (Oral Physiol.)

vocal c. Membranous structures in the throat that produce sound; the thyroarytenoid ligaments of the larynx. The inferior cords are called the true vocal cords, and the superior cords are called the false vocal cords. (Anesth.)

core A section of a mold, usually of plaster, made over assembled parts of a dental restoration or construction to record and maintain the relationships of the parts so that the parts can be reassembled in their original positions; e.g., to hold a tooth in position on a denture for the purpose of repair or replacement. Also a section of gypsum material used for eliminating undercuts from casts when dies are made for swaging metal bases. (Comp. Prosth.; Fixed Part. Prosth.; Remov. Part. Prosth.)

cast c. A metal casting, usually with a post in the canal or a root, designed to retain an artificial crown. (Fixed Part. Prosth.; Remov. Part. Prosth.)

corium, gingival (kō'rē-ŭm) The most stable, inert, and mature phase of connective tissue elements of the gingiva lying between the periosteum and the lamina propria mucosae. (Periodont.)

cornea The transparent anterior part of the eye. (Anesth.)

cornification Conversion of epithelium to a horn-like substance, e.g., at the surface of a corn or leukoplakia. Keratinization is a more specific term implying the formation of true keratin. (Oral Diag.)

coronoid process (see **process, coronoid**)

coronoidectomy (kor"ō-noid-ĕk'tō-mē) Surgical removal of the coronoid process of the mandible. (Oral Surg.)

corpuscle(s) Any small body, mass, or organ. (Oral Physiol.)

   blood c. A formed element in the blood. (Oral Physiol.) (see also **erythrocyte, leukocyte, lymphocyte, monocyte**)

   Golgi's c. Small spindle-shaped proprioceptive end-organ located in tendons and activated by stretch. (Oral Physiol.)

   Krause's c. Bulboid encapsulated nerve endings located in mucous membranes and activated by cold. (Oral Physiol.)

   Meissner's c. Medium encapsulated nerve endings found in the skin and activated by light touch. (Oral Physiol.)

   Merkel's c. Specialized sensory nerve endings located in the submucosa of the mouth and activated by light touch. (Oral Physiol.)

   Pacini's c. Large sensory nerve endings, scattered widely in subcutaneous tissues, joints, tendons, etc. and activated by deep pressure. (Oral Physiol.)

   Ruffini's c. Specialized sensory nerve organs in the skin and mucous membranes for perceiving heat. Temperature variations of less than 5° C are not readily received by these end organs. (Oral Physiol.)

corrected master cast (see **cast, master, corrected**)

correction, occlusal Correction of malocclusion, by whatever means is employed. Elimination of disharmony of occlusal contacts. (Comp. Prosth.; Fixed Part. Prosth.; Remov. Part. Prosth.)

corrective A prescription ingredient designed to compensate for or nullify undesirable effects of the basis and the adjuvant. (Oral Med.; Pharmacol.)

correspondence Written or typed communication between two individuals or groups of individuals. (Pract. Man.)

corrosion Electrolytic or chemical attack of a surface. Usually refers to the attack of a metal surface. (D. Mat.)

— Disintegration of a metallic surface by some medium in contact with it. (Oper. Dent.)

cortex The outer layer of an organ or other structure. (Oral Physiol.)

   adrenal c. The outer layer of the adrenal gland, the site of secretion of the adrenocortical hormones. (Oral Physiol.)

   cerebral c. The outer gray matter of cerebrum, where many of the higher functions—volition, consciousness, conceptualization, sensation, etc.—are carried out. (Oral Physiol.)

corticalosteotomy (kor"tǐ-kahl-ŏs'tō-mē) An osteotomy through the cortex at the base of the dentoalveolar segment, which serves to weaken the resistance of the bone to the application of orthodontic forces. (Oral Surg.)

corticoid, adrenal (kor'tē-koid) An adrenal corticosteroid hormone, e.g., 11-dehydrocorticosterone (compound A), corticosterone (compound B), 11-deoxycorticosterone (cortexone, DOC), cortisone (compound E), cortisol (compound F), 17-ochydroxy, 11-deoxycortisol (substance S), aldosterone, androgen, progesterone, estrogen, and many other inactive steroids. (Oral Med.) (see also **aldosterone, androgen, corticosterone, cortisone, estrogens, hydrocortisone, progesterone**)

corticosteroid (kor"tǐ-kō-ster'oid) (see **steroid, adrenocortical**)

corticosterone (Kendall's compound B) (kor"tǐ-kō-ster'ōn; kor"tǐ-kos'ter-ōn) An adrenal corticosteroid hormone that is necessary for the maintenance of life in adrenalectomized animals; protects against stress, influences muscular efficiency, and influences carbohydrate and electrolyte metabolism. (Oral Med.)

corticotropin (kor"tǐ-kō-trō'pǐn) A purified preparation of adrenocorticotropic hormone derived from the pituitary gland of animals. (Oral Med.) (see also **ACTH**)

cortin General term for the hormonal secretions of the adrenal cortex. (Oral Med.)

cortisol (see **hydrocortisone**)

cortisone (17-hydroxy-11-dehydrocorticosterone, Kendall's compound E) An adrenal corticosteroid with effects similar to corticosterone in adrenalectomized animals; used in the treatment of adrenal insufficiency, the collagen diseases, and arthritis. (Oral Med.)

— A hormone produced by the adrenal cortex;

a glucocorticoid, 17-hydroxy-11-dehydrocorticosterone; useful in the treatment of rheumatoid arthritis, lupus erythematosis, some allergic conditions, etc. Has marked anti-inflammatory properties. Excess production or administration produces signs of hyperadrenocorticalism (Cushing's syndrome) with hyperlipemia and obesity hyperglycemia, edema, etc. (Periodont.)

Costen's syndrome (see **syndrome, Costen's**)

cothromboplastin (kō-thrahm″bō-plăs′tĭn) (see **thromboplastin, extrinsic**)

cotton, absorbent Fibers or hairs of the seed of cultivated varieties of *Gossypium herbaceum,* so prepared that the cotton readily absorbs liquid. (Oper. Dent.)

cotton pliers (see **pliers, cotton**)

cotton roll rubber dam clamp (see **clamp, rubber dam, cotton roll**)

cough A sudden noisy expulsion of air from the lungs. (Anesth.)

gander c. The characteristic clanging, brassy cough of tracheal obstruction. (Anesth.)

count, blood, complete Determination of the number of red blood cells (erythrocytes), white blood cells, and platelets in an accurately measured volume of blood. It usually includes the quantity of hemoglobin per cubic millimeter of blood. A normal count is 4 to 5.5 million cells per cubic millimeter of blood. (Oral Diag.)

count, platelet Determination of the number of platelets in a cubic millimeter of blood. The normal count is 200,000 to 500,000. (Oral Diag.)

count, reticulocyte (rē-tĭk′ū-lō-sīt″) The number of reticulocytes in the circulating blood, giving some indication of bone marrow activity. The number is increased after acute blood loss and after recovery from anemia. The number is decreased in anemias associated with defective red cell or hemoglobin production (nutritional, endocrine, toxic, or displacement anemias). The normal range is 0.5% to 1.5% of the erythrocytes. (Oral Med.)

count, white blood cell Determination of the number of white blood cells in an accurately measured volume of blood. The normal value is from 4,000 to 9,000 per cubic millimeter of blood. (Oral Diag.)

differential w.b.c.c. Determination of the number of each type of white blood cell in the peripheral blood. The relative count is obtained by counting the number of each type of cell in every 100 cells. The results are expressed in percentages. The normal figure for neutrophils is 60% to 70%, lymphocytes 20% to 35%, monocytes 2% to 8%; basophils 0% to 1%, and eosinophils 2% to 4%. (Oral Diag.)

counter A device for enumerating ionizing events. Term is sometimes used loosely to include the associated detector. (Oral Radiol.)

Geiger-Müller c. (G-M c., Geiger c.) A highly sensitive gas-filled radiation-measuring device operating at voltages sufficiently high to produce avalanche ionization. (Oral Radiol.)

proportional c. A gas-filled radiation detection tube in which the pulse produced is proportional to the number of ions formed in the gas by the primary ionizing particle. (Oral Radiol.)

scintillation c. The combination of phosphor, photomultiplier tube, and associated circuits for counting light emissions produced in the phosphor. (Oral Radiol.)

counterdie The reverse image of a die, usually made of a softer and lower fusing metal than the die. It is used to swage metal, wax, or other material over a die. (Comp. Prosth.; Oper. Dent.) (see also **die**)

counterirritant An irritant that blocks perception of pain by diverting attention to the sensation that it itself produces. (Oral Med.; Pharmacol.)

coupling fitness test A laboratory test of a pair of hand-held artificial molars to see if they can be joined in a nonrocking centric occlusion without changing their forms. An occlusal fitness test of a pair of natural molars that consists of determining whether their casts can be coupled in a nonrocking centric occlusion. (Gnathol.)

courses, refresher Postgraduate study offered either in institutions of higher learning, by groups with an organized dental program, or by individuals especially qualified in certain areas; usually does not involve graduate credit. (Pract. Man.)

coverage (see **denture coverage**)

Coxsackie A disease (see **herpangina**)

Crane-Kaplan pocket marker (see **pocket marker, Crane-Kaplan**)

cranial prosthesis An artificial replacement for a portion of the skull. (M.F.P.)

craniofacial appliance (see **appliance, craniofacial**)

craniofacial dysostosis (krā″nē-ō-fā′shŭl dĭs″ostō′sĭs) (see **dysostosis, craniofacial**)

craniometry (krā″nē-ahm′ĕ-trē) Study of the measurements of the skull. (Orthodont.)

craniopharyngioma (krā″nē-ō-fah-rĭn″jē-ō′mah) A tumor, histologically identical to ameloblastoma, that arises from remnants of the craniopharyngeal duct. (Oral Path.)

craniotabes (krā″nē-ō-tā′bēz) A soft, yielding skull; shallow pitting and thinning of skull bones of infants due to congenital syphilis or rickets. (Oral Med.)

crater formation Formation of interdental depressions in the gingival tissues and/or subjacent bone; often associated with the destructive effects of necrotizing ulcerative gingivitis. The buccal and lingual tissues usually are not destroyed to the same extent as the tissues interposed between them. (Periodont.)

crazing Formation of small cracks on the surface of structures induced by release on internal stress. Generally associated with acrylic resin denture bases and teeth. (D. Mat.)

  c. of plastic teeth Minute cracks appearing on the surface of plastic teeth. (Comp. Prosth.; Remov. Part. Prosth.)

creasote (see **creosote, N.F. XI**)

credit rating Evaluation of any person's responsibility toward meeting his financial obligations. (Pract. Man.)

creditor A person to whom a debt is owed by another person. (D. Juris.)

crenation (krē-nā′shŭn) Wrinkling of the surface of cells as a result of shrinkage in their volume. (Oral Med.; Pharmacol.)

  c. of tongue Scalloping along the lingual periphery of the tongue caused by the tongue's lying against the lingual surface of the mandibular teeth. (Pedodont.)

creosote, N.F. XI (wood creosote) A mixture of phenols obtained from wood tar and occasionally used to treat root canals. (Endodont.)

crepitus (krĕp′ĭ-tŭs) A crackling sound such as that produced by the rubbing together of fragments of a fractured bone or by air moving in a tissue space. (Oral Surg.)

  bony c. The crackling sound noted during auscultation; also the sensation noted during palpation when the fragments of a fractured bone are rubbed together. (Oral Surg.)

crescent, sublingual The crescent-shaped area on the floor of the mouth formed by the lingual wall of the mandible and the adjacent part of the floor of the mouth. (Comp. Prosth.; Fixed Part. Prosth.)

crest A projecting ridge or structure.

  alveolar c. (see **bone crest**)

gingival c. The coronal margin of the gingival tissue. (Periodont.)

cretin A thyroid-deficient dwarfed individual with mental subnormality. (Pedodont.)

cretinism (krē′tĭ-nĭzm) **(congenital hypothyroidism)** Marked retardation of physical and mental development caused by congenital lack of secretion of thyrotropic hormone by the pituitary gland. Slow tooth eruption is one of the results. (Oral Diag.)

— Effects of fetal or early childhood hypothyroidism, characterized by idiocy; dwarfism; dry skin; a coarse, puffy face; a protruding abdomen; and a broad, thickened tongue. (Oral Med.)

— A thyroid deficiency that results in retardation of physical and mental development. (Oral Path.)

crib, Jackson A removable orthodontic appliance retained in position by crib-shaped wires. (Orthodont.)

crib, lingual An orthodontic appliance consisting of a wire framework suspended lingually to the maxillary incisor teeth; used to obstruct thumb and tongue habits. (Orthodont.)

crib splint (see **splint, crib**)

cricoid cartilage (krī′koid) (see **cartilage, cricoid**)

cricoidynia (krī″koi-dĭn′ē-ah) Pain in the cricoid cartilage. (Anesth.)

cricothyrotomy (krī″kō-thī-rot′ō-mē) An incision between the cricoid and thyroid cartilages for the purpose of maintaining a patent airway. (Oral Surg.)

cri-du-chat syndrome (krē-doo-shăt′) (see **syndrome, cri-du-chat**)

crisis, adrenal Acute adrenocortical insufficiency, with clinical manifestations of headache, nausea, vomiting, diarrhea, confusion, costovertebral angle pain, circulatory collapse, and coma. May occur in relation to stress of dental or medical procedures in patients with latent adrenal disease or in patients who have undergone prior ACTH or cortisone therapy, especially without control or termination of therapy. (Oral Med.)

crisis, thyroid A complication occurring after thyroidectomy, or prior to or during other surgical procedures where even mild hyperthyroidism is present. It is characterized by tachycardia, high temperature, nervousness, and occasionally delirium. (Oral Med.)

cristobalite (krĭs-tō′bah-līt) A form of crystalline silica used in dental casting investments because of its relatively high capacity for thermal expansion. (D. Mat.; Oper. Dent.)

Crooke's tube (see **tube, Crooke's**)

cross arch bar splint (see **connector**)

cross arch bar splint connector (see **connector, cross arch bar splint**)

cross arch fulcrum line (see **line, fulcrum, cross arch**)

cross arch splinting (see **splinting, cross arch**)

cross-bite Abnormal relation of a tooth or teeth of one arch to the opposing tooth or teeth in the other arch due to buccal, labial, or lingual deviation of tooth position or to abnormal jaw position. (Comp. Prosth.; Orthodont.) (see also **occlusion, cross-bite**)

— An occlusion with the line of occlusion of the mandibular teeth anterior and/or buccal to the maxillary teeth. (Periodont.)

   anterior c.-b. Primary or permanent maxillary incisors locked lingual to mandibular incisors. (Periodont.)

   posterior c.-b. Primary permanent maxillary posterior teeth in lingual position in relation to the mandibular teeth. (Pedodont.)

cross-examination Questioning of a witness by the party against whom he has been called and examined. (D. Juris.)

cross linkage (see **polymerization, cross**)

cross polymerization (see **polymerization, cross**)

cross-resistance (see **resistance, cross-**)

cross-section form (see **clasp, flexibility of**)

cross-tolerance (see **tolerance, cross-**)

cross tooth contact stability Multiple use of tripodism, provided in the premolars, for instance, by the upper lingual cusp coupling of the lingual fossae of the lower premolars and by the lower buccal cusp coupling in fossae of the upper premolars. Each stamp cusp gains stability by its three-point contact. (Gnathol.)

Crouzon's disease (kroo-zahnz′) (see **dysostosis, craniofacial**)

Crouzon's syndrome (see **dysostosis, craniofacial**)

crowding of teeth A condition in which teeth assume altered positions in such a manner as to produce bunching of the teeth, resulting in overlapping, displacement in various directions, torsoversion, etc. (Periodont.)

crown That portion of a human tooth covered by enamel. (Endodont.; Oper. Dent.)

   anatomic c. That portion of dentin covered by enamel; it performs the function usually attributed to teeth. (Periodont.)

   — The portion of a natural tooth extending from its cementoenamel junction to the occlusal surface or incisal edge. (Fixed Part. Prosth.; Remov. Part. Prosth.)

   artificial c. A dental prosthesis restoring the anatomy, function, and esthetics of part or all of the coronal portion of the natural tooth. (Fixed Part. Prosth.)

   —A fixed restoration of the major part or of the entire coronal part of a natural tooth; usually of gold, porcelain, or acrylic resin. (Remov. Part. Prosth.)

   clinical c. That portion of enamel visibly present in the oral cavity. (Periodont.)

   — The portion of a tooth that is occlusal to the deepest part of the gingival crevice. (Oper. Dent.)

      extra-alveolar c. c. The portion of a tooth that extends occlusally or incisally from the junction of the tooth root and the supporting bone. (Oper. Dent.)

   complete c. A restoration that reproduces the entire surface anatomy of the clinical crown and fits over a prepared tooth stump. (Fixed Part. Prosth.)

      c. veneer c. A restoration that reproduces the entire surface anatomic form of the clinical crown and fits over a prepared tooth or root. It may be made of porcelain, acrylic resin, metal, or a combination of these materials. (Fixed Part. Prosth.)

         c. v. c., acrylic resin A restoration that usually restores the clinical crown of a tooth with acrylic resin. (Fixed Part. Prosth.)

         c. v. c., porcelain A restoration that usually restores the clinical crown of a tooth with porcelain. (Fixed Part. Prosth.

   dowel c. A restoration that replaces the entire coronal portion of a tooth and derives its retention from a dowel extending into a treated (filled) root canal. (Fixed Part. Prosth.)

   faced c. (see **crown, veneered metal**)

   faulty c. An imperfect partial or full restoration. It may act as a gingival irritant because of overextension or underextension of margins, imperfect fit (permitting food and calculus to collect in the sulcal area), or a poor deflecting contour. It may also act as an occlusal irritant by introducing interceptive occlusal contacts into the path of closure or into the various excursions. (Periodont.)

full c. restoration (see **crown, complete veneer**) An individual tooth prosthesis encompassing the entire prepared clinical crown; designed to possess accurate marginal fit, occlusal sluiceways, harmonious axial contours, ridge conformity, contouring of proximal surfaces for embrasures, deflecting contours on buccal and lingual surfaces, and correct supragingival or subgingival location of the cervical extension of the complete crown. A series of connected full crowns, encompassing a series of adjacent teeth, is employed for provisional or permanent stabilization of teeth. (Periodont.)

jacket c. (see **crown, complete veneer, porcelain; crown, complete veneer, acrylic resin**)

partial c. A restoration that covers three or more, but not all, surfaces of a tooth. Used as a retainer or a single-unit restoration. The surfaces involved are usually the lingual, proximal, and occlusal or incisal. (Fixed Part. Prosth.)

porcelain-faced c. An artificial crown that makes use of porcelain inlayed in or veneered onto the labial or buccal surface. (Fixed Part. Prosth.)

c.-root ratio Relation of the clinical crown to the clinical roots of the teeth—an important consideration in diagnosis, prognosis, and treatment planning. (Periodont.)

steel c. A preformed steel crown used for the restoration of badly broken-down primary teeth and first permanent molars. Also used for the temporary restoration of fractured permanent incisors. (Pedodont.)

three-quarter c. Term frequently used to designate a partial veneer crown. (Fixed Part. Prosth.)

veneered metal c. A complete crown that has one or more surfaces prepared for and covered by a tooth-colored substance such as porcelain or resin. (Fixed Part. Prosth.)

crown and bridge prosthodontics The division of prosthodontics that deals with crown restorations and the fixed type of tooth-borne partial denture prosthesis. (Remov. Part. Prosth.) (see also **prosthodontics, fixed**)

Crozat appliance, clasp (see under appropriate noun)

crucible (kroo′sĭ-bl) A vessel or container that will withstand high heat and is used for melting or holding material. (D. Mat.)

c. former (sprue base) The stand or base into which a sprued pattern is placed. It establishes the shape or form of the hollowed-out end of the investment in the casting ring, which will receive the molten metal on its course through the sprue hole. (Oper. Dent.) (see also **sprue former**)

crushing strength (see **strength, compressive**)

cryolite (krī′ō-līt) (**sodium aluminum fluoride [Na₃AlF₆]**) A fluoride often used as a flux in the manufacture of silicate cements. (D. Mat.)

crystal(s) A naturally produced solid. The ultimate units of the substance from which it was formed are arranged systematically.

c. gold (see **gold, mat**)

platinocyanide c. A chemical substance used in the manufacture of fluorescent screens. Barium platinocyanide was first used by Roentgen for this purpose. (Oral Radiol.)

silver halide c. Silver compounds, usually silver bromide and silver iodide, that are impregnated in the photographic emulsion of film. These compounds, when acted on by actinic rays, are disintegrated, with the formation of metallic silver in a finely divided state. The photographic image results when the film is subjected to processing. (Oral Radiol.)

cubic centimeter (cc) Unit of volume sometimes used in prescription writing. For that purpose it may be considered identical with the milliliter (ml). (Oral Med.; Pharmacol.) (see also **milliliter**)

cubital (kū′bĭ-tal) Pertaining to the forearm. (Anesth.)

cubitus (kū′bĭ-tŭs) The forearm. (Anesth.)

cuboid (kū′boid) (**cuboidal**) Resembling a cube in form. (Oper. Dent.)

cuboidal (see **cuboid**)

culture Growth of microorganisms or other living cells on artificial media. (Endodont.)

bacterial c. Bacterial growth on or in an artificial medium. The medium used may be selective for a given type or genus of organism, e.g., tomato juice agar for lactobacilli. (Oral Diag.)

endodontic c. Growth of microorganisms obtained from root canals or periapical tissues. (Endodont.)

c. medium A substance, liquid or solid, used for cultivating bacteria. (Endodont.)

endodontic c. m. A specific medium used for endodontic cultures. (Endodont.)

Cummer's guideline (see **guideline, Cummer's**)

cumulative Increasing in effect. (Anesth.)

cup, chin An orthopedic device that directs a posterior and/or vertical force to the mandible, through the attachment of a cup fitting over the chin to a headcap. (Orthodont.)

cup, suction A thin rubber disk, usually with a hole in its center to fit over a button that is larger in diameter than the hole. This causes the disk to assume a cup shape. When applied on the tissue surface of a denture, the cup attaches itself to the mucous membrane by suction. (Comp. Prosth.)

— A flexible rubber cup that, when moistened, will attach to a flat, exposed surface of a cast to facilitate the removal of the cast from a duplicating impression. (Remov. Part. Prosth.)

curare (koo-rah′rē) A nondepolarizing, peripherally acting, skeletal muscle relaxant. (Anesth.)

— A drug used to cause muscle relaxation during anesthesia by blocking acetylcholine at the neuromuscular and synaptic junctions. (Oral Physiol.)

cure Successful treatment of a disease or wound.

— A procedure or reaction that changes a plastic material to a hard material, e.g., vulcanization or polymerization. (Comp. Prosth.) (see also **process**)

curet, curette (kū-rět′) A periodontal or surgical instrument having a sharp, spoon-shaped working blade; used for debridement. The periodontal curet, available in many sizes and shapes, is used for root and gingival curettage. (Periodont.)

curettage (kū″rě-tahzh′) Scraping or cleaning with a curet. (Oral Surg.)

   apical c. (apoxesis) Curettement of diseased periapical tissue and smoothing of the apical surface of a tooth without excision of the root tip. (Endodont.)

   gingival c. A procedure involving debridement of the inner wall of the pocket, the objective of which is the conversion of a pathologic gingival attachment (pocket) to a state of health. (Periodont.)

      g. c., objectives Therapeutic results, clinical and histologic, expected within the tissues of the gingivae as a consequence of exacting gingival curettage. The expected results include remission of edema and inflammation; complete epithelial débridement of the pocket; removal of the subepithelial zone of connective tissue inflammation, characterized by the presence of intense inflammatory infiltrate; shrinkage of the tissues, with elimination of the pocket; and restoration of physiologic tissue contours. (Periodont.)

   infrabony pocket c. Enucleation, by means of suitable instrumentation, of the inflammatory soft tissue elements lying within and surrounding the crest of an infrabony resorptive defect; also includes the débridement and planing of the root surface of the pocket. (Periodont.)

   pocket epithelium in c. Epithelial tissue in which a pocket, or recess, has been created by means of curettage. In gingival curettage

the entire inner epithelial lining and the epithelial attachment are removed in conjunction with removal of subjacent connective tissue that is inflamed and that contains profuse inflammatory cell infiltrate. The sulcal epithelium and epithelial attachment must be removed to provide access to the underlying inflamed connective tissue and to promote ideal healing. (Periodont.)

   root c. Debridement and planing to smoothness of the root surface of a tooth in order to eliminate accretions on the root and to provide a suitable environment for the return of the gingival tissues to a state of health. (Periodont.)

   subgingival c. The process of debridement of the epithelial attachment, the ulcerated and entire (pocket) epithelium, and subjacent inflamed and altered gingival corium; usually results in resolution of the inflammatory process and desirable shrinkage and repair of the edematous tissue. (Periodont.)

   surgical, apical c. Removal of tissue and debris surrounding the apex of a root. (Endodont.)

curette (see **curet**)

curie (kū′rē) A measurement of radioactivity produced by the disintegration of unstable elements. The curie is that quantity of a radioactive nuclide in which the number of disintegrations per second is 3.700×10^{10}. Since the curie is a relatively large unit, the millicurie (0.001 curie) and the microcurie (one millionth of a curie) are more often used. It is important to note that the curie is based on the number of nuclear disintegrations and not on the number or amount of radiations emitted. The quantity (grams) of radon in equilibrium with 1 g of radium was an earlier definition of the curie. (Oral Radiol.)

curing The act of polymerization. (Comp. Prosth.; D. Mat.; Remov. Part. Prosth.)

   denture c. (see **denture curing**)

current A measure of the number of electrons per second that pass a given point on a conductor. (Oral Radiol.)

   alternating c. A current that alternately changes its direction of flow. The current flows for a given length of time in one direction and then immediately flows in the opposite direction for the same length of time. It usually consists of 60 complete cycles/sec. This current (AC) is one that varies in sine and progresses through both positive and negative values. (Oral Radiol.)

   coagulating c. An electrical current, delivered

by a needle, ball, or other variously shaped points, that coagulates tissue. (Oral Surg.)

direct c. An electrical current in which the electron flow is in only one direction. A current may be intermittent or pulsating and still be called a direct current. Direct current (DC) is a current that does not vary in sine, i.e., from positive to negative values. (Oral Radiol.)

galvanic c. A direct current created by a battery. An electromotive force of 500 mv may exist in the mouth. (D. Mat.)

saturation c. The maximum current in a roentgen ray tube that fully utilizes all electrons that are available at the cathode for the production of roentgen rays. (Oral Radiol.)

curvature, occlusal (see **curve of occlusion**)

curve Nonangular deviation from a straight line or surface. (Comp. Prosth.; Remov. Part. Prosth.)

alignment c. (see **alignment**)

anti-Monson c. (see **curve, reverse**)

compensating c. The curvature of alignment of the occlusal surfaces of the teeth that is developed to compensate for the paths of the condyles as the mandible moves from centric to eccentric positions. A means for maintaining posterior tooth contacts on the molar teeth and providing balancing contacts on dentures when the mandible is protruded. Corresponds to the curve of Spee of natural teeth. (Comp. Prosth.; Remov. Part. Prosth.)

dose-effect c. A curve relating the dose of radiation with the effect produced. (Oral Radiol.)

milled-in c. (see **path, milled-in**)

Monson c. The curve of occlusion, described by Monson, in which each cusp and incisal edge touch or conform to a segment of the surface of a sphere 8 inches in diameter, with its center in the region of the glabella. (Comp. Prosth.; Remov. Part. Prosth.) (see also **curve, compensating**)

c. of occlusion (occlusal curvature) A curved occlusal surface that makes simultaneous contact with the major portion of the incisal and occlusal prominences of the existing teeth. (Comp. Prosth.)

— The curve of a dentition on which the occlusal surfaces of the teeth lie. (Remov. Part. Prosth.)

Pleasure c. An occlusal curve described by Pleasure. (Comp. Prosth.; Remov. Part. Prosth.) (see also **curve, reverse**)

reverse c. A curve of occlusion that is convex

upward when viewed in the frontal plane. (Comp. Prosth.; Remov. Part. Prosth.)

sine c. The wave form of an alternating current, characterized by a rise from zero to maximum positive potential, then descending to zero to its maximum negative value, and then rising to its maximum positive potential, to fall to zero again. (Oral Radiol.)

c. of Spee Anatomic curvature of the occlusal alignment of teeth, beginning at the tip of the lower canine, following the buccal cusps of the natural premolars and molars, and continuing to the anterior border of the ramus, as described by von Spee. (Comp. Prosth.; Oper. Dent.; Remov. Part. Prosth.)

— An imagined circular relation between the curvatures of the articular eminences and those of the occlusal surfaces of the postcanine teeth. Observed by von Spee on selected profile photographs of cadaver heads. Three points—the tip of the lower canine, a tip of a rear cusp, and a point on the edge of the articular eminence—were selected. From these points he located a center around which he drew an arc to show that it coincided with the curvature of the eminence and that of the much-worn buccal teeth. (Gnathol.)

— The curve of the occlusal surfaces of the arches in vertical dimension, brought about by a dipping downward of the mandibular premolars, with a corresponding adjustment of the upper premolars. (Orthodont.)

survival c. A curve obtained by plotting the number or percentage of organisms surviving at a given time against a given dose of radiation. A curve showing the percentage of individuals surviving at different intervals after a particular dosage of radiation. (Oral Radiol.)

c. of Wilson By-product term of the thinking that supported the theory that occlusion should be spherical. The curvature of the cusps as projected on the frontal plane is expressed in both arches. The curve in the lower arch is concave, whereas the one in the upper arch is convex. The curvature in the lower arch is effected by an equal lingual inclination of the right and left molars so that the tip points of the corresponding cross-aligned cusps can be put into the circumference of a circle. The transverse cuspal curvature of the upper teeth is effected by the equal buccal inclinations of their long axes. Natural unworn dentitions display such inclinations but not enough to satisfy what Wilson prescribed for denture teeth. (Gnathol.)

Cushing's syndrome (see **syndrome, Cushing's**)

cusp A notably pointed or rounded eminence on or near the masticating surface of a tooth. (Oper. Dent.)

    c. angle (see **angle, cusp**)

    c. height The shortest distance between the deepest part of the central fossa of a posterior tooth and a line connecting the points of the cusps of the tooth. The shortest distance between the tip of a cusp and its base plane. (Comp. Prosth.; Oper. Dent.; Remov. Part. Prosth.)

    —- The vertical distance between two parallel planes passing at right angles to the long axis of the tooth through the crown so that one plane has in it the highest point of the cusp and the other has in it the lowest point of the fossa. (Gnathol.)

    shoeing c. (see **restoration of cusps**)

cuspal interference (see **contact, deflective occlusal**)

cusp-fossa relations Organic relations between a stamp cusp and its fossa. They are coupled in the intergnathic space in stances and crown rotational relations so that the cross and oblique grooves of the fossa are mere arcs about the condylar axes. The cusp is thus allowed to leave its fossa by either of these grooves and return to its three contact points without a sliding landing. Such relations form centrically related centric occlusion. (Gnathol.)

cuspid (see **canine**)

cuticle The outer layer of the skin. Also, a layer that covers the free surface of an epithelial cell. (Oper. Dent.)

    primary c. The transitory remnants of the enamel organ and oral epithelium covering the enamel of a tooth after eruption. Also called Nasmyth's membrane. (Periodont.)

    — Believed to be the last substance formed by ameloblasts, mediating the attachment of ameloblasts to the enamel. (Periodont.)

    secondary c. The second cuticle formed when the ameloblasts are replaced by the oral epithelium. It then covers the primary cuticle on the enamel and is the only cuticle on the cementum. (Periodont.)

    — A keratinized pedicle found between the gingival epithelium and the surface of a tooth. (Periodont.)

cuticula dentis (kū-tĭk'ū-lah děn'tĭs) (see **cuticle, primary**)

cutting instrument (see **instrument, cutting**)

cutting stream In the airbrasive technique, the stream of abrasive aluminum oxide traveling under pressure from the nozzle of the handpiece to the tooth. (Oper. Dent.)

CVA (see **accident, cerebrovascular**)

cyanocobalamin (sī″ah-nō-kō-băl'ah-mĭn) (see **vitamin B$_{12}$**)

cyanosis (sī-ah-nō'sĭs) Term applied to a characteristic bluish tinge or color of the skin and mucous membranes associated with reduction in hemoglobin brought about by inadequate respiratory change (5 gm/100 ml are necessary for color to be perceptible). (Anesth.; Oral Diag.)

cycle A succession of events.

    chewing c. A complete course of movement of the mandible during a single masticatory stroke. (Comp. Prosth.; Remov. Part. Prosth.)

    masticating c. Three-dimensional patterns of mandibular movements formed during the chewing of food. (Comp. Prosth.; Remov. Part. Prosth.)

    — The movements of the mandible during the chewing of food; controlled by its associated neuromuscular mechanism. Modified by the character of the food being chewed and, to some extent, by the person's pain threshold. (Periodont.)

cyclothymia (sī″klō-thī'mē-ah) (see **psychosis, manic-depressive**)

cyclotron (sī'klō-trahn) A device for accelerating charged particles to high energies by means of an alternating electrical field between electrodes placed in a constant magnetic field. (Oral Radiol.)

cylindroma (sĭl-ĭn-drō'mah) An adenocystic basal cell carcinoma of the salivary glands. A malignant tumor that may occur in the sublingual, submandibular, parotid, or labial salivary glands. (Oral Diag.) (see also **carcinoma, adenocystic**)

cyst (sĭst) A pathologic space in bone or soft tissue containing fluid or semifluid material and, in the oral regions, almost always lined by epithelium. (Oral Diag.; Oral Path.)

    branchial c. (branchial cleft c.) A fluid-filled sac formed along the side of the neck; results from the trapping of epithelium between the branchial arches. (Oral Diag.)

    — Soft tissue cyst usually seen on the lateral side of the neck. Formerly believed to be derived from branchial arch remnants, it has since been shown to be a cyst that arises from epithelial inclusions within the cervical lymph nodes. Microscopic examination shows the epithelial lining of stratified squamous epithelium surrounded by lymphoid tissue. (Oral Path.)

calcifying and keratinizing odontogenic c. A cyst arising from odontogenic epithelium, with abundant production of keratin-containing ghost cells and areas of dystrophic calcification. This lesion has no age or sex distribution. (Oral Diag.)

dental c. (see **cyst, periodontal**)

dentigerous c. An epithelium-lined sac filled with fluid or semifluid material that surrounds the crown of an unerupted tooth or odontoma. (Oral Diag.)

— An odontogenic cyst surrounding the crown of an unerupted tooth or an odontoma. (Oral Path.)

dentoalveolar c. (see **cyst, periodontal**)

dermoid c. An epithelium-lined sac with one or more skin appendages (hair follicles, sweat glands, sebaceous glands) in its wall. It may be found in the floor of the mouth. This lesion should not be confused with the teratomatous dermoid cyst of the ovary. (Oral Diag.)

— A cyst of developmental origin consisting of a fibrous connective tissue wall containing ectodermal appendages and having a lining of stratified squamous epithelium. The lumen may contain keratin, the products of the appendages, or both. (Oral Path.)

— A form of cystic teratoma derived principally from the embryonic germinal epithelium and often containing structures of other germ layers; derived from the enslavement of epithelial debris in the midline during closure of the mandibular and hyoid branchial arches. Often contains keratin, sebaceous glands, hair follicles, sweat glands, and teeth surrounded by a connective tissue wall lined on its inner surface by a stratified squamous epithelium. (Periodont.)

epidermoid c. An epithelium-lined sac containing fluid; possesses characteristics of the epidermis but does not have the skin appendages seen in dermoid cysts. (Oral Diag.)

— A cyst consisting of a fibrous connective tissue wall and lined by keratinized stratified squamous epithelium. The lumen often contains keratin. (Oral Path.)

eruption c. A dentigerous cyst that causes a clinically evident bulging of the overyling alveolar ridge. (Oral Path.)

extravasation c. (see **cyst, traumatic**)

fissural c. A cyst that arises from the enslaved epithelium in maxillary suture lines due to fusion of the embryonic processes of the facial bones. (Oral Path.)

follicular c. An epithelium-lined cyst formed in or from the follicle of the tooth. The term follicular cyst is sometimes considered to be a synonym for primordial cyst, sometimes a synonym for dentigerous cyst, and sometimes a synonym for both. (Oral Diag.)

— An odontogenic cyst that arises from the epithelium of the tooth bud and dental lamina. Follicular cysts include dentigerous, primordial, and multilocular cysts. (Oral Path.)

    lateral f. c. A follicular cyst occurring on the lateral surface of a tooth, usually near the cementodentinoenamel junction. (Oral Path.) (see also **cyst, follicular**)

globulomaxillary c. An epithelium-lined sac formed at the junction point of the globular (median nasal) and maxillary processes. It is seen as a pear-shaped radiolucency between the maxillary lateral incisor and cuspid, and it separates their roots. (Oral Diag.)

— A fissural cyst that develops from epithelial inclusions in the line of fusion of the globular and maxillary processes between the maxillary lateral incisor and the canine. (Oral Path.)

hemorrhagic c. An extravasation cyst or lesion; traumatic bone cyst or lesion. This is not a true cyst but is probably a defect in the bone produced by trauma and repair. It appears as a definite radiolucent area with a sharply marked radiopaque border. It contains air and is lined by a thin endosteum. (Oral Diag.) (see also **cyst, solitary bone**)

incisive canal c. (see **cyst, nasopalatine**)

indefinite bone c. (see **cyst, extravasation**)

lateral c. (see **cyst, periodontal**)

median palatal c. An epithelium-lined sac containing fluid; appears as a radiolucency in the midline of the palate. It is of developmental origin. (Oral Diag.)

mucous c. (mucocele) An epithelium-lined sac containing mucus. Mucous cysts in the sinus may appear as spherical, radiopaque areas. (Oral Diag.)

multilocular c. A follicular cyst containing many loculi, or spaces, and not associated with a tooth. (Oral Path.)

nasoalveolar c. A fluid-containing sac lined by epithelium and located at the ala of the nose. A developmental cyst, it may simulate a nasal or periapical abscess. (Oral Diag.)

—A soft tissue fissural cyst arising at the junction of the globular lateral nasal and maxillary processes. (Oral Path.)

nasopalatine c. (nasopalatine duct) An epithelium-lined sac containing fluid and located in the nasopalatine canal or the incisive canal. (Oral Diag.)

— A cyst arising within the nasopalatine canal. Radiographically it may appear as a heart-shaped radiolucency between the maxillary central incisors. Histologically it may show mucous cells and nerve bundles in addition to a lining of stratified squamous or respiratory epithelium. The incisive canal cyst and the cyst of the papilla incisiva are the recognized subtypes. (Oral Path.)

odontogenic c. An epithelium-lined sac produced from the tooth-forming tissues; e.g., primordial, dentigerous, and periodontal cysts. (Oral Diag.)

— A cyst arising from and lined by odontogenic epithelium. (Oral Path.)

periapical c. (see **cyst, radicular**)

periodontal c. (dental root c., dentoalveolar c., lateral c., periapical c.) An epithelium-lined sac containing fluid. Usually found at the apex of a pulp-involved tooth. Lateral types occur less frequently along the side of the root. (Oral Diag.)

primordial c. An epithelium-lined sac containing fluid and appearing as a radiolucency in the jaws. It is derived from an enamel organ before any hard tissue is formed. (Oral Diag.)

— An odontogenic cyst arising from an enamel organ in lieu of a tooth. (Oral Path.)

radicular c. (periapical c., root end c.) A cyst that has a fibrous connective tissue wall and a lining of stratified squamous epithelium and that is attached to the apex of the root of a tooth with a nonvital pulp or a defective root canal filling. (Oral Path.)

residual c. An odontogenic cyst that remains within the jaw after the removal of the tooth with which it was associated. May be radicular or follicular. (Oral Path.)

root end c. (see **cyst, radicular**)

solitary bone c. A pathologic bone space of disputed origin that may be either empty or filled with fluid. It may have a delicate connective tissue lining. (Oral Path.)

thyroglossal duct c. An epithelium-lined sac containing fluid formed in portions of the incompletely involuted thyroglossal duct, which connects the primitive pharynx with the tongue in embryonic life. These cysts may appear in the midline at any region from the subhyoid to the base of the tongue. (Oral Diag.)

— A developmental cyst arising from remnants of the embryonic thryoglossal duct between the foramen cecum of the tongue and the thyroid gland. (Oral Path.)

traumatic c. (extravasation c., extravasation lesion, traumatic bone lesion) A radiolucent lesion appearing chiefly in the mandible as a well-defined area with a radiopaque border; clinically it appears as a cavity lined by extremely thin periosteum and filled with air. Assumed to be caused by injury to young spongy bone, hemorrhage resorption, and then walling off by cortical bone. (Oral Diag.) (see also **cyst, solitary bone**)

cystadenoma (sĭs-tăd″ĕ-nō′mah) An adenoma with the development of cystic spaces due to dilation of acinar or ductal structures. (Oral Diag.)

papillary c. lymphomatosum (Warthin's tumor) A benign tumor of the parotid gland characterized by cystlike spaces with papillary projections and a lymphoid stroma. (Oral Diag.)

— A benign salivary gland tumor that consists of numerous cystic spaces lined by a double layer of epithelium. A dense aggregate of lymphocytes containing germinal centers surrounds the cystic spaces. (Oral Path.)

cytology, exfoliative (sī-tahl′ō-jē) Study of desquamated cells. (Oral Path.)

cytomegalic inclusion disease (see **disease, salivary gland**)

cytozyme (sī′tō-zīm) (see **thromboplastin**)

D

Dalton's law (see **law, Dalton's**)

dam A barrier to the passage of moisture or saliva. (Endodont.; Oper. Dent.)

post-d. (see **seal, posterior palatal**)

rubber d. A thin sheet of latex rubber used to isolate a tooth or teeth and keep them dry during a dental procedure. (Endodont.; Oper. Dent.)

r. d. punch A hand punch instrument with progressively larger openings, used to make a hole(s) in the rubber dam. (Endodont.)

damages Compensation or indemnity that may be recovered at law by any person who has suffered loss, detriment, or injury to his person, property, or rights through the unlawful act or negligence of another. (D. Juris.)

compensatory d. A sum that compensates the injured party for his injury only. (D. Juris.)

exemplary d. (punitive d.) Damages awarded to the plaintiff over those that will barely compensate him for his property loss. Such compensation may be awarded when the wrong done to the plaintiff involved violence, malice, or fraud by the defendant. The objective is to provide compensation for mental suffering or loss of pride. It may be employed as punishment of the defendant. (D. Juris.)

nominal d. A trifling sum awarded to a plaintiff in an action in which there is no substantial loss or injury to be compensated but in which the law still recognizes a technical invasion of his rights or a breach of the defendant's duty. Also awarded in cases in which, although there has been a real injury, the plaintiff's evidence is not sufficient to show its amount. (D. Juris.)

punitive d. (see **damages, exemplary**)

Darier's disease (see **disease, Darier's**)

darkroom A completely lightproof room or cubicle that is utilized in the processing of photographic, medical, and dental films. (Oral Radiol.) (see also **safe-light**)

datum (dā'tŭm) (plural, data) A fact.

datum symptom The tracings on the gnathic projection plane that do not record condyle motions but are distant effects of movements and furnish data indicative of the positions, movements, and motion directions of points in the axes of the condyle. (Gnathol.)

daughter (decay product) A nuclide formed from the radioactive decay of another nuclide called the parent. (Oral Radiol.)

day sheet A form that permits systematic record keeping of treatment of patients and of monies received and expended. (Pract. Man.)

Day's syndrome (see **syndrome, Riley-Day**)

dead Without life; destitute of life. (Anesth.)

d. space (see **space, physiologic dead; anatomic dead space**)

deaf Without usable hearing. (Cleft Palate)

deafen To make deaf; to cause the loss of all usable hearing. (Cleft Palate)

deafness Impaired hearing.

central d. Impaired hearing due to interference with cerebral auditory pathways or in the auditory centers in the brain (e.g., cerebrovascular accidents and other degenerative brain diseases). May also be found in functional disorders (e.g., conversion hysteria, in which sounds sent over normal pathways appear distorted to the patient). Hearing aids are of little benefit. (Oral Path.; Oral Physiol.)

conduction d. (see **deafness, transmission**)

nerve d. Impaired hearing due to pathology in the auditory nerve or the hair cells of the organ of Corti in the inner ear (e.g., high-tone deafness, which comes with age, damage to the organ of Corti by noise, or a tumor of an auditory nerve). Hearing aids are usually of little benefit. (Oral Physiol.)

transmission d. (conduction d.) Impaired hearing due to interference with passage of sound waves through the external ear (e.g., wax) or the middle ear (e.g., otitis media, aerotitis media, or otosclerosis). May (or may not) be characterized by greater interference with hearing of low tones. Hearing aids that amplify may help. (Oral Physiol.)

deanesthesiant (dē″an-ĕs-thē′zē-ănt) Anything that will arouse a patient from a state of anesthesia. (Anesth.)

death Cessation of life; the stoppage of life beyond the possibility of resuscitation. (Anesth.)
— The cause or occasion of loss of life. (D. Juris.)

debility (dē-bĭl′ĭ-tē) Weakness; lack of strength; asthenia. (Oral Physiol.)

débridement (dā-brēd-maw′) Removal of intracanal material from the root canal system. (Endodont.)

— Removal of foreign material and or devitalized tissue from the vicinity of a wound. Medication and insulation procedures are used. The term has been suggested as a euphemism for the phrase "toilet of the cavity." (Oper. Dent.)

— A technique of scaling and root planing to resolve edema and inflammation and to shrink the gingival tissues. (Periodont.)

epithelial d. (deepithelization) Removal of the entire inner lining and the epithelial attachment from a gingival or periodontal pocket; a phase of gingival curettage. Deepithelization is necessary not only to remove ulcerated sulcate epithelium, which provides an avenue of ingress into the subjacent connective tissue for bacteria and their toxins, but also to remove any vestiges of epithelium that could act as a barrier to the reattachment of newly formed connective tissue to the tooth. (Periodont.)

debris (dĕ-brē′) Foreign material or particles loosely attached to a surface. (Oper. Dent.)

d. of Malassez (măl-ah-sā′) Remnants of Hertwig's epithelial root sheath within the periodontal ligament. (Oral Path.)

debt A sum of money due by agreement; the contract may or may not be express and does not necessarily fix the precise amount to be paid. (D. Juris.)

decalcification (dē-kăl″sĭ-fĭ-kā′shŭn) Loss or removal of calcium salts from calcified tissues. (Oral Diag.; Oper. Dent.)

decay (objectionable as a synonym for **area of decay, caries,** or **carious lesion**) Chemically decomposed dentin or enamel. (Oper. Dent.)

d. product (see **daughter**)

radioactive d. Disintegration of the nucleus of an unstable nuclide by the spontaneous emission of charged particles and/or photons. (Oral Radiol.)

secondary d. (see **caries, dental, secondary**)
senile d. (see **caries, dental, senile**)

decibel (dĕs′ĭ-bĕl) A logarithmic ratio unit that indicates by what proportion one intensity level differs from another. One decibel is equal to the least intensity of sound at which any given tone can be heard. It is sometimes inaccurately called a sensation unit. (Cleft Palate)

deciduous (dē-sĭd′ū-ŭs) That which will be shed. Term pertains specifically to the first dentition of man or animal. Given preference over the terms primary and temporary. (Oper. Dent.)

d. dentition Term that refers to the first teeth. (Oper. Dent.)

d. teeth The teeth constituting the first dentition. (Oper. Dent.)

declaration and provision for affairs A systematic statement of the affairs and estate of a person, in which all of his assets and property are listed. (Pract. Man.)

decompression, nerve Release of pressure on a nerve trunk by surgical widening of the bony canal. (Oral Surg.)

decuspation (dē-kŭsp-ā′shŭn) Removal or complete reduction of the cusp of a tooth. (Endodont.)

deep bite (see **overbite, deep**)
deep sensibility (see **sensibility, deep**)
deepithelization (dē-ĕp″ĭ-thē″lĭ-zā′shŭn) (see **débridement, epithelial**)
DEF rate (see **rate, DEF**)

defamation (dĕf-ah-mā′shŭn) The act of detracting from the reputation of another. The offense of injuring a person's reputation by false and malicious statements. (D. Juris.)

default Omission or failure to fulfill an obligation or a promise; failure to accomplish an agreement. (D. Juris.)

defect Absence of some legal requisite; an imperfection. (D. Juris.)

operative d. Incomplete repair of bone after root resection or periapical curettage. (Endodont.)

osseous d. A concavity in the bone surrounding one or more teeth, resulting from periodontal disease. (Periodont.)

speech d. Any deviation of speech that is outside the range of acceptable variation in a given environment. (Cleft Palate)

defective, mental A mentally subnormal individual. A person in whom a basic nervous system defect may be assumed because of social and intellectual deficiencies; e.g., persons afflicted with microcephaly, hydrocephalus, or mongolism. (Periodont.)

defendant (dē-fĕnd′ănt) The person denying; the party against whom recovery is sought in a court of law. (D. Juris.)

defense The reason that is offered and alleged by the party processed against in an action or suit as to why, in law or fact, the plaintiff should not recover or establish what he seeks. It may be a denial, justification, confession, or avoidance of the facts affirmed as a ground of action or an exception to their sufficiency in point of law. (D. Juris.)

d. cell (see **cell, defense**)

defibrillation (dē-fĭ″brĭ-lā′shŭn) The arrest of

fibrillation, usually that of the cardiac ventricles. An intense alternating current is briefly passed through the heart muscle, throwing it into a refractory state. (Anesth.)

defibrillator (dē-fǐ′brǐ-lā″tor) An apparatus for defibrillating the ventricles of the heart. (Anesth.)

deficiency A lack or defect.

ac-globulin d. (see **parahemophilia**)

dietary d. An inadequate amount of food intake or an insufficiency of any of the food elements necessary for proper nutrition. (Comp. Prosth.)

mineral d. A form of nutritional deficiency produced by the inadequate ingestion, absorption, utilization, and/or overexcretion of essential inorganic elements such as calcium, magnesium, or phosphorus. (Periodont.)

nicotinic acid d. Deficiency of nicotinic acid in the diet, resulting in acute erythematous stomatitis, papillary atrophy of the tongue, and ulcerative gingivitis. (Periodont.)

plasma thromboplastic antecedent d. (see **hemophilia C**)

protein d. A malnutritive state produced by inadequate ingestion, absorption, utilization, and/or overexcretion of essential protein elements. Degenerative lesions produced in the periodontium include osteoporosis of the alveolar and supporting bone and disappearance of fibroblasts and connective tissue fibers of the periodontal membrane. Gingival changes occur only after the introduction of local etiologic factors capable of inducing local inflammatory changes. (Periodont.)

PTA d. (see **hemophilia C**)

vitamin A d., gingival hyperplasia in Hyperplastic and hyperkeratotic gingival changes occurring with decreased ingestion, diminished absorption, faulty utilization, or overexcretion of vitamin A; e.g., in diabetes the liver often cannot effectively convert carotene to vitamin A. (Periodont.)

definition (image) The property of projected images relating to their sharpness, distinctness, or clarity of outline. Penumbra width is a measure of definition. (Oral Radiol.) (see also **resolution**)

deflective occlusal contact (see **contact, deflective occlusal**)

deformation (dē″for-mā′shŭn) Distortion; disfigurement.

elastic d. Term applied when the alteration

in shape of a material disappears as the causative load is removed. (Oper. Dent.)

inelastic d. Deformation occurring when a material is stressed beyond its elastic limit. (D. Mat.)

permanent d. Deformation occurring beyond the yield point so that the structure will not return to its original dimensions after removal of the applied force. (Oper. Dent.)

deformity Distortion or disfigurement of a portion of the body; may be congenital, familial, hereditary, acquired, pathologic, or surgical. (Oral Surg.)

bone d. Interdental defect. (Periodont.)

gingival d. Deviation from the normal gingival topographic and architectural pattern occurring as a result of inflammatory, degenerative, or neoplastic diseases; e.g., gingival cleft, gingival crater, and hyperplasia associated with the ingestion of diphenylhydantoin sodium (Dilantin sodium). (Periodont.)

macromandibular d. Overdeveloped mandible. (Orthodont.)

macromaxillary d. Overdeveloped maxillae. (Orthodont.)

micromandibular d. Underdeveloped mandible. (Orthodont.)

micromaxillary d. Underdeveloped maxillae. (Orthodont.)

degeneration, ballooning A condition seen in vesicles of viral origin, in which epithelial cells are washed from the vesicle wall. The cells swell and their nuclei undergo amitotic division, resulting in multinucleated giant cells that may be seen floating in vesicular fluid. (Oral Path.)

degeneration, basophilic granular (bā″sō-fĭl′ĭk) (see **basophilia**)

degloving Intraoral surgical exposure of the bony mandibular anterior region. This procedure can be performed in the posterior region if necessary. (Oral Surg.)

deglutition (dĕg″loo-tĭsh′ŭn) **(swallowing)** The act of swallowing, mediated by a complex neuromuscular mechanism controlling the actions of the tongue the mandible, the soft palate, the uvula, the pharyngeal musculature, etc. (Anesth.; Periodont.)

— A succession of muscular contractions from above downward or from the front backward; propels food from the mouth toward the stomach. The action is generally initiated at the lips; it proceeds back through the oral cavity, and the food is moved automatically along the dorsum of the tongue. When the food is ready for swallowing, it is passed back through the fauces. Once the food is beyond the fauces and in the pharynx, the soft palate closes off the nasopharynx, and the hyoid bone and larynx are elevated upward and forward. This action keeps food out of the larynx and dilates the esophageal opening so that the food may be passed quickly toward the stomach by peristaltic contractions. The separation between the voluntary and the involuntary characteristics of this wave of contractions is not sharply defined. At birth the process is already well established as a highly coordinated activity, i.e., the swallowing reflex. (Oral Physiol.)

degradation (dĕg-rah-dā'shŭn) Reduction of a chemical compound to a less complex compound, e.g., when one or more groups are split off. (Anesth.)

dehiscence (dē-hĭs'ĕns) A fissural defect in the facial alveolar plate extending from the free margin apically. (Orthodont.)

dehiscent (dē-hĭs'ĕnt) Opened wide; fissured.

   d. mandibular canal A condition caused by bone resorption, which leaves the mandibular canal without a covering or roof of bone. The contents are found in a trough or sometimes merely lying in the soft tissues at the crest of the ridge. (Oral Implant.)

dehydration (dē"hī-drā'shŭn) Removal of water, e.g., from the body or tissue. (Anesth.)

— Decrease in serum fluid coupled with the loss of interstitial fluid from the body. Dehydration is associated with disturbances in fluid and electrolyte balance. (Oral Physiol.)

   d. of gingivae The drying of gingival tissue, leading to a lowered tissue resistance, which can result in gingival inflammation; seen in mouth breathing. (Periodont.)

delayed expansion (see **expansion, delayed**)

delict (dē-lĭkt') A wrong or an injury; an offense; a violation of public or private obligation. (D. Juris.)

delinquent, *adj.* (dē-lĭng'kwĕnt) Pertaining to a debt or claim that is due and unpaid at the time due. (D. Juris.)

delirium A condition of mental excitement, confusion, and clouded sensorium, usually with hallucinations, illusions, and delusions; precipitated by toxic factors in diseases or drugs. (Anesth.)

   d. tremens A delirious state marked by distressing delusions, illusions, and hallucinations, constant tremor, fumbling movements of the hands, insomnia, and great exhaustion. (Anesth.)

delivery Transfer of the possession of personal property from one person to another. (D. Juris.)

dementia (dē-mĕn'shē-ah) Progressive deterioration of judgment and memory associated with brain damage; e.g., senile psychosis. (Oral Med.)

   d. precox Term formerly used to refer to mental deterioration at an early age but now outmoded in favor of the term schizophrenia. (Oral Med.) (see also **schizophrenia**)

Demerol (dĕm'er-ahl) Proprietary brand of meperidine hydrochloride. (Pharmacol.)

demurrer (dē-mĕr'ĕr) An admission of the facts charged by the opponent while maintaining that those facts are legally insufficient to establish liability. (D. Juris.)

denasality (dē-nā-săl'ĭ-tē) The quality of the voice when the nasal passages are obstructed, preventing adequate nasal resonance during speech. (Cleft Palate)

dendrite (dĕn'drīt) The process of a neuron that carries the nerve impulse to the cell body. (Anesth.)

— Fingerlike projections formed during the solidification of crystalline materials. (D. Mat.)

— A branched, treelike protoplasmic process of a neuron that carries nerve impulses toward the cell body. (Oral Physiol.) (see also **axon**)

denervation (dē"ner-vā'shŭn) Sectioning or removal of a nerve to interrupt the nerve supply to a part. (Anesth.)

dens in dente (dĕnz ĭn dĕn'tā) (**dens invaginatus, gestant odontoma**) Anomaly of the tooth found chiefly in upper lateral incisors; characterized by invagination of the enamel at the incisal edge, giving a radiographic appearance that suggests a "tooth within a tooth." (Oral Diag.)

— Invagination of the enamel organ into the dental papilla before calcification has occurred. (Oral Path.)

dens invaginatus (dĕnz ĭn-văj-ĭn-ā'tŭs) (see **dens in dente**)

Densite (dĕn'sīt) Proprietary name for a form of alpha-hemihydrate with a low setting expansion and greater hardness; used for dies, models, and casts; sometimes referred to as a Class II stone. (D. Mat.)

densitometer (dĕn"sĭ-tŏm'ĕ-ter) An instrument for determining the degree of darkening of developed photographic or x-ray film, based on the use of a photocell to measure the light transmission through a given area of the film. (Oral Radiol.)

density Concentration of matter, measured by mass per unit volume. (D. Mat.)

— The quality or condition of compactness. (Remov. Part. Prosth.)

radiographic d. The degree of darkening of exposed and processed photographic or x-ray film, expressed as the logarithm of the opacity of a given area of the film. (Oral Radiol.) (see also **opacity**)

dental Relating to the teeth.

d. arch (see **arch, dental**)

d. assistant (see **assistant, dental**)

d. caries (see **caries, dental**)

d. cement (see **cement, dental**)

d. chart (see **chart, dental**)

d. dysfunction (see **dysfunction, dental**)

d. engine (see **engine, dental**)

d. floss Waxed or plain thread of nylon or silk; used to carry a rubber dam through contact areas, to test contacts, or to disengage loose debris or plaque from contact areas or interproximal spaces. (Oper. Dent.)

— Wax-impregnated or wax-covered nylon string, generally flattened, used to clean the interdental areas; an aid in oral physiotherapy. (Periodont.)

d. geriatrics (see **geriatrics, dental**)

d. granuloma (see **granuloma, dental**)

d. handpiece (see **handpiece**)

d. history (see **history, dental**)

d. hygienist (see **hygienist, dental**)

d. implant (see **implant, dental**)

d. jurisprudence (see **jurisprudence, dental**)

d. laboratory technician (see **technician, dental laboratory**)

d. material (see **material, dental**)

d. porcelain (see **porcelain, dental**)

d. prosthetic restoration (see **prosthesis, dental**)

d. senescence (see **senescence, dental**)

d. stone (see **stone, dental**)

d. tape (see **tape, dental**)

d. unit (see **unit, dental**)

dentate (den'tāt) Having teeth. (Remov. Part. Prosth.)

denticle (den'tĭ-kl) (**endolith, pulp nodule, pulpstone**) A calcified deposit in the dental pulp. (Endodont.)

— Focal nodules of dentin within the pulp chamber or root canal. They may be free in the pulp or attached to the dentinal wall. (Oral Path.)

— A calcified body found in the pulp chamber of a tooth; it may be composed either of irregular dentin (true denticle) or an ectopic calcification of pulp tissue (false denticle). (Periodont.)

dentifrice A pharmaceutical compound utilized in conjunction with the toothbrush to clean and polish the teeth. Contains a mild abrasive, a detergent, flavoring agent, binder, and occasionally deodorants and various medicaments designed as caries preventives, e.g., antiseptics. (Periodont.)

d. abrasion (see **abrasion, dentifrice**)

dentin (den'tĭn) (**dentine**) The portion of the tooth that lies subjacent to the enamel and cementum. Consists of an organic matrix on which mineral (calcific) salts are deposited; pierced by tubules containing filamentous protoplasmic processes of the odontoblasts that line the pulpal chamber and canal. It is of mesodermal origin. (Oper. Dent.; Periodont.)

carious d. Dentin that is involved in or affected by the carious process. (Oper. Dent.)

residual c. d. (see **caries, dental, residual**)

d. dysplasia (see **dysplasia, dentinal**)

d. eburnation (ē-bŭr-nā'shŭn) A change in carious teeth in which the softened and decalcified dentin assumes a hard, brown, polished appearance. (Oral Path.)

hereditary opalescent d. (see **dentinogenesis imperfecta**)

hyperesthesia of d. Excessive sensibility of dentin. (Oper. Dent.)

sclerotic d. (see **dentin, transparent**)

secondary d. Dentin formed or deposited on the walls of pulp chambers and canals subsequent to the complete formation of the tooth; due to certain metabolic disturbances that result in irritation and stimulation of the odontoblasts to renewed activity. (Oper. Dent.)

transparent d. (**sclerotic d.**) Dentin formed as a defense mechanism in reaction to various stimuli. Dental tubules are obliterated by deposits of calcium salts that are harder and denser than normal dentin. This dentin appears transparent in ground sections. (Oper. Dent.)

d. wall The portion of the wall of a prepared cavity that consists of dentin. (Oper. Dent.)

dentine (see **dentin**)

dentinocemental junction (den-tē"nō-sē-men'tal) (see **junction, dentinocemental**)

dentinoenamel junction (see **junction, dentinoenamel**)

dentinogenesis imperfecta (den"tĭ-nō-jen'ĕ-sĭs im-per-fĕk'tah) (**hereditary opalescent dentin**) Disturbance of the dentin of genetic origin; characterized by early calcification of the pulp chambers and root canals, marked attrition, and an opalescent hue to the teeth. (Oral Diag.)

— A localized form of mesodermal dysplasia affecting the dentin of the tooth. It may be hereditary and may be associated with osteogenesis imperfecta. (Oral Path.)

— A hereditary condition associated with a defect in dentin formation; the enamel remains normal. (Pedodont.)

dentinoma (děn″tĭ-nō′mah) An odontogenic tumor composed of regular or irregular dentin. (Oral Path.)

dentist One whose profession is to treat diseases and injuries of the teeth and oral cavity and to construct and insert restorations of and for teeth. (D. Juris.)

dentistry The department of medicine that is concerned with the teeth, oral cavity, and associated parts, including the prevention, diagnosis, and treatment of their diseases and the restoration of defective and missing tissue; the work done by dentists, such as fillings, crowns, and partial and complete dentures; the dental profession collectively.

— The science and art of preventing, diagnosing, and treating diseases, injuries, and malformations of the teeth, jaws, and mouth and of replacing lost or absent teeth and associated structures. (Comp. Prosth.)

faulty d. Improperly executed dental restorations (e.g., rough fillings, overextended crowns, improperly contoured restorations, and faulty clasps on partial dentures) that often cause food impaction and retention and/or periodontal inflammation and destruction; may contribute to additional adverse changes in the tooth substance. Also, improperly planned or executed dental therapy, e.g., overhanging restorations, faulty contact, and ill-fitting dentures, any or all of which may contribute to the destruction of the teeth or their supporting structures. (Periodont.)

forensic d. (see **jurisprudence, dental**)

four-handed d. The technique of chairside operating in which four hands are kept busy working in the oral cavity simultaneously. (Pract. Man.)

operative d. The branch of oral health service concerned with operations to restore or reform the hard dental tissues; e.g., operations that are necessitated by caries, trauma, impaired function, and the improvement of appearance. (Oper. Dent.)

prosthetic d. (see **prosthodontics**)

psychosomatic d. Dentistry that concerns itself with the mind-body relationship. (Comp. Prosth.)

washed-field d. Constant flushing of the operative field with an irrigant (usually water) and the evacuation of the washing (debris, etc.) from the mouth by vacuum airstream. (Oper. Dent.) (see also **technique, hydroflow**)

dentition (děn-tĭsh′ŭn) The natural teeth in position in the dental arches. (Comp. Prosth.)

— The kind, number, and arrangement of the teeth of an animal. (Oper. Dent.)

artificial d. Artificial substitutes for the natural dentition. (Comp. Prosth.; Remov. Part. Prosth.) (see also **denture**)

deciduous d. (see **dentition, primary**)

mixed d. The complement of teeth in the jaws after the eruption of some of the permanent teeth but before all the deciduous teeth are absent. (Remov. Part. Prosth.)

natural d. The natural teeth, as considered collectively, in the dental arch; may be deciduous, permanent, or mixed. (Comp. Prosth.)

permanent d. (secondary d., permanent teeth) The thirty-two teeth of adulthood that either replace or are added to the complement of deciduous teeth. (Comp. Prosth.; Oper. Dent.; Remov. Part. Prosth.)

d., physiologic forces affecting The forces developed by the muscles of mastication, facial muscles, and tongue muscles, which normally exist in functional equilibrium, counteracting one another. (Periodont.)

primary d. The teeth that erupt first and are usually replaced by the permanent teeth. (Comp. Prosth.; Remov. Part. Prosth.)

prognosis of d. Evaluation by the dentist of the prospect of recovery from dental, periodontal, or other disease, combined with a forecast of the probability of maintaining the dentition and associated structures in function and health. (Periodont.)

secondary d. (see **dentition, permanent**)

Dentocoll Proprietary elastic reversible hydrocolloid introduced as a dental impression material. (Remov. Part. Prosth.)

dentode (děn-tōd) An exact reproduction of a tooth on a gnathographically mounted cast. (Gnathol.)

dentoenamel junction (see **junction, dentinoenamel**)

dentoform A mock-up of the dentition and alveolar structures; used as a teaching aid or for display purposes. (Orthodont.)

dentulism (děnt′ū-lĭzm) (see **dentulous**)

dentulous (děnt′ū-lŭs) (**dentulism**) Having the natural teeth present in the mouth. (Comp.

Prosth.; Fixed Part. Prosth.; Remov. Part. Prosth.)

denture An artificial substitute for missing natural teeth and adjacent tissues. (Fixed Part. Prosth.; Comp. Prosth.; Remov. Part. Prosth.)

acrylic resin d. A denture made of acrylic resin. (Comp. Prosth.)

artificial d. (see **denture**)

basal surface of d. (impression surface of d., foundation surface of d.) The part of a denture base that is shaped to conform to that of the basal seat for the denture. The impression surface of a denture; the portion that has its contour determined by the impression. It includes the denture borders and extends to the polished surface. (Comp. Prosth.; Remov. Part. Prosth.)

d. brush A brush designed especially for cleaning dentures. (Comp. Prosth.; Remov. Part. Prosth.)

d. characterization Modification of the form and color of the denture base and teeth to produce a more lifelike appearance. (Comp. Prosth.; Remov. Part. Prosth.)

complete d. (complete dental prosthesis) A dental prosthesis that replaces the lost natural dentition and associated structures of the maxillae or mandible. (Comp. Prosth.; Remov. Part. Prosth.)

    implant c. d. A complete prosthodontic appliance consisting of (1) a fixed part, called the substructure or the implant proper, that is placed under the mucoperiosteum and (2) a removable part, called the superstructure, that bears the teeth. (Oral Implant.)

continuous gum d. An artificial denture consisting of porcelain teeth and tinted porcelain denture base material, fused to a platinum base. (Comp. Prosth.; Remov. Part. Prosth.)

d. coverage The extent to which the oral tissue is covered by the denture base. (Remov. Part. Prosth.)

d. curing The process by which the denture-base materials are hardened in a denture mold to the form of a denture. (Comp. Prosth.; Remov. Part. Prosth.) (see also **process**)

d. design A planned visualization of the form and extent of a denture. It is arrived at after a study of all factors involved. (Comp. Prosth.)

d. dislodging force (see **force, denture dislodging**)

duplicate d. A second denture intended to be a copy of the first denture. (Comp. Prosth.; Remov. Part. Prosth.)

d. edge (see **border, denture**)

d. esthetics (see **esthetics, denture**)

d., finish of The final perfection of the form of the polished surfaces of a denture. (Comp. Prosth.; Remov. Part. Prosth.)

d. flange (see **flange, denture**)

d. foundation The portion of the oral structures that is available to support a denture; the basal seat. (Comp. Prosth.; Remov. Part. Prosth.)

    d. f. area The portion of the basal seat that supports the complete or partial denture base under occlusal load. (Comp. Prosth.; Remov. Part. Prosth.) (see also **area, basal seat**)

    d. f., surface of (see **denture, basal surface of**)

full d. (see **denture, complete**)

heel of d. (see **distal end**)

immediate d. (immediate-insertion d.) A removable dental prosthesis constructed for placement immediately after removal of the remaining natural teeth. (Comp. Prosth.; Remov. Part. Prosth.)

implant d. A denture that gains its support, stability, and retention from a substructure that is implanted under the soft tissues of the basal seat of the denture and is in contact with bone. (Comp. Prosth.; Remov. Part. Prosth.)

    i. d. substructure (see **substructure, implant**)

    i. d. superstructure (see **superstructure, implant**)

impression surface of d. (see **denture, basal surface of**)

interim d. A dental prosthesis to be used for a short interval of time for reasons of esthetics, mastication, occlusal support, or convenience, or to condition the patient to the acceptance of an artificial substitute for missing natural teeth until more definitive prosthodontic treatment can be provided. (Comp. Prosth.; Remov. Part. Prosth.)

maintenance of d. An important part of prosthodontic treatment and a major factor in the longevity of the service that the restoration can be expected to give. (Comp. Prosth.; Remov. Part. Prosth.)

metal base d. A denture with a base of gold, chrome-cobalt alloy, aluminum, or other metal. (Comp. Prosth.; Remov. Part. Prosth.)

model d., wax (see **denture, trial**)

occlusal surface of d. The portion of the surface of a tooth, denture, or dentition that makes contact or near contact with the corresponding surface of the opposing tooth, denture, or dentition. (Comp. Prosth.; Remov. Part. Prosth.)

d. packing (see **packing, denture**)

partial d. (partial dental prosthesis) A prosthesis that replaces one or more, but less than all, of the natural teeth and associated structures and that is supported by the teeth and/or mucosa; may be removable or fixed. (Fixed Part. Prosth.; Remov. Part. Prosth.)

bilateral p. d. A dental prosthesis that supplies teeth and associated structures on both sides of a semiedentulous arch. (Fixed Part. Prosth.; Remov. Part. Prosth.)

cantilever p. d. (see **denture, partial, fixed, cantilever**)

components of p. d. The units that compose a removable partial denture; e.g., the base, the artificial teeth, direct and indirect retainers, and major and minor connectors. (Remov. Part. Prosth.)

construction of p. d. The science and technique of designing and constructing partial dentures. (Remov. Part. Prosth.)

extension p. d. A removable partial denture that is retained by natural teeth at one end of the denture base segments only; a portion of the functional load is carried by the residual ridge. (Remov. Part. Prosth.)

fixed p. d. A partial denture that cannot be readily removed by either the patient or dentist; it is intended to be permanently attached to the teeth or roots that furnish support to the restoration. (Comp. Prosth.; Fixed Part. Prosth.; Remov. Part. Prosth.)

cantilever f. p. d. A fixed dental prosthesis that has one or more abutments at one end of the fixed partial denture supporting pontic(s) at its other end. (Fixed Part. Prosth.; Remov. Part. Prosth.)

p. d., instruction to patient Instruction to the patient undergoing treatment with removable partial dentures, to increase the patient's knowledge of the oral cavity, its care, and maintenance procedures for the restoration. (Remov. Part. Prosth.)

removable p. d. A partial denture that can be readily placed in the mouth and removed by the wearer. (Fixed Part. Prosth.; Remov. Part. Prosth.)

temporary p. d. (see **denture, partial, treatment**)

tissue-borne p. d. A removable partial denture that is vertically supported entirely by the structure subadjacent to its base. (Fixed Part. Prosth.; Remov. Part. Prosth.)

tooth-borne p. d. A partial denture that is supported entirely by the teeth that bound the edentulous area covered by the base. (Remov. Part. Prosth.)

tooth-borne/tissue-borne p. d. A partial denture that gains support from both an abutment tooth or teeth and from the structures of an edentulous area covered by the base. (Remov. Part. Prosth.)

treatment p. d. (temporary p. d.) A dental prosthesis used for the purpose of treating or conditioning the tissues that are called on to support and retain a denture base. (Remov. Part. Prosth.)

unilateral p. d. A dental prosthesis that restores lost or missing teeth on one side of the arch only. (Remov. Part. Prosth.)

d. periphery (see **border, denture**)

polished surface of d. The portion of the surface of a denture that extends in an occlusal direction from the border of the denture and includes the palatal surface. It is the part of the denture base that is usually polished and includes the buccal and lingual surfaces of the teeth. (Comp. Prosth.)

d. processing (see **processing, denture**)

d. prognosis (see **prognosis, denture**)

d. retention (see **retention, denture**)

d. space The space between the residual ridges and between the cheeks and the tongue that is available for dentures. (Comp. Prosth.) (see also **distance, interarch**)
— The portion of the oral cavity that is or may be occupied by a maxillary and/or mandibular denture(s). (Remov. Part. Prosth.)

d. stability (see **stability, denture**)

d.-supporting structure (see **structure, denture-supporting**)

temporary d. A denture intended to serve a very short time in a temporary or emergency situation. (Comp. Prosth.; Remov. Part. Prosth.)

transitional d. A removable partial denture that serves as a temporary prosthesis to which teeth will be added as more teeth are lost and that will be replaced after postextraction tissue changes have occurred. A transitional denture may become an interim denture when all the teeth have been removed from the dental arch. (Remov. Part. Prosth.)

trial d. (model d., wax) A temporary denture, usually made of wax on a baseplate, that is used for checking jaw relation records, occlusion, and the arrangement and observation of teeth for esthetics. (Comp. Prosth.; Remov. Part. Prosth.)

denture-bearing area (see **area, basal seat**)

denture-sore mouth (see **mouth, denture-sore**)

denture-supporting area (see **area, basal seat**)

dependency Addiction to drugs. The quality of being dependent on another—a significant and important human characteristic. The human organism requires a long period of physical, emotional, and social dependency from infancy to adulthood. Dependency appropriate to infancy, childhood, and adolescence may be fixed and retained in adulthood because of some emotional trauma early in life. In the normal mature adult there is a degree of acceptable dependency. This dependency is modified so that he lives more in a world of interdependence between individuals. Therefore, mature adults regard neither independence as isolation nor dependence as helplessness, but rather regard both as symbiotic mechanisms wherein they support each other. (Oral Physiol.)

overt d. Behavior that is demanding, urgent, and repetitious—that is, childish. A patient exhibiting such behavior wants immediate and continuous attention by the dentist, the hygienist, and the assistant. When it is not available, he may be aggressive and abusive. (Oral Physiol.)

depletion, salt (dē-plē'shŭn) A condition resulting from inadequate water intake, low intake of sodium and chlorides in the alimentary tract, and secretion of sweat and urine. The most significant of these losses are the gastrointestinal fluid losses resulting from vomiting, diarrhea, and fistulas. (Oral Physiol.)

depolarization (dē-pō"lar-ĭ-zā'shŭn) Neutralization of polarity; the breaking down of polarized semipermeable membranes, as in nerve or muscle cells in the induction of impulses. (Anesth.)

deponent (dē-pō'nĕnt) One who testifies or makes oath in writing to the truth of certain facts. (D. Juris.)

deposit, bismuth (see **stomatitis, bismuth**)

deposit, calcareous (see **calculus**)

deposition (dĕp-ō-zĭ'shŭn) Evidence given by a witness under interrogatories, oral or written, and usually written down by an official person and intended to be used on the trial of an action in court. (D. Juris.)

depot (dē'pō) In physiology, the site of accumulation, deposit, or storage of body products not immediately or actively involved in metabolic processes; e.g., a fat depot. (Anesth.)

depreciation The annual monetary loss of value of dental equipment. (Pract. Man.)

depressant (dē-prĕs'ănt) A medicine that diminishes functional activity. (Anesth.)

depression (dē-prĕsh'ŭn) Decrease of functional activity. (Anesth.)

— Absence of cheerfulness or hope; dejection. (Oral Physiol.)

emotional d. A state of mental dejection, often resulting in such consequences as poor oral hygiene due to neglect, indifference anorexia with subsequent vitamin and other dietary deficiencies, adverse oral habits (e.g., thumbsucking and bruxism), decrease in blood circulation with lowering of tissue tone, and diminution of resistance to infection. (Periodont.)

derivative (dē-rĭv'ah-tĭv) A chemical substance that is the result of a chemical reaction. (Anesth.)

dermatalgia (der-mah-tăl'jē-ah) Pain, burning, and other sensations of the skin unaccompanied by any structural change; probably caused by some nervous disease or reflex influence. (Anesth.)

dermataneuria (der"mat-ah-nū're-ah) Derangement of the nerve supply of the skin, causing disturbance of sensation. (Anesth.)

dermatitis (der-mah-tī'tĭs) Inflammation of the skin. (Oral Path.)

d. herpetiformis Dermatitis characterized by grouped, erythematous, papular, vesicular, pustular, or bullous lesions occurring in various combinations, often accompanied by vesicobullous and ulcerative lesions of the oral mucous membranes. (Periodont.)

d. infectiosa eczematoides (Engman's disease) A pustular eczematous eruption that frequently follows or occurs coincidentally with some pyogenic process. (Oral Path.)

radiation d. Inflammation of the skin resulting from a high dose of radiation. The reaction varies with the quality and quantity of radiation used and is usually transitory. (Oral Radiol.)

dermatomyositis (der"mah-tō-mī"ō-sī'tĭs) **(polymyositis, dermatomucosomyositis)** A form of collagen disease related to scleroderma and lupus erythematosus. The skin lesions are diffuse erythematous desquamations, or rashlike lesions. The skin symptoms are related to a variety of patterns of myositis. (Oral Diag.)

dermatosclerosis (der″mah-tō-sklĕ-rō′sĭs) (see **scleroderma**)

dermatosis (der″mah-tō′sĭs) Any disease of the skin. (Oral Med.)

desaturation (dē-săt″ŭr-ā′shŭn) Conversion of a saturated compound (e.g., stearin) into an unsaturated compound (e.g., olein) by the removal of hydrogen. (Anesth.)

desensitization (dē-sĕn″sĭ-tĭ-zā′shŭn) A condition of insusceptibility to infection or an allergen; established in experimental animals by the injection of an antigen that produces sensitization or an anaphylactic reaction. After recovery, a second injection of the antigen is made, bringing about no reaction and thus producing desensitization. (Anesth.)

desiccate (dĕs′-ĭ-kāt) To dry by chemical or physical means; e.g., electrocoagulation can produce deep desiccation in tissues; usually accomplished by the insertion of a monoterminal electrode into the tissues, producing dehydration and coagulation. (Oral Surg.)

desiccation (dĕs″ĭ-kā′shŭn) Excessive loss of moisture; the process of drying up. (Oper. Dent.) (see also **electrocoagulation**)

design, *n.* An outline and/or drawing of a proposed prosthesis. (Remov. Part. Prosth.)

—, *v.* To plan and/or delineate by drawing the outline of a proposed prosthesis. (Remov. Part. Prosth.)

desmolysis (dĕs-mol′ĭ-sĭs) Destruction and disintegration of connective tissue. Some authorities connect this desmolytic process with the destruction of connective tissue lying between the enamel and oral epithelium, which thus permits proliferation of the oral epithelium and fusion of enamel and oral epithelium. (Periodont.)

desmosomes (see **epithelium, desmosomes of**)

detail, radiographic A component portion of some larger image, its visibility being dependent on the factors of definition and radiographic contrast. (Oral Radiol.)

detector, radiation (see **radiation detector**)

detention Restraint; custody; confinement. (D. Juris.)

detergent A cleanser. Also applied in a more specific sense to chemicals that possess surface-active properties in water and whose solutions are therefore able to wet surfaces that are normally water-repellant and thereby assist in the mechanical dispersion and emulsification of fatty or oily material and other substances that soil the surface. (Oral Med.; Pharmacol.)

anionic d. A detergent in which the cleansing action resides in the anion. Soaps and many synthetic detergents are anionic. (Oral Med.; Pharmacol.)

cationic d. A detergent in which the cleansing action resides in the cation. Many such detergents are strong germicides; e.g., those that contain quaternary ammonium compounds. (Oral Med.; Pharmacol.)

nonionic d. A cleanser that acts by depressing the surface tension of water but does not ionize. (Oral Med.; Pharmacol.)

synthetic d. A cleanser, other than soap, that exerts its effect by lowering the surface tension of an aqueous cleansing mixture. (Oral Med.; Pharmacol.)

detoxicate (dē-tok′sĭ-kāt) (see **detoxify**)

detoxify (detoxicate) To remove the toxic quality of a substance. (Anesth.)

developer A chemical solution that converts the invisible (latent) image on a film into a visible one composed of minute grains of metallic silver. (Oral Radiol.)

developing, time-temperature method Procedure of developing dental films; a solution of fixed temperature is used, and the films are immersed in the solution for a specific length of time. (Oral Radiol.)

developing, visual method Procedure of developing dental films in which the films are placed in the developing solution and watched by holding them from time to time before a safelight. Correct development has occurred when the film becomes so dark that it is difficult to distinguish between tooth and bone structure. (Oral Radiol.)

development The process by which the individual reaches maturity. (Orthodont.)

development of film The reaction of a chemical reducer with the invisible latent image in the silver halide emulsion of an exposed x-ray or photographic film to produce (when fixed) a visible and stable image composed of minute grains of metallic silver. (Oral Radiol.)

deviation (dē″vē-ā′shŭn) Turning from a regular course; deflection. (Anesth.)

devital tooth (see **tooth, pulpless**)

dextran A water-soluble polymer of glucose of high molecular weight. A purified form, having an average molecular weight of 75,000, is used in 6% concentration in isotonic sodium chloride solution to expand plasma volume and maintain blood pressure in emergency treatment of hemorrhagic and traumatic shock. (Anesth.)

dextro- Prefix designating that an aqueous solution of a substance rotates the plane of polarized light to the right. (Oral Med.; Pharmacol.) (see also **isomers, optical**)

dextrorotatory (děk″strō-rō′tah-tor″ē) Turning the plane of polarization, or rays of polarized light, to the right. (Anesth.)

dextrose ($C_6H_{12}O_6 \cdot H_2O$) A dextrorotatory monosaccharide occurring as a white, crystalline powder; colorless and sweet; soluble in about 1 part water. (Anesth.)

diabetes (dī-ah-bē′tēz) A deficiency condition involving carbohydrate metabolism and characterized by the habitual discharge of an excessive amount of urine. (Oral Path.)

 bronzed d. The combination of hemochromatosis and diabetes mellitus. The skin takes on a bronzed appearance due to the deposition of an iron-containing pigment in the skin. (Oral Med.)

 d. insipidus A metabolic disturbance characterized by marked urinary excretion and great thirst but no elevation of sugar in the blood or urine. (Oral Diag.)

 — A pituitary dysfunction characterized by an insufficient output of the antidiuretic hormone and leading to polyuria and polydipsia. (Oral Path.)

 juvenile d. Diabetes mellitus occurring in children and adolescents, usually of a more severe and rampant nature than diabetes mellitus in adults, with consequent difficulty of regulation. (Periodont.)

 d. mellitus A metabolic disturbance characterized by excessive passage of urine, excessive thirst, and high blood and urine sugar levels; caused by a disturbance in insulin production. (Oral Diag.)

 — A disorder of carbohydrate metabolism characterized by hyperglycemia and glycosuria. An important factor is a deficiency of insulin. Several processes are involved, however: failure of body tissues to oxidize carbohydrates, liberation of glucose from the liver, and the production and liberation of pituitary and adrenocortical hormones. Manifestations include dysphagia, polydipsia, weakness, loss of weight, increased susceptibility to infection (e.g., multiple periodontal abscesses), and, in advanced stages, acidosis and coma. Degenerative changes occur later in life. (Oral Med.)

 — A metabolic disorder, due primarily to a defect in the production of insulin by the islet cells of the pancreas, with resultant inability to utilize carbohydrates. Characterized by hyperglycemia, glycosuria, polyuria, hyperlipemia (due to imperfect catabolism of fats), acidosis, ketonuria, a lowered resistance to infection, etc. Periodontal manifestations may include recurrent and multiple periodontal abscesses, osteoporotic changes in alveolar bone, fungating masses of granulation tissue protruding from periodontal pockets, a lowered resistance to infection, and delay in healing after periodontal therapy. (Periodont.)

 phlorizin d. Glycosuria due to inhibition of phosphorylation of phlorizin. It is not related to an endochine disturbance. (Oral Med.)

diadochokinesia (dī″ah-dō″kō-kǐ-nē′zē-ah) The act or process of repeating at maximum speed some simple cyclical reciprocating movement such as raising and lowering of the mandible, or protrusion and retraction of the tongue. (Oral Physiol.)

diagnosis Scientific evalution of existing conditions. (Comp. Prosth.; Oper. Dent.; Orthodont.; Remov. Part. Prosth.)

 — The process by which one recognizes or identifies any condition that may be a departure from normal. (Oral Diag.)

 — Determination of the nature of a disease process and the distinguishing of one disease from another. Based on an accurate compilation of facts acquired from the medical and dental history, from an expression of symptoms by the patient, from an observation of the signs of the disease by the clinician, and from physical examination of the patient, with subsequent recognition of the disease process. (Periodont.)

 — Translation of data gathered by clinical and radiographic examination into an organized, classified definition of the conditions present. (Pract. Man.)

 clinical d. Determination of the specific disease or diseases involved in producing symptoms and signs by examination of the patient and use of analogy. (Oral Diag.)

 differential d. The process of identifying a condition by differentiating all pathologic processes that may produce similar lesions. (Oral Diag.)

 final d. The diagnosis arrived at after all the data have been collected, analyzed, and subjected to logical thought. Treatment may be necessary in some instances before the final diagnosis is made. (Oral Diag.)

radiographic d. Limited term used to indicate those radiologic interpretations that cannot be verified or disproved by clinical examination. (Oral Radiol.)

diagnostic cast (see **cast, diagnostic**)

diagnostic equilibration A measuring method of determining and recording on dentodes the amount and the direction that deflective cusps anteriorize or lateralize the closure direction of the mandible, as can be seen in mountings. (Gnathol.)

dialysis (dī-ăl'ĭ-sĭs) Diffusion through a membrane. (Anesth.)

diameter, buccolingual, grinding of (see **tooth, grinding of buccolingual diameter of**)

diaphragm (dī'ah-frăm) A musculotendinous partition that separates the thorax and abdomen. (Anesth.)

— A metal barrier plate, often of lead, pierced with a central aperture so arranged as to limit the emerging, or useful, beam of roentgen rays to the smallest practical diameter for making radiographic exposures. (Oral Radiol.) (see also **collimation; collimator; distance, cone, long; source-collimator distance**)

Potter-Bucky d. (see **grid, Potter-Bucky**)

diaphysis (dī-ăf'ĭ-sĭs) Shaft of a long bone. (Oral Physiol.)

diarthrosis (dī"ăr-thrō'sĭs) A freely movable joint enclosed in a fluid-filled cavity and limited variously by muscles, ligaments, and bone. (Oral Physiol.)

diastema (dī"ah-stē'mah) A space between two adjacent teeth in the same dental arch. (Comp. Prosth.; Orthodont.; Periodont.; Remov. Part. Prosth.)

— A space between the primary or permanent teeth unrelated to the physiologic development of the dentition. (Pedodont.)

diastole (dī-ăs'tō-lē) The rhythmic period of relaxation and dilation of a chamber of the heart during which it fills with blood. (Anesth.)

— The period after the contraction of the heart muscle, during which the aorta releases the potential energy stored in its elastic tissue. The energy is converted into kinetic energy and sustains the pressure necessary for steady flow of blood in the vessels. The pressure measured at this period is the lowest attained during the cardiac pumping cycle and is called the diastolic pressure. The normal pressure in the adult is approximately 120/80 mm Hg (systolic/diastolic) and increases with age from 128/85 at 45 years of age to 135/89 at 60 years of age. (Oral Physiol.)

diathermy (di'ah-ther"mē) A generalized rise in tissue temperature produced by a high-frequency alternating current between two electrodes. The temperature rise is produced without causing tissue damage. (Oral Surg.)

diathesis (dī-ăth'ĕ-sĭs) A condition of the body that causes the tissues to react in an abnormal way to certain stimuli. As a result, the person is more susceptible to a certain disease or diseases than are others. (Oral Diag.)

— A tendency, based on body makeup; constitutional, hereditary, or acquired states of the body that cause a predisposition or susceptibility to diseases. (Oral Med.; Pharmacol.)

hemorrhagic d. A condition that may be due to defects in the coagulation mechanism, defects in the blood vessel wall, or both. (Oral Diag.)

Dick's test (see **test, Dick's**)

die The positive reproduction of the form of a cast in any suitable hard substance, usually in metal or specially prepared artificial stone. (Comp. Prosth.) (see also **counterdie**)

— A cast or reproduction. A working model on which dental appliances are fabricated. (D. Mat.)

— The positive reproduction of the form of a prepared tooth in any suitable hard substance, usually in metal or specially prepared (improved) artificial stone. (Fixed Part. Prosth.; Oper. Dent.; Remov. Part. Prosth.)

d. lubricant A material applied to a die to serve as a separating medium so that the wax pattern will not adhere to the die but may be withdrawn from it without sticking. (Oper. Dent.)

stone d. A positive likeness in artificial (dental) stone; used in the fabrication of a dental restoration, and usually formed in polysulfide rubber (Thiokol) or a silicone rubber base, or hydrocolloid, or modeling compound–copper band impressions of prepared teeth. (Comp. Prosth.; Fixed Part. Prosth.; Remov. Part. Prosth.)

waxing d. A mold into which wax is forced for the production of standardized wax patterns. (Remov. Part. Prosth.)

diet The food and drink consumed by a given person from day to day. Not all the diet is necessarily utilized by the body. For this reason diet and nutrition must be differentiated. (Comp. Prosth.; Oral Diag.; Periodont.; Remov. Part. Prosth.)

alkaline d. A diet that is basic in reaction; produced by the addition of alkaline salts, including sodium bicarbonate. (Periodont.)

lysine-poor d. A diet deficient in lysine, an essential amino acid. It is necessary that all the essential amino acids be present in the diet; should one or more be absent, proper utilization of the others cannot occur. Periodontal changes described in experimental animals with lysine deficiency include osteoporosis of supporting bone, disintegration and failure of replacement of periodontal fibers, etc. (Periodont.)

dietary analysis (see **analysis, dietary**)

dietary consistency The physical character of the diet. It may tend to produce or modify periodontal disease. (Periodont.)

diethylstilbestrol (dī-ĕth″ĭl-stĭl-bĕs′trol) An estrogenic substance, $C_{18}H_{20}O_2$, that has an estrogenic activity considered to be greater than that of estrone. Useful in treating menopausal symptoms and occasionally used in the therapy of chronic desquamative gingivitis associated with artificial or natural menopause. (Periodont.)

difficult eruption (see **teething**)

diffusibility (dĭ-fūz″ĭ-bĭl′ĭ-tē) Capable of being diffused. (Anesth.)

diffusion (dĭ-fū′zhŭn) The process of becoming widely spread, as when gasses emanating from a small jet spread throughout a room. In liquids, the velocity of the molecules of two solutions will cause them to diffuse, the diffusion varying in rate according to their molecular weight and temperature. (Anesth.)

— A property of ions or molecules of a solute that permits them to pass through a membrane or to intermingle by rapid or gradual permeation with the molecules of a solvent. This process may be qualified by the descriptive properties of rate, magnitude, and direction that may be applied to a specific solute-solvent relationship. For example, there is a difference in intrinsic rate of diffusion between substances such as O_2 or CO_2, between various anesthetic agents, and between the various salt ion electrolytes and the associated water balance. (Oral Physiol.)

digitalization (dĭj″ĭ-tăl-ĭ-zā′shŭn) Administration of digitalis in sufficient amount by any of several types of dosage schedules to build up the concentration of digitalis glycosides in the body of a patient. (Anesth.)

dilaceration (dī-lăs″er-ā′shŭn) Displacement of some portion of a developing tooth that continues its development in its new position. A curvature of a tooth root. (Endodont.)

— Severe angular distortion in the root of a tooth or at the junction of the root and crown. It results from trauma during tooth development. (Oral Diag.; Oral Path.)

Dilantin enlargement (see **hyperplasia, gingival, Dilantin**)

Dilantin gingival hyperplasia (see **hyperplasia, gingival, Dilantin**)

Dilantin sodium (dī-lăn′tĭn sō′dē-ŭm) Proprietary name for diphenylhydantoin sodium. (Pharmacol.)

dilation (dī-lā′shŭn) The act of stretching or dilating. (Anesth.)

diluent (dĭl′ū-ĕnt) An agent that dilutes the strength of a solution or mixture; medication that dilutes any one of the body fluids. (Anesth.)

dilute To make weaker the strength of a solution or mixture. (Anesth.)

dimension, vertical A vertical measurement of the face between any two arbitrarily selected points that are conveniently located one above and one below the mouth, usually in the midline. (Comp. Prosth.; Orthodont.; Remov. Part. Prosth.) (see also **relation, vertical**)

— The vertical height of the face with the teeth in occlusion or acting as stops. (Periodont.)

v. d., decrease Decrease of the vertical distance between the mandible and the maxillae by modifications of teeth or of the positions of teeth or occlusion rims, or through alveolar or residual ridge resorption. (Comp. Prosth.; Remov. Part. Prosth.)

v. d., increase Increase of the vertical distance between the mandible and the maxillae by modifications of teeth and the positions of teeth or occlusion rims. (Comp. Prosth.; Remov. Part. Prosth.)

— The process of increasing the distance between the occlusal surfaces of the teeth and the alveolar or residual ridges in one or both dental arches. (Comp. Prosth.; Fixed Part. Prosth.; Remov. Part. Prosth.)

decreasing occlusal v. d. The process of reducing the distance between the maxillae and the mandible when the teeth are in contact. (Comp. Prosth.; Remov. Part. Prosth.)

increasing occlusal v. d. The process of increasing the distance between the maxillae and the mandible when the teeth are in contact. (Comp. Prosth.; Fixed Part. Prosth.; Remov. Part. Prosth.)

occlusal v. d. The vertical dimension of the face when the teeth or occlusion rims are in contact in centric occlusion. (Comp. Prosth.; Remov. Part. Prosth.)

— The height of the face measured from the

nasion to the gnathion when the mandibular teeth are in maximum occlusal contact with the maxillary teeth. (Periodont.)

o. v. d., decrease May result from modification of the tooth form by attrition or grinding, drifting of teeth, or, in edentulous patients, resorption of residual ridges. (Comp. Prosth.; Remov. Part. Prosth.)

o. v. d., increase May result from modification of the tooth form, tooth position, height of the occlusion rims, relining, or occlusal splints. (Comp. Prosth.; Remov. Part. Prosth.)

rest v. d. The vertical dimension of the face with the jaws in the rest relation. (Comp. Prosth.; Remov. Part. Prosth.)

r. v. d., decrease May or may not accompany a decrease in occlusal vertical dimension. It may occur without a decrease in occlusal vertical dimension in patients with a preponderant activity of the jaw-closing musculature, as in chronic gum-chewers or patients with muscular hypertension. (Comp. Prosth.; Remov. Part. Prosth.)

r. v. d., increase May or may not accompany an increase in occlusal dimension. It sometimes occurs after the removal of remaining occlusal contacts, perhaps as a result of the removal of noxious reflex stimuli. (Comp. Prosth.; Remov. Part. Prosth.)

dimensional stability (see **stability, dimensional**)

dimethylbenzene (dī-mĕth″ĭl-bĕn′zēn) (see **xylene**)

Dimitri's disease (dē-mē′trēz) (see **disease, Sturge-Weber-Dimitri**)

diphenylhydantoin sodium (dī-fĕn″ĭl-hī-dăn′tō-ĭn) **(Dilantin sodium)** A drug used for the control of convulsive grand mal and petit mal epileptic seizures; often associated with the production of a profuse gingival hyperplasia. (Periodont.)

diphtheria (dĭf-thē″rē-ah) An acute disease caused by *Corynebacterium diphtheriae* and resulting in swelling of the pharynx and larynx with fever. (Oral Diag.)

diplopia (dĭ-plō′pē-ah) Seeing of a single object as two images. May occur after fracture of the bony orbital cavity as a result of displacement of the globe of the eye inferiorly. (Oral Surg.)

direct (dī-rĕkt′) Relating to any restorative procedure performed directly on a tooth without the use of a die, e.g., a wax pattern or platinum matrix formed in the prepared cavity, or one of the powdered, granular, or foil golds compacted into a prepared cavity. (Oper. Dent.)

d. gold Any of the forms of pure gold that may be compacted directly into a prepared cavity to form a restoration, e.g., gold foil, powdered gold, mat gold, Goldent. (Oper. Dent.)

d. pulp capping (see **capping, pulp, direct**)

d. retainer (see **retainer, direct**)

d. retention (see **retention, direct**)

disability Want of legal qualification to do a thing; legal incompetency. (D. Juris.)

denial of d. A symptom in which patients deny the existence of a disease or disability. A patient who is edentulous may insist he eats better, looks better, and speaks better than if he had teeth. Another may insist that filthy, carious, periodontally involved teeth are beautiful and healthy, and enhance his appearance. Denial by these patients is a nonrealistic attempt to maintain their predisease status. These patients regard ill health and disability as an imperfection, a weakness, and even a disgrace. (Oral Physiol.)

disarticulation (dĭs″ăr-tĭk″ū-lā′shŭn) Amputation or separation of joint parts, as in hemimandibulectomy, with inclusion of the condyloid process of the mandible. (Oral Surg.)

disc (see **disk**)

discharge To release; liberate; annul; unburden. To cancel a contract; to make an agreement or contract null and void. (D. Juris.)

purulent d. (see **pus**)

disclosing solution A material, usually some form of dye, applied to the teeth to stain bacterial and mucinous plaque on the tooth surface. (Oral Diag.)

disclusion (dĭs-klū′zhŭn) Separation of the occlusal surfaces of the teeth directly and simply by opening the jaws, or indirectly in excursions by the anterior teeth, which aids the downward- and forward-moving condyles to keep the ridged tooth surfaces from having sliding contacts. In procursion the slopes of the eminences and the slopes of the skidways of the incisors enforce a physiologic separation of all postincisor teeth. In laterocursion a condyle-oriented pair of coupled canines plus the sloping eminence of the orbiting (balancing side) condyle enforce a physiologic separation of all incisors, the other canines, and all other postcanine teeth. In unworn dentitions, organically occluded, most of the occlusal areas of the postcanine teeth are kept out of occlusal contact even in centrically related centric closure because the stamp cusps make contact at only three points in the brims of their fossae. Disclusion of the occlusal surfaces is also maintained physiologically during the chewing of tough food fibers. Ankylosed teeth are pathologically separated from occlusion by their lack of eruptivity. Thumb-sucking develops pathologic disclusion of the anterior teeth. (Gnathol.)

discoid (dĭs'koid) A carving instrument with a blade of circular form that has a cutting edge around the entire periphery except where it meets the shank. Resembles a disk in shape. (Oper. Dent.)

discoloration, enamel (see **tetracycline**)

discoloration, gingival (see **gingiva, discoloration**)

discount An allowance or deduction made from a gross sum. (D. Juris.)

— The procedure of reducing the amount of a professional fee. (Pract. Man.)

discrimination, tactile The ability to perceive two simultaneous touch stimuli; two-point discrimination. When the distance between the two stimuli is diminished to the amount that only one stimulus is perceived, a value is determined for the two-point discrimination capacity of a special part. Thus correspondence is noted between the mobility of a structure and its discriminatory ability. The manual dexterity of a man is also concomitant with the high specific activity of the lips and tongue and the facial and masticatory musculture. Thus the hands and the orofacial complex of structures complement each other, particularly in the masticatory function. When patients are anesthetized by local agents, they have diminished tactile sense and frequently bite their lips rather severely without being aware of it. (Oral Physiol.)

disease(s) A definite deviation from the normal state; characterized by a series of symptoms. Disease may be caused by developmental disturbances, genetic factors, metabolic factors, living agents, and physical, chemical, or radiant energy, or the cause may be unknown. (Oral Diag.)

Adams-Stokes d. (Adams-Stokes syndrome) A disease characterized by a slow and perhaps irregular pulse, vertigo, syncope, occasional pseudoepileptic convulsions, and Cheyne-Stokes respiration. (Anesth.)

adaptation d. (adaptation syndrome) Metabolic disorders occurring as the result of adaptation or resistance to severe physical or psychologic stress. (Oral Med.) (see also **syndrome, general adaptation**)

Addison's d. A disease characterized by atrophy of the adrenal gland; often shows associated intraoral pigmentation. (Oral Diag.)

— Chronic adrenocortical insufficiency due to bilateral tuberculosis, aplasia, atrophy, or degeneration of the adrenal glands. Symptoms include muscular weakness, hypotension, dehydration, loss of weight, hypoglycemia, gastrointestinal disturbances, and progressive brownish pigmentation of the skin and mucosa. (Oral Med.)

— An insidious, progressive disease caused by hypofunction of the adrenal cortex and characterized by weakness, bronzing of the skin, and brown pigmentation of the mucous membrane. (Oral Path.)

— A progressive, debilitating condition due to hypofunction of the adrenal cortex; produces severe weakness, weight loss, low blood pressure, digestive disturbances, hypoglycemia, lowered resistance to infection, and abnormal pigmentation (bronzelike) of the skin, with associated melanotic pigmentation of the oral mucous membranes, particularly of the gingival tissues. The most common etiology is tuberculosis of the adrenal gland. (Periodont.)

adrenocortical d. Disorders of adrenocortical function, giving rise to Addison's disease, Cushing's syndrome, adrenogenital syndrome, and primary aldosteronism. (Oral Med.)

Albers-Schonberg d. (see **osteopetrosis**)

autoallergic d. (see **disease, autoimmune**)

autoimmune d. (autoallergic d., autoimmunization syndrome, chronic hypersensitivity d., hypersensitivity d.) Any one of the diseases that are believed to be caused in part by reactions of hypersensitivity of the host tissue (antigens). Includes various hemolytic anemias, idiopathic thrombocytopenias, rheumatoid arthritis, systemic lupus erythematosus, glomerulonephritis, scleroderma, Hashimoto's thyroiditis, and Sjögren's syndrome. (Oral Med.)

Barlow's d. (see **scurvy, infantile**)

Basedow's d. (see **goiter, exophthalmic**)

Behçet's d. (see **syndrome, Behçet's**)

Besnier-Boeck-Schaumann d. (see **sarcoidosis**)

bleeder's d. (see **hemophilia**)

blood d. A disease affecting the hematologic system, e.g., anemia, leukemia, agranulocytosis purpura, and infectious mononucleosis. Such a disease often presents lesions of the oral structures, particularly of the mucosal surfaces. (Periodont.)

Bowen's d. (carcinoma in situ, intraepithelial carcinoma) A dysplastic epithelial disease involving the skin and mucous membrane and considered to be precancerous. (Oral Med.)

— Precancerous lesions, usually occurring on the skin. Dyskeratosis is evident, but there is no invasion. (Oral Path.)

Brill-Symmers d. (see **lymphoblastoma, giant follicular**)

brittle bone d. (see **osteogenesis imperfecta**)

Caffey's d. (see **hyperostosis, infantile cortical**)

cardiac d. A disease affecting the heart. (Periodont.)

cat-scratch d. (see **fever, cat-scratch**)

Cheadle's d. (see **scurvy, infantile**)

Christmas d. (see **hemophilia B**)

collagen d. (group d., visceral angiitis) Term describing collectively a group of diseases affecting the collagenous connective tissue of several organs and systems. These diseases have in common similar biochemical structural alterations and include rheumatic fever, scleroderma, rheumatoid arthritis, systemic lupus erythematosus, periarteritis, and serum sickness. (Oral Med.)

— Disease characterized by degeneration of collagen of the various tissues, e.g., scleroderma, lupus erythematosus, and dermatolysis. Continuity of the fiber bundles is broken in the periodontal membrane, and there is derangement of the normally orderly arrangement of the fiber apparatus; inflammatory changes are conspicuously absent. Basic etiology is unknown. Adverse progress of collagen diseases may be controlled by the administration of the corticosteroids. (Periodont.)

combined system d. Pernicious anemia in which there is central nervous system damage associated with the hematologic findings. (Oral Med.)

communicable d. Any disease that may be transmitted directly or indirectly to a well person or animal from an infected person or animal. Any disease with the capacity for maintenance by natural modes of spread; e.g., by contact, by airborne routes, through drinking water or food, or by means of arthropod vectors. (Oral Med.)

congenital d. Any disease present at birth. More specifically, one that is acquired in utero. (Oral Med.)

Coxsackie A d. (see **herpangina**)

Crouzon's d. (see **dysostosis, craniofacial**)

Cushing's d. (see **syndrome, Cushing's**)

cytomegalic inclusion d., generalized (see **disease, salivary gland**)

Darier's d. (keratosis follicularis) An apparently genetic dermatologic disease that also involves mucous membranes. The oral lesions are whitish papules of gingiva, tongue, or palate. (Oral Diag.)

— A hereditary dermatologic disease that may affect the oral cavity, minute whitish papules appearing on the gingiva, tongue, and palate. It is characterized histologically by the presence of "corps ronds." (Oral Path.)

deficiency d. Disturbance produced by lack of nutritional or metabolic factors. Term is used chiefly in reference to avitaminosis. (Oral Diag.)

— Any disease resulting from a true or relative lack of minerals, proteins, fatty acids, or vitamins in the diet. (Oral Med.)

nutritional d. d. The bodily manifestations, usually of a regressive nature, produced by decreased intake, diminished absorption, poor utilization, or overexcretion of an essential nutritional element. Some of the vital elements are ascorbic acid, necessary for the hydroxylation of amino acids and thus for collagen formation; calcium, necessary for the formation and maintenance of bone and other mineralized structures; protein, necessary for the formation of collagen; and the vitamins, e.g., riboflavin, which is essential as a coenzyme in intermediary metabolism of carbohydrates. (Periodont.)

degenerative joint d. (see **osteoarthritis**)

demyelinating d. The diseases that have in common a loss of myelin sheath, with preservation of the axis cylinders; e.g., multiple sclerosis and Schilder's disease. (Oral Med.)

dental d., hereditary Heritable defects of the dentition without generalized disease; e.g., amelogenesis imperfecta, dentinogenesis imperfecta, dentinal dysplasia, localized and generalized hypoplasia of enamel, peg-shaped lateral incisors, familial dentigerous cysts, missing teeth, giantism, and fused primary mandibular incisors. Dental defects occurring with generalized disease include dentinogenesis imperfecta with osteogenesis imperfecta, missing teeth with ectodermal dysplasia, enamel hypoplasia with epidermolysis bullosa dystrophia, retarded eruption with cleidocranial dysostosis, missing lateral incisors with ptosis of the eyelids missing premolars with premature whitening of the hair, and enamel hypoplasia in vitamin D–resistant rickets. (Oral Med.)

dermatologic d. Any one of the diseases affecting the skin; often accompanied by pathologic manifestations of various mucosal surfaces of the body, e.g., the oral mucosa, the genital mucosa, and the conjunctiva. (Periodont.)

Engman's d. (see **dermatitis infectiosa eczematoides**)

exanthematous d. Any one of a group of diseases caused by a number of viruses but having as a prominent feature a skin rash; e.g., smallpox, chickenpox, cowpox, measles, and rubella. (Oral Med.)

familial d. A disease occurring in several members of the same family. Term is often used to mean members of the same generation and is occasionally used synonymously with hereditary disease. (Oral Med.)

Feer's d. (see **erythredema polyneuropathy; acrodynia**)

fibrocystic d. (mucoviscidosis) A hereditary defect of most of the exocrine glands in the body, including the salivary glands. The secretion of the affected mucous glands is abnormally viscous. (Oral Path.)

foot-and-mouth d. (aphthous fever, epidemic stomatitis, epizootic stomatitis) The virus disease transmitted by animals or animal secretions, producing vesicles on the lips, on the fingers and toes, and intraorally. (Oral Diag.; Oral Med.)

—Primarily a disease of animals caused by a filtrable virus that may be transmitted to man and that occasionally produces symptoms. Human form is characterized by fever, nausea, vomiting, malaise, and ulcerative stomatitis. Skin lesions consisting of vesicles may appear, usually on the palms of the hands and soles of the feet. Spontaneous regression usually occurs within two weeks. (Oral Path.)

Fordyce's d. (see **spots, Fordyce's**)

functional d. A disease that has no observable or demonstrable cause. (Oral Med.)

Gaucher's d. Disturbance of metabolism usually classified with the xanthomatoses. In addition to leukopenia, skin pigmentation, anemia, and thrombocytopenia, osteoporosis is a symptom. On radiographic examination the jaw defects may be seen as radiolucencies, with the excessive teeth appearing to be unsupported by bone. Kerasin is

stored in the reticuloendothelial system. (Oral Diag.)

— A disorder of cerebroside metabolism in which kerasin accumulates in the reticuloendothelial system. Manifestations include enlargement of the spleen, liver, and lymph nodes, anemia, thrombocytopenia, and occasionally bone lesions. The disease is congenital, frequently familial, and may not be manifest until adult life. (Oral Med.)

— A constitutional defect in the metabolism of the cerebroside kerasin. This glycoprotein accumulates in the reticuloendothelial system and leads to splenomegaly, hepatomegaly, lymph node enlargement, and bone defects. (Oral Path.) (see also **cell, Gaucher's**)

Graves' d. (see **goiter, exophthalmic**)

group d. (see **disease, collagen**)

Hand-Schüller-Christian d. (chronic disseminated histiocytosis X) A disease characterized by defects (radiolucencies) of membranous bones, including the skull, and by exophthalmos and diabetes insipidus. Teeth may be loosened and exfoliated. (Oral Diag.)

— A chronic granulomatous, inflammatory disease of unknown etiology characterized by diabetes insipidus, exophthalmos, and bone lesions, principally in the skull. It is usually manifest in children but may persist into adult life. The Hand-Schüller-Christian complex includes also Letterer-Siwe disease and eosinophilic granuloma. (Oral Med.)

— A type of cholesterol lipoidosis characterized clinically by defects in membranous bones, exophthalmos, and diabetes insipidus. (Oral Path.)

Hansen's d. (see **leprosy**)

heart d. Any abnormal condition of the heart (organic, mechanical, or functional) that causes difficulty.

arteriosclerotic h. d. A variety of functional changes of the myocardium that result from arteriosclerosis. (Oral Med.)

congenital h. d. Defective formation of the heart or defective formation of the major vessels of the heart. (Oral Med.)

rheumatic h. d. Scarring of the endocardium resulting from involvement in acute rheumatic fever. The process most often involves the mitral valve. (Oral Med.)

thyrotoxic h. d. Cardiac failure occurring as the result of hyperthyroidism or its superimposition on existing organic heart disease. Thyrotoxicosis is an important cause of auricular fibrillation. (Oral Med.)

hemoglobin C d. A disease due to an abnormal hemoglobin (hemoglobin C); occurs primarily in Negroes and causes a mild normochromic anemia, target cells, and vague, intermittent arthralgia. (Oral Med.)

hemolytic d. of newborn Hemolysis due to isoimmune reactions associated with Rh incompatibility or with blood transfusions in which there is an incompatibility of the ABO blood system. Several forms of the disease occur: erythroblastosis fetalis, congenital hemolytic disease, icterus gravis neonatorum, and hydrops fetalis. (Oral Med.)

hemophilioid d. Hemophilic states (conditions) that clinically resemble hemophilia; e.g., parahemophilia and hemophilia B (Christmas disease). (Oral Med.)

hemorrhagic d. of newborn A hemorrhagic tendency in newborn infants occurring usually on the third or fourth day of life; thought to be due to defects of prothrombin and factor VII, resulting from a deficiency of vitamin K. (Oral Med.)

hereditary d. A disease transmitted from parent to offspring through genes. Three main types of mendelian heredity are recognized: dominant, recessive, and sex-linked. (Oral Med.)

hidebound d. (see **scleroderma**)

Hodgkin's d. A neoplastic disease that usually is fatal; characterized by proliferation of cells of the reticuloendothelial system. Marked enlargement of the cervical lymph nodes may be the first or an early symptom. (Oral Diag.)

— A generally fatal lymphomatous disorder of unknown etiology that has neoplastic and granulomatous characteristics. Chiefly involves the lymph nodes, but sometimes the spleen, liver, bone marow, and other organs are involved. Three variants include Hodgkin's paragranuloma, Hodgkin's granuloma (classical or common type), and Hodgkin's sarcoma. All have in common the presence of Sternberg-Reed, or Dorothy Reed, cells and lymph node enlargement. Cervical lymph nodes are often the first to be affected. (Oral Med.)

— A painless, progressive, and fatal enlargement of lymphoid tissues. Many forms are recognized but all involve the Sternberg-Reed cell. (Oral Path.) (see also **cell, Sternberg-Reed**)

hypersensitivity d. (see **disease, autoimmune**) **chronic h. d.** (see **disease, autoimmune**)

iatrogenic d. A disease arising as a result of the actions or words of a physician or dentist; e.g., an obsession of having heart disease or bruxism as a result of a misunderstanding on the part of a patient. (Oral Med.)

idiopathic d. (ĭd″ē-ō-păth′ĭk) A disease in which the cause is not recognized or determined. (Oral Med.)

infectious d. Pathologic alterations induced in the tissues by the action of microorganisms and/or their toxins. Some of the infectious diseases involving the oral tissues are herpes zoster, herpetic gingivostomatitis, moniliasis, syphilis, and tuberculosis. (Periodont.)

"kissing d." (see **mononucleosis, infectious**)

Letterer-Siwe d. (sĕ′veh) (**acute disseminated histiocytosis X, nonlipid histiocytosis, nonlipid reticuloendotheliosis**) A metabolic disturbance found primarily in young children. Characterized by an increase in histiocytosis in nearly all organs, including the skull, and by a rapid, fatal course. (Oral Diag.)

— A fatal febrile disease of unknown cause occurring in infants and children; characterized by focal granulomatous lesions of the lymph nodes, spleen, and bone marrow. Results in enlargement of the lymph nodes, spleen, and liver, defects of the flat and long bones, anemia, and sometimes purpura. (Oral Med.)

— An acute fatal disease of infants and young children characterized by proliferation of the cells of the reticuloendothelial system. Results in splenomegaly, hepatomegaly, lymphadenopathy, and diffuse bone lesions. (Oral Path.)

lipoid storage d. (**lipoidosis, reticuloendothelial granuloma**) Any one of a group of diseases in which lipid substances accumulate in the fixed cells of the reticuloendothelial system. Included are Gaucher's disease, Niemann-Pick disease, and the Hand-Schüller-Christian complex. Other storage diseases include lipochondrodystrophy (gargoylism) and cerebral sphingolipidosis. (Oral Med.)

Lobstein's d. (see **osteogenesis imperfecta**)

Marie's d. (see **acromegaly**)

Mediterranean d. (see **thalassemia major**)

Mikulicz' d. (mĭk′ū-lĭch) A pathologic disturbance of the parotid, submandibular, sublingual, and lacrimal glands characterized by swelling. The disease is not neoplastic and should be treated conservatively. (Oral Diag.)

— Diffuse enlargement of the parotid glands and frequently the submandibular glands in association with a benign lymphoepithelial lesion. (Oral Med.)

— A benign hyperplasia of the lymph nodes of the parotid or other salivary glands and/or the lacrimal glands. (Oral Path.)

Moeller's d. (see **scurvy, infantile**)

molecule d. A disease associated with genetically determined abnormalities of protein synthesis at the molecular level. (Oral Med.)

muscle d. Pathologic muscle tissue changes. Such changes reveal few structural alterations, and the highly differentiated contents of muscle fibers tend to react as a whole. The pathologic features that distinguish one muscle disease from another are the age and character of changes within a muscle, the distribution of those changes within one or several muscles, the presence of inflammatory cells and parasites, and the coexistence of pathologic changes in other organs. Muscles undergo a number of degenerative changes. There are alterations in the striation in certain pathologic states, caused by cloudy swelling, granular degeneration, waxy or hyaline degeneration, and other cellular modifications, such as multiplication of the sarcolemmic nuclei and phagocytosis of muscle fibers. (Oral Physiol.)

neuromuscular d. A condition in which various areas of the central nervous system are affected; results in dysfunction or degeneration of the musculature and disabilities of the organ. (Pedodont.)

Niemann-Pick d. (nē'măn) A rapidly fatal disease characterized by disturbed phosphatic metabolism, enlarged spleen and liver, and often oral manifestations. (Oral Diag.)

— A congenital, familial disorder of lipid metabolism, probably sphingomyelin; occurs chiefly in Jewish female infants, terminating fatally before the third year. (Oral Med.)

— A fatal disease of infants characterized by the accumulation of the phospholipid sphingomyelin in the cells of the reticuloendothelial system. (Oral Path.)

oral d., hereditary Heritable defects of oral and paraoral structures (excluding the dentition) without generalized defects; includes ankyloglossia, hereditary gingivofibromatosis, and possible cleft lip and cleft palate. Many oral and paraoral defects are associ-

ated with generalized defects; e.g., Peutz-Jeghers, Franceschetti, Ehlers-Danlos, Pierre Robin, and Sturge-Weber syndromes, hemorhagic telangiectasia, Crouzon's disease, sickle cell disease, acatalasemia, white spongy nevus, xeroderma pigmentosum, gargoylism, neurofibromatosis, familial amyloidosis, and achondroplasia. (Oral Med.)

organic d. A disease in which actual structural changes have occurred in the organs or tissues. (Oral Med.)

Osler's d. (see **erythremia**)

Owren's d. (see **parahemophilia**)

Paget's d. (see **osteitis deformans**)

periodic d. (see **disorders, periodic**)

periodontal d. Any disturbance of the periodontium, including periodontitis, periodontosis, gingivitis, gingival enlargement, atrophy, and traumatism. (Oral Diag.)

— A pathologic alteration affecting the investing and supporting structures of the teeth. Diseases affecting the periodontium may be loosely divided into two types: inflammatory and dystrophic. Etiologic factors may be local or systemic or may involve an interplay between the two. (Periodont.)

etiologic factors of p. d. The local and systemic factors, singly or in combination, that initiate periodontal lesions. (Periodont.)

local factors of p. d. The environmental conditions within the oral cavity that initiate, perpetuate, or alter the course of diseases of the periodontium; e.g., calculus, diastemata between teeth, food impaction, prematurities in centric path of closure, and tongue habits. (Periodont.)

peripheral vascular d. A disease of arteries, veins, and/or lymphatic vessels. (Oral Med.)

pink d. (see **acrodynia**)

Pott's d. Spinal curvature (kyphosis) resulting from tuberculosis. (Oral Med.)

psychosomatic d. A disease that appears to have been precipitated or prolonged by emotional stress; manifested largely through the autonomic nervous system. Various conditions may be included; e.g., certain forms of asthma, dermatoses, migraine headache, hypertension, peptic ulcer, rheumatoid arthritis, and ulcerative colitis. Occlusal trauma associated with bruxism is often considered to be a disease of this type. (Oral Med.) (see also **disorder, psychophysiologic, autonomic, and visceral**)

Quincke's d. (see **edema, angioneurotic**)

Recklinghausen's d. (von Recklinghausen's disease) (see **hyperparathyroidism; osteitis; generalized fibrosa cystica; neurofibromatosis**)

Rendu-Osler-Weber d. (ron'dū) (see **telangiectasia, hereditary hemorrhagic**)

rheumatic d. (see **rheumatism**)

rickettsial d. A disease caused by microorganisms of the family Rickettsiaceae; e.g., Rocky Mountain spotted fever, rickettsialpox, typhus, and Q fever. (Oral Med.)

Riga-Fede d. (rĕ'gah-fā'dā) Ulceration of the lingual frenum of infants due to abrasion by natal or neonatal teeth. (Oral Path.)

Sainton's d. (see **dysostosis, cleidocranial**)

salivary gland d. (generalized cytomegalic inclusion d.) A generalized infection in infants caused by intrauterine or postnatal infection with a cytomegalovirus of the group of herpesviruses. Manifestations include jaundice, purpura, hemolytic anemia, vomiting, diarrhea, chronic eczema, and failure to gain weight. (Oral Med.; Oral Path.)

Schüller's d. (shĭl'erz) (see **osteoporosis**)

Selter's d. (see **acrodynia**)

sex-linked d. A hereditary disorder transmitted by the gene that also determines sex; e.g., hemophilia. (Oral Med.)

sickle cell d. A hematologic disorder due to the presence of an abnormal hemoglobin (hemoglobin S) that permits the formation or results in the formation of sickle-shaped red blood cells. Two forms of the disease occur: sickle cell trait and sickle cell anemia. (Oral Med.) (see also **anemia, sickle cell; trait, sickle cell**)

Simmonds' d. (pituitary cachexia, hypophyseal cachexia, hypopituitary cachexia) Panhypopituitarism due to destruction of the pituitary gland, usually from hemorrhage or infarction. (Oral Med.)

"students' d." (see **mononucleosis, infectious**)

Sturge-Weber-Dimitri d. (encephalotrigeminal angiomatosis) A congenital condition characterized by venous angioma of the meninges and cerebral cortex and ipsilateral angiomatous lesions of the face and jaws. (Oral Diag.)

subclinical d. A latent, incipient, or mild form of a disease that does not produce known, clinically detectable manifestations. Abuse of the term occurs by including diseases deduced to be present only on the basis of borderline laboratory values. (Oral Med.)

Sutton's d. (see **periadenitis mucosa necrotica recurrens**)

Swift's d. (see **acrodynia**)

systemic d. Any disease involving the whole body. (Oral Med.)

— Disease affecting the body as a whole. Diseases of the oral mucosa, gingivae, attachment apparatus, bony mandibulomaxillary structures, etc. may be reflections of disease of systemic origin. (Periodont.)

oral manifestations of s. d. The lesions occurring within the stomatologic system in association with systemic diseases, often influenced by the local environmental factors within the oral cavity. (Periodont.)

Takahara's d. (tah"kah-hăr'ahz) A form of rare progressive oral gangrene occurring in childhood and seen only in Japan. Apparently related to a congenital lack of enzyme catalase (acatalasemia). Characterized by a mild to severe form of a peculiar type of oral gangrene that may develop at the roots of the teeth or the tonsils. Loss of teeth occurs, with necrosis of the alveolar bone. Patients become symptom free after puberty. (Oral Med.)

transmissible d. Any disease capable of being transmitted from one individual to another; any disease capable of being maintained in successive passages through a susceptible host, usually under experimental conditions, e.g., by injection. (Oral Med.) (see also **disease, communicable**)

Vaquez' d. (vah-kāz') (see **erythremia**)

von Recklinghausen's d. of bone (see **hyperparathyroidism; osteitis fibrosa cystica, generalized**)

von Recklinghausen's d. of skin (see **neurofibromatosis**)

Weil's d. (vīlz) **(epidemic jaundice)** An acute febrile disease caused by *Leptospira icterohaemorrhagiae* or *Leptospira canicola*. Manifestations include fever, petechial hemorrhage, myalgia, renal insufficiency, hepatic failure, and jaundice. (Oral Med.)

Werlhof's d. (verl'hofs) (see **purpura, thrombocytopenic**)

disharmony, occlusal A phenomenon in which contacts of opposing occlusal surfaces of teeth are not in harmony with other tooth contacts and with the anatomic and physiologic controls of the mandible. Occlusions that do not coincide with their respective jaw relation. (Comp. Prosth.; Fixed Part. Prosth.; Orthodont.; Remov. Part. Prosth.) (see also contact, deflective occlusal; contact, interceptive occlusal; malocclusion)

disinfect To destroy pathogenic microorganisms. (Oral Surg.; Pharmacol.)

disinfectant A chemical especially for use on instruments to destroy most pathogenic microorganisms. (Oral Med.; Oral Surg.; Pharmacol.)

disintegration, nuclear A spontaneous nuclear transformation (radioactivity) characterized by the emission of energy and/or mass from the nucleus. When numbers of nuclei are involved, the process is characterized by a definite half-life. (Oral Radiol.)

   induced n. d. Disintegration resulting from artificial bombardment of a material with high-energy particles such as alpha particles, deuterons, protons, neutrons, or gamma rays. (Oral Radiol.)

disk (disc) A thin, flat, circular object. A circular piece of material that serves as a carrier for abrasive or polishing agents bonded to its surface or impregnated in its structure; it is fastened on a mandrel that is mounted on a handpiece, thus becoming a rotary instrument for cutting, smoothing, or polishing. (Oper. Dent.)

   abrasive d. A disk with abrasive particles attached to one or both of its surfaces or its edge. (Oper. Dent.)

   diamond d. A disk of steel with diamond chips bonded to its surface. (Oper. Dent.)

   garnet d. A disk with particles of garnet as the abrading medium. (Oper. Dent.)

   Jo-dandy d. Proprietary name of a separating disk. (Oper. Dent.) (see also **disk, separating**)

   lightning d. A steel separating disk. (Oper. Dent.)

   Merkel's d. (see **corpuscle, Merkel's**)

   polishing d. A disk with an extremely fine abrasive; used to finish and polish a surface. (Oper. Dent.)

   safe-side d. A separating disk with abrasive on one side only; the other side is smooth. (Oper. Dent.)

   sandpaper d. An abrasive disk with sandpaper as the abrading medium. (Oper. Dent.)

   separating d. A disk of steel or hard rubber. (Oper. Dent.)

   d. of temporomandibular joint A plate of fibrous tissue that divides the temporomandibular joint into an upper and a lower cavity. The disk is attached to the articular capsule and moves forward with the condyle in free opening and protrusion. (Oral Physiol.)

dislocation Displacement of any part, especially a bone or bony articulation. (Oral Surg.)

dislodgment Movement or removal of a prosthesis from its established position. (Remov. Part. Prosth.)

disorder(s) Derangement of function.

   coagulation d. Any one of the hemorrhagic diseases caused by a deficiency of plasma thromboplastin formation (deficiency of antihemophilic factor, plasma thromboplastic antecedent, Hageman factor, Stuart factor), deficiency of thrombin formation (deficiency of prothrombin, factor V, factor VII, Stuart factor), and deficiency of fibrin formation (afibrinogenemia, fibrinogenopenia). (Oral Med.)

   periodic d. A variety of disorders of unknown cause that have in common periodic recurrence of manifestations. Such disorders are usually benign, resist treatment, often begin in infancy, and occasionally have a hereditary pattern. Included are periodic sialorrhea, neutropenia, arthralgia, fever, purpura (anaphylactoid purpura), edema (angioneurotic edema), abdominalgia, and periodic parotitis (recurrent parotitis). (Oral Med.)

   platelet d. Hemorrhagic disease due to an abnormality of the blood platelets; e.g., thrombocytopenia and thrombasthenia. (Oral Med.)

   psychophysiologic, autonomic, and visceral d. Diseases due to overactivity or underactivity of organs and viscera innervated by the autonomic nervous system; related to exaggerated forms of the normal physiologic organic components of emotion; e.g., peptic ulcer. (Oral Med.) (see also **disease, psychosomatic**)

   visual d. Disorders that may result from injury or disease to the eyeball and its adnexa, the retina, or the cornea; e.g., contusions of the orbit and eyelids, opacities of the lens, corneal scars, and vascular changes to the retina. These peripheral disorders are effective in causing partial or total loss of vision in one or both eyes. They are simple, concrete, and fundamental. One sees or one does not see, and gray visions are generally quantitative differences that affect the perception of light and shadow, color and form. Visual disorders may also result from injury or disease to the optic tract fibers, the optic chiasma, the cerebral pathways, and the visual cortex in the occipital region of the cerebrum. These disorders are qualitative deviations from the normal, and the symptoms include visual field defects such as tubular vision found in hysteria, complete blindness in one or both eyes due to optic nerve injury, and hemianopsia, in which vision may be lost in one half of the visual field of one or both eyes. Other visual disorders include night and day blindness, color blindness, and the serious visual agnosia that results from trauma, tumor, or vascular disorders in the visual cortex of the cerebrum. (Oral Physiol.)

displaceability of tissue (see **tissue, displaceability**)

disprove To refute or to prove to be false by affirmative evidence to the contrary. (D. Juris.)

dissection, neck Removal of the lymph nodes and contiguous tissues from a primary site in the mandibular and/or maxillofacial area as treatment of neoplastic cells that have involved the regional cervical lymphatic system. (Oral Surg.)

dissolve To terminate, cancel, annul, disintegrate. To release the obligation of anything, as to dissolve a partnership. (D. Juris.)

distal Away from the median sagittal plane of the face and following the curvature of the dental arch. (Comp. Prosth.; Oper. Dent.; Orthodont.; Remov. Part. Prosth.)

d. end The most posterior part of a removable dental restoration or denture flange. (Comp. Prosth.; Remov. Part. Prosth.)

distance The measure of space intervening between two objects or two points of reference.

anode-film d. (see **distance, target-film**)

cone d. The distance between the focal spot and the outer end of the cone; usually expressed in inches or centimeters. Modern dental roentgen-ray units usually have cone distances of from 5 to 20 inches. (Oral Radiol.)

long c. d. A tubular extension made of either plastic or metal. When properly diaphragmed for its length, it restricts the beam of x radiation to the part of the object under immediate examination and thus minimizes the secondary radiation by limiting the size of the exposed area. Increased cone distance results in decreased geometric haziness, making radiographic detail more plainly visible. Long (extended) cone distance is usually 14 to 20 inches. (Oral Radiol.)

short c. d. A focal-skin distance of 9 inches or less; usually refers to the distance as determined by the cone supplied by the manufacturer in the basic x-ray unit. (Oral Radiol.)

focal-film d. (see **distance, target-film**)

interarch d. (interridge d.) The vertical distance between the maxillary and mandibular arches (alveolar or residual) under conditions of vertical relations that must be specified. (Comp. Prosth.; Remov. Part. Prosth.)

large i. d. A large distance between the maxillary and mandibular arches. (Comp. Prosth.; Remov. Part. Prosth.)

reduced i. d. (overclosure) An occlusal vertical dimension that results in (1) an excessive interocclusal distance when the mandible is in rest position and (2) a reduced interridge distance and shortened face length when the teeth are in contact. (Comp. Prosth.; Remov. Part. Prosth.)

small i. d. A small distance between the maxillary and mandibular aches. (Comp. Prosth.; Remov. Part. Prosth.)

interocclusal d. (interocclusal gap, free-way space) The distance between the occluding surfaces of the maxillary and mandibular teeth when the mandible is in its physiologic rest position. This can be determined by calculating the difference between the rest vertical dimension and the occlusal vertical dimension of the face. (Comp. Prosth.; Fixed Part. Prosth.; Remov. Part. Prosth.)

interridge d. (see **distance, interarch**)

object-film d. The distance, usually expressed in centimeters or inches, between the object being radiographed and the cassette or film. (Oral Radiol.)

target-film d. (anode-film d., focal-film d.) The distance between the focal spot of the tube and the film; usually expressed in inches or centimeters. (Oral Radiol.)

distention A state of dilation. (Anesth.)

distocclusion Posterior malrelation of lower jaw to upper jaw. (Orthodont.)

bilateral d. Distocclusion on both sides. (Orthodont.)

unilateral d. Distocclusion on one side. (Orthodont.)

distomolar A supernumerary (fourth) molar located posterior to the third molar. (Oral Diag.)

— An accessory tooth located distal to the third molar. (Oral Path.)

distortion Permanent deformation of an object. (Comp. Prosth.; Remov. Part. Prosth.)

— Modification of the speech sound in some way so that the acoustic result only approximates the standard sound and is not accurate. (Cleft Palate)

— Twisting or deformation. Loss of accuracy in reproduction of cavity form. (Oper. Dent.)

film-fault d. Change in the size or shape of an object upon projection, by either magnification, elongation, or foreshortening. Distortion is brought about by malalignment of the cone relative to the object and/or film and may be influenced by cone distance and/or object-film distance. (Oral Radiol.)

horizontal d. Disproportional change in size and shape in the horizontal plane due to oblique horizontal angulation. (Oral Radiol.)

magnification d. Proportional enlargement of a radiographic image. It is always present to some degree in oral radiography but is minimized with extended focal-film distances. (Oral Radiol.)

vertical d. (foreshortening) Disproportional change in size, either elongation or foreshortening, due to incorrect vertical angulation or improper film placement. (Oral Radiol.)

distoversion Placement of a tooth farther than normal from the median plane or midline. Also, placement of the maxilla or mandible in a position posterior to its normal position. (Orthodont.)

distraction Placement of teeth or other maxillary or mandibular structures farther than normal from the median plane. (Orthodont.)

disturbances, nutritional Alterations of the processes and structural components of the body produced by dietary deficiencies or excesses of essential nutritional substances. For example, vitamin deficiency may result in hypocalcification of the teeth (during tooth formation) and in skeletal deformities associated with insufficient calcification; hypervitaminosis D results in weakness, fatigue, loss of weight, etc. (Periodont.)

disturbances, occlusal Derangements in the patterns of occlusion that may produce disturbances in the periodontium; e.g., faulty centric relation with a positive habit pattern or plunger cusps that contribute to food impaction. (Periodont.)

ditch (ditching) Undesirable loss of tooth substance in the region of a restoration margin (usually gingival). (Oper. Dent.)

ditching (see **ditch**)

diuretic, *n.* (dī″ū-rĕt′ĭk) A drug that increases the formation of urine. (Pharmacol.)

—, *adj.* Pertaining to the increased formation of urine. (Oral Med.)

dizziness An unpleasant sensation of disturbed relations to surrounding objects in space. (Anesth.)

DMF index rate (see **rate, DMF index**)

doctor A learned person; one qualified in a science or art; one who has received the highest academic degree in a particular field. (D. Juris.)

dolichocephalic (dol′ĭ-kō-sĕ-făl′ĭk) Descriptive term applied to a long and narrow head (with a cephalic index below 75). (Orthodont.)

dolor (dō′lor) Pain. (Anesth.)

Donders, space of (see **space of Donders**)

donor site The portion of the body from which a skin, tooth, bone, or other graft or implant is taken. (Oral Implant.; Oral Surg.) (see also **recipient site**)

Donovan body (see **body, Donovan**)

dope Any drug, taken temporarily or habitually, that is administered to stimulate or to stupefy.

dorsal (dor′săl) Pertaining to the back or to the posterior part of an organ. (Anesth.)

dorsum sella (dŏr′sŭm sĕl′ah) Most posterior point on the internal contour of sella turcica. (Orthodont.)

dosage (dō′sĭj) The amount of a medicine or other agent administered for a given case or condition. (Anesth.)

dose The quantity of drug necessary to produce a desired effect. (Anesth.; Oral Med.; Pharmacol.)

— The total radiation delivered to a specified area or volume or to the whole body. In radiology the dose may be specified in air, on the skin, or at some depth beneath the surface; no statement of dose is complete without specification of location. Dose can be expressed in terms of roentgens (or curies in the case of particulate energy), which would be an expression of the exposure dose, but the more modern and informative method is to express dose in terms of energy absorbed by tissue (e.g., ergs per gram). Dose in oral radiology is still properly expressed as roentgens—usually roentgens in air. (Oral Radiol.) (see also **dose, radiation absorbed**)

absorbed d. (symbol D) The amount of energy imparted by ionizing particles to unit mass of irradiated material at a place of interest. The unit of absorbed dose is the rad (100 ergs/g). (Oral Radiol.)

air d. X-ray dose delivered at a point in free air; expressed in roentgens. It consists only of the radiation of the primary beam and the radiation scattered from surrounding air; does not include backscatter from radiated matter, e.g., tissue. (Oral Radiol.)

booster d. Portion of an immunizing agent given at a later time to stimulate the effects of a previous dose of the same agent. (Anesth.)

cumulative d. The total accumulated dose resulting from a single or repeated exposure to radiation of the same region or of the whole body. If used in area monitoring, it represents the accumulated radiation exposure over a given period of time. (Oral Radiol.)

depth d. The absorbed dose of radiation imparted to matter at a particular depth below the surafce, usually expressed as percentage depth dose. (Oral Radiol.) (see also **dose, percentage depth**)

d. distribution A representation of the variation of dose with position in any region of an irradiated object. The dose distribution may be measured using detectors small enough to avoid disturbing the distribution; or it may be calculated and expressed in mathematical form. (Oral Radiol.)

doubling d. The amount of ionizing radiation, absorbed by the gonads of the average person in a population over a period of several generations, that will result in a doubling of the current rate of spontaneous mutations. (Oral Radiol.)

d. equivalent (DE) The product of absorbed dose and modifying factors, namely the quality factor (QF), distribution factor (DF), and any other necessary factors. The unit of dose equivalent is the rem (rads × qualifying factors). (Oral Radiol.)

erythema d. The dose of radiation necessary to produce a temporary redness of the skin. This dose varies with the quality of radiation. (Oral Radiol.)

exit d. The absorbed dose delivered by a beam of radiation at the surface through which the beam emerges from a phantom or patient. (Oral Radiol.)

exposure d. (see **exposure**)

fractionation d. A dose given by a number of shorter exposures over a longer period than would be required if the dose was given by a continuous exposure in one session at the same dose rate. (Oral Radiol.)

gonadal d. The dose of radiation absorbed by the gonads. (Oral Radiol.)

integral d. (integral absorbed dose, volume dose) The total energy absorbed by a part or object during exposure to radiation. The

unit of integral dose is the gram rad (100 ergs). (Oral Radiol.)

LD$_{50}$ (see **median lethal dose**)

lethal d. The amount of a drug that would prove fatal to the majority of persons. (Anesth.)

— The amount of radiation that will be or may be sufficient to cause the death of an organism. (Oral Radiol.)

median l. d. (LD$_{50}$) The amount of ionizing radiation required to kill, within a specified period, 50% of the individuals in a large group or population of animals or organisms. (Oral Radiol.)

minimum l. d. (MLD) The minimal amount of a drug that will kill an experimental animal. (Oral Med.; Oral Radiol.; Pharmacol.)

maintenance d. The quantity of drug necessary to sustain a normal physiologic state or a desired blood or tissue level of drug. (Anesth.; Oral Med.; Pharmacol.)

maximum permissible d. (MPD) The maximum relative biologic effect dose that the body of a person or specific parts thereof shall be permitted to receive in a stated period of time. In most instances, for the x radiation used in dental radiography, it is satisfactory to consider the RBE dose in rems numerically equal to the absorbed dose in rads; and the absorbed dose in rads numerically equal to the exposure dose in roentgens. (Oral Radiol.) (see also **dose, weekly permissible**)

median effective d. (ED$_{50}$) A dose that, under standard conditions, is effective in 50% of a randomly selected group of subjects. (Oral Med.; Pharmacol.)

percentage depth d. The ratio (expressed as a percentage) of the absorbed dose at a given depth in an irradiated body, to the absorbed dose at a fixed reference point on the central ray, usually the surface-absorbed dose. (Oral Radiol.)

priming d. A quantity several times larger than the maintenance dose; used at the initiation of therapy to establish rapidly the desired blood and tissue levels of the drug. (Anesth.; Oral Med.; Pharmacol.)

d. protraction A method of radiation administration delivered continuously over a relatively long period at a relatively low dosage rate. (Oral Radiol.)

radiation d. The amount of energy absorbed per unit mass of tissue at a site of interest. Note: This definition limits the use of "dose" to conform with the 1962 recommendations of the International Commission on Radiological Units and Measurements (ICRUM). The following terms therefore become obsolete. They will be found in this glossary under the general heading of exposure: air dose, cumulative dose, exposure dose, and threshold dose. (Oral Radiol.)

radiation-absorbed d. (rad) The unit of absorbed dose, with a value of 100 ergs per gram. (Oral Radiol.)

d. rate The time rate at which radiation dose is applied, expressed in either roentgens per unit time or rads per unit time. (Oral Radiol.)

skin d. (see **dose, surface-absorbed**)

surface-absorbed d. The absorbed dose delivered by a radiation beam at the point where the central ray passes through the superficial layer of the phantom or patient. (Oral Radiol.)

therapeutic d. A quantity several times larger than the maintenance dose; used in vitamin therapy where a marked deficiency exists. (Anesth.; Oral Med.; Pharmacol.)

threshold d. The minimum dose that will produce a detectable degree of any given effect. (Oral Radiol.)

tissue d. The dose absorbed by a tissue or the tissues in a region of interest. (Oral Radiol.)

tolerance d. (see **dose, maximum permissible**)

toxic d. The amount of a drug that causes untoward symptoms in the majority of persons. (Anesth.)

transit d. A measure of the primary radiation transmitted through the patient and measured at a point on the central ray at some point beyond the patient. (Oral Radiol.)

U.S.P. d. (see **dose, median effective [ED$_{50}$]; dose, lethal, median [LD$_{50}$]; dose, lethal, minimum [MLD]; drug, official**)

volume d. (see **dose, integral**)

weekly permissible d. A dose of ionizing radiation accumulated in 1 week and of such magnitude that, in the light of present knowledge, exposure at this weekly rate for an indefinite period of time is not expected to cause appreciable bodily injury to a person at any time during his lifetime. (Oral Radiol.)

dose-effect curve (see **curve, dose-effect**)

dosimetry (dō-sĭm′ĕ-trē) The accurate and systematic determination of the amount of radiation to which an animal or person has been exposed during a given period of time. (Oral Radiol.)

dovetail A widened or fanned-out portion of a prepared cavity, usually established deliberately to increase the retention form and the resistance form. (Oper. Dent.)

lingual d. A dovetail established as a step portion, with lingual approach, in some Class 3 and Class 4 preparations; used to supplement the retention form and the resistance form. (Oper. Dent.)

occlusal d. A dovetail established at the terminal of the occlusal step of a proximal cavity. (Oper. Dent.)

dowel A post or pin, usually made of metal, fitted into a prepared root canal of a natural tooth. When combined with an artificial crown, it gives added retention to the prosthesis. (Fixed Part. Prosth.)

drachm (drăm) (see **dram**)

draft (see **draw**)

drag The lower, or cast, side of a denture mold or flask, to which the cope is fitted. The base of the cast is embedded in plaster or stone, with the remainder of the denture pattern exposed to be engaged by the plaster or stone in the cope (the upper part of the flask). (Comp. Prosth.)

drain Any substance that provides a channel for release or discharge from a wound. (Oral Surg.)

cigarette d. (see **drain, Penrose**)

Penrose d. (cigarette d.) A thin-walled rubber tube through which a piece of gauze has been pulled. (Oral Surg.)

dram (drachm) A unit of weight that equals the eighth part of the apothecaries' ounce. Symbol ℥. (Anesth.)

draught (drăft) (see **draw**)

draw (draft, draught) The taper or divergence of the walls of a preparation for a cemented restoration. (Oper. Dent.)

drepanocythemia (drĕp″ah-nō-sī-thē′mē-ah) (see **anemia, sickle cell**)

dressing, Kirkland cement A surgical dressing applied to the tissues after periodontal surgery; consists of zinc oxide, tannic acid, and powdered rosin, admixed with a liquid composed of lump rosin, sweet almond oil, and eugenol. (Periodont.)

dressing, postoperative surgical A surgical cement dressing applied to the teeth and tissues after surgical periodontal therapy. Possesses supportive, protective, hemostatic, analgesic, and other properties. (Periodont.)

drift (see **tooth, drifting**)

drill A cutting instrument for boring holes by rotary motion. (Oper. Dent.)

bibevel d. A drill with two flattened sides and and the end cut in two beveled planes. (Oper. Dent.)

spear-point d. A drill with a tribeveled, or three-planed, point. (Oper. Dent.)

twist d. A drill with one or more deep spiral grooves that extend from the point to the smooth part of the shaft. (Oper. Dent.)

drilling (objectionable as a term describing the general preparation of cavities with rotary instruments) Boring a hole with a rotary cutting instrument; used in reference to pinholes. (Oper. Dent.)

drip The continuous slow intravenous introduction of fluid containing nutrients or drugs. (Anesth.)

droplet spread Transmission of an infection through the projection of oral and nasal secretions by coughing, sneezing, or talking. (Oral Med.)

dropsy (drahp′sē) (see **anasarca**)

drug(s) A substance used in the prevention, cure, or alleviation of disease or pain, or as an aid in some diagnostic procedures. (Oral Med.; Periodont.; Pharmacol.)

d. abuse Excessive or improper use of drugs, especially through self-administration for nonmedical purposes. This term has increased significance because of the enactment of the Comprehensive Drug Abuse Prevention and Control Act of 1970, which replaces the Harrison Narcotic Act. (D. Juris.; Pharmacol.)

antibiotic d. Chemical compounds obtained from certain living cells of lower plant forms such as bacteria, yeasts, and molds, and from synthesis. They are antagonistic to certain pathogenic organisms and have a lethal effect on them. (Periodont.)

antiseptic d. A chemical compound used to reduce the number of microorganisms in the oral cavity. (Periodont.)

autonomic d. A drug that mimics or blocks the effects of stimulation of the autonomic nervous system. (Oral Med.; Pharmacol.)

desensitizing d. A pharmaceutical utilized to diminish or eliminate sensitivity of teeth to physical, chemical, thermal, or other irritants; e.g., strontium chloride, silver nitrate (ammoniacal), sodium fluoride, formalin, zinc chloride. (Periodont.)

endodontic d. Any one of the drugs used in treating the dental pulp and dental periapical tissues. (Endodont.)

nonofficial d. A drug that is not listed in the *United States Pharmacopeia* (U.S.P) or the *National Formulary* (N.F.). (Oral Med.; Pharmacol.)

official d. A drug that is listed in the U.S.P. or N.F. (Oral Med.; Pharmacol.)

officinal d. (of-ĭs′ĭn-al) Drugs that may be purchased without a prescription. More commonly called over-the-counter (OTC) drugs. (Oral Med.; Pharmacol.)

over-the-counter (OTC) d. A drug that may be purchased without a prescription. Sometimes called a nonlegend drug because its label does not bear the prescription legend required on all drugs that may be dispensed only on prescription. (Oral Med.; Pharmacol.)

parasympathetic d. Belladonna alkaloids that inhibit glandular secretions of the nose, mouth, pharynx, and bronchi. This is the chief reason for using atropine and scopolamine for preanesthetic medication. In contrast to atropine, scopolamine in therapeutic doses normally causes drowsiness, euphoria, amnesia, and dreamless sleep. In combination with pentobarbital, a less profound but more pleasant and longer-acting sedation is provided than when the barbiturate is used alone. (Oral Physiol.)

parasympatholytic d. (par″ah-sĭm″pah-thō-lĭt′ĭk) A drug that blocks nerve impulses passing from parasympathetic nerve fibers to postganglionic neuroeffectors. (Anesth.)

parasympathomimetic d. (par″ah-sĭm″pah-thō-mĭ-met′ĭk) A drug that has an effect similar to that produced when the parasympathetic nerves are stimulated. (Anesth.)

proprietary d. A drug that is patented or controlled by a private organization or manufacturer. (Oral Med.; Pharmacol.)

dry socket (see **socket, dry**)

Dry-foil Proprietary form of tinfoil that is supplied with an adhesive powder or coating on one side. (Oper. Dent.)

dual impression technique (see **technique, impression, dual**)

duct A small passage.

nasopalatine d. (see **cyst, nasopalatine**)

Stensen's d. The excretory duct of the parotid gland; it passes lateral to the masseter muscle and enters the oral cavity through the buccal tissues adjacent to the maxillary first and second molars. (Oral Surg.; Periodont.)

Wharton's d. The excretory duct of the submaxillary glands; opens into the oral cavity at the sublingual papillae of the mucous membrane of the floor of the mouth behind the lower incisor teeth. (Oral Surg.; Periodont.)

ductility (dŭk-tĭl´ĭ-tē) Ability of a material to withstand permanent deformation under a tensile load without rupture. It is assessed by percentage elongation, cold bend, or reduction in area tests. Generally a reflection or indication of brittleness. (D. Mat.)

— The property of a material that allows permanent deformation under tension without rupture. It is measured as percentage increase in length on rupture compared with original length and is termed percentage elongation or elongation. (Oper. Dent.)

— The property of a metal that allows bending, burnishing, or drawing without danger of breakage. (Remov. Part. Prosth.)

Duke's test (see **test, Duke's**)

Dunlop file (see **file, Hirschfeld-Dunlop**)

duplication The procedure of accurately reproducing a cast or other object. (Remov. Part. Prosth.)

    d. impression (see **duplication**)

duty That which is due from a person; that which a person owes to another. An obligation. (D. Juris.)

dwarf, pituitary (pĭ-tū´ĭ-tār˝ē) An individual who is of small stature as a result of a deficiency of growth hormones. Such dwarfs usually are well proportioned. (Oral Diag.)

dwarfism Deficient growth and development leading to small stature and often skeletal deformity. It may be associated with ovarian agenesis, pituitary insufficiency, mongolism, progeria, rickets, renal disease, dietary deficiency, achondroplasia, cleidocranial dysostosis, osteogenesis imperfecta, microcephaly, hydrocephaly, sexual precocity, delayed adolescence. (Oral Diag.; Oral Med.; Oral Path.)

dye, occlusal registration A water-soluble dye used as an aid in the detection of deflective occlusal contacts or interferences. Particularly a valuable aid in effecting the fine adjustments in the final phases of the selective grinding procedure. (Periodont.)

dyes, treatment The dyes used in medicine and dentistry in the treatment of diseased states, the most useful of which are the rosanilin dyes (e.g., gentian violet and crystal violet) and the fluorescein dyes (e.g., Mercurochrome), which possess antiseptic and protective properties. (Periodont.)

dynamic relation (see **relation, dynamic**)

dysautonomia, familial (dĭs˝aw-tō-nō´mē-ah) (see **syndrome, Riley-Day**)

dyscrasia (dĭs-krā´zē-ah) A morbid condition, especially one that involves an imbalance of component elements. (Anesth.)

— Abnormal composition of the blood, e.g., in leukemias and anemias. (Oral Diag.)

dysdiadochokinesia (dĭs˝dī-ah-dō˝kō-kĭ-nē´zē-ah) Disturbance of musculoskeletal function. There is a disorganization in the reciprocal innervation of agonists and antagonists and a loss of the ability to stop one act in terms of rate, magnitude, and the direction of movement and immediately to follow it with another act diametrically opposite, e.g., alternately elevating and depressing the mandible. Another example is observed in the inappropriate use of the tongue during mastication when it is necessary to change, reverse, and modify the energy and direction of movement. (Oral Physiol.)

dysesthesia (dĭs˝ĕs-thē´zē-ah) Impairment of the senses, especially of the sense of touch. Painfulness of any sensation not normally painful. (Anesth.)

dysfunction (dĭs-fŭnk´shŭn) **(malfunction)** Any abnormality or impairment of function. (Anesth.)

— Impairment or abnormality in the functioning of a part or organ. (Periodont.)

    dental d. Abnormal functioning of dental structures. Partial disturbance or impairment of the functioning of the dental organ. (Comp. Prosth.; Remov. Part. Prosth.)

    endocrine d. Abnormality in the function of an endocrine gland, either by hypofunction or hyperfunction of the secretory elements of the gland. Endocrine dysfunction may produce oral manifestations; e.g., hypoestrogenism associated with diminution of keratinization and desquamation of areas of the oral mucosal surface. (Periodont.)

dysgnathia (dĭs-nā´thē-ah) Those abnormalities that extend beyond the teeth and include the maxillae, the mandible, or both. (Oral Surg.; Orthodont.) (see also **anomaly, dysgnathic**)

dyskeratosis (dĭs˝ker-ah-tō´sis) An irreversible alteration in the maturation of stratified squamous epithelium. Term refers to an increase of abnormal mitosis, individual cell keratinization, epithelial pearls within the spinous layer, loss of polarity of the cells, hyperchromatism, nuclear atypia, and basilar hyperplasia. (Oral Path.)

dysmenorrhea (dĭs˝mĕn-ō-rē´ah) Painful menstruation. (Oral Diag.)

dysmetria (dĭs-mē'trē-ah) Loss of ability to gauge distance, speed, or power of movement associated with muscle function; e.g., the patient is unable to control the force of closure and strikes the opposite occluding teeth with greater vigor than necessary. This either wears the teeth by abrasion or causes periodontal disease. (Oral Physiol.)

dysostosis (dĭs-ŏs-tō'sĭs) Defective ossification. (Oral Path.)

cleidocranial d. (klī"dō-krā'nē-al) (**Sainton's disease**) A familial disease or congenital disorder characterized by failure to form, or retarded formation of, the clavicles; delayed closure of the sutures and fontanels; and delayed eruption of teeth, with formation of supernumerary teeth. It is characterized by underdevelopment of the maxillae; agnesis or aplasia of the clavicle; abnormalities in other skeletal bones and muscles; and irregularities of the dentition. The syndrome may be mutational or transmitted on an autosomal dominant basis. (Oral Diag.; Oral Med.; Oral Path.; Pedodont.)

craniofacial d. (Crouzon's disease, Crouzon's syndrome) A condition of unknown etiology that is similar to cleidocranial dysostosis but differs in that the clavicles are not affected. (Oral Path.) (see also **dysostosis, cleidocranial**)

faciomandibular d. Developmental disturbance of the cranial bones and hypoplasias of the upper part of the face. The mandibular body is underdeveloped, but the ramus is hyperplastic. The teeth are crowded and malposed. (Oral Path.)

d. multiplex (see **syndrome, Hurler's**)

dysphagia (dĭs-fă-jē-ah) Difficulty in swallowing. It may be due to lesions in the mouth, pharynx, or larynx, neuromuscular disturbances, or mechanical obstruction of the esophagus; e.g., dysphagia of Plummer-Vinson syndrome (sideropenic dysphagia), peritonsillar abscess, Ludwig's angina, and carcinoma of the tongue, pharynx, or larynx. (Oral Diag.; Oral Med.)

dysphoria (dĭs-for'ē-ah) A feeling of discomfort or restlessness. (Oral Med.; Pharmacol.) (see also **euphoria**)

dysplasia (dĭs-plā'zē-ah) Developmental abnormality. (Oral Diag.) (see also **dysplasia, dentinal**)

— Reversible, regressive alteration in adult cells, seen as alterations in their size, shape, orientation, and functions; leads to change in tissue architecture and is related to chronic inflammation or protracted irritation. Abnormality of development. (Oral Path.)

— Disharmony between component parts. (Orthodont.)

anteroposterior d. (anteroposterior facial d.) An abnormal anteroposterior relationship of the maxillae and mandible to each other or to the cranial base. (Orthodont.)

craniofacial d. Disharmony between the cranium and the face. (Orthodont.)

dentinal d. A genetic disturbance of the dentin; characterized by early calcification of the pulp chambers and root canals and by root resorption. It is differentiated from dentinogenesis imperfecta by the latter's characteristics of attrition and relative freedom from root resorption. ·(Oral Diag.)

dentofacial d. Disharmony between teeth and bones of the face, e.g., crowding or spacing. (Orthodont.)

ectodermal d. A disease of genetic origin characterized by failure to form ectodermal derivatives. Sweat glands and teeth may be missing (anhidrosis and anodontia, respectively), and there may be scant hair, faulty fingernails, and malformation of the iris. (Oral Diag.)

— A condition, usually hereditary, in which there is partial or complete absence of ectodermal structures, including skin, sweat glands, sebaceous glands, hair, teeth, and portions of teeth. (Oral Path.)

— A hereditary disorder in which ectodermal derivations are arrested in development during the first trimester of pregnancy. (Pedodont.)

fibro-osseous d. (see **dysplasia, fibrous**)

fibrous d. (fibro-osseous d.) A metabolic disturbance characterized by replacement of the bone marrow with fibrous tissue and slow, progressive remolding and enlargement of the bone. It may be monostotic (limited to one bone) or polyostotic (present in many bones). Albright's syndrome shows polyostotic fibrous dysplasia and other symptoms. The monostotic lesions may be identical with ossifying fibroma or with osseous dysplasia. (Oral Diag.)

— Disease of bone in which there is a central proliferation of fibrous connective tissue that may contain bone spicules. Causes localized replacement of bone marrow and thinning and distortion of cortex. The lesions may be monostotic or polyostotic (ossifying fibroma and Albright's syndrome, respectively). (Oral Path.) (see also **osteofibroma; syndrome, Albright's**)

polyostotic f. d. Fibrous dysplasia occurring in more than one bone. (Oral Path.) (see also **dysplasia, fibrous; osteofibroma; syndrome, Albright's**)

maxillomandibular d. Disharmony between one jaw and the other. (Orthodont.)

osseous d. A chronic reaction of the bone to injury; characterized by replacement of the bone marrow with fibrous connective tissue, unilateral enlargement of the maxillae or mandible, and characteristic radiographic findings. It is similar to or identical with monostotic fibrous dysplasia and ossifying fibroma. (Oral Diag.)

focal o. d. (see **fibroma, periapical**)

dyspnea (dǐsp-nē'ah) Difficult, labored, or gasping breathing; inspiration, expiration, or both may be involved. (Anesth.; Oral Diag.; Oral Med.)

dysrhythmia (dǐs-rǐth'mē-ah) Disordered rhythm. (Anesth.)

dystonia (dǐs-tō'nē-ah) Disorder or lack of tonicity. (Anesth.)

dystrophy (dǐs'trō-fē) Faulty nutrition. Often used to refer to the results of faulty nutrition, i.e., wasting away. (Oral Diag.)

muscular d. Defective nutrition of the muscles, leading to weakness and atrophy. (Oral Diag.)

— A chronic, degenerative, noncontagious, progressive disorder of unknown etiology manifested by weakness and wasting away of the voluntary muscles. (Pedodont.)

E

Eames' technique (ēmz) (see **technique, Eames'**)

eburnation (ē″ber-nā′shŭn) Increased bony density at the ends of ununited fractures. (Oral Surg.) (see also **osteitis, condensing; dentin eburnation**)

eccentric (ĕk-sĕn′trĭk) Deviation from the normal or conventional, or away from the central or reference position. (Comp. Prosth.)

> **e. checkbite** (see **record, interocclusal, eccentric**)
>
> **e. jaw relation** (see **relation, jaw, eccentric**)
>
> **e. occlusion** (see **occlusion, eccentric**)
>
> **e. position** (see **position, eccentric**)

ecchymosis (ĕk″ĭ-mō′sĭs) Discoloration of mucous membranes caused by a diffuse extravasation of blood. Frequently called a bruise. (Oral Diag.)

— Blotchy discoloration of the skin, mucous membrane, or serosal surface caused by extravasation of blood; over 1 cm. in diameter. (Oral Path.)

economics In dentistry, a broad term that covers all the business aspects of dental practice. (Pract. Man.)

ectomorph (ĕk′tō-morf) A constitutional body type (Sheldon's classification) characterized by long, fragile bones and a highly developed nervous system. (Oral Med.)

ectopic eruption (see **eruption, ectopic**)

ectropion (ĕk-trō′pē-on) Eversion, or rolling outward, of the eyelid margin. (Oral Diag.)

eczema (ĕk′zē-mah) An inflammatory skin disease characterized by vesiculation, inflammation, watery discharge, and the development of scales and crusts. The large variety of types can be distinguished according to location and etiology. (Oral Diag.)

ED₅₀ (see **dose, median effective**)

edema (ĕ-dē′mah) Excessive accumulation of fluid in the tissue spaces due to a disturbance in the mechanism of fluid exchange. (Anesth.)

— Presence of abnormally large quantities of fluid in the intercellular regions, resulting in swelling. (Oral Diag.)

— Accumulation of fluid in the tissues or in the peritoneal or pleural cavities. Primary factors favoring edema are increased capillary hydrostatic pressure (increased venous pressure), decreased osmotic pressure of plasma (hypoproteinemia), decreased tissue tension, increased osmotic pressure of tissue fluids, lymphatic drainage, and increased capillary permeability. Additional renal and hormonal factors are important. Clinical manifestations may consist of a steady weight gain or localized or generalized swelling. (Oral Med.; Oral Physiol.)

— Extravasation of fluid components of the blood into the intercellular tissue spaces of the body, a phenomenon often associated with inflammation, increased hydrostatic pressure of the blood, and/or gradient in colloid osmotic pressure between the circulatory system and the surrounding extravascular areas. (Periodont.)

> **angioneurotic e. (angioedema, giant urticaria, Quincke's disease)** Spontaneous swelling of the lips, cheeks, eyelids, tongue, soft palate, pharynx, and glottis, frequently associated with allergy to foods or drugs and lasting from several hours to several days. Involvement of the glottis results in obstruction of the airway. (Oral Diag.; Oral Med.)
>
> — A smooth, diffuse swelling that usually occurs around the lips, eyes, and chin but may involve any body area. It is characterized as giant urticaria and occurs in a hereditary form and also in a nonhereditary form that is usually associated with food allergy. (Oral Path.)
>
> — A sudden, painless swelling affecting the cheeks, lips, tongue, eyelids, soft palate, pharynx, etc. Produced by hypersensitivity to certain substances or by a predisposing neurotropic background. Such swelling does not pit on pressure, and there is a conspicuous absence of erythema. (Periodont.)
>
> **cardiac e.** Edema due to venous congestion in association with congestive heart failure; tends to appear first in such dependent parts as the legs. (Oral Med.)
>
> **dependent e.** Edema that changes its position with the posture of dependent parts; e.g., edema of the legs in progressive heart failure. (Oral Med.)
>
> **periorbital e.** Edematous swelling of the eyelids in association with local injury, allergic reactions, hypoproteinemia, trichinosis, myxedema, etc. (Oral Med.)
>
> **pitting e.** Persistent indentation of the skin when pressure is applied to an edematous area. (Oral Med.)

edentate (ē-děn′tāt) Without teeth. (Comp. Prosth.; Remov. Part. Prosth.)

edentulate (ē-děn′tū-lāt) (see **edentulous**)

edentulism (ē-děn′tū-lĭzm) The condition of being edentulous, without teeth. (Comp. Prosth.; Remov. Part. Prosth.)

edentulous (ē-děn′tū-lŭs) Without teeth; lacking teeth. (Comp. Prosth.)

edge strength (see **strength, edge**)

edge-to-edge bite (see **occlusion, edge-to-edge**)

edge-to-edge occlusion (see **occlusion, edge-to-edge**)

edgewise appliance (see **appliance, edgewise**)

Edtac Proprietary chelating agent used to soften calcified tissue. (Endodont.)

education of patient Effective communication between the dentist (and/or his auxiliaries) and the patient concerning dentistry and the principles of treatment and prevention. The procedure of increasing the patient's knowledge of the oral cavity and its care to the point where he can understand the reasons for proposed dental services. (Pract. Man.)

effect The result of an action.

   e. of external radiation on bone (see **osteoradionecrosis**)

   e. of function on bone (see **law, Wolff's**)

   heel e. (anode heel effect) Varation of intensity over the cross section of a useful x-ray beam, due to the angle at which x rays emerge from beneath the surface of the focal spot, which causes a differential attenuation of photons comprising the useful beam. (Oral Radiol.)

   lysing e. The disintegrating action on tissue components produced by the toxic and compressive products of inflammation. In gingival inflammation, lysis of the gingival fibers must occur before apical migration of the epithelial attachment can occur. In microbiology, the presence of complement in the antigen-antibody complex is necessary for bacterial lysis. Hemolysis occurs with coexistence of erythrocyte, antibody, and complement. (Periodont.)

   wedging e. An effect produced by food impaction that forces the teeth apart. (Periodont.)

effective half-life (see **life, radioactive**)

effector (ě-fěk′tor) A motor or secretory nerve ending in an organ, gland, or muscle; consequently called an effector organ. (Anesth.)

— An on-the-job organ of the body that responds to stimulations asking for corrections. It is the opposite term for receptor. (Oral Physiol.)

efferent (ěf′er-ěnt) Conveying away from a center toward the periphery. (Anesth.)

efficiency Operation of a dental practice in such a way that both business and professional services are performed in a minimum amount of time without sacrificing quality of work, sympathetic attitude, and kindliness. (Pract. Man.)

eH Symbol for oxidation-reduction potential, which is regarded as a significant factor in the protection of the body against anaerobic bacteria. The eH of living tissue of pH 7.4 is about 0.12 volt. (Oral Med.)

Ehlers-Danlos syndrome (ā′lerz dăn′lōs) (see **syndrome, Ehlers-Danlos**)

ejector By common usage, a device used to remove debris and fluids by negative pressure. Correct term for such a device, however, is aspirator. (Oper. Dent.) (see also **aspirator**)

   saliva e. A device (containing a removable tip) that is attached to a water supply to create negative pressure to remove saliva from a dental field of operation. (Oper. Dent.)

     s. e. tip A removable tip made of metal, glass, rubber, plastic, or a combination of these, which is attached to a saliva ejector and bent to fit over lower teeth and reach the floor of the oral cavity. (Oper. Dent.)

elastic, *adj.* Referring to property of a solid substance permitting recovery of its shape after a deformation resulting from force application. (Comp. Prosth.; Remov. Part. Prosth.)

   e. deformation (see **deformation, elastic**)

   e. impression (see **impression, elastic**)

   e. limit (see **limit, elastic**)

   e. memory The property of a material (e.g., wax), enabling it, after being warmed, bent, and cooled, to return to its original form on rewarming. (Oper. Dent.)

—, *n.* A rubber elastic band used to apply force to the teeth. (Orthodont.)

   intermaxillary e. (see **elastic, maxillomandibular**)

   intramaxillary e. An elastic band within either the maxillary or mandibular arch. (Orthodont.)

   maxillomandibular e. An elastic band used between the maxillary and mandibular dentitions. (Orthodont.)

   rubber dam e. An elastic band of rubber dam latex, available in various sizes, that is utilized in the orthodontic movement of teeth. (Periodont.)

elasticity The quality or condition of being elastic. (Comp. Prosth.; Oper. Dent.; Remov. Part. Prosth.)

   modulus of e. (Young's modulus) A measurement of elasticity obtained by dividing stress below the proportional limit by its corresponding strain value. A measure of stiffness. (D. Mat.)

— A measurement of the elasticity of a material, arrived at by dividing the stress by the corresponding strain value. (Oper. Dent.)

elastomer (ē-lăs'tō-mer) A soft, rubberlike material; synthetic rubber. A rubber base impression material; e.g., silicone and mercaptan. (D. Mat.)

elastosis (ē"lăs-tō'sĭs) Degeneration of the elastic tissues; found particularly in the lips and associated with senile or actinic cheilitis. (Oral Diag.)

senile e. A dermatologic disease, the result of degeneration of the elastic connective tissue. (Oral Path.)

electroanesthesia (ē-lěk"trō-ăn-es-thē'zē-ah) Local or general anesthesia induced by electric current. (Anesth.)

electrocoagulation (ē-lěk"trō-kō-ăg"ū-lā'shŭn) The use of electrically generated heat to destroy tissue by coagulation necrosis. Usually a platinum wire electrode or loop is used. (Oral Surg.)

electrocortin (ē-lěk"trō-kor'tĭn) (see **aldosterone**)

electrode An instrument with a point or a surface from which a current can be discharged into or received from the body of a patient. (Endodont.)

electroencephalograph (ē-lěk"trō-ĕn-sĕf'ah-lō-grăf) An instrument for recording the electrical activity of the brain. (Anesth.)

electrogalvanism (ē-lěk-trō-găl'văn-ĭzm) **(galvanism)** The flow of electric current between two different metals in an electrolyte solution. Various metals used in different intraoral restorations (even two gold alloys of different composition) and saliva supply the elements for an electric current; under certain conditions such current may be produced. On relatively rare occasions it may cause pulpal pain or even mucosal lesions. (Oral Diag.; Oral Implant.)

electrolyte (ē-lěk'trō-līt) A solution that conducts electricity by means of its ions. (Anesth.; Endodont.)

— A substance which, in solution, will conduct an electric current. The electrolyte composition of the plasma includes Na, K, Mg, and Ca as cations, and Cl, HCO_3, HPO_4, and SO_4 as anions. (Oral Med.)

e. affinity The attraction of the electrolytes in the body to the different fluid compartments of the intracellular and extracellular

environments. Sodium is the predominant cation in the extracellular fluid; potassium is the predominant cation within the cells; chlorine and bicarbonate are the predominant anions in the plasma and interstitial fluids; and phosphates and proteins are the chief anions in the cells. (Oral Physiol.)

e. balance, fluid and (see **fluid and electrolyte balance**)

electrolyzer (ē-lěk'trō-lī"zer) **(ionizer)** An electric apparatus designed for use in a root canal to break down a treatment chemical into its various ions by direct current. (Endodont.) (see also **electrosterilizer**)

electromallet, McShirley's (see **condenser, electromallet**)

electromedication (see **electrosterilization**)

electrometer (ē"lěk-trom'ě-ter) An electrostatic instrument for measuring the potential difference between two points. In radiology, electrometers are used to measure changes in the potential of charged electrodes due to ionization occasioned by radiation. (Oral Radiol.)

electromyography (ē-lěk"trō-mī-ŏg'rah-fē) The recording of the electric current set up by muscular activity. (Comp. Prosth.)

— Detection, recording, and interpretation of electric voltage generated by the skeletal muscles. (Oral Physiol.)

electron (ē-lěk'tron) (symbol e) A negatively charged elementary particle constituent in every neutral atom, with a mass of 0.000549 amu, or 9.1×10^{-28} g. (Particles with an equal but opposite charge are called positrons.) (Oral Radiol.)

e. beam (see **electron stream**)

e. stream (**e. beam, cathode ray, cathode stream**) A stream of electrons emitted from the negative electrode (cathode) in a roentgen ray tube; their bombardment of the glass wall of the tube or of the anode gives rise to the roentgen rays. (Oral Radiol.)

electronic knife (see **knife, electronic**)

electroplating Plating by electrolysis; covering or coating with a layer of silver or copper. Impressions are plated in dentistry to form metalized working dies. (D. Mat.)

electropolishing Removal of a minute layer of metal by electrolysis to produce a bright surface. (D. Mat.)

electrosection An incision created by electrosurgery, ideally by using a fully rectified, alternating high-frequency current and producing minimal cellular injury. (Oral Surg.)

electrosterilization Sterilization of a prepared root canal by use of an electrosterilizer. (Endodont; Pharmacol.)

electrosterilizer An electric apparatus designed for use in root canal treatment for the electrolysis of a halide such as sodium iodide in order to release iodine in the cleaned root canal for the purpose of destroying residual organisms. (Endodont.; Pharmacol.) (see also **electrolyzer**)

electrosurgery The use of electrically generated energy from high-frequency alternating currents to cut or alter tissue within definite limits and without undesirable postsurgical sequelae. (Oral Surg.)
— The surgical technique of utilizing the electric knife, cautery, or a suitably shaped electrode. Removal and/or contouring of soft tissues may be accomplished by this method. (Periodont.)

element A simple substance that cannot be decomposed by chemical means and that is made up of atoms that are alike in their peripheral electronic configuration and chemical properties but differ in their nuclei, atomic weights, and radioactive properties. (Anesth.)
— A substance all of whose atoms have the same atomic number (i.e., same number of orbital electrons). The atomic weight (mass) of an element may vary (i.e., the number of neutrons in the nucleus), thus producing a mixture of isotopes of the same element. (Oral Radiol.)

elephantiasis (ĕl″ĕ-făn-tī′ah-sĭs) Enlargement of the gingivae due to genetic factors. Technically, elephantiasis is a specific disease caused by filariasis, but the term is used for enlargement of tissue from other causes, e.g., gingival elephantiasis. (Oral Diag.)
e. gingivae (see **fibromatosis gingivae**)

elevator An instrument used to raise or lift something. (Oral Surg.)
dental e. One of a variety of blades used for engaging teeth and/or roots to remove them from their alveoli. (Oral Surg.)
malar e. An instrument used to elevate or reposition the zygomatic bone. (Oral Surg.)
periosteal e. A thin blade used to lift periosteum from bone. (Oral Surg.)

elixir (ē-lĭk′ser) A pleasantly flavored, sweetened hydroalcoholic solution of a drug intended for oral administration. (Oral Med.; Pharmacol.)

elliptocytosis (ē-lĭp″tō-sī-tō′sĭs) (**ovalocytosis, oval cell anemia**) A hereditary anomaly in which the red blood cells are elliptical, or oval shaped, and are predisposed to hemolysis. (Oral Med.)

Elon (ē′lŏn) Proprietary chemical; one of the two chemicals used as a reducing agent in film-developing solutions. Its action controls the detail of the film and brings the image up quickly. (Oral Radiol.)

elongation (ē″long-gā′shŭn) The process or condition of increasing in length before breaking; indicates the ductility of, for example, a metal. (Remov. Part. Prosth.)
e., % The increase in length of a material after fracture in tension; a mechanical test usually employed to measure ductility. (D. Mat.)

embedded Referring to a tooth, root tip, or foreign body that is deep in bone. (Oral Surg.)

embolism (ĕm′bō-lĭzm) The clogging of a vessel by solid matter (e.g., a clot or mass of vegetation) that is carried by the bloodstream to some point where the lumen of the vessel narrows; in contradistinction to thrombosis, in which the clotting mechanism is organized in situ. (Oral Physiol.)
air e. (see **aeroembolism**)

embolus (ĕm′bō-lŭs) A blood clot or other material that travels in the bloodstream and then lodges in a vessel and obstructs circulation. (Oral Surg.)

embrasure (ĕm-brā′zhūr) The space between the curved proximal surfaces of the teeth. (Oper. Dent.)
— The space sloping occlusal to the contact area on either side of the proximal surfaces of adjacent teeth. (Remov. Part. Prosth.)
buccal e. An embrasure that opens toward the cheeks. (Oper. Dent.)
e. clasp (see **clasp, embrasure**)
e. hook An extension into the embrasure above the contact area between two adjacent teeth. It engages the buccal or labial angles of each tooth so as to resist movement in a cervical direction. Generally used for the support of a unit of a removable prosthesis. (Remov. Part. Prosth.)
interdental e. The spaces formed by the interproximal contours of adjoining teeth, beginning at the contact area and extending lingually, facially, occlusally, and apically. The flatter the proximal surfaces of the teeth, the smaller the embrasures. (Periodont.)
labial e. An embrasure that opens toward the lips. (Oper. Dent.)

lingual e. An embrasure that opens toward the tongue. (Oper. Dent.)

occlusal e. An embrasure that opens toward the occlusal surface or plane. (Oper. Dent.)

— The wedge-shaped spaces between the contact point and the buccal and lingual line angles whose forms determine whether the portion of the interdental tissue under them will receive adequate stimulation in use or whether it will be flaccid and broad because of an obstructed embrasure above it. (Periodont.)

— The space sloping occlusal to the contact area on either side of the proximal surfaces of adjacent teeth. (Remov. Part. Prosth.)

emergency An unforeseen occurrence or combination of circumstances that calls for immediate action or remedy; pressing necessity; exigency. (D. Juris.)

e. treatment Treatment that must be rendered to the patient immediately because of acute infection or pain. (Pract. Man.)

emesis (ĕm′ĕ-sĭs) The sudden expulsion of gastric contents through the esophagus into the pharynx. The act is partly voluntary and partly involuntary. (Anesth.)

emetic (ē-mĕt′ĭk) A drug that induces vomiting. (Anesth.; Oral Med.; Pharmacol.)

emetine hydrochloride (ĕm′ĕ-tēn) An alkaloid, $C_{33}H_{44}O_4N_2 \cdot 2HCl$, regarded as a protozoacide and formerly used in the treatment of periodontitis as well as in the treatment of amebic dysentery. (Periodont.)

EMF (erythrocyte-maturing factor) (see **vitamin B₁₂**)

eminence, retromylohyoid (ĕm′ĭ-nĕns, ret″-rō-mī-lō-hī′oid) The distal end of the lingual flange of a lower denture. It occupies the retromylohyoid space and usually turns laterally toward the ramus. Its anterior boundary is the lingual tuberosity (the distal end of the mylohyoid ridge), and its posterior boundary is the retromylohyoid curtain and the superior constrictor muscle. It is bounded above by the retromolar pad and below by the alveolo-lingual sulcus. (Comp. Prosth.)

eminenectomy (ĕm″ĭ-nĕn-ĕk′tō-mē) Operative removal of the anterior articular surface of the glenoid fossa. (Oral Surg.)

emollient (ē-mol′yĕnt) An agent that is soothing to the skin or mucous membrane; makes the skin softer or smoother. (Oral Med.)

emotiometabolic (ē-mō″shē-ō-mĕt″ah-bol′ĭk) Modifying metabolism as a result of emotion. (Anesth.)

emotion (ē-mō′shŭn) A mental feeling or sentiment. (Anesth.)

empathy (ĕm′pah-thē) Sensing and entering into the feelings of another person. (Comp. Prosth.; Pract. Man.)

emphysema (ĕm″fĭ-sē′mah) Presence of air in the intra-alveolar tissue of the lungs due to distention or rupture of the pulmonary alveoli with air. Interstitial (interlobular) emphysema is caused by the escape of air from the lungs into the interstitial tissue between the alveoli; vesicular (alveolar) emphysema is caused by distention of the alveoli with air. (Anesth.)

— A swelling due to air in the tissue spaces. In the oral and facial regions it may be caused either by air introduced into a tooth socket or gingival crevice with the air syringe or by blowing of the nose. (Oral Diag.)

— Permanent dilation of the respiratory alveoli. (Oral Med.)

empyema (ĕm″pī-ē′mah) Term used to indicate the presence of pus in a cavity, hollow organ, or space, e.g., the pleural cavity. (Anesth.)

emulsion (ē-mul′shŭn) A colloidal dispersion of one liquid in another. (Oral Med.; Pharmacol.) (see also **suspension**)

double e. A suspension of sensitive silver halide salts impregnated in gelatin and coated on both sides of a radiographic film base. (Oral Radiol.)

silver e. A suspension of sensitive silver halide salts impregnated in gelatin and used for coating photographic plates, radiographic films, etc. (Oral Radiol.)

single e. A suspension of sensitive silver halide salts impregnated in gelatin and coated on only one side of a radiographic film base. (Oral Radiol.)

enamel (ē-năm′ĕl) The vitreous covering tissue of the anatomic crowns of the teeth; consists of enamel rods, or prism rod sheaths, and a cementing interrod substance. It is cleavable along the general direction of the rods. (Oper. Dent.)

— The outermost layer or covering of the coronal portion of the tooth that overlies and protects the dentin. (Periodont.)

mottled e. (see **fluorosis, chronic endemic dental**)

e. pearl (see **pearl, enamel**)

enameloma (see **pearl, enamel**)

enanthem (ĕn-ăn′thĕm) (see **enanthema**)

enanthema (ĕn″ăn-thē′mah) **(enanthem)** Lesions involving the mucous membrane. (Oral Med.)

end section The distal portion of a twin-wire labial arch wire, consisting of a tube in which the anterior section of the labial arch is engaged. (Orthodont.)

end-bulb (see **end-feet**)

end-feet (boutons terminaux, end-bulb) Small terminal enlargements of nerve fibers that are in contact with the dendrites or cell bodies of other nerve cells. The synaptic ending of a nerve fiber. (Anesth.)

ending A termination; the point at which something is concluded.

annulospiral e. A nerve ending, associated with an intrafusal muscle fiber, that is stimulated by a stretch impulse resulting from the extension of a muscle. The ending is in the form of a gradual spiral around the length of the intrafusal muscle fiber in the muscle spindle and is connected to the coarse myelinated fibers. When the fibers are stretched, the distorted intrafusal fibers send impulses to the central nervous system in order to reorganize the muscle and prevent further stretching that might possibly injure joints, tendons, and muscle fibers. (Oral Physiol.)

flower spray e. A sensory nerve ending that is attached to the distal end of an intrafusal muscle fiber and that is stimulated when the muscle fiber contracts, pulling on the nerve ending. The ending has the appearance of a flower spray—a short stem with multiple buds—that seems to function principally when a muscle organ is contracting with maximum effort. The stimulus of the flower spray sends information to the central nervous system, causing it to reorganize the stimuli that are contracting the muscle organ. (Oral Physiol.)

free nerve e. The peripheral terminal of the sensory nerve. (Anesth.)

endocarditis, subacute bacterial (ĕn″dō-kar-dī′tĭs) **(S.B.E.)** Bacterial infection involving the endocardium that occurs primarily following bacteremia and the establishment of bacterial vegetation on an area of defective endocardium such as is found in patients with rheumatic or congenital heart disease. (Oral Med.)

endochondral bone (see **bone, endochondral**)

endocrine dysfunction (ĕn′dō-krīn dĭs-fŭnk′shŭn) (see **dysfunction, endocrine**)

endodontally involved (ĕn″dō-dŏn′tah-lē) Pertaining to the dental pulp and dental periapical tissues. (Endodont.)

endodontia (ĕn″dō-don′shē-ah) (see **endodontology**)

endodontic implant The lengthening of the root of a pulpless tooth by means of a metallic implant extending through the root canal into the periapical bone structure. (Endodont.)

endodontic techniques Procedures used in pulpless teeth or teeth that are to be made pulpless. (Endodont.)

endodontics (ĕn″dō-don′tĭks) The branch of dental practice that applies the knowledge of endodontology. (Endodont.)

endodontist (ĕn″dō-don′tĭst) A dentist who practices endodontics as a specialty. (Endodont.)

endodontology (ĕn″dō-don-tahl′ō-jē) **(endodontia, pulp canal therapy, root canal therapy)** The division of dental science that deals with the etiology, diagnosis, prevention, and treatment of diseases of the dental pulp and their sequelae. (Endodont.)

endolith (ĕn′dō-lĭth) (see **denticle**)

end-organ The expanded termination of a nerve fiber in muscle, skin, mucous membrane, or other structure. (Anesth.)

proprioceptor e.-o. End-organ situated in a muscle, tendon, or joint. Because the proprioceptors are associated with body sense and body movement, the term kinesthetic (*kin-,* movement; *-esthetic,* sensation) is applied to this group of receptors. These receptors respond to physical stimulation (e.g., pressure or stretch) and to sensations of pain. Some receptors arouse no conscious sensation because sensations are referred to the subconscious or subcortical level of the central nervous system function. There are four specific end-organs: the muscle spindles; the Golgi corpuscles, stimulated by tension; the pacinian corpuscles, stimulated by pressure; and the bare nerve endings, stimulated by pain. (Oral Physiol.)

sensory e.-o. Sensory nerve fibers that end peripherally as either unmyelinated fibers or special structures called receptors. They are highly specialized to respond most effectively to one type of stimulus or another. Receptors are situated in the skin, mucous membranes, muscles, tendons, joints, and other structures and also in such special sense organs as those for vision, hearing, smell, and taste. The receptors are organized into a system that relates them to the environment: exteroceptors, interoceptors, and proprioceptors. (Oral Physiol.)

endosteum (ĕn-dos′tē-ŭm) A thin layer of connective tissue that lines the walls of the bone marrow cavities and of the haversian canals of compact bone and covers the trabeculae of cancellous bone. It is a condensed peripheral layer of the stroma of the bone marrow and, in some respects, resembles the periosteum. It has both osteogenic and hematopoietic potencies and, like the periosteum, takes an active part in the healing of fractures. (Oral Physiol.)

endothelioma (ĕn″dō-thē″lē-ō′mah) (see **tumor, Ewing's**)

endotoxin (ĕn′dō-tahk′sĭn) A nondiffusible lipid-polysaccharide-polypeptide complex formed within bacteria (some gram-negative bacilli and others); when released from the destroyed bacterial cells, it is capable of producing a toxic manifestation within the host. (Periodont.)

end-plate A complex hypolemmal terminal arborization of a motor nerve fiber in a bed of specailized sarcoplasm; it transmits nerve impulses to muscle. (Anesth.)

   motor e.-p. The end-plate by which impulses from nerves are transmitted to the muscle fibers. In the terminal plate there is a specialized region of muscle fibers where each axon loses its myelin sheath and ends in a delicate and intricate arborization. The end-plate is a modification of the sarcolemma and is continuous with it. The end-plate potential generated by the nerve impulse activates the muscle impulse. (Oral Physiol.)

end-to-end bite (see **occlusion, edge-to-edge**)

end-to-end occlusion (see **occlusion, edge-to-edge**)

energy Capacity for doing work. (Oral Radiol.)

   atomic e. Energy that can be liberated by changes in the nucleus of an atom (as by fission of a heavy nucleus or fusion of light nuclei into heavier ones, with accompanying loss of mass). (Oral Radiol.)

   binding e. Energy represented by the difference in mass between the sum of the component parts and the actual mass of the nucleus of an atom. (Oral Radiol.)

   e. dependence The characteristic response of a radiation detector to a given range of radiation energies or wavelengths as compared with the response of a standard free-air chamber. Emulsions also show energy dependence. (Oral Radiol.)

   excitation e. Energy required to change a system from its ground state to an excited state. With each excited state there is associated a different excitation energy. (Oral Radiol.) (see also **excitation**)

   ionizing e. The average energy lost by ionizing radiation in producing an ion pair in a

gas. (For air it is about 33 eV.) (Oral Radiol.)

   kinetic e. Energy possessed by a mass because of its motion. (Oral Radiol.)

   nuclear e. (see **energy, atomic**)

   photon e. (symbol hv) Electromagnetic energy in the form of photons, with a value in ergs equal to the product of their frequency in cycles per second and Planck's constant ($E = hv$). (Oral Radiol.)

   potential e. Energy inherent in a mass because of its position with reference to other masses. (Oral Radiol.)

   radiant e. The energy of electromagnetic waves, such as radio waves, visible light, x rays, and gamma rays. (Oral Radiol.)

engine, dental An electric motor that, by means of a continuous-cord drive over pulleys, actuates a handpiece that holds a rotary instrument. (Oper. Dent.)

engineering, dental The application of physical, mechanical, and mathematical principles to dentistry. (Comp. Prosth.; Remov. Part. Prosth.)

Engman's disease (see **dermatitis, infectiosa eczematoides**)

enlargement Increase in size.

   Dilantin e. (see **hyperplasia, gingival, Dilantin**)

   idiopathic e. Gingival enlargement, of unknown causation, clinically characterized by a firm, rounded thickening of the gingival tissues and histologically presenting connective tissue hyperplasia of the gingival corium. (Periodont.)

enostosis (ĕn″os-tō′sĭs) A bony growth located within a bone cavity or centrally from the cortical plate; e.g., bone sclerosis. (Oral Diag.)

— An osteoma arising within a bone. (Oral Path.) (see also **osteoma**)

Entamoeba gingivalis (ĕn″tah-mē′bah) A genus of protozoan amoeba found in the mouth; repeatedly, but not conclusively, associated with the initiation and/or perpetuation of periodontitis. (Periodont.)

enteric coating (ĕn-ter′ĭk) (see **coating, enteric**)

entropion (ĕn-trō′pē-on) Inversion, or infolding, of the eyelid margin. (Oral Diag.)

enucleate (ĕ-noo′klē-āt) To remove a lesion in its entirety. (Oral Surg.)

enunciation An auxiliary function of teeth, particularly those in the anterior sector of the dental arch; the formation of sounds as in speech. (Remov. Part. Prosth.)

enuresis (ĕn-ū-rē′sĭs) Involuntary urination; e.g.,

during general anesthesia or at night. (Oral Diag.)

environment (ĕn-vī'ron-mĕnt) The aggregate of all the external conditions and influences affecting the life and development of an organism. (Comp. Prosth.)

extracellular e. External, or interstitial, environment provided and maintained for the tissue cells. The extracellular environment must provide physical and chemical activity required for cellular integrity. The body has many self-regulatory mechanisms to maintain the optimal environment, particularly for such conditions as temperature control, acid-base balance, and electrolyte and fluid balance. Providing and maintaining the extracellular environment constitutes a major activity of the body. (Oral Physiol.)

oral e. The aggregate of all oral conditions and influences affecting the life and development of an organism. (Remov. Part. Prosth.)

enzyme (ĕn'zīm) A substance, elaborated by living cells, that possesses catalytic properties. (Anesth.)

— An organic catalyst, usually protein in nature, that facilitates biochemical reaction. (Oral Med.; Pharmacol.)

— A protein substance that acts as a catalyst to speed up metabolic and other processes involving organic materials. Some enzymes function within cells; others function in the extracellular fluids and tissue spaces and organs. They are active in all major tissue functions, such as cellular respiration, muscle contraction, digestive processes, and energy consumption, and are produced intracellularly. (Oral Physiol.)

— A polypeptide substance capable of catalysis in a biochemical reaction. Both constructive and destructive activities within organic systems are modified by enzymes. (Periodont.)

— An organic compound capable of causing or accelerating the transformation of materials in plants and animals. (Remov. Part. Prosth.)

eosinophil (ē''ō-sĭn'ō-fĭl) (see **leukocyte, eosinophilic**)

eosinophilia (ē''ō-sĭn''ō-fĭl'ē-ah) An absolute or relative increase in the normal number of eosinophils in the circulating blood. Various limits are given; e.g., absolute eosinophilia if the total number exceeds 500/mm³ and relative if greater than 3% but total less than 500 mm³. It may be associated with skin diseases, infestations, hay fever, asthma, angioneurotic edema, adrenocortical insufficiency, and Hodgkin's disease. (Oral Diag.; Oral Med.)

eosinophilic granuloma (see **granuloma, eosinophilic**)

ephelis (ĕh-fē'lĭs) **(freckle)** Circumscribed macular collection of pigment in the epidermis or oral mucosa. Increased amount of melanin pigment is seen in the region of the basal layer of cells. (Oral Path.)

epidemiology (ĕp''ĭ-dĕm''ē-ol'ō-jē) The science of epidemics and epidemic diseases, which involve the total population rather than the individual. Its aim is to determine those factors in the group environment that make the group more or less susceptible to disease. (Periodont.)

epidermolysis bullosa (ĕp''ĭ-der-mahl'ĭ-sĭs) A disease of the skin characterized by bullae, vesicles, cysts, and, often, associated mandibular enlargement. (Oral Diag.; Oral Med.; Oral Path.) (see also **syndrome, Goldscheider's; syndrome, Weber-Cockayne**)

epiglottis (ĕp''ĭ-glot'ĭs) An elastic cartilage, covered by mucous membrane, that forms the superior part of the larynx and guards the glottis during swallowing. (Anesth.)

epilepsy (ĕp'ĭ-lĕp''sē) General term for a variety of disorders characterized by abnormalities of consciousness and convulsions due to brain damage. Drugs used in the treatment of symptoms (e.g., hydantoin sodium or diphenylhydantoin sodium) promote gingival hyperplasia. (Oral Med.)

— A condition characterized by recurrent seizures of various types, disturbances of consciousness, and electrical discharge from the cortical cells. (Pedodont.)

epiloia (ĕp-ĭ-loi'yah) (see **syndrome, Bourneville-Pringle**)

epinephrine (ĕp''ĭ-nĕf'rĭn) The active principle of the medullary portion of the suprarenal gland. It exerts its influence on the structures that are innervated by the sympathetic nerves. (Anesth.; Oral Physiol.; Pharmacol.)

— A hormone secreted by the adrenal medulla. It stimulates hepatic glycogenolysis, causing an elevation in the blood sugar, vasodilation of blood vessels of the skeletal muscles, vasoconstriction of the arterioles of the skin and mucous membranes, relaxation of bronchiolar smooth muscles, and stimulation of heart action. (Oral Med.)

epiphysis (ē-pĭf'ĭ-sĭs) Terminal portion of a long bone. It is separated from the diaphysis during growth by a cartilaginous zone that serves as a growth center. Once ossification unites the epiphysis with the diaphysis, growth is completed. (Oral Physiol.)

epispinal (ĕp-ĭ-spī'nal) Located on the spinal column. (Anesth.)

epistaxis (ĕp″ĭ-stăk′sĭs) (**nosebleed**) Bleeding from the nose. (Anesth.; Oral Diag.)

epithelial (ĕp-ĭ-thē′lē-al) Pertaining to the epithelium. (Periodont.)

e. attachment (see **attachment, epithelial**)

e. cuff, attached The attachment of the gingival epithelium to the enamel, including the close approximation of the free gingiva to the tooth. (Periodont.)

e. cuff, implant The band of tissue that is constricted around an implant abutment post. (Oral Implant.)

e. inclusion Bits of epithelial tissue introduced into bone crypts during perforation osteotomies. (Oral Implant.) (see also **osteotomy, perforation**)

epithelioma (ĕp″ĭ-thē′lē-ō′mah) An epithelial cancer.

e. adenoides cysticum (**Brooke's tumor, trichoepithelioma**) A form of basal cell carcinoma believed to arise from the epithelium of hair follicles. Regarded as a less invasive form of basal cell carcinoma. (Oral Diag.; Oral Path.)

basal cell e. (see **carcinoma, basal cell**)

epithelium (ĕp″ĭ-thē′lē-ŭm) The structural arrangement of the various cellular components of epithelium characterized by two basic forms: medium suprapapillary width with medium-length rete pegs, and narrow suprapapillary width with long rete pegs. (Periodont.)

basement membrane of e. (see **membrane, basement**)

desmosomes of e. An electromicroscopic finding of intercellular bridges that serve to attach adjacent epithelial cells to each other. (Periodont.)

enamel e., inner The innermost layer of cells (ameloblasts) of the enamel organ that deposit the organic matrix of the enamel on the crown of the developing tooth. Also the innermost layer of Hertwig's epithelial root sheath. (Periodont.)

enamel e., outer The outermost layer of cells of the enamel organ. It is separated from the inner enamel epithelium in the area of the developing crown by the stratum intermedium and stellate reticulum and lies immediately adjacent to the inner enamel epithelium in the area of the developing root. (Periodont.)

enamel e., reduced Combined enamel epithelium; the remains of the enamel organ after enamel formation is complete. After eruption of the tip of the crown, that part of the combined epithelium remaining on the enamel surface is called the epithelial attachment. (Periodont.)

gingival e. A stratified squamous epithelium consisting of a basal layer; it is keratinized or parakeratinized when comprising the attached gingiva. (Periodont.)

hyperplastic e. Increase in thickness, with alterations in structure, produced by proliferation of cellular elements of epithelium. The stratum spinosum epidermidis is usually the layer of cells that becomes thickened, resulting in acanthosis. (Periodont.)

intercellular tonofibrils of e. Structures that course from cell to attachment plaque and, together with desmosomes, appear to make up a supporting system for the epithelium. (Periodont.)

oral e. The epithelial covering of the oral mucous membranes. Composed of stratified squamous epithelium of varying thickness and varying degrees of keratinization. (Periodont.)

pocket e. The epithelium that lines the gingival or periodontal pocket. Its most prominent characteristics are the presence of hyperplasia and ulceration, with exposure to the corium of the gingiva. (Periodont.)

squamous e. Epithelium consisting of flat, scalelike cells. (Periodont.)

stratified s. e. The variety of epithelium prevalent as the covering of the oral mucous membrane and of dermal surfaces; composed of layers of cells oriented parallel to the surface. The various layers of cells in order of ascent from basement membrane to surface are stratum germinativum, stratum spongiosum, stratum granulosum, stratum lucidum (in dermal epithelium), and stratum corneum. The gingival epithelium generally exhibits some degree of keratinization, variable from parakeratosis to hyperkeratosis. (Periodont.)

sulcal e. The stratified squamous epithelium forming the covering of the soft tissue wall of the gingival sulcus, or crevice. Extends from the gingival margin to the line of attachment of the epithelium to the tooth surface. It becomes hyperplastic and ulcerative when a gingival or periodontal pocket exists. (Periodont.)

epithelization (ĕp″ĭ-thē″lē-zā′shŭn) The natural act of healing by secondary intention; the proliferation of new epithelium into an area devoid of it but which naturally is covered by it. (Oral Implant.)

epoxy resin (ē-pahk′sē) (see **resin, epoxy**)

Epstein's pearls (see **nodules, Bohn's**)

epulis (ĕp'ū-lĭs) A tumor (tumescence) of the gingiva. (Oral Diag.)

    congenital e. of newborn A raised or pedunculated lesion located on the anterior gingivae of the newborn. It is histologically similar to the granular cell myoblastoma. (Oral Path.) (see also **myoblastoma, granular cell**)

    e. fissurata (inflammatory fibrous hyperplasia, redundant tissue) Enlargement in the mucobucal fold produced by dentures that have outworn their usefulness. (Oral Diag.)

    — A curtainlike fold of excess tissue associated with the flange of a denture. (Comp. Prosth.; Oral Path.)

    giant cell e. (see **granuloma, giant cell reparative, peripheral**)

    e. granulomatosa A tumorlike mass of red, easily bleeding, infected granulation tissue that occurs due to exuberant reparative phenomena. It is seen arising from tooth sockets or is associated with exfoliating necrotic bone. (Oral Path.)

equilibration (ē″kwĭ-lĭ-brā'shŭn) The act of placing a body in a state of equilibrium. (Comp. Prosth.)

— Achievement of equalized pressure. (Comp. Prosth.; Remov. Part. Prosth.)

    e., diagnostic (see **diagnostic equilibration**)

    mandibular e. The act or acts performed to place the mandible in a state of equilibrium. (Comp. Prosth.)

    e. of mounted casts Equilibration of the occlusion of the dentodes and gnathodes made of a patient for the purpose of observing and recording what must be done to adjust the occlusion. Such equilibrated casts are used and followed in adjusting the patient's occlusion. (Gnathol.)

    occlusal e. Modification of occlusal forms of teeth by grinding, with the intent of equalizing occlusal stress or of harmonizing cuspal relations. (Comp. Prosth.; Remov. Part. Prosth.)

equilibrator (ē″kwĭ-lĭ-brā'tor) An instrument or device used in achieving or maintaining a state of equilibrium. (Comp. Prosth.)

equilibrium (ē″kwĭ-lĭb're-ŭm) A state of balance between two opposing forces or processes. (Anesth.)

— The state of a body in which the forces acting on it are so arranged that their resultant at every point is zero. (Comp. Prosth.)

    functional e. The equalization of the counteraction of antagonistic forces acting on the masticatory apparatus. The forces originat-

ing from the facial and labial muscles are equalized by the forces exerted by the tongue. A lack of neutralization of these antagonistic forces leads, for example, to directional changes in the arrangement of the dentition. Also, the state of homeostasis within the oral cavity existing when all the local environmental factors, including the forces of mastication, are in a state of balance. (Periodont.)

equipment The nonexpendable items used by the dentist in the performance of his professional duties. (Pract. Man.)

equity (ĕk'wĭ-tē) A free and reasonable claim or right; fairness; impartiality. (D. Juris.)

equivalent Equal in force, value, measure, or effect; corresponding in function. (Oral Radiol.)

    aluminum e. The thickness of pure aluminum affording the same radiation attenuation, under specified conditions, as the material or materials being considered. (Oral Radiol.)

    concrete e. The thickness of concrete having a density of 2.35 g/cm^3 that would afford the same radiation attenuation, under specified conditions, as the material or materials being considered. (Oral Radiol.)

    lead e. The thickness of pure lead that would afford the same radiation attenuation, under specified conditions, as the material or materials under consideration. (Oral Radiol.)

erg A unit of energy (equal to a force of 1 dyne acting through a distance of 1 cm) equal to 2.4×10^{-8} calories, or $6.24 \times 10^6 \text{eV}$. (Oral Radiol.)

ergotoxine A potent alkaloid that paralyzes the motor and secretory nerves of the sympathetic system but has no effect on the inhibitory or parasympathetic nerves. (Oral Physiol.)

erosion (ē-rō'zhŭn) Chemical or mechanicochemical destruction of tooth substance of nonoccluding surfaces. (Oper. Dent.)

— Progressive loss of hard dental tissues by a chemical process, without bacterial action. Acid erosion may be caused by a specific action, e.g., sucking lemons or regurgitating gastric fluids. Idiopathic erosion is more common and is of unknown cause, although many causes have been proposed. (Oral Diag.)

— A process, the mechanism of which is incompletely known, that leads to the creation of concavities of many shapes in the enamel of a tooth near the cementoenamel junction. The surface of the cavity, unlike dental caries, is hard and smooth. (Oral Path.)

error Violation of duty; fault; a mistake in the proceedings of a court in matters of law or of fact. (D. Juris.)

eruption The appearance of a tooth in the oral cavity. (Oper. Dent.)

continuous e. Extrusion or occlusal progression of a tooth. The tendency to continuous eruption may increase the length of the clinical crown, or the periodontium may extrude with the tooth. A change that may occur when a tooth loses its antagonist. A compensation for the wear of occlusal and incisal surfaces of the teeth. (Periodont.)

difficult e. (see **teething**)

ectopic e. Eruption of a maxillary first permanent molar mesial to its normal position, resulting in the resorption of the roots of the second primary molar. The condition also occurs occasionally in the mandibular permanent lateral incisor area, causing premature resorption of the root of the adjacent primary cuspid. (Pedodont.)

passive e. Gingival recession as the result of a physiologic process, the atrophy of the gingival margin being associated with apical proliferation of the epithelial attachment as well as with a slow, steady resorption of the crestal bone. The stages of passive eruption, according to Gottlieb, are as follows: (1) the most apical limit of the epithelial attachment is at the cementoenamel junction; (2) the most apical limit of the attachment is on the cementum, with the base of the gingival sulcus still on the enamel surface; (3) the most apical limit of the epithelial attachment is on the cementum, with the base of the sulcus at the cementoenamel junction; (4) both the base of the sulcus and the epithelial attachment are on the surface of the cementum. (Periodont.)

surgical e. Uncovering of an unerupted tooth to permit further eruption; done surgically by removing overlying scar tissue, bone, a cyst, and/or a tumor. (Oral Surg.)

eruptive gingivitis (see **gingivitis, eruptive**)

erythema (er″ĭ-thē′mah) Patchy, circumscribed, or marginated macular redness of the skin or mucous membranes due to hyperemia, or inflammation. (Oral Diag.; Oral Med.)

e. multiforme complex An acute inflammation of unknown cause characterized by a variety of skin and mucosal lesions. The multiform lesions include bullae, vesicles, ulceration, and erythema. (Oral Diag.)

— An acute, inflammatory dermatologic disease of uncertain etiology (although occasionally related to drug administration) characterized by erythematous macules, papules, vesicles, and bullae that appear on the skin and not infrequently on the oral mucosa. (Oral Med.)

— Term used to indicate any one of a group or series of dermatologic symptoms that always include an initial red macule and range from vesicle formation through bulla and ulcer formation. Numerous combinations of lesions occurring in various anatomic locations have been described as subtypes and syndromes. Essentially, the term refers to a nonspecific, erythematous macule formation that is of unknown etiology but is associated with drug allergy, viruses, and bacteria. (Oral Path.)

— An acute inflammatory disease of the skin and mucous membranes characterized by a rash of erythematopapular or vesicobullous nature. Its etiology has not been established, although virus infection and hypersensitivity have been offered as possible factors. (Periodont.) (see also **syndrome, Stevens-Johnson**)

erythredema polyneuropathy (ĕ-rĭth″rĕ-dē′mah pol″ĭ-noo-rop′ah-thē) **(acrodynia, Feer's disease, pink disease, Selter's disease, Swift's disease)** A disease of childhood characterized by intense pain that may cause the child to bite off the tip of the tongue and also to grind the teeth, resulting in their loosening and exfoliation. (Oral Diag.)

— A disease of infancy thought to be due to mercury poisoning. It is manifested by itching of the hands and feet, profuse sweating, hypertension, vasomotor disturbances, bruxism, and precocious shedding of the teeth. (Oral Med.)

erythremia (er″ĭ-thrē′mē-ah) **(Osler's disease, polycythemia rubra, polycythemia vera, primary polycythemia, Vaquez' disease)** A myeloproliferative disease characterized by a marked increase in the circulating red blood cell mass. It may represent a neoplastic growth of erythropoietic tissue. Neutrophilia, thrombocytopenia, and splenomegaly are common. Manifestations include plethora, vertigo, headache, and thrombosis. (Oral Med.)

— A disease of unknown etiology characterized by a persistent increase in the number of red blood cells due to excessive erythropoiesis. (Oral Path.)

erythroblastosis fetalis (ĕ-rĭth″rō-blăs-tō′sĭs fē-tăl′ĭs) Excessive destruction of red blood cells begun before or shortly after birth. It may be due to an Rh factor reaction. The skin is yellow, and the teeth may be markedly discolored. (Oral Diag.)

— Hemolytic anemia of the fetus or newborn infant due to sensitization of a pregnant Rh-negative mother by Rh agglutinogens via an Rh-positive fetus or by incompatible blood transfusion. The manifestations, which vary, include icterus, mental deficiency, hydrops, intrinsic staining of the teeth, nucleated red blood cells, and stillborn infants. (Oral Med.)

erythrocyte (ĕ-rĭth'rō-sīt) Red blood cell; a non-nucleated, circular, biconcave, discoid, hemoglobin-containing, oxygen-carrying formed element circulating in the blood. (Oral Physiol.)

erythrocytosis (ĕ-rĭth″rō-sī-tō'sĭs) **(secondary polycythemia)** An increased circulating red blood cell mass due to compensatory effort to meet reduced oxygen content. May be seen in persons living at high altitudes, as well as in emphysema, pulmonary insufficiency, and heart failure. (Oral Med.)

erythroplasia of Queyrat (ĕ-rĭth″rō-plā'zē-ah of kuh-răt') A form of intraepithelial carcinoma. The oral lesions are usually seen as plaques with a bright, velvety surface. (Oral Path.)

escharotic (ĕs-kah-rot'ĭk) A caustic or corrosive agent that has the strength to burn tissue. (Oral Surg.)

essence An alcoholic solution of an essential oil. (Oral Med.; Pharmacol.)

essential oil (see **oil, essential**)

Essig-type splinting (see **splinting, Essig-type**)

estate One's interest in land or other property. (D. Juris.)

e. planning A detailed, written-out plan (usually arrived at with the advice of estate counselors), in which all the financial affairs of the dentist are clearly stated and provisions are made for alterations when changing conditions warrant it. (Pract. Man.)

ester Any compound formed from alcohol and an acid. (Anesth.)

esterase (es'ter-ās) An enzyme that catalyzes the hydrolysis of an ester into its alcohol and acid. (Anesth.)

esthetics (ĕs-thĕt'ĭks) The branch of philosophy dealing with beauty, especially with the components thereof; i.e., color and form. The qualities involved in the appearance of a given restoration. (Comp. Prosth.; Fixed Part. Prosth.; Oper. Dent.; Remov. Part. Prosth.)

denture e. The cosmetic effect, produced by a denture, that affects the desirable beauty, charm, character, and dignity of the individual. (Comp. Prosth.; Fixed Part. Prosth.; Oper. Dent.; Remov. Part. Prosth.)

d. base e. (gingival tissue e.) The esthetically proper tinting, contouring, and festooning of the gingival tissue portion of a denture base—one of the most important factors in attaining a pleasing result in a restoration. (Comp. Prosth.; Remov. Part. Prosth.)

gingival tissue e. (see **esthetics, denture base**)

estimate The anticipated fee for dental services to be performed. (Pract. Man.)

Estlander's operation (see **operation, Abbé-Estlander**)

estoppel (ĕ-stop'ĕl) A preclusion, in law, that prevents a person from alleging or denying a fact because of his own previous act or allegation. (D. Juris.)

estradiol benzoate (ĕs″trah-dī'ol bĕn'zō-āt) A topical steroid (β-estradiol-3-benzoate) with estrogenic activity, useful in the treatment of lesions produced by diminution of bodily production of estrogens. Experimental administration to aged laboratory mice has resulted in an increased downgrowth of epithelial attachment along the root surface of teeth and subsequent production of periodontal disease. (Periodont.)

estrin Generic term for the ovarian estrogens: estriol, estrone, and estradiol. (Periodont.)

estrogens (ĕs'trō-jĕnz) Collective term for substances capable of producing estrus. It is also applied to the estrogenic hormones in women. Estriol is the principal estrogen found in the urine of pregnant women and in the placenta. Synthetic estrogens include diethylstilbestrol, hexestrol, and ethynyl estradiol. (Oral Med.)

ether, divinyl (ē'ther, dī-vī'nĭl) **(divinyl oxide, $CH_2:CH_2O$)** A highly volatile saturated ether used as an inhalation anesthetic for short operations. (Anesth.)

etherization (ē″ther-ĭ-zā'shŭn) Administration of ether to produce anesthesia. (Anesth.)

ethics (ĕth'ĭks) The science of moral obligation; a system of moral principles, quality, or practice. (D. Juris.)

— The moral obligation to render to the patient the best possible quality of dental service and to maintain an honest relationship with other members of the profession and mankind in general. (Pract. Man.)

ethyl chloride (ĕth'ĭl klō'rĭd) **(C_2H_5Cl)** A colorless liquid that boils between 12° and 13° C. It acts as a local anesthetic of short duration through the superficial freezing produced by its rapid vaporization from the skin. It is used occasionally in inhalation therapy as a rapid fleeting general anesthetic, comparable to nitrous oxide but somewhat more dangerous. (Anesth.)

ethylene (ĕth′ĭ-lēn) (**olefiant gas, CH₂CH₂**) A colorless gas of slightly sweet odor and taste; used as an inhalation anesthetic. (Anesth.)

etiology (ē″tē-ol′ō-jē) Causative factors. (Orthodont.)

— The factors implicated in the causation of disease; the study of the factors causing disease. (Periodont.)

   e., local factors The environmental influences that may be implicated in the causation and/or perpetuation of a disease process. (Periodont.)

   e., systemic factors Factors that are implicated in the causation, modification, and/or perpetuation of a disease entity. Within the oral cavity, the actions of the systemic factors are modified by interaction with local factors. (Periodont.)

eudaemonic (ū-dē-mon′ĭk) Pertaining to a drug that brings about a feeling of normal well-being in a previously depressed patient. (Anesth.)

eugenol (ū′jĕ-nol) An allyl guaiacol obtainable from oil of cloves. Used with zinc oxide in a paste for temporary restorations, for bases under restorations, and for impression materials. Believed to have a palliative effect on dental pulp and possibly a limited germicidal effect. (D. Mat.)

— Colorless or pale yellow liquid obtained from clove oil; has a clove odor and pungent, spicy taste. Used as the liquid portion of zinc oxide and eugenol cements and in toothache medications. (Oper. Dent.)

eugnathia (ū-nā′thē-ah) Those abnormalities which are limited to the teeth and their immediate alveolar supports. (Oral Surg.)

euphoria (ū-for′ē-ah) A sense of well-being or normalcy. Pleasantly mild excitement. (Oral Med.; Pharmacol.)

euphoric (ū-for′ĭk) A substance that produces an exaggerated sense of well-being. (Anesth.)

eupnea (ūp-nē′ah) Easy or normal respiration. (Anesth.)

eutaxia (ū-tăk′sē-ah) Muscular coordination in good order. Good physical organization. Opposite of ataxia. (Oral Diag.)

eutectoid (ū″tĕk′toid) Usually referring to an alloy of carbon and iron; also known as pearlite. (D. Mat.)

euthyroidism (ū-thī′roid-ĭzm) A state of normal thyroid function. (Oral Med.)

evidence Any kind of proof of probative matter legally presented at a trial by the act of the

parties and through witnesses, records, documents, and objects, for the purpose of inducing belief in the minds of the court or jury. (D. Juris.)

   radiographic e. The shadow images depicted in radiographs. (Oral Radiol.)

Evipal (ĕ′vĭ-pahl) Proprietary brand of hexobarbital, a rapid-acting barbiturate. (Anesth.)

   E. sodium Proprietary brand of hexobarbital sodium. An ultrashort-acting barbiturate of the N-methyl type whose pharmacologic actions, from a clinical standpoint, are essentially similar to thiopental (Pentothal). (Anesth.)

evulsed tooth (see **tooth, evulsed**)

evulsion (**avulsion**) The sudden tearing out, or away, of tissue due to a traumatic episode. (Oral Surg.)

— Displacement of a tooth from its alveolar housing; may be partial or complete. (Endodont.)

   nerve e. The operation of tearing a nerve from its central origin by traction. (Oral Surg.)

Ewing's sarcoma (see **tumor, Ewing's**)

Ewing's tumor (see **tumor, Ewing's**)

examination Scrutiny or investigation for the purpose of making a diagnosis using visual, radiographic, digital, and other means. (Comp. Prosth.; Remov. Part. Prosth.)

— Inspection; search; investigation; inquiry; scrutiny; testing. (D. Juris.)

— Investigation of a patient, using the techniques of inspection, palpation, auscultation, and percussion; these techniques are supplemented by special clinical, laboratory, and radiographic evaluations. (Oral Surg.)

— Inspection and/or investigation of part or all of the body in order to measure and evaluate the parameters of a disease. The examination may include visual inspection, percussion, palpation, auscultation, and measurement of mobility, as well as various laboratory and radiographic procedures. (Periodont.)

   clinical e. Visual and tactile scrutiny of the tissues of and surrounding the oral cavity. (Pract. Man.)

   gingival e. Observation of the primary visual symptoms of periodontal disease, including color changes, changes in surface texture, deviations from normal contour and structure, tissue tone and vitality, presence or absence of clefts, and the depth of the pocket. (Periodont.)

   intraoral e. Examination of all the structures contained within the oral cavity. Includes inspection, palpation, percussion, transillumination, radiography, biopsy, etc. (Periodont.)

radiographic e. Production of the number of radiographs necessary for the radiologic interpretation of the part or parts in question. (Oral Radiol.)
— Study and interpretation of radiographs of the mouth and associated structures. (Pract. Man.)

extraoral r. e. Examination of the teeth and bones of the head by means of a radiograph made by placing a large film exposure holder or cassette against the side of the head or face under survey and projecting the roentgen rays from a position at various angles to the opposite side of the head or face and to the film. (Oral Radiol.)

anteroposterior e. r. e. Examination in which the film is placed at the posterior, with the rays passing from the anterior to the posterior direction to record images. An examination for exploration of the posterior skull. (Oral Radiol.)

body section e. r. e. (**tomogram**) A radiographic procedure whereby shadows of various internal layers of the head and body are separated for the purpose of obtaining a radiograph showing distinct shadows of a certain layer and at the same time blurring out everything above and below the layer. This is accomplished by the synchronized movement of the roentgen-ray tube and film in parallel planes but in opposite directions from each other. Also known as tomography, laminagraphy, planigraphy, and stratigraphy. (Oral Radiol.)

bregma-mentum e. r. e. Examination in which the film is placed beneath the chin, with the rays directed downward through the junction of the coronal and sagittal sutures (bregma) to the chin (mentum). An examination for the temporomandibular articulator and a topographic view of the mandible. (Oral Radiol.)

cephalometric e. r. e. Examination by means of film placed to obtain lateral and posteroanterior views of the head. Used in orthodontics and, to some degree, in prosthodontics to measure and study maxillofacial growth and jaw relationships. The head is held in position by means of a cephalometer. (Oral Radiol.)

lateral facial e. r. e. Examination by means of a lateral head film. The film size and bundle of radiation are designed to record the images of the facial bones. An examination for exploration and localization in the superior-inferior plane. (Oral Radiol.)

lateral head e. r. e. Examination in which the film is placed parallel to the sagittal plane of the head, with the rays directed at right angles to the plane of the film and the sagittal plane. An examination showing the entire skull. (Oral Radiol.)

lateral jaw e. r. e. Examination in which the film is placed adjacent to the ramus or the body of the mandible, with the rays directed obliquely upward from the oppostie side and the central beam directed at the point of interest. The horizontal angulation will be such as to cast the image of the opposite mandible superior and/or anterior to the area of interest. (Oral Radiol.)

mental e. r. e. Examination in which the film is placed beneath the chin and the radiation is directed through the long axis of the lower central incisors while the mouth is open. An examination for viewing the mental process. (Oral Radiol.)

posteroanterior e. r. e. Examination in which the film is placed anteriorly, with the rays passing from the posterior to the anterior direction to record the images. An examination for exploration and localization of the facial bones. (Oral Radiol.)

profile. e. r. e. Lateral head examination to show the profile of bone and soft tissue outline. It utilizes a decrease in milliampere seconds or an increase in target-film distance for recording the soft tissue image. (Oral Radiol.)

stereoscopic e. r. e. Radiographic examination used in conjunction with a stereoscope for localization. Exposures of two films are made, with identical placement of each film adjacent to the part in question and with a different angulation for each exposure. The angulation for each exposure is directed through the part with a tube shift of 65 mm (the interpupillary distance). (Oral Radiol.)

temporomandibular e. r. e. Examination in which the film is placed adjacent to the area to be examined, with the rays directed through a point 2½ inches above the tragus of the opposite external ear with a vertical angulation of 15° and a horizontal angulation of 5° downward. Various other techniques and angulations are used (including laminagraphy) in examining this area. (Oral Radiol.)

Waters e. r. e. Posteroanterior examination of the paranasal sinuses. The film is placed in contact with the nose and chin, with the rays directed at right angles to the plane of the film. (Oral Radiol.)

intraoral r. e. Examination of the teeth and facial bones by placing films within the oral cavity and directing roentgen rays at various angles through the area of interest. (Oral Radiol.)

bite-wing i. r. e. Examination in which an intraoral radiograph records on a single film the shadow images of the outline, position, and mesiodistal extent of the crowns, necks, and coronal third of the roots of both the maxillary and mandibular teeth and the alveolar crests. (Oral Radiol.)

extradental i. r. e. Examination in which the film is placed between the teeth and the tissue of the cheek or lip for the exploration or localization of the internal structures of these tissues. (Oral Radiol.)

oblique occlusal i. r. e. Exploratory examination of the maxillae or mandible using an occlusal type of film placed between the teeth. The rays are directed obliquely downward or upward (usually 60° to 75° in the vertical) and parallel to the sagittal plane. (Oral Radiol.)

periapical i. r. e. The basic extraoral examination, showing all of a tooth or part of it, the surrounding periodontium, and, in the instance of pathologic or questionable change, normal bone beyond its borders. (Oral Radiol.)

topographic i. r. e. (see **examination, radiographic, intraoral, true occlusal topographic**)

true occlusal topographic i. r. e. A localizing examination of the maxillae or mandible using an occlusal type of film placed between the teeth, with the rays directed at right angles to the plane of the film or through the long axis of the

teeth adjacent to the part in question. (Oral Radiol.)

excavator, spoon (ĕks′kah-vā″tor) A paired hand instrument intended primarily to remove carious material from a cavity; lateral cutting blade is curet shaped, discoid shaped, or spoon shaped, and the entire periphery is sharpened. (Preferable to restrict this term to this type of instrument rather than to include the cutting instrument.) (Oper. Dent.)

excess More than is necessary, useful, or specified. (Oper. Dent.)

marginal e. A condition in which the contour of a restoration is greater than desired in the region of its margin(s). (Oper. Dent.)

e. overhang Gingival margin excess. (Oper. Dent.)

excipient (ĕk-sĭp′ē-ĕnt) An ingredient included in a pharmaceutical preparation for the purpose of improving its physical qualities. (Oral Med.; Pharmacol.) (see also **binder; filler; vehicle**)

excision (ĕk-sĭzh′ŭn) The act of cutting away or taking out.

local e. An excision limited to the immediate area of the lesion in question. (Oral Surg.)

radical e. An excision involving not only the lesion in question but also anatomic parts removed from the site. (Oral Surg.)

wide e. An excision involving the lesion in question and immediately adjacent anatomic structures. (Oral Surg.)

excitant (ĕk-sīt′ănt) An agent that stimulates the activity of an organ. (Anesth.)

excitation (ĕk-sī-tā′shŭn) The addition of energy to a system, thereby transferring it from its ground state to an excited state. Excitation of a nucleus, an atom, or a molecule can result from absorption of photons or from inelastic collision with other particles. (Oral Radiol.)

excursion, lateral Movement of the mandible from the midline, the path being produced by the action of the external pterygoid muscle on the nonfunctioning (balancing) side, and regulated by the shape of the inner curvature of the glenoid fossa on the balancing side, the amount and direction of the Bennett (direct lateral) shift, the occlusal relationship of the teeth on both working and balancing sides during lateral movement, etc. (Periodont.)

execute To finish; accomplish; fulfill. To carry out according to its terms. (D. Juris.)

exercise prosthesis (see **prosthesis, exercise**)

exercises, myotherapeutic (see **therapy, myofunctional**)

exfoliation (ĕks-fō″lē-ā′shŭn) (**shedding**) Physiologic loss of the primary dentition. (Pedodont.)

— Movement of a tooth beyond the natural occlusal plane, with resultant loss of a normal relationship between the tooth and its investing tissues. (Remov. Part. Prosth.)

exhalation (ĕks-hah-lā′shŭn) Giving off or sending forth in the form of vapor; expiration. (Anesth.)

exhaustion (ĕg-zawst′yŭn) Loss of vital and nervous power from fatigue or protracted disease. (Anesth.)

exhibit (ĕg-zĭb′ĭt) A paper, document, or object presented to a court during a trial or hearing as proof of facts, or as otherwise connected with the subject matter, and which, on being accepted, is marked for identification and considered a part of the case. (D. Juris.)

    dental e. Visual aids illustrated and arranged to disseminate knowledge about dentistry; displayed anywhere that a maximum number of people can see them. (Pract. Man.)

exodontics (ĕk″sō-don′tĭks) The science and practice of removing teeth from the oral cavity as performed by dentists. (Oral Surg.)

exolever (ĕks′ō-lē″ver) An instrument that uses the principles of leverage for extracting and removing teeth or roots of teeth from the oral cavity. (Oral Surg.)

exophthalmos (ĕk″sof-thăl′mos) Abnormal protrusion of the eyeball. It is characteristic of toxic (exophthalmic) goiter. (Oral Diag.)

exostosis (ĕk″sŏs-tō′sĭs) (**hyperostosis**) A bony growth projecting from a bony surface. (Oral Diag.)

— An osteoma projecting outward from the surface of a bone. (Oral Path.)

exotoxin (ĕk″sō-tok′sĭn) The toxic material formed by micro-organisms and subsequently released into their surrounding environments. Exotoxins are protein in nature, are heat labile, and possess pyrogenic properties. The release of the toxic substance into the environment of the host by live microorganisms results in toxic responses on the part of the host. (Periodont.)

expanded duty auxiliary A person trained to carry out dental procedures more complex than the responsibilities usually delegated to dental auxiliaries. (Pract. Man.)

expansile infrastructure endosteal implant An intraosseous implant device designed to enlarge or open after its insertion into the bone to provide retention. (Oral Implant.)

expansion Increase in extent, size, volume, or scope. (Oper. Dent.)

— Increase in circumference of the dental arch by buccal and/or labial movement of the teeth. (Orthodont.)

    delayed e. (secondary e.) Expansion occurring in amalgam restorations due to moisture contamination. (D. Mat.)

— Expansion exhibited by amalgam that has been contaminated by moisture during trituration or insertion. (Oper. Dent.)

    hygroscopic e. Expansion (usually of a gypsum material) due to the absorption of moisture. (Comp. Prosth.; Remov. Part. Prosth.)

—Expansion caused by absorption of water during setting of an investment. The amount of expansion may be governed by the amount and size of the silica particles and by the quantity of water absorbed. Hygroscopic expansion is employed in the so-called low heat techniques in order to provide additional compensation. It is probably a prolongation of the normal setting expansion. (D. Mat.)

— Expansion of a gypsum product that results when a mixture of the material is in contact with water during its setting. (Oper. Dent.)

    secondary e. (see **expansion, delayed**)

    setting e. Dimensional increase that occurs concurrently with the hardening of various materials, such as plaster of paris. (Comp. Prosth.; Remov. Part. Prosth.)

— Expansion that occurs during the setting or hardening of a material such as amalgam and gypsum products. (D. Mat.)

    thermal e. Expansion caused by heat. (Comp. Prosth.)

— Dimensional change induced by temperature change. (D. Mat.; Oper. Dent.)

— Expansion due to heat. One of the important factors in achieving adequate compensation for the contraction of cast metal, when it resolidifies, is the necessary thermal expansion of the mold, which must be obtained before the casting is made. (Remov. Part. Prosth.)

    t. e., coefficient In dentistry, the dimensional change induced in a tooth as compared to that produced in the restorative material; a ratio. (D. Mat.)

experiment A trial or special observation made to confirm or disprove something doubtful; an act or operation undertaken in order to discover some unknown principle or effect or to test, establish, or illustrate some suggested or known truth. (D. Juris.)

expert One who has special skill or knowledge in a particular subject, such as a science or art, whether acquired by experience or study; a specialist. (D. Juris.)

expiration Act of breathing forth or expelling air from the lungs. (Anesth.)

— Cessation; termination; the expiration of a lease. (D. Juris.)

exploration Examination by touch, either with or without instruments. For example, a carious lesion is explored with a special explorer, but the mucobuccal fold may be explored with the finger. (Oral Diag.)

— The process of examination of a surface, with or without the use of instruments, in order to determine the condition or the surface depth of a defect or other, similar diagnostic parameters. (Periodont.)

explore To investigate. (Pract. Man.)

explosion A violent, noisy outbreak due to a sudden release of energy. (Anesth.)

exposure (formerly **exposure dose**) (symbol X) A measure of the x or gamma radiation to which a person or object, or a part of either, is exposed at a certain place, this measure being based on its ability to produce ionization. The unit of x or gamma radiation exposure is the roentgen (R). (Oral Radiol.)

acute e. Radiation exposure of short duration; usually referring to radiation of relatively high intensity. (Oral Radiol.)

air e. Radiation exposure measured in a small mass of air under conditions of electronic equilibrium with the surrounding air, that is, excluding backscatter from irradiated parts or objects. (Oral Radiol.)

chronic e. Radiation exposure of long duration, either continuous (protraction exposure) or intermittent (fractionation exposure); usually referring to exposure of relatively low intensity. (Oral Radiol.)

cumulative e. The total accumulated exposure resulting from repeated radiation exposures of the whole body or of a particular region. (Oral Radiol.)

double e. Two superimposed exposures on the same radiographic or photographic film. (Oral Radiol.)

entrance e. Exposure measured at the surface of an irradiated body, part, or object. It includes both primary radiation and backscatter from the irradiated underlying tissue or material. (Oral Radiol.)

erythema e. The radiation exposure necessary to produce a temporary redness of the skin. The exposure required will vary with the quality of the radiation to which the skin is exposed. (Oral Radiol.)

protraction e. Exposure to radiation continuously over a relatively long period at a low exposure rate. (Oral Radiol.)

pulp e. An opening through the wall of the pulp chamber uncovering the dental pulp. (Oper. Dent.)

> **accidental p. e.** Pulp exposure unintentionally created during instrumentation. (Oper. Dent.)
>
> **carious p. e.** Pulp exposure occasioned by extension of the carious process to the pulp chamber wall. (Oper. Dent.)
>
> **mechanical p. e.** (see **exposure, pulp, surgical**)
>
> **surgical p. e.** (**mechanical p. e.**) Pulp exposure created intentionally or unintentionally during instrumentation. (Oper. Dent.)

e. rate, output Exposure to radiation at a specified point per unit of time, usually expressed in roentgens per minute. (Oral Radiol.)

surface e. (see **exposure, entrance**)

threshold e. The minimum exposure that will produce a detectable degree of any given effect. (Oral Radiol.)

e. time The time during which a person or object is exposed to radiation, expressed in one of the conventional units of time. (Oral Radiol.)

express Stated distinctly and explicitly and not left to inference. Set forth in words. (D. Juris.)

exsufflation (ĕk″sŭf-flā′shŭn) Forced discharge of the breath. (Anesth.)

extension Enlargement in boundary, breadth, or depth. (Oper. Dent.)

— The process of increasing the angle between two skeletal levers having end-to-end articulation with each other. The opposite of flexion. (Oral Physiol.)

e. base (see **base, extension**)

gingiva e., attached Gingival extension operation; a surgical technique designed to broaden the zone of attached gingiva by repositioning the mucogingival junction apically. (Periodont.)

groove e. Enlargement of a cavity preparation outline to include a developmental groove. (Oper. Dent.)

e. for prevention A principle of cavity preparation laid down by G. W. Black in 1891. To prevent the recurrence of decay, the cavity outline form is extended beyond that boundary essential to include incipient lesions. This additional extension provides smoothly finished margins that either are self-cleansing or may be readily cleaned, or they are placed under the free gingival margin. (Oper. Dent.)

ridge e. An intraoral surgical operation for deepening the labial, buccal, and/or lingual sulci. It is performed to increase the intraoral height of the alveolar ridge in order to assist denture retention. (Oral Surg.)

extenuate To lessen; to mitigate. (D. Juris.)

external oblique line (ō-blĕk') (see **line, external oblique**)

external pin fixation (see **appliance, fracture**)

external traction (see **traction, external**)

exteroceptors (ek″ster-ō-sĕp'tors) Sensory nerve end receptors that respond to external stimuli; located in the skin, mouth, eyes, ears, and nose. (Oral Physiol.)

extirpation, pulp (ĕk″ster-pā'shŭn) (see **pulpectomy**)

extracoronal (ĕk″strah-kor'ō-năl) Pertaining to that which is outside, or external to, the body of the coronal portion of a natural tooth; usually refers to the form of both the tooth preparation and the subsequent restoration; e.g., extracoronal preparation, extracoronal restoration, or partial or complete crown. (Fixed Part. Prosth.)

e. retainer (see **retainer, extracoronal**)

extract A concentrate obtained by treating a crude material, such as plant or animal tissue, with a solvent, evaporating part or all of the solvent from the resulting solution, and standardizing the resulting product. (Oral Med.; Pharmacol.) (see also **fluidextract**)

extraction A method of removing a tooth from the oral cavity by means of elevators and/or forceps. (Oral Surg.)

serial e. Extraction of selected primary teeth over a period of years (often ending with removal of the first premolar teeth) to relieve crowding of the dental arches during eruption of the lateral incisors, canines, and premolars. (Orthodont.)

extrahazardous In the law of insurance, an action attended by circumstances or conditions of unusual danger. (D. Juris.)

extraoral anchorage (see **anchorage, extramaxillary**)

extrapolate (ĕk-străp'ō-lāt) To infer values beyond the observable range from an observed trend of variables; to project by inference into the unexplored. (Oral Radiol.)

extrasystole (ĕk″strah-sĭs'tō-lē) A heartbeat occurring before its normal time in the rhythm of the heart and followed by a compensatory pause. (Anesth.)

extravasation (ĕk-străv″ah-zā'shŭn) The escape of a body fluid out of its proper place; e.g., blood into surrounding tissues after rupture of a vessel, or urine into surrounding tissues after rupture of the bladder. (Anesth.)

extrinsic coloring Coloring from without; e.g., coloring of the external surface of a prosthesis. (M.F.P.)

extroversion A tendency of the teeth or other maxillary structures to become situated too far from the median plane. (Orthodont.)

extrude To elevate. To move a tooth coronally. (Orthodont.)

extrusion Movement of teeth beyond the natural occlusal plane that may be accompanied by a similar movement of investing tissues. (Remov. Part. Prosth.)

— Migration of a tooth beyond the normal or natural occlusal plane. (Endodont.)

tooth e. Supraocclusal migration of teeth due to absence of opposing occlusal force (i.e., tooth migration in the absence of a functional tooth antagonist). (Periodont.) (see also **eruption, continuous**)

extubate (ĕks'tū-bāt) To remove a tube, usually an endotracheal anesthesia tube or a Levin gastric suction tube. (Oral Surg.)

extubation (ĕks″tū-bā'shŭn) Removal of a tube used for intubation. (Anesth.)

exudate (ĕks'ū-dāt) The outpouring of a substance onto the surface, such as exudated pus or tissue fluid. (Oral Diag.)

— Any adventitious substance deposited in or on a tissue by a vital process or disease. (Oral Path.)

gingival e. The outpouring of an exudate from the gingival tissues, particularly that exuding through the ulcerated sulcal epithelium during gingival inflammation. (Periodont.)

exudation (ĕks″ū-dā'shŭn) (see **exudate**)

eye-ear plane (see **plane, Frankfort horizontal**)

F

fabrication (făb″rĭ-kā′shŭn) Construction or building up of a restoration. (Oper. Dent.)

face-bow A caliper-like device that is used to record the relationship of the maxillae to the temporomandibular joints (or opening axis of the mandible) and to orient the casts in this same relationship to the opening axis of an articulator. (Comp. Prosth.)

adjustable axis f.-b. (see **face-bow, kinematic**)

kinematic f.-b. (**hinge-bow**) A face-bow whose caliper ends (condyle rods) can be adjusted to permit the accurate location of the axis of rotation of the mandible by observation of the movement of the condyle rods while the mandible is moved up and down in its most posterior position. (Comp. Prosth.)

face, changeable area of The part of the face from the nose to the chin. (Orthodont.)

face form (see **form, face**)

facet (făs′ĕt) A flattened, highly glazed wear pattern as noted on a tooth. (Comp. Prosth.; Periodont.)

facial cleft (see **cleft, facial**)

facial profile (see **profile, facial**)

facies (fā′shē-ēz) The features, general appearance, and expression of a face. (Oral Diag.; Oral Surg.)

facilitation Reinforcement of a lower-level nerve stimulus by a higher-level nerve stimulus. Thus a reflex that cannot be elicited by a subliminal impulse may be reinforced by an additional stimulus from a higher center. The combined effect of the two stimuli may cause a reflex response. (Oral Physiol.)

facsimile (făk-sĭm′ĭ-lē) A true copy that preserves all the markings and contents of the original. (D. Juris.)

fact A thing done; an action performed; an event; an actual happening. (D. Juris.)

factor(s) A constituent, element, cause, or agent that influences a process or system; a gene; a dietary substance. (Oral Med.)

f. I (**fibrinogen, profibrin**) (see **fibrinogen**)

f. II (**prothrombin, component A, prothrombase, prothrombin B, thrombogen, thrombozyme**) Considered to be the only essential precursor of thrombin. (Oral Med.)

f. III (**thromboplastin [tissue], thrombokinase, cytozyme [platelet], thrombokinin [blood], thromboplastic protein**) (see **thromboplastin**)

f. IV (**calcium, Ca^{++}**) Ionized and/or bound(?) calcium, which is generally required for the coagulation of blood, although some early phases of coagulation and the thrombin-fibrinogen reaction can take place without calcium. (Oral Med.)

f. V (**labile f., proaccelerin, accelerin, acceleration f., cofactor of thromboplastin, component A of prothrombin, plasma ac-globulin, plasma prothrombin conversion f. [PPCF], prothrombinase, prothrombin accelerator, prothrombin conversion accelerator I, thrombogen, thrombogene, proaccelerin-accelerin system**) A factor apparently necessary for the formation of a prothrombin converting substance in blood and tissue extracts, i.e., intrinsic and extrinsic prothrombin activators. A deficiency results in parahemophilia (hypoproaccelerinemia). (Oral Med.)

f. VI Term formerly used as indicating an intermediate product in the formation of thromboplastin and also used synonymously with accelerin and activated factor V. It has no designation at the present time. (Oral Med.)

f. VII (**stable f., serum prothrombin conversion accelerator [SPCA], proconvertin, autoprothrombin I, cofactor V, component B of prothrombin, cothromboplastin, kappa f., precursor of serum prothrombin conversion accelerator [pro-SPCA], prothrombin conversion f., prothrombin converting f., prothrombin conversion accelerator II, proconvertin-convertin system, prothrombinogen, serozyme, stabile f.**) A factor that accelerates the conversion of prothrombin to thrombin in the presence of factors III, IV, and V; a serum factor necessary for the formation of extrinsic prothrombin activator. A deficiency may be congenital, or it may be acquired in liver disease, vitamin K deficiency, or from prothrombinopenic agents used in anticoagulation therapy; it results in a prolonged (quantitative) one-stage prothrombin time test. (Oral Med.)

f. VIII (**antihemophilic f. [AHF], antihemophilic globulin, antihemophilic globulin A, antihemophilic f. A, plasma thromboplastin f. A [PTF-A], plasma thromboplastin f. [PTF], plasmokinin, platelet cofactor I, pro-**

145

thrombokinase, thrombocatalysin, thrombocytolysin, thrombokatilysin, thromboplastic plasma component [TPC], thromboplastinogen) A factor essential for the formation of blood thromboplastin. A deficiency results in classic hemophilia (hemophilia A); the clotting time is prolonged, and thromboplastin and prothrombin conversion is diminished. (Oral Med.)

f. IX (**Christmas f., plasma thromboplastin component [PTC], antihemophilic f. B, antihemophilic globulin B, autoprothrombin II, beta prothromboplastin, plasma f. X, plasma thromboplastin f. B [PTF-B], platelet cofactor II**) A factor that is active in the formation of intrinsic blood thromboplastin. A deficiency results in Christmas disease (hemophilia B), which is caused by a decrease in the amount of thromboplastin formed. (Oral Med.)

f. X (**Stuart-Prower f., Stuart f., Prower f.**) A factor influencing the yield of intrinsic (plasma) thromboplastin. A deficiency results in a prolonged one-stage prothrombin time—brain tissue or Russell's viper venom are used to test for thromboplastin deficiency. (Oral Med.)

f. XI (**plasma thromboplastin antecedent [PTA], antihemophilic f. C, PTA f., plasma thromboplastin f. C [PTF-C]**) A factor related to intrinsic (plasma) thromboplastin activation, which occurs when blood is exposed to a foreign surface. A deficiency results in hemophilioid states due to poor utilization of prothrombin. (Oral Med.) (see also **hemophilia C**)

f. XII (**Hageman f., antihemophilic f. D, clot-promoting f., fifth plasma thromboplastin precursor, glass f.**) A factor whose absence results in a long clotting time and abnormal prothrombin consumption and thromboplastin generation tests when the tests are carried out in glass tubes. No abnormal bleeding tendency occurs with a deficiency of the factor. (Oral Med.)

acceleration f. (see **factor V**)
antihemophilic f. (AHF) (see **factor VIII**)
antihemophilic f. A (see **factor VIII**)
antihemophilic f. B (see **factor IX**)
antihemophilic f. C (see **factor XI**)
antihemophilic f. D (see **factor XII**)
antipernicious f. (see **vitamin B₁₂**)
bone f. A hypothetical systemic influence thought to regulate the bone-formative and bone-resorptive response of the alveolar bone to functional forces or to inflammation associated with local irritation. (Oral Med.)

negative b. f. Excessive bone loss for age and severity of local factors present. (Oral Med.)

positive b. f. Slight loss of bone in the presence of severe local factors. (Oral Med.)

f. C (**contact f., contact activation product, third thromboplastic f.**) A coagulation accelerator product formed by the interaction of active factor XII and factor XI. (Oral Med.)

Castle's intrinsic f. (**intrinsic f.**) A factor produced by the gastric mucosa and possibly the duodenal mucosa, and considered to be responsible for the absorption of vitamin B₁₂. (Oral Med.) (see also **anemia, pernicious**)

Christmas f. (see **factor IX**)
clot-promoting f. (see **factor XII**)
clotting f. "Trace" proteins (excluding calcium) present in normal blood in such small amounts (except fibrinogen) that their presence is usually established by deductive reasoning and by genetic and biochemical characteristics. They are associated with thromboplastic activity and the conversion of prothrombin to thrombin. (Oral Med.)

contact f. (see **factor C**)
environmental f. Local causative agents that have allowed a lesion to occur or those conditions that have secondarily become involved. Examples include narrow interdental spaces, saddle areas, cleft formations, complications of frenula, oblique ridges, etc. (Periodont.)

erythrocyte-maturation f. (EMF) (see **vitamin B₁₂**)

etiologic f. The element or influence that can be assigned as the cause or reason for a disease or lesion. (Comp. Prosth.; Orthodont.; Remov. Part. Prosth.)

extrinsic f. (see **vitamin B₁₂**)
familial f. A characteristic derived through heredity. (Orthodont.)

glass f. (see **factor XII**)
glucocorticoid f. (see **hormone, "S"**)
Hageman f. (see **factor XII**)
Hr f. Blood factors that are reciprocally related to the Rh factors. They are present in agglutinogens when the corresponding Rh factor is absent from the gene. (Oral Med.)

hyperglycemic f. (see **glucagon**)
hyperglycemic-glycogenolytic f. (see **glucagon**)
intrinsic f. (see **factor, Castle's intrinsic**)
kappa f. (see **factor VII**)
labile f. (see **factor V**)
local f. Includes dental and bacterial plaques,

bacterial toxins and irritants, calculus, food impaction, and other surface and locally placed irritants that are capable of producing injury to the periodontium. (Oral Med.)

pellagra-preventive f. (see **acid, nicotinic**)

plasma f. X (see **factor IX**)

plasma prothrombin conversion f. (PPCF) (see **factor V**)

plasma thromboplastin f. (PTF) Substances with thromboplastic activity contributed by the plasma. Included are the antihemophilic factor, Christmas factor, plasma thromboplastin antecedent, and Hageman factor. (Oral Med.) (see also **factor VIII**)

plasma thromboplastin f. A (PTF-A) (see **factor VIII**)

plasma thromboplastin f. B (PTF-B) (see **factor IX**)

plasma thromboplastin f. C (PTF-C) (see **factor XI**)

plasma thromboplastin f. D (PTF-D) Considered by some to be a fourth plasma substance with thromboplastic activity. Not well characterized. (Oral Med.)

platelet f. Any one of the substances on or within the surface of blood platelet necessary for coagulation in the absence of extravascular thromboplastic substances. (Oral Med.)

platelet f. 1 (platelet ac-globulin, citrin) Either factor V or a factor with factor V activity; absorbed on platelets and accelerates conversion of prothrombin to thrombin. (Oral Med.)

platelet f. 2 (platelet thrombin accelerator, platelet thromboplastic activity) A substance that accelerates the conversion of fibrinogen to fibrin. (Oral Med.)

platelet f. 3 (thromboplastic cellular component [TCC], thromboplastinogenase, platelet activator) A substance associated with thromboplastin-generation activity. (Oral Med.)

platelet f. 4 An antiheparin factor. (Oral Med.)

P.-P. f. (pellagra-preventive f.) (see **acid, nicotinic**)

prothrombin conversion f. (see **factor VII**)

prothrombin converting f. (see **factor VII**)

Prower f. (see **factor X**)

psychosomatic f. Psychic, mental, or emotional factors that play a role in determining the initiation, course, and extent of a physical process, either directly or indirectly. Psychosomatic factors have been implicated in necrotizing ulcerative gingivitis (NUG),

bruxism, clenching, oral habits, etc. (Periodont.)

PTA f. (plasma thromboplastin antecedent f.) (see **factor XI**)

radiographic f. Kilovoltage, exposure time, milliamperage, and focal-film distance—the primary radiographic factors considered when making an exposure. (Oral Radiol.)

reparative f. The ability of the tissues to heal or regenerate when they have been subjected to injury, disease, etc. (Periodont.)

Rh f. Agglutinogens of red blood cells responsible for isoimmune reactions such as occur in erythroblastosis fetalis and incompatible blood transfusions. (Oral Med.)

spreading f. An enzyme that increases the permeability of ground substance. (Oral Med.; Pharmacol.)

stabile f. (see **factor VII**)

stable f. (see **factor VII**)

Stuart f. (see **factor X**)

Stuart-Prower f. (see **factor X**)

third thromboplastic f. (see **factor C**)

failure Deficiency; ineffectualness; an unsuccessful effort. (D. Juris.)

faint A state of syncope, or swooning. (Anesth.)

fall back (see **reversion**)

falsify To forge; to give a false appearance to anything, as to falsify a record. (D. Juris.)

family A body of persons who live in one house and under one head; a father, mother, and children; a husband and wife living together. (D. Juris.)

fascitis (fah-si′tis) A tumorlike growth occurring in subcutaneous tissues in the mouth, usually in the cheek. A benign lesion sometimes mistaken for fibrosarcoma, it consists of young fibroblasts and numerous capillaries. It grows rapidly and may regress spontaneously. (Oral Path.)

fate Synonym for the more modern term biotransformation. (Oral Med.; Pharmacol.) (see also **biotransformation**)

fatigue A condition of cells or organs resulting in a diminution or loss of the power or capacity of an individual to respond to stimulation. (Anesth.)

muscle f. A peripheral phenomenon due to the failure of the muscle to contract when stimuli from the nervous system reach it. Muscular work is accomplished by the body at the expense of increased metabolism. The potential energy of foodstuffs is transformed into the free energy of work and the energy of heat. When the activity of the muscle fiber is too great or too continuous, efficient utilization of glycogen does not take place, and the fibers retain considerable amounts of lactic acid. The accrual of catabolites interferes with the contractile mechanisms of muscle. In addition, the replenishment of oxygen and other nutrient anabolites is required. The catabolic and anabolic aspects of muscle function thus depend on the circulatory mechanisms. (Oral Physiol.)

fauces (faw′sēz) The archway between the pharyngeal and oral cavities; formed by the tongue, the anterior tonsillar pillars, and the soft palate. (Oral Physiol.)

fear A negative reaction on the part of the patient to the pain or cost or to an unknown aspect of dental care. On the part of the dentist, fear is manifested by apprehension of the patient's reaction to proposed dental services and their resulting cost. (Pract. Man.)

Fede's disease (see **disease, Riga-Fede**)

fee Compensation for services rendered or to be rendered; payment for professional services. (D. Juris.)

— Remuneration received by the dentist for professional services. (Pract. Man.)

feeblemindedness Mental deficiency that incapacitates an individual to the extent that supervision and control are necessary. Customarily, the IQ is below 70, and the mental age is that of a child 11 years of age or younger. (Oral Med.)

feedback The constant flow of sensory information back to the brain. The basis for control over the motor activity associated with muscle contraction depends on a constant return to the brain of information on the state of motion and energy consumption in the musculature. This return from the exteroceptors, the proprioceptors, and the chemoreceptors provides not only information on the state of activity of muscles but also the information necessary for corrections and adjustments in order to sustain smooth, coordinated muscle function. Where feedback mechanisms are deficient because of sensory deprivation, motor function becomes distorted, aberrant, and uncoordinated. (Oral Physiol.)

Feer's disease (fairz) (see **erythredema polyneuropathy**)

feldspar (fĕld′spahr) A crystalline mineral of aluminum silicate with potassium, sodium, barium, or calcium—$NaAlSi_3O_8$ or $KAlSi_3O_8$. Feldspar melts over a range of 1100° F. to 2000° F. An important constituent of dental porcelain. (D. Mat.)

f., orthoclase ceramic A clay found in large quantity in the solid crust of the earth. It acts as a filler and imparts body to the fused dental porcelain. (Fixed Part. Prosth.)

fenestration (fĕn-ĕs-trā′shŭn) Opening, window, interstice. (Oral Implant.)

f. in alveolar plate A round or oval defect or opening in the alveolar cortical plate of bone over the root surface. Found particularly where the alveolus is thin. May be seen when soft tissue is reflected and may be a result of occlusal trauma. (Periodont.)

Ferrier's separator (fer′ē-erz) (see **separator, Ferrier's**)

festoon(s) (fĕs-toon′) A carving in the base material of a denture that simulates the contours of the natural tissues being replaced by the denture. (Comp. Prosth.; Remov. Part. Prosth.)

gingival f. The distinct rounding and enlargement of the margins of the gingival tissue found in early gingival involvement. (Periodont.)

McCall's f. Enlargements of the gingival margins that may be associated with occlusal trauma. (Oral Diag.)

festooning (fĕs-toon′ĭng) The process of carving the base material of a denture or denture pattern to simulate the contours of the natural tissues to be replaced by the denture. (Comp. Prosth.)

fetor ex ore (fē′tor ĕks ō′rē) (see **halitosis**)

fetor oris (fē′tor ō′rĭs) Bad breath, a common characteristic of ANUG. The degree of seriousness may be correlated with the amount of destruction present. (Periodont.)

fever (**pyrexia**) Elevation of the body temperature. (Anesth.; Oral Diag.; Oral Surg.)

acute necrotizing ulcerative gingivitis (ANUG) and acute primary keratotic gingivostomatitis (APKG) f. A moderate-to-high elevation of temperature is not a symptom of ANUG; however, the presence of a significantly elevated temperature might suggest the presence of APKG, a viral disease accompanied by a bleeding and tender gingiva, marked fetor oris, and lymphadenopathy. (Periodont.)

aphthous f. (see **disease, foot-and-mouth**)

cat-scratch f. (benign inoculation lymphoreticulosis, cat-scratch disease) A granulomatous process that occurs at the site of a scratch or bite of a house cat. Local lesions occur at the site of injury, with a regional adenitis that is out of proportion to the primary lesion occurring within one to three weeks. Systemic symptoms of infection may occur. Diagnosis is confirmed by reaction to cat-scratch antigen or the antigen of lymphogranuloma venereum, which is a related form of disease. (Oral Diag.)

hay f. Rhinitis and conjunctivitis resulting from allergy; frequently caused by allergy to pollens. (Oral Med.)

rheumatic f. An inflammatory disease with multiple joint involvement that occurs frequently in young children and may affect the entire course of their lives. Rheumatic fever is characterized by a rapid onset, and the systemic and articular symptoms are almost simultaneous. The joint involvement is intense and subsides after a short period of activity. Because there is no pannus formation, no articular or bone damage ensues. When the disease subsides, there are no residual clinical, junctional, or pathologic alterations in the joint. The metabolic, chemical, and pathologic symptoms are similar to those of the first stage of rheumatoid arthritis. The difficulties in rheumatic fever are associated with cardiac involvement by the precipitating agent. However, not all patients with rheumatic fever have cardiac involvement. (Oral Physiol.)

— An apparently infectious disease produced by hemolytic streptococci or associated with their presence in the body; characterized by upper respiratory tract inflammation, cervical lymphadenopathy and lymphadenitis, polyarthritis, cardiac involvement, subcutaneous nodules, etc. The disease may be produced by an autoantibody reaction. A severe disease, apparently related to hypersensitive reaction to the hemolytic streptococci and characterized by polyarthritis, cardiac involvement, cervical lymphadenopathy, subcutaneous nodules, and low-grade fever. (Periodont.)

scarlet f. (scarlatina) An acute disease caused by a specific type of streptococcus and characterized by a rash and a strawberry tongue. (Oral Diag.)

uveoparotid f. (Heerfordt's syndrome, uveoparotitis) A disease characterized by inflammation of the parotid gland and of the uveal regions of the eye. (Oral Diag.)

— Firm, nodular enlargement of the parotid glands, uveitis, and cutaneous lesions may be present. Considered to be a form of sarcoidosis. (Oral Med.)

— Term used to indicate a syndrome consisting of sarcoidosis affecting the parotid glands, inflammation of the lacrimal glands, and inflammation of uveal tract of the eye. (Oral Path.)

fiber(s) An elongated, threadlike structure of organic tissue. (Anesth.)

adrenergic f. Those nerve fibers, including most of the postganglionic sympathetic fibers, that transmit their impulses across synapses or neuroeffector junctions through the local release of the neurohormone more recently identified as norepinephrine and formerly designated "sympathin." (Oral Med.; Pharmacol.)

alveolar f. White collagenous fibers of the periodontal membrane (ligament) that extend from the alveolar bone to the intermediate plexus, where their terminations are interspersed with the terminations of the cemental group of fibers. (Periodont.)

alveolar crest f. Collagenous fibers of the periodontal membrane that extend from the cervical area of the tooth to the alveolar crest. (Periodont.)

apical f. Fibers of the periodontal ligament radiating apically from tooth to bone. (Periodont.)

association f. Extensions of nerve cells that are neither efferent nor afferent neurons but that furnish a pathway of connection between them. (Oral Physiol.)

bundle f. The gathering together of collagen fibers in a group, particularly the collagen fiber bundles of the periodontal membrane. (Periodont.)

cemental f. Fibers of the periodontal membrane extending from the cementum to the zone of the intermediate plexus, where their terminations are interspersed with the terminations of the alveolar group of periodontal fibers. (Periodont.)

circular f. Fibers in the free gingiva that encircle the tooth in a ringlike fashion. (Periodont.)

collagen f. The most conspicuous part of the gingival connective tissue. Some fibers are distributed haphazardly throughout the connective tissue ground substance, and others are arranged in coarse bundles that exhibit a distinct orientation. (Periodont.)

crestal f. One group of periodontal ligament fibers extending from the cervical area of the tooth to the alveolar crest. (Periodont.)

dentogingival f. Part of a fan-shaped fiber system that emerges from the supra-alveolar part of the cementum and terminates in the free gingiva. (Periodont.)

dentoperiosteal f. A fiber system emerging from

the supra-alveolar part of the cementum of the tooth and passing outward beyond the alveolar crest in an apical direction into the mucoperiosteum of the attached gingiva. (Periodont.)

gingival f. That group of fiber systems belonging to the gingival and supra-alveolar connective tissue and composed of circular, dentogingival, dentoperiosteal, and transseptal fiber groups. (Periodont.)

horizontal f. Collagen fibers of the periodontal membrane that extend horizontally from the cementum to the alveolar bone. (Periodont.)

nerve f., myelinated A nerve fiber that is covered with a protective, or insulating, medullary sheath. The medullated fiber that lies both inside and outside the brain and spinal cord has relay stations (nodes of Ranvier) distributed at intervals along the fiber. These medullary sheaths facilitate the passage of impulses, increasing by ten times the speed of passage and reducing the energy required for transmission to one tenth of that of an equivalent nonmedullated fiber. Myelination of the nerve fibers is associated with volitional function. At birth, the fibers to and from the brain are not myelinated, and stimulation of the motor areas of the brain of an infant elicits no response. After the first year, the pyramidal cells in the motor area become myelinated, and motor functions are improved to such an extent that the child can perform motor skills such as walking, talking, and chewing. As the size of the nerve fiber increases, the conduction velocity increases. The association fibers that are the machinery of memory are the last to be myelinated. (Oral Physiol.)

nonmedullated f. A nerve fiber that is not covered by an insulating medullary sheath and is thus exposed to other tissue fluids and their respective electric potentials. In nonmedullated fibers, the impulse is relayed from point to contiguous point. Most of the nonmedullated fibers are within the substance of the central nervous system, and the distances between the cells are short. The general environment of nerve tissue is favorable to impulse transmission, and the bulk of nerve tissue is reduced, thus preventing the total volume of nerve structure from becoming disproportionate to the volume of the rest of the body tissue. (Oral Physiol.)

oblique f. The group of the collagen fibers in bundle arrangement in the periodontal ligament that are obliquely situated, with insertions in the cementum, and that extend more occlusally in the alveolus (approximately two thirds of the periodontal fibers fall into this group). (Periodont.)

principal f. The numerous bundles of collagenous tissue fibers arranged in groups that function as the mode of attachment of the tooth to the alveolus. (Periodont.)

Sharpey's f. Collagenous fibers that become incorporated into the cementum. (Periodont.)

transseptal f. A part of the gingival fiber system that extends from the supra-alveolar cementum of one tooth horizontally through the interdental attached gingiva above the septum of the alveolar bone to the cementum of the adjacent tooth. (Periodont.)

fibrillation (fĭ″brĭ-lā′shŭn) A local quivering of muscle fibers. (Anesth.)

atrial f. Cardiac arrhythmia due to disturbed spread of excitation through atrial musculature. (Anesth.)

auricular f. (aw-rĭk′ū-lar) An uncoordinated, independent contraction of the heart that results in marked irregularity of heart action. (Oral Med.)

ventricular f. Uncoordinated, independent contraction of the ventricular musculature resulting in cessation of cardiac output. (Oral Med.)

fibrinogen (fi-brĭn′ō-jĕn) **(factor I, profibrin)** A plasma protein (globulin) that is acted on by thrombin to form fibrin. The normal level is 200 to 400 mg/100 ml in plasma. Coagulation is impaired if the concentration is less than 100 mg/100 ml. (Oral Med.)

— A soluble protein in the blood plasma that is converted into fibrin by the action of thrombin, thus producing clotting of the blood. Another form of fibrinogen, called tissue fibrinogen, which has the power of clotting the blood without the presence of thrombin, occurs in body tissues. (Oral Path.)

fibrinokinase (fĭ″brĭ-nō-kĭ′nās) **(fibrinolysokinase, lysokinase)** An activator of plasminogen found in many animal tissues. (Oral Med.)

fibrinolysin (fĭ″brĭ-nol′ĭ-sĭn) (see **plasmin**)

fibrinolysokinase (see **fibrinokinase**)

fibroblast (fi′brō-blăst) A spindle-shaped cell of both loose and dense connective tissue with the capacity to form fibers of these tissues; opinion differs as to its ability to form bone. (Oral Physiol.)

— A cell found within fibrous connective tissue, varying in shape from stellate (young) to fusiform and spindle shaped. Associated with the formation of collagen fibers and ground substance of connective tissue. (Periodont.)

fibroblastoma (fi″brō-blăs-tō′mah) A tumor arising from an ordinary connective tissue cell or fibroblast. The tumor may be a fibroma or a fibrosarcoma. (Oral Path.)

neurogenic f. (see **neurofibroma**)

perineural f. (see **neurilemoma; neurofibroma**)

fibrocystic disease (see **disease, fibrocystic**)

fibroma (fi-brō′mah) A benign neoplasm of connective tissue elements. (Oral Diag.)

— A benign mesenchymal tumor composed primarily of fibrous connective tissue. (Oral Path.)

ameloblastic f. A mixed tumor of odontogenic origin characterized by the simultaneous proliferation of both the epithelial and mesenchymal component of the tooth germ without the production of hard structure. (Oral Path.)

calcifying f. (see **osteofibroma**)

cementifying f. An intrabony lesion not associated with teeth, composed of a fibrous connective tissue stroma containing foci of calcified material resembling cementum; a rare odontogenic tumor composed of varying amounts of fibrous connective tissue with calcified material resembling cementum. Central lesion of the jaws. (Oral Path.)

irritation f. A localized peripheral, tumorlike enlargement of connective tissue due to prolonged local irritation and usually seen on the gingiva or buccal mucosa. (Oral Path.)

f. with myxomatous degeneration (see **fibromyxoma**)

neurogenic f. (see **neurilemoma; neurofibroma**)

odontogenic f. A benign connective tissue neoplasm derived from fibroblasts; associated with tooth formation. (Oral Diag.)

— Central odontogenic tumor of the jaws, consisting of connective tissue in which small islands and strands of odontogenic epithelium are dispersed. A mesodermal odontogenic tumor composed of active dense or loose fibrous connective tissue; contains inactive islands of epithelium. (Oral Path.)

peripheral o. f. A fibrous connective tissue tumor associated with the gingival margin and believed to originate from the periodontium. Often contains areas of calcification. Localized form of fibromatosis gingivae. (Oral Path.)

ossifying f. (see **osteofibroma**)

periapical f. (**benign periapical f., fibrous dysplasia, first-state cementoma, focal osseous dysplasia, traumatic osteoclasia**) A benign connective tissue mass formed at the apex of a tooth with a normal pulp. (Oral Diag.)

fibromatosis (fi″brō-mah-tō′sĭs) The production of excessive connective (fibrous) tissue that has an appearance similar to a neoplasm. (Oral Diag.)

— Gingival enlargement believed to be a hereditary condition that is manifested in the permanent dentition and characterized by a firm hyperplastic tissue that covers the surfaces of the teeth. Differentiation between this and diphenylhydantoin (Dilantin) hyperplasia is based on a history of drug ingestion. (Periodont.)

f. gingivae (elephantiasis gingivae, idiopathic f., idiopathic gingival hyperplasia) Generalized enlargement of the gingivae due to fibrous hyperplasia. Idiopathic in nature and similar in appearance to Dilantin hyperplasia. (Oral Path.)

hereditary gingival f. A condition possessing a familial attribute of distribution, in which there is gingival enlargement due to marked fibroplasia. (Periodont.)

idiopathic f. (see **fibromatosis, gingivae**)

fibromyxoma (fi″brō-mĭk-sō′mah) **(fibroma with myxomatous degeneration)** A fibroma that has certain characteristics of a myxoma; a fibroma that has undergone myxomatous degeneration. Combination of both fibrous and myxomatous elements. (Oral Path.)

fibro-osteoma (fi″brō-ahs″tē-ō′mah) (see **osteofibroma**)

fibropapilloma (fi″brō-păp″ĭ-lō′mah) A lesion that resembles a benign neoplasm and shows fibroblastic and epithelial proliferation. Such lesions occur in regions of cheek chewing or other trauma. Since they are not true neoplasms, they may be better designated as irritation fibroses or fibrous hyperplasias. (Oral Diag.)

fibrosarcoma (fi″brō-săr-kō′mah) A malignant connective tissue neoplasm characterized by fibroblasts. (Oral Diag.)

— Malignant mesenchymal tumor, the basic cell type being a fibroblast. Most fibrosarcomas are locally infiltrative and persistent but do not metastasize. (Oral Path.)

odontogenic f. An extremely rare malignant form of odontogenic fibroma. (Oral Path.)

fibrosis (fi-brō′sĭs) The process of forming fibrous tissue, usually by degeneration; e.g., fibrosis of the pulp. (Oral Diag.; Oral Path.)

hereditary gingival f. An uncommon form of severe gingival hyperplasia that may begin with the eruption of the deciduous or permanent teeth and is characterized by a firm, dense, pink gingival tissue with little tendency toward bleeding. (Periodont.)

diffuse h. g. f. An uncommon form of severe gingival hyperplasia considered to be of genetic origin. The tissue is pink, firm, dense, and insensitive and has little tendency to bleed. (Periodont.)

fibrous gold (see **foil, gold**)

fiduciary (fĭ-doo'shē-ăr'ē) A person who has a duty to act primarily for another's benefit, as a trustee. Also, pertaining to the good faith and confidence involved in such a relationship. (D. Juris.)

field An area, region, or space.

f. block (see **block, field**)

operating f. The area immediately surrounding and directly involved in a treatment procedure; e.g., all the teeth included in a rubber dam application for the restoration of a single tooth or portions thereof. (Oper. Dent.)

radiation f. The region in which radiant energy is being propagated. (Oral Radiol.)

file, *n.* An instrument that cuts with a rasping action. Used to enlarge the root canal and smooth its surface. (Endodont.)

— A metal tool of varying size and form with numerous ridges or teeth on its cutting surfaces; may be push-cut or pull-cut; used for smoothing or dressing down metals and other substances. (Oper. Dent.)

— An instrument that has a serrated working area; in reality, a series of miniature hoes on a single-blade face. Used with a pull stroke in the removal of calcareous accretions from the teeth. (Periodont.)

gold f. A file designed for removing surplus gold from gold restorations; may be pull-cut or push-cut. (Oper. Dent.)

Hirschfeld-Dunlop f. A variety of periodontal file used with a pull stroke for the removal of calculus; available in various angulations for approach to different surfaces of teeth. (Oper. Dent.)

root canal f. A small metal hand instrument with tightly spiraled blades used to clean and shape the canal. (Endodont.)

—, *v.* To reduce by means of a file. (Oper. Dent.)

filled resin (see **resin, composite**)

filler An ingredient present in a pharmaceutical preparation for the purpose of providing bulk. (Oral Med.; Pharmacol.)

filling Term that is more correctly applied to

restorations of a temporary nature, such as one used for sealing in treatment or for protecting an inlay cavity until cementation of the cast restoration. (Objectionable as a synonym for restoration.) (Oper. Dent.; Pract. Man.) (see also **restoration**)

"ditched" f. Refers to the marginal failure of amalgam restorations due to fracture of either the material or the tooth structure itself in that area. (D. Mat.)

f. material (see **material, filling**)

f. method (see **method, filling**)

postresection f. (see **filling, retrograde**)

retrograde f. (postresection f., retrograde obturation) A filling placed in the apical portion of a tooth root after surgical removal of a periapical lesion. The filling of a root canal through the apex of the tooth after surgical approach through the alveolar bone. (Endodont.)

root canal f. Material placed in the root canal system to seal the space previously occupied by the dental pulp. (Endodont.)

f. technique (see **technique, filling**)

treatment f. A temporary filling, usually of a sedative nature, used to allay sensitive dentin prior to the final preparation of the cavity. Said of a temporary filling when the extent of the carious process cannot be determined until the demineralized dentin is first "hardened" to facilitate its removal with less chance of pulp exposure. (Remov. Part. Prosth.)

film Plaque accumulated on the surface of teeth. It may be the cariogenic or calculus-producing dentobacterial plaque or an organic precipitate from the saliva. (Oral Diag.)

— A thin, flexible, transparent sheet of cellulose acetate or similar material coated with a light-sensitive emulsion. (Oral Radiol.)

f. badge A pack of x ray–sensitive film used for the detection and approximate measurement of radiation exposure for personnel-monitoring purposes; the badge may contain two or three films of differing sensitivity, and it may contain a filter that shields part of the film from certain types of radiation. (Oral Radiol.)

f. base (see **base, film**)

bite-wing f. (interproximal f.) A type of dental x-ray film that has a central tab or wing on which the teeth close to hold the film in position; a valuable aid in verifying the fit of restorations before cementation, removing marginal excess and proximal contours, and observing the progress of carious lesions; invaluable in detecting proximal lesions and caries under restorations. (Oper. Dent.)

f. fault A defective result in a radiograph; usually caused by a chemical, physical, or electrical error in its production. (Oral Radiol.)

f. f., black spots Spots caused by dust particles or developer on the films before development; also caused by outdated (expired) film. (Oral Radiol.)

blurred f. f. A fault caused by film movement during exposure, bent films during exposure, double exposures, or flowing of emulsion during processing in excessively warm solution. (Oral Radiol.)

dark f. f. A fault caused by overexposure of the film to radiation, film fog from extended development, accidental exposure to light (light leaks in film packet or dark room), or an unsafe darkroom light. (Oral Radiol.)

distorted f. f. (see **distortion, film-fault**)

dyschroic fog f. f. A fogging of the radiograph, characterized by the appearance of a pink surface when the film is viewed by transmitted light and a green surface when the film is seen by reflected light. It usually is caused by an exhaustion of the acid content of the fixing solution (incomplete fixation). (Oral Radiol.)

fogged f. f. A fault caused by stray radiation, use of expired film, or an unsafe darkroom light. (Oral Radiol.)

light f. f. A fault caused by underexposure, underdevelopment (expired or diluted developing solution), development in temperatures that are too cold, or accidental use of a wrong film speed. (Oral Radiol.)

reticulation f. f. A network of corrugations produced accidentally or intentionally by a treatment that causes rapid expansion and shrinkage of the swollen gelatin during the processing of a film. This occurs because of an excessive difference in temperature between any two of the three darkroom solutions. (Oral Radiol.)

stained f. f. A fault caused by contaminated solutions, improper rinsing, exhausted solutions, improper washing, contamination by improper handling of the emulsions during or after processing, or film hangers containing dried fixer on the clips. (Oral Radiol.)

static electricity f. f. Image in the emulsion that has the appearance of lightning.

Caused by rapid opening of the film pocket or transfer of static electricity from the technician to the film. (Oral Radiol.)

white spots f. f. A fault caused by air bubbles clinging to the emulsion during development or by fixing solution spotted on the emulsion before development. (Oral Radiol.)

f. hanger An instrument or device for holding x-ray film during processing procedures. (Oral Radiol.)

f. holder, cardboard A light-tight film container made of heavy cardboard and paper; used in extraoral radiography for direct exposure without the use of intensifying screens. Usually backed by a thin sheet of lead to absorb the secondary radiation. (Oral Radiol.)

f. identification Recognition of tube side of film. Intraoral films can be oriented by means of an embossed dot in one corner, the convexity of the dot indicating the tube or tissue side. (Oral Radiol.)

f. image The shadow of a structure as depicted on a radiographic or photographic emulsion. (Oral Radiol.)

interproximal f. (see **film, bite-wing**)

f. mounting Placement of radiographs in an orderly sequence on a suitable carrier for illumination and study. The radiographs are arranged on the carrier with the patient's right side to the examiner's left. (Oral Radiol.)

f. packet A small, light-proof, moisture-resistant, sealed paper or plastic envelope containing an x-ray film (or two x-ray films) and a lead-foil backing designed for use in the making of intraoral radiographs. (Oral Radiol.)

f. placement Positioning of the x-ray film to receive the image cast by the roentgen rays. (Oral Radiol.)

f. processing Chemical transformation of the latent image, produced in a film emulsion by exposure to radiation, into a stable image visible by transmitted light. The usual procedure is basically a selective reduction of affected silver halide salts to metallic silver grains (development), followed by the selective removal of unaffected silver halide (fixation), washing to remove the processing chemicals, and drying. (Oral Radiol.)

rapid f. p. The use of high-speed developers or the removal of the film from the fixing solution after clearing so that the film can be viewed immediately. (Oral Radiol.)

f. speed (film sensitivity) The amount of exposure to light or roentgen rays required to produce a given image density. It is expressed as the reciprocal of the exposure in roentgens necessary to produce a density of 1.0 above base and fog; films are classified on this basis in six speed groups, between each of which is a twofold increase in film speed. (Oral Radiol.)

f. on teeth Mucinous deposits on teeth, containing microorganisms, desquamated tissue elements, blood cellular elements, etc.; usually thin and adherent. (Periodont.)

f. thickness Refers to thickness of a layer of material, particularly in reference to dental cements. In standardization tests it is the minimal thickness or layer obtained under a specific load. (D. Mat.)
— Dimension of a thin coating or layer; A.D.A. specification No. 8 for cement. (Oper. Dent.)

x-ray f. (see **x-ray film**)

filter A material placed in the useful beam to absorb preferentially the less energetic (less penetrating) radiations. (Oral Radiol.) (see also **filtration**)

added f. Filter added to the inherent filter. (Oral Radiol.)

compensating f. A filter designed to shield less dense areas so that a more uniform image quality will be produced. (Oral Radiol.)

inherent f. Filtration introduced by the glass wall of the x-ray tube, any oil used for tube immersion, or any permanent tube enclosure in the path of useful beam. (Oral Radiol.)

total f. Sum of inherent and added filters. (Oral Radiol.)

filtration The use of absorbers for the selective attenuation of radiation of certain wavelengths from a useful primary beam of x radiation. (Oral Radiol.)

added f. Supplemental filtration by means of an absorber or absorbers deliberately interposed in the beam additional to the inherent filtration. Added filtration is usually positioned immediately beneath or at the base of the collimating device. (Oral Radiol.)

built-in f. Filtration effected by nonremovable absorbers deliberately built into the tube-head assembly to increase the inherent beam filtration. (Oral Radiol.)

external f. The action of absorbers external to

the tube-head assembly, consisting of added filtration (see above) plus the attenuating effect of materials of which any closed-end cone such as a pointer-cone may be made. (Oral Radiol.)

inherent f. The filtration effect of tube-head components in the path of the useful beam, such as the glass wall of the x-ray tube, oil (if any) used for insulation and heat dissipation, material used to contain the oil behind the tube-head port, and any other materials permanently situated between the target and the collimator. It is often expressed as the equivalent thickness of a given substance which, if inserted as a filter immediately in front of the target, would produce a radiation beam of the same quality and intensity as that which emerges from the apparatus. (Oral Radiol.)

total f. The sum total of the inherent and built-in filtration (nonremovable) and filtration added externally (supplemental filters and/or pointer-cones), usually expressed in terms of equivalence to the filtration effected by a stated thickness of pure aluminum (measured in mm or aluminum equivalent). (Oral Radiol.)

findings, radiographic (roentgenographic f.) The recorded radiographic evidence of normal anatomic structures and deviations therefrom. (Oral Radiol.)

fineness A means of grading alloys with regard to gold content. The fineness of an alloy is designated in parts per thousand of pure gold, pure gold being 1000 fine. (D. Mat.)

finger Any one of the five digits of the hand.

clubbed f. A condition seen in hypertrophic osteoarthropathy where the base angle between the base of the fingernail and adjacent dorsal surface of the terminal phalanx is obliterated and becomes 180° or greater. The base of the nail projects downward, and the area of nail is increased. (Oral Med.)

f. positions The positions of the fingers when operating; refers not only to the fingers grasping the instrument but also to the fingers used for rests, support, and holding the tissues out of the way. (Oper. Dent.)

f. rest A support for the hand holding an instrument; may be teeth, instruments such as clamps and separators firmly attached to teeth, or soft tissues. (Oper. Dent.)
— An integral part of instrumentation, in which the fingers of the working hand are allowed to rest on the teeth, adjacent tis-

sues, fingers of the opposing hand, etc., in order to limit the working stroke of an instrument, provide an arc of movement for the instrument, increase tactile acuity, or provide a fulcrum for movement of the working fingers and instruments. (Periodont.)

f. strut A bar or similar component of the infrastructure of a subperiosteal or endosteal implant that projects from it, being attached only at one side. (Oral Implant.)

finish line (see **line, finish**)

finish, satin The degree of finish of a polished surface that has been made very smooth but is without a high sheen. (Oper. Dent.)

finishing and polishing Removal of excess restoration material from the margins and contours of a restoration, and polishing of the restoration. (Oper. Dent.)

first surgical stage (subperiosteal) The operation performed to obtain a direct bone impression. (Oral Implant.)

fission (fĭsh'ŭn) The splitting of a nucleus into two fragments. Fission may occur spontaneously or may be induced artificially. In addition to the fission fragments, particulate radiation energy and gamma rays are usually produced during fission. (Oral Radiol.)

nuclear f. The splitting of an atomic nucleus (as by bombardment with neutrons), especially into approximately equal parts, resulting in the release of enormous quantities of energy when certain heavy elements (such as uranium and plutonium) are split. (Oral Radiol.)

n. f. products Elements (nuclides) or compounds resulting from nuclear fission. (Oral Radiol.)

f. products The nuclides produced by the fission of a heavy-element nuclide. (Oral Radiol.)

fissure A deep groove or cleft; a developmental linear fault usually found in the occlusal or buccal surface of a tooth; commonly the result of the imperfect fusion of the enamel or adjoining dental lobes. (Oper. Dent.)

gingival f. (see **cleft, gingival**)

pterygomaxillary f. The most posterior point in the anterior contour of the maxillary tuberosity. (Orthodont.)

retrocuticular f. An intraepithelial split. When the oral epithelium is broken by the tooth at the time of tooth eruption, most of the epithelial cells keep their connection with the basal layer of epithelium, but a few cells remain with the cuticle (Weske's the-

ory of formation of gingival sulcus and the epithelial attachment). (Periodont.)

fissured tongue (see **tongue, fissured**)

fistula (fĭs'tū-lah) A patent sinus tract leading from a chronic alveolar involvement to an epithelial surface. (Endodont.)

— A small opening leading from a pathologic or natural internal cavity to the surface. (Oral Diag.)

— A tract connecting two body surfaces; e.g., a tract between two anatomic body cavities or between an anatomic cavity and the skin. The tract may be lined with epithelium. (Oral Surg.)

alveolar f. A fistula communicating with the cavity of an alveolar abscess. More properly called alveolar sinus. (Endodont.) (see also **sinus, alveolar**)

arteriovenous f. (see **shunt, arteriovenous**)

branchial f. A fistula associated with a branchial cyst; usually seen on the lateral surface of the neck. (Oral Path.)

dental f. A passage or channel extending from an abscess cavity to the outer surface of the gingivae. (Periodont.)

f. of lip Congenital malformation in which there is a deep pit or fistula on the mucosa of the lip; often bilateral and usually found on the lower lip. (Oral Path.)

oroantral f. An opening between the maxillary sinus and the oral cavity, most often through a tooth socket. (Oral Surg.) (see also **fistula**)

orofacial f. An opening between the cutaneous surface of the face and the oral cavity. (Oral Surg.)

oronasal f. An opening between the nasal cavity and the oral cavity. (Oral Surg.)

salivary f. An opening between a salivary duct and/or gland and the cutaneous surface or into the oral cavity through other than the normal anatomic pathway. (Oral Surg.)

fit Adaptation of any dental restoration. Adaptation of a denture to its basal seat, a clasp to a tooth, an inlay to a cavity preparation, etc. (Comp. Prosth.; Remov. Part. Prosth.)

fix To make firm, stable, immovable; to place in a desired position and hold there. In dentistry, to secure in position, usually by means of cementation, a prosthesis such as a crown or a fixed partial denture. (Fixed Part. Prosth.)

fixation Act or result of fixing. In dentistry, the act of securing in position, usually by means of cementation, some treatment appliance such as a crown or fixed partial denture when willful removal of the restoration by the patient is not intended. (Fixed Part. Prosth.)

— Retention of a part in a fairly immobile position, as in the treatment of fractures. (Oral Surg.)

— In photographic and radiographic film processing, the chemical removal of all the undeveloped salts of the film emulsion, so that only the developed (reduced) silver will remain as a permanent image. (Oral Radiol.)

biphase pin f. (see **appliance, fracture**)

elastic band f. Stabilization of fractured segments of the jaws by means of intermaxillary or maxillomandibular elastic bands applied to splints or appliances. (Oral Surg.)

f. of elements by the skeleton Fixation of many elements for long periods of time in the bone matrix due to a special affinity of the elements for the matrix. Recent work with radioactive isotopes has firmly established the concept of the skeleton as a dynamic system. In addition to the changes in structure and in distribution of the bone mineral mediated by cellular activity, every ionic grouping in the mineral is capable of replacement. (Oral Physiol.)

external pin f. (see **appliance, fracture**)

intermaxillary f. (objectionable except in reference to the two maxillae) (see **fixation, maxillomandibular**)

intraosseous f. Reduction and stabilization of fractured bony parts by direct fixation to one another with surgical wires, screws, pins, and/or plates. (Oral Surg.)

mandibulomaxillary f. (see **fixation, maxillomandibular**)

maxillomandibular f. (mandibulomaxillary f.) Retention of fractures of the maxillae or mandible in the functional relations with the opposing dental arch through the use of elastic wire ligatures and interdental wiring and/or splints. (Oral Surg.)

nasomandibular f. Mandibular immobilization, especially for edentulous jaws, using mandibulomaxillary splints, circummandibular wiring, and intraoral interosseous wiring through the nasal process of the maxillae. (Oral Surg.)

Roger-Anderson pin f. An appliance used in extraoral fixation of mandibular fractures and prognathisms. (Oral Surg.) (see also **appliance, fracture**)

fixed partial denture (see **denture, partial, fixed**)

fixed saddle bridge A fixed prosthesis with distal extension pontics designed with a ridge-hugging saddle (denture base). (Oral Implant.)

flabby tissue (see **tissue, hyperplastic**)

flaccid (flăk′sĭd) A relaxed or flabby state, as in a flaillike condition or paralysis of a muscle. (Oral Physiol.)

flange (flănj) The part of the denture base that extends from the cervical ends of the teeth to the border of the denture. (Comp. Prosth.; Remov. Part. Prosth.)

—**(guide appliance)** An appliance (prosthesis) with a lateral vertical extension designed to direct a resected mandible into centric occlusion. (M.F.P.)

buccal f. The portion of the flange of a denture that occupies the buccal vestibule of the mouth and that extends distally from the buccal notch. (Comp. Prosth.; Remov. Part. Prosth.)

contour of f. The design of the flange of a denture. (Comp. Prosth.; Remov. Part. Prosth.)

denture f. The essentially vertical extension from the body of the denture into one of the vestibules of the oral cavity. Also, on the lower denture, the essentially vertical extension along the bucal side of the alveololingual sulcus. The buccal and labial denture flanges have two surfaces; the buccal or labial surface and the basal seat surface. The lower lingual flange has two surfaces: the basal seat surface and the lingual surface. (Comp. Prosth.; Remov. Part. Prosth.)

labial f. The portion of the flange of a denture that occupies the labial vestibule of the mouth. (Comp. Prosth.; Remov. Part. Prosth.)

lingual f. The portion of the flange of a mandibular denture that occupies the space adjacent to the residual ridge and next to the tongue. (Comp. Prosth.; Remov. Part. Prosth.)

flap A partly detached sheet of soft tissue to be used in repairing defects in an adjacent or a remote part of the body. (Oral Surg.)

envelope f. Mucoperiosteal tissue retracted from a horizontal linear incision (as along the free gingival margin), with no vertical component of the incision. (Oral Surg.)

lingual tongue f. A flap used to repair a fistula of the hard palate, which combines the raising of a palatal flap to form the floor of the nose with a flap taken from the back or edge of the tongue to form the palatal surface. (Oral Surg.)

mucoperiosteal f. A flap of mucosal tissue, including the periosteum, reflected from a bone. (Oral Surg.)

pedicle f. A detached mass of tissue containing cutaneous and subcutaneous components, along with an adequate blood supply maintained at its base. (Oral Surg.)

sliding f. A flap that is advanced from its original location in a direction away from its base, to close a defect. (Oral Surg.)

V-Y f. A flap in which the incision is shaped like a V and after closure like a Y, to lengthen a localized area of tissue. (Oral Surg.) (see also **flap, Y-V**)

Y-V f. A flap in which the incision is shaped like a Y and after closure like a V, to shorten a localized area of tissue. (Oral Surg.) (see also **flap, V-Y**)

flash Excess material that is squeezed out of the mold; e.g., during packing of a denture by compression technique. (D. Mat.)

flask A metal case or tube used in investing procedures. (Comp. Prosth.)

casting f. (see **flask, refractory**)

f. closure The procedure of bringing the parts of a flask together to form a complete mold. (Comp. Prosth.; Fixed Part. Prosth.; Remov. Part. Prosth.)

final f. c. The last closure of a flask before curing and after trial packing of the mold with a denture base material. (Comp. Prosth.; Remov. Part. Prosth.)

trial f. c. Preliminary closures made for the purpose of eliminating excess denture base or other plastic material and of ensuring that the mold is completely filled. (Comp. Prosth.; Fixed Part. Prosth.; Remov. Part. Prosth.)

crown f. A small, sectional, metal boxlike case in which a sectional mold of plaster of paris or artificial stone is made for the purpose of compressing and curing plastics on small dental restorations. (Comp. Prosth.; Fixed Part. Prosth.)

denture f. A sectional, metal boxlike case in which a sectional mold of plaster of paris or artificial stone is made for the purpose of compressing and curing dentures or other resinous restorations. (Comp. Prosth.; Fixed Part. Prosth.; Remov. Part. Prosth.)

injection f. A special flask designed to permit the filling of the mold after the flask is closed or to permit the addition of denture base material to that in the flask after the flask is closed. (Comp. Prosth.; Remov. Part. Prosth.)

refractory f. (casting f., casting ring) A metal tube in which a refractory mold is made for casting metal dental restorations or appli-

ances. (Comp. Prosth.; Fixed Part. Prosth.)

flasking The act of investing a pattern in a flask. The process of investing the cast and a wax denture in a flask preparatory to molding the denture base material into the form of the denture. (Comp. Prosth.; Fixed Part. Prosth.; Remov. Part. Prosth.)

flexibility The property of elastic deformation under loading. (Remov. Part. Prosth.)

flexion The bending of a joint between two skeletal members in order to decrease the angle between the members; opposite of extension. (Oral Physiol.)

f.-extension reflex (see **reflex, flexion-extension**)

flexure The quality or state of being flexed.

clasp f. The flexure of a retentive clasp arm to permit passage over the surveyed height of contour, thus permitting the seating or removal of the clasp. (Remov. Part. Prosth.)

floor of cavity (see **cavity, floor**)

flora The bacteria living in various parts of the alimentary canal. (Oral Med.; Oral Path.; Periodont.)

fusospirochetal f. The microorganisms *Fusobacterium fusiforme* and *Borrelia vincentii*. Present in most individuals as normal inhabitants of the oral cavity. Believed by some to be the primary cause of necrotizing ulcerative gingivitis (NUG); believed by others to be secondary invaders, the primary infectious agent being unknown. Stress and fatigue have been shown to play a role in the genesis of NUG, possibly acting to decrease tissue resistance and antibody formation, thus permitting the fusospirochetal organisms to assume a pathogenic role. (Periodont.)

oral f. The microorganisms inhabiting the oral cavity of an individual. They are usually saprophytic in nature and live together in a symbiotic relationship. Some are potentially pathogenic, assuming a pathologic role when adverse local and/or systemic factors influence the symbiotic balance of the microorganic flora. (Periodont.)

floss tape A silk tape often incorporated with pumice and used to polish the proximal surfaces of teeth. (Periodont.)

flow Continued deformation or change in shape under a static load. Used in conjunction with waxes and amalgam. (D. Mat.)

— Any continuous movement; the property of continuous deformation under a given load without an increase in the magnitude of the applied force. (Oper. Dent.)

traffic f. The pattern of conducting patients from one area within the office to another. (Pract. Man.)

flowmeter A physical device for measuring the rate of flow of a gas or liquid. (Anesth.)

fluctuation A wavelike motion produced in soft tissues in response to palpation or percussion. Due to a collection of fluids or exudates in the tissues. (Oral Surg.)

fluid A liquid or gaseous substance.

f. distribution and transport The phenomenon in which intracellular and extracellular fluids are distributed throughout the body by various modes of transport. The factors that control fluid distribution in the various water compartments of the body are the barriers of the compartments, the hydrostatic pressures in the circulatory and interstitial fluids, and the osmotic pressures determined by the chemical composition of the fluids. The principal physical barriers to fluid transfer are the cell membrane and the capillary walls, both of which possess highly selective permeability to the passage of ions and salts. (Oral Physiol.)

f. and electrolyte balance Maintenance by the body fluids of a constancy of salt ion concentration appropriate to the function of the specific tissues or organ systems. The body fluids are thus essentially composed of water, which is the most abundant component of the body, and electrolytes, which are composed of organic and inorganic salts and ions. (Oral Physiol.)

extracellular f. Body fluid that is outside the cells. Extracellular fluid is divided into two general subdivisions: intravascular fluid and extravascular fluid. The blood plasma constitutes the bulk of the intravascular fluid. The extravascular fluid is compartmentalized according to anatomic areas and spaces. The interstitial fluid, which includes the lymph, composes the largest proportion of the extracellular fluid. The other major extravascular fluids include the cerebrospinal fluid, the vitreous humor of the eye, synovial fluids, biles, secretions, water in the gastrointestinal tract, and excretory fluids such as urine in the bladder. (Oral Physiol.)

synovial f. The small amount of fluid occurring in normal joints. Its content is approximately 95% water, with only 1% to 2% protein concentration. The cell content varies considerably and includes up to 200 white blood cells per cubic millimeter of fluid. The principal function of the fluid is to lubricate the joint surfaces and to nourish the articular cartilage. The synovial membrane is easily permeable to electrolytes and small colloidal particles. Larger colloidal substances, however, are transferred by a more complex mechanism. Microorganisms gain access to synovial fluid more readily than to cerebrospinal fluid. (Oral Physiol.)

total body f. All the fluids contained in the body. There are two main types: the intracellular fluid, which is contained totally within the cells, and the extracellular fluid, which is contained entirely outside the cells. (Oral Physiol.)

f. wax (see **wax, fluid**)

fluidextract The liquid that results from the treatment of a crude material, such as plant tissue, with solvents and from the adjustment of the volume of the resulting solution so that each milliliter contains the extractives from 1 g of crude material. (Oral. Med.; Pharmacol.)

fluorescence (flū-ō-rĕs′ĕns) Emission of radiation of a particular wavelength by certain substances as the result of absorption of radiation of a shorter wavelength. Essentially, the emission occurs only during the irradiation. (Oral Radiol.)

fluorescent screen (see **screen, intensifying**)

fluoridate (flū-or′ĭ-dāt) To add fluoride to a water supply. (Pedodont.)

fluoridation The use of a fluoride to reduce caries activity; may be by means of communal water supplies, oral hygiene preparations for home use, or topical applications for the purpose of prophylaxis. (Oper. Dent.)

fluoridization (flū-or″ĭ-dī-zā′shŭn) The topical application of a solution of a fluoride to teeth. (Pedodont.)

fluoroscope (flū-or′ō-skōp) A device consisting of a fluorescent screen mounted in a metal frame covered with lead glass. In the presence of a roentgen ray, the screen glows in direct proportion to the intensity of the remnant x radiation, producing visual impressions of the densities traversed. (Oral Radiol.)

fluorosis (flū-ō-rō′sĭs) General term for chronic fluoride poisoning. (Oral Diag.) (see also **fluorosis, chronic endemic dental**)

— Enamel hypoplasia due to the ingestion of water containing excess fluorine during the time of enamel formation. (Oral Path.)

chronic endemic dental f. (mottled enamel) An enamel defect caused by excessive ingestion of fluoride in the water supply (usually 2 to 8 ppm) during the period of tooth calcification. Affected teeth appear chalky white on eruption and later turn brown. (Oper. Dent.; Oral Diag.; Oral Path.)

Fluothane Proprietary term for halothane. (Pharmacol.)

flush Blush, as the cheeks; due to vasodilation of small arteries and arterioles. (Anesth.)

flutter A quick, irregular motion. (Anesth.)

flux A substance used in the casting of metals to increase fluidity and to assist in preventing oxidation of the surface of molten metal. In soldering, flux is applied to the surfaces to be joined in order to remove oxides. In silicates, flux is used to promote fusion of the metals. (D. Mat.)

— Any substance or mixture used to promote fusion, especially the fusion of metals or minerals. Used principally in dentistry as an inclusion in ceramic materials and in soldering and casting metals. (Fixed Part. Prosth.)

— A substance mixed with or added to minerals or metals to promote fusion. (Oper. Dent.)

casting f. A flux that increases fluidity of the metal and helps to prevent oxidation. (Oper. Dent.)

ceramic f. A flux used in the manufacture of porcelain and silicate powders. (Oper. Dent.)

reducing f. A flux that contains powdered charcoal to remove oxides. (Oper. Dent.)

soldering f. A ceramic material such as borax, boric acid, or a combination of them, in paste, liquid, or granular form; used to keep metallic parts clean while they are being heated during a soldering procedure. It is a solvent for metallic oxides and will flow over the parts to be soldered at temperatures well below the fusion temperature of solder, but it becomes separated from the solid metal by the molten solder. (Oper. Dent.)

F.M.I.A. (see **angle, Frankfort-mandibular incisor**)

focal-film distance (see **distance, target-film**)

focal infection (see **infection, focal**)

focal spot (see **spot, focal**)

fog (fogging) Darkening of the whole or part(s) of a developed radiograph from sources other than the radiation of the primary beam to which the film was exposed. (Oral Radiol.)

chemical f. Film darkening due to imbalance or deterioration of processing solutions. (Oral Radiol.)

dyschroic f. (see **film fault, dyschroic fog**)

light f. Film darkening due to unintentional exposure to light, to which the emulsion is sensitive, either before or during processing. (Oral Radiol.)

radiation f. Film darkening due to radiation from sources other than intentional exposure to the primary beam; e.g., film may be exposed to scatter radiation, or accidental exposure may occur if stored film is not protected from radiation. (Oral Radiol.)

foil An extremely thin, pliable sheet of metal. (Comp. Prosth.; Remov. Part. Prosth.)

— A very thin, flexible sheet of metal, usually gold, platinum, or tin; in operative dentistry, the term refers to gold foil, unless otherwise specified. (Oper. Dent.)

adhesive f. Tinfoil that is covered on one side with powdered gum arabic or karaya gum. When moistened on the gummed side and applied over the teeth, gingival tissues, and/ or postoperative surgical periodontal dressing, the foil serves to protect the area it covers. (Periodont.)

f. assistant (see **foil holder**)

f. cylinder A cylinder of gold foil formed by repeatedly folding a sheet of foil into a narrow ribbon, which is then rolled into cylindrical form; used in a noncohesive state to line the surrounding walls of a Class 5 preparation or to fill the gingival portion of the proximal box of a Class 2 preparation. (Oper. Dent.)

gold f. (fibrous gold) Pure gold rolled into extremely thin sheets. A precious-metal foil used in the restoration of carious or fractured teeth. (Comp. Prosth.; Remov. Part. Prosth.)

— Pure gold that has been rolled and beaten from ingots into a very thin sheet. Thickness usually varies from 1/40,000 inch (No. 2 foil) to 1/20,000 inch (No. 4 foil). Classified as cohesive, semicohesive, or noncohesive. One of the oldest restorative materials, the most permanent if used properly, and the yardstick by which all others are measured. It is compacted or condensed into a retentive cavity form piece by piece, utilizing this metal's property of cold welding. (D. Mat.; Oper. Dent.)

cohesive g. f. A foil prepared by rolling gold into a thin sheet, which is then beaten until it is extremely thin. It has the ability to weld to itself at room temperature when subjected to condensation pressure. Used for dental restorations. (D. Mat.)

— Gold foil that has been annealed or whose surface is completely pure so that it will cohere or weld at room temperature. (Oper. Dent.)

corrugated g. f. A gold foil made by burning

gold-foil sheets between paper in the absence of air. (Oper. Dent.)

noncohesive g. f. Gold foil that will not cohere at room temperature due to the presence on its surface of a protecting or contaminating coating. If the coating is a volatile substance, such as ammonia, the foil may be rendered cohesive by heating or annealing it to remove the protection. If annealing will not drive off the coating, the gold is said to be permanently noncohesive. (D. Mat.; Oper Dent.)

platinized g. f. A form rolled or hammered from a "sandwich" made of platinum placed between two sheets of gold; used in portions of foil restorations where greater hardness is desired. (Oper. Dent.)

semicohesive g. f. A gold foil in which the degree of cohesiveness is controlled by the annealing. (D. Mat.; Oper. Dent.)

f. holder (foil assistant) An instrument used to retain a foil pellet in place while it is being condensed or to retain a bulk of gold while additions to it are made. (Oper. Dent.)

lingual approach f. (invisible foil) A type of Class 3 gold-foil restoration in which the labial outline is markedly restricted to avoid visual detection of the metal; all the foil is placed in the cavity from the lingual surface of the tooth. (Oper. Dent.)

f. passer (f. carrier) A pointed or forked instrument used to carry pellets of gold foil through an annealing flame or from the annealing tray to the prepared cavity for compaction. (Oper. Dent.)

f. pellet (see **pellet, foil**)

platinum f. Pure platinum rolled into extremely thin sheets. A precious-metal foil whose high fusing point makes it suitable as a matrix for various soldering procedures; also suitable for providing the internal form of porcelain restorations during fabrication. (Comp. Prosth.; Oper. Dent.; Remov. Part. Prosth.)

tin-f. Tin rolled into extremely thin sheets. A base-metal foil used as a separating material, for example, between the cast and denture base material during flasking and curing procedures. (Comp. Prosth.; D. Mat.; Remov. Part. Prosth.)

t. substitute (see **substitute, tinfoil**)

fold A doubling back of a tissue surface.

mucobuccal f. (mucobuccal reflection) The line of flexure of the oral mucous membrane as it passes from the mandible or maxillae to the cheek. (Comp. Prosth.; Orthodont.; Remov. Part. Prosth.)

mucolabial f. The line of flexure of the oral mucous membrane as it passes from the mandible or maxillae to the lip. (Comp. Prosth.)

sublingual f. The crescent-shaped area on the floor of the mouth following the inner wall of the mandible and tapering toward the molar regions. It is formed by the sublingual gland and the submaxillary duct beneath the mucous membrane of the alveololingual sulcus. (Comp. Prosth.; Fixed Part. Prosth.; Remov. Part. Prosth.)

folder Usually a heavy paper envelope in which the patient's records are kept. (Pract. Man.)

Fones' method (see **method, Fones'**)

food Ingested solids and liquids that supply the body with nutriment and energy.

comminution of f. (kom′ĭ-noo′shŭn) Reduction of food into small parts. (Comp. Prosth.; Remov. Part. Prosth.)

f. impaction (see **impaction, food**)

physical character of f. The consistency, as the firmness, viscosity, or density, of food substances. Soft, adhesive, and nonabrasive foods tend to cling to the teeth, whereas coarse foods leave little debris and create a frictional effect on the tissues, thus cleansing them. A soft diet can thus lead to calculus formation. (Periodont.)

foramen (fō-rā′mĕn) A natural opening in a bone or other structure.

— A natural opening in the root, usually at or near the apical end. (Endodont.)

incisive f. (ĭn-sī′sĭv) **(nasopalatine f.)** The opening of the nasopalatine canal. (Comp. Prosth.)

— The foramen, or opening, in the midline of the palate in the region where the premaxilla and maxillae join, which is situated palatal to the upper central incisors; contains nasopalatine vessels and nerve. (Periodont.)

mandibular f. The opening on the medial aspect of the vertical ramus of the mandible approximately midway between the mandibular and gonial notches; may be located posterior to the middle of the ramus. It contains interior alveolar vessels and the inferior alveolar nerve. (Periodont.)

mental f. A circular opening on the lateral aspect of the body of the mandible either below the apex of the first premolar or below the apex of the second premolar but usually between the first and second premolars inferior to their apices. The mental vessels and nerve pass through this foramen to supply the lip. In edentulous mandibles, the bone may have been resorbed, so that it is in such a position that the denture base will cover it. (Comp. Prosth.; Periodont.)

nasopalatine f. (see **foramen, incisive**)

force An influence that changes or tends to change motion in a body. (Comp. Prosth.; Remov. Part. Prosth.)

— Any push or pull on matter, either internal or external to its structure; that which initiates, changes, or arrests motion. (Oper. Dent.)

— Energy produced and transmitted to the teeth and their supporting and investing structures by tooth-to-tooth contact through an intervening bolus of food, by the application and progress of food to and over the gingivae, etc. (Periodont.)

centrifugal f. Force that tends to recede from the center. (Oper. Dent.)

chewing f. The degree of force applied by the muscles of mastication during the mastication of food. (Comp. Prosth.; Remov. Part. Prosth.)

component of f. One of the factors from which a resultant force may be compounded or into which it may be resolved. (Comp. Prosth.; Remov. Part. Prosth.)

— One of the parts of a force into which it may be resolved. (Oper. Dent.)

condensing f. The force required to compress gold-foil pellets, facilitating their cohesion, to fabricate or build up a gold-foil restoration. (Oper. Dent.)

— The force required to compact or condense a plastic material, e.g., amalgam or wax. (Oper. Dent.)

constant f. Continuous force or pressure applied to the teeth. (Orthodont.)

denture-dislodging f. An influence that tends to displace a denture from its intended position on supporting structures. (Comp. Prosth.; Remov. Part. Prosth.)

denture-retaining f. An influence that tends to maintain a denture in its intended position on its supporting structures. (Comp. Prosth.; Remov. Part. Prosth.)

electromotive f. The difference in potential in a roentgen-ray tube between the cathode and anode; usually expressed in kilovolts. (Oral Radiol.)

intermittent f. A force or pressure applied to the teeth that is alternated with a period of passiveness or rest. (Orthodont.)

line of f. The direction of the power exerted on a body. (Comp. Prosth.; Oper. Dent.; Remov. Part. Prosth.)

masticatory f. The force applied by the mus-

cles attached to the mandible during mastication. (Comp. Prosth.; Remov. Part. Prosth.)

occlusal f. (occlusal load) The resultant of muscular forces applied on opposing teeth. (Comp. Prosth.; Remov. Part. Prosth.)

— The force transmitted to the teeth and their supporting structures by tooth-to-tooth contact or through a bolus of food or other interposed substance. (Periodont.)

f. and stress Pressure forcibly exerted on the teeth and on their investing and supporting tissues that is detrimental to tissue integrity. In occlusal trauma the production of lesions of the attachment apparatus depends on an interrelationship of the strength, duration, and frequency of the application of the force. (Periodont.)

forceps An instrument used for grasping or applying force to teeth, tissues, or other instruments.

— An instrument used for grasping and holding tissues or specific structures. (Oral Surg.)

— Objectionable term in restorative dentistry because of its association with the extraction of teeth. (Oper. Dent.)

bone f. Forceps used for grasping or cutting bone. (Oral Surg.)

chalazion f. A thumb forceps with a flattened plate at the end of one arm and a matching ring on the other. Originally used for isolation of eyelid tumors. It is useful for isolation of lip and cheek lesions (e.g., a mucocele) to facilitate removal. (Oral Surg.)

dental extracting f. Forceps used for grasping teeth. (Oral Surg.)

hemostatic f. An instrument for grasping blood vessels to control hemorrhage. (Oral Surg.)

insertion f. (see **forceps, point**)

lock f. (see **forceps, point**)

mosquito f. A small hemostatic forceps. (Oral Surg.)

point f. (lock f., insertion f.) A device used in filling root canals that securely holds the filling cones during their placement. (Endodont.)

rubber dam clamp f. (see **forceps; holder, rubber dam clamp**)

suture f. (see **needle holder**)

thumb f. Forceps used for grasping soft tissue; used especially during suturing. (Oral Surg.)

tissue f. A thumb forceps; an instrument with one or more fine teeth at the tip of each blade for controlling tissues during surgery, especially during suturing. (Oral Surg.)

Fordyce's spots, disease (see under appropriate noun)

foreign body (see **body, foreign**)

forensic dentistry (see **jurisprudence, dental**)

foreshortening (see **distortion, vertical**)

forging Working or shaping heated metal; hot-working a metal. (D. Mat.)

fork, face-bow The part of the face-bow assembly used to attach an occlusion rim or transfer record of maxillary teeth to the face-bow proper. (Comp. Prosth.; Remov. Part. Prosth.)

form The configuration, shape, or particular appearance of anything. (Oper. Dent.)

acquaintance f. A registration sheet for new patients on which data (e.g., the patient's name and address) are recorded and which contains a statement of the policies of the specific dentist's office and the responsibilities of the dentist to the patient. (Pract. Man.)

anatomic f. The natural shape of a part. (Oper. Dent.)

— The surface form of the edentulous ridge at rest or when it is not supporting a functional load. Also, the contour of the crown of a tooth. (Remov. Part. Prosth.)

arch f. The shape of the dental arch. (Comp. Prosth.; Orthodont.; Remov. Part. Prosth.)

— The shape of the residual ridge of an edentulous jaw as viewed from the occlusal plane. (Comp. Prosth.; Remov. Part. Prosth.) (see also **arch, dental**)

convenience f. The modifications necessary, beyond basic outline form, to facilitate proper instrumentation for the preparation of the cavity or insertion of the restorative material; also the placing of starting points or slight undercuts to retain the first portions of restorative material while succeeding portions are placed. (Oper. Dent.)

face f. The outline form of the face from an anterior frontal view. (Comp. Prosth.; Remov. Part. Prosth.)

f. and function The interdependent relationship that exists in all dental therapy in which proper function can be expected to follow proper form. Physiologically, form and function are related: proper form tends to make an organ function better, and function, in turn, will preserve the proper form of the organ. (Periodont.)

functional f. The shape that permits optimal performance. (Oper. Dent.)

message f. A checklist form, by means of which auxiliary personnel can quickly make a record of telephone communications for the dentist to persue later. (Pract. Man.)

occlusal f. The form of the occlusal surface of a tooth, a row of teeth, or dentition. (Comp.

Prosth.; Fixed Part. Prosth.; Remov. Part. Prosth.)

outline f. The shape of the area of the tooth surface included within the cavosurface margins of a prepared cavity of a restoration. (Oper. Dent.)

registration f. A form used to gather personal data about a patient other than professional information. (Pract. Man.)

resistance f. The shape given to a prepared cavity to enable the restoration *and remaining tooth structure* to withstand masticatory stress. (Oper. Dent.)

retention f. The provision made in a cavity preparation to prevent displacement of the restoration by lateral or tipping forces as well as masticatory stress. (Oper. Dent.)

root f. The shape of the root of the tooth; it is capable of being modified by such factors as resorption and cemental apposition. (Periodont.)

tooth f. The characteristics of the curves, lines, angles, and contours of various teeth that permit their identification and differentiation. (Comp. Prosth.; Fixed Part. Prosth.; Remov. Part. Prosth.)

anterior t. f. The outline form and other contours of an anterior tooth. (Comp. Prosth.; Fixed Part. Prosth.; Remov. Part. Prosth.)

posterior t. f. The distinguishing contours of the occlusal surface of the various posterior teeth. (Comp. Prosth.; Fixed Part. Prosth.; Remov. Part. Prosth.)

former, angle (see **angle former**)

former, crucible (see **sprue former**)

former, sprue (see **sprue former**)

fortified Containing additives more potent than the principal ingredient. (Oral Med.; Pharmacol.)

forward protrusion (see **protrusion, forward**)

Foshay's test (see **test, Foshay's**)

fossa (fahs'ah) A pit, hollow, or depression.

canine f. The concavity, or depression, in the maxilla superior to the apex of the canine tooth. (Periodont.)

depth of f. The extent or measurement of the fossa from the top of the shorter cusp downward into the bottom of the fossa. If all cusps were of equal length, the fossa depth would be the same as the cusp height. Since the cusps of lower bicuspids are so unequal in size and height, the depth of the fossa is determined by the height of the shorter cusp. (Gnathol.)

nasal f. (see **cavity, nasal**)

foundation A structure added to a remaining tooth structure to enhance stability and retention of a cast restoration placed over it. May be pin retained of amalgam, plastic cement, or a cast. (Oper. Dent.)

four-handed dentistry (see **dentistry, four-handed**)

Fournier's glossitis (foor-nē-āz′) (see **glossitis, interstitial sclerous**)

Fox scissors (see **scissors, Fox**)

Fox's knife (see **knife, Goldman-Fox**)

fracture A break or rupture of a part. In the oral region it is most frequently seen in teeth and bones. (Oral Diag.)
— A break of a hard object as opposed to a rupture, which applies to soft objects. (Oral Surg.)
— The action or fact of breaking or of being broken. (Remov. Part. Prosth.)

  avulsion f. Loss of a section of bone. (Oral Surg.)

  blow-out f. A fracture involving the orbital floor, its contents, and the superior wall of the maxillary antrum, in which orbital contents are incarcerated in the fracture area, producing diplopia. (Oral Surg.)

  cementum f. The tearing of fragments of the cementum from the tooth root at the cementodentinal junction, especially a fracture occurring in association with occlusal trauma. (Periodont.)

  clasp f. Failure of a clasp arm because of stresses that have exceeded the elastic limit of the metal from which the arm was made. (Remov. Part. Prosth.)

  closed reduction of f. Reduction and fixation of fractured bones without making a surgical opening to the fracture site. Intraoral maxillofacial and mandibular techniques and external skeletal fracture devices may be used. (Oral Surg.)

  comminuted f. A fracture in which the bone has several lines of fracture in the same region; a fracture in which the bone is crushed and splintered. (Oral Surg.)

  compound f. A fracture in which the bony structures are exposed to an external environment. May be extraoral, intraoral, intrasinal, or intranasal. (Oral Surg.)

  craniofacial dysjunction f. (transverse facial f.) A complex fracture in which the facial bones are separated from the cranial bones; a LeFort III fracture. (Oral Surg.)

  f. dislocation A fracture of a bone near an articulation, with dislocation of the condyloid process. (Oral Surg.)

  fissured f. A fracture that extends partially through a bone, with no displacement of the bony fragments. (Oral Surg.)

  greenstick f. A fracture in which the bone appears to be bent; usually only one cortex of the bone is broken. (Oral Surg.)

  Guérin's f. A LeFort I fracture of the facial bones in which there is a bilateral horizontal fracture of the maxillae. (Oral Surg.)

  impacted f. A fracture in which one fragment is driven into another portion of the same or an adjacent bone. (Oral Surg.)

  indirect f. A fracture at a point distant from the primary area of injury due to secondary forces. (Oral Surg.)

  intra-articular f. A fracture of the articular surface of the condyloid process of a bone. (Oral Surg.)

  intracapsular f. A fracture of the condyle of the mandible occurring within the confines of the capsule of the temporomandibular joint. (Oral Surg.)

  LeFort f. A transverse fracture involving the orbital, malar, and nasal bones. (Oral Diag.; Oral Surg.)

  midfacial f. Fractures of the zygomatic, maxillary, nasal, and associated bones. (Oral Surg.)

  pyramidal f. A fracture of the midfacial bones, with the principal fracture lines meeting at an apex in the area of the nasion; a LeFort II fracture. (Oral Surg.)

  root f. A microscopic or macroscopic cleavage of the root in any direction. (Endodont.; Periodont.)

  simple f. Linear fractures that are not in communication with the exterior. (Oral Surg.)

  transverse facial f. (see **fracture, craniofacial dysjunction**)

fragilitas ossium (frah-jĭl′ĭ-tās os′ē-ŭm) (see **osteogenesis imperfecta**)

frambesia (frăm-bē′zē-ah) (see **yaws**)

frame A structure, usually rigid, designed to give support or attachment to a part, or to immobilize a part.

  implant f. (see **substructure, implant**)

  occluding f. A device for relating casts to each other for the purpose of arranging teeth or for use in making an index of the occlusion of dentures; an articulator. (Comp. Prosth.; Remov. Part. Prosth.) (see also **articulator**)

  rubber dam f. (see **holder, rubber dam**)

framework The skeletal metal portion of a removable partial denture around which and to which the remaining units are attached. (Remov. Part. Prosth.)

Frankfort horizontal plane (see **plane, Frankfort horizontal**)

Frankfort-mandibular incisor angle (see **angle, Frankfort-mandibular incisor**)

fraud Intentional perversion of truth for the purpose of inducing another, in reliance on it, to part with something valuable belonging to him or to surrender a legal right; deliberate deception; deceit; trickery. (D. Juris.)

freckle (see **ephelis**)

free-end (see **base, extension**)

free gingiva (see **gingiva, free**)

free gingival margin (see **margin, gingival, free**)

free mandibular movement (see **movement, mandibular, free**)

free-way space (see **distance, interocclusal**)

Frei's test (frīz) (see **test, Frei's**)

fremitus (frĕm′ĭ-tŭs) Palpable vibrations of nonvascular origin that can be noted by placing the hand on the chest. (Oral Diag.) (see also **thrill**)

frenectomy (frē-nĕk′tō-mē) Excision of a frenum. (Oral Surg.; Orthodont.)
— Surgical detachment and/or excision of a frenum from its attachment into the mucoperiosteal covering of the alveolar processes. (Periodont.)

frenotomy (frē-not′ō-mē) The cutting of a frenum; especially the release of tongue-tie, or ankyloglossia. (Oral Surg.)

frenoplasty (frĕn″ō-plăs′tē) Correction of an abnormal frenum by repositioning it. (Oral Surg.)

frenulum (frĕn′ū-lŭm) (see **frenum**)

frenum (frē′nŭm) (frenulum) A fold of mucous membrane attaching the cheeks and lips to the mandibular and maxillary mucosa and limiting the motions of the lips and cheeks. (Oral Diag.; Orthodont.)
    abnormal f. (enlarged labial f.) A labial frenum appearing to be unusually heavy, broad, or attached too near the crest of the ridge. (Orthodont.)
    — A frenum that may be an etiologic factor in the production, perpetuation, and/or modification of lesions of the marginal gingivae. (Periodont.)
    buccal f. A fold or folds of mucous membrane connecting the residual alveolar ridge to the cheek in the bicuspid region. They exist in both the upper and lower jaws and separate the labial vestibule from the buccal vestibule. (Comp. Prosth.)
    — A band of tissue connecting the mucous membrane of the buccal mucosa with the gingival tissue. (Periodont.)
    labial f. The fold of mucous membrane connecting the lip of the residual alveolar ridge near the midline of both the upper and lower ridges. (Comp. Prosth.)
    — A band of tissue connecting the mucous membrane of the lip with the gingival tissue. (Periodont.)
    enlarged l. f. (see **frenum, abnormal**)
    lingual f. The vertical band of mucous membrane connecting the tongue with the floor of the mouth and the alveolar or residual alveolar ridge. (Comp. Prosth.; Periodont.)

frequency The number of cycles per second of a wave or other periodic phenomenon. (Cleft Palate)

Frey's syndrome (frīz) (see **syndrome, auriculotemporal**)

fricative (frĭk′ah-tĭv) Any speech sound made by forcing the airstream through such a narrow orifice or opening that audible high-frequency air currents or vibrations are set up. (Cleft Palate; Oral Physiol.)

Friedman splint (frēd′măn) (see **splint, cast bar**)

Friedman's test (frēd′mănz) (see **test, pregnancy**)

frit (frĭt) A partly or wholly fused porcelain that is plunged into water while hot. The mass cracks and fractures, and it is from this "frit" that dental porcelain powders are made. (D. Mat.)
— The semifused mass of porcelain before complete vitrification, fusion, or glazing. (Fixed Part. Prosth.)

Fröhlich's syndrome (frā′lĭks) (see **syndrome, Fröhlich's**)

fulcrum line (see **line, fulcrum**)

fulguration (ful-gū-rā′shŭn) Destruction of soft tissue by an electric spark that jumps the gap from an electrode to the tissue without the electrode's touching the tissue. (Oral Surg.) (see also **electrocoagulation**)

function The normal or special action of a part. As a noun, function has the following synonyms: role, capacity, task, use, purpose, service, activity, and direction. As a verb, function has the following synonyms: act, operate, work, perform, go, take effect, and serve. Use of the term function to express intended purpose may be misleading. (Gnathol.; Oper. Dent.)
— The activities, primary or auxiliary, that are performed by a part or organ and that contribute to the performance of the whole. (Remov. Part. Prosth.)
    auxiliary f. A function that is supplementary or additional to the function for which the

part or organ is primarily intended. (Remov. Part. Prosth.)

dental f., normal The correct action of opposing teeth in the process of mastication; sometimes referred to as normal occlusion. (Orthodont.)

form and f. (see **form and function**)

group f. The simultaneous contact of opposing teeth in a segment or a group. (Periodont.)

heavy f. (occlusal f.) An increase in functional activities of the tooth, which may result in compensatory changes in the attachment apparatus, e.g., a stronger periodontal ligament, with an increase in the number of fibers; a reinforcement of the supporting bone by formation of new bone; and the formation of cemental spikes, which are calcifications of the cemental fibers. Such changes take place so that the increased stress may be withstood wtihout damage. (Periodont.)

impaired f. Diminished, weakened, or less-than-optimal work or action. (Oper. Dent.)

insufficiency of f. Hypofunction of the tooth, which may lead to regressive changes in the attachment apparatus and supporting bone. The severity of lesions varies with the degree of hypofunction. (Periodont.) (see also **atrophy of disuse**)

muscle f. The action of muscle—principally contraction. A contracting muscle shortens, and it may pull a bone, a skeletal structure, or another muscle or organ to which it is attached. The contraction of muscle affects pumping of the blood, motility of the digestive tract, sphincter action, respiratory movements, and the posture and locomotion of the body. Ultimately the activities of the nervous system and the endocrine system are organized to externalize their combined function in the single phenomenon of muscle contractility and movement. Thus, all behavior that relates to the external environment of an organism is ultimately the result of neuromuscular function. (Oral Physiol.)

occlusal f. (see **function, heavy**)

physiologic f. The degree of activity that stimulates the physical structures but that is so limited as to stop short of irritation of those tissues. (Remov. Part. Prosth.)

skeletal f. The role of the skeleton in relation to the maintenance of body functions. The skeleton is a relatively inert organ system when viewed from a physiologic standpoint. The bony skeleton welds together and protects the softer vital visceral organs, supports

and maintains the body form, and accomplishes body movement for locomotion, respiration, manual skills, and the functions associated with mandibular motion. (Oral Physiol.)

subcortical f. Function controlled by all the structures of the brain except the outer cortical rim of the cerebrum. These structures—the thalamus, the basal ganglion, the hypothalamus, and the massive nerve tracts that pass between them—mediate most of the nonconscious activities of a sensory and motor nature. The basal ganglion plays an important part in the regulation of muscle tone and motor control. The thalamus is a large sensory impulse integrator. (Oral Physiol.)

substitution of sensory f. The taking over of one or more functions of a sensory apparatus by another sensory apparatus. The intimacy of relationships among the sensory projection systems in the cerebral cortex establishes a basis for learning experiences and for the organization of action and of adaptive behavior. This is also true, in part, for the general senses but is of great significance in relationships between special senses. Thus, under circumstances in which the vestibular apparatus or its related cerebellar mechanisms for maintaining balance are impaired, the patient must use his visual sense to maintain spatial position. Gradually, with experience, the visual system takes over the functional role of providing the cues for postural balance. This substitution is also observed when persons become blind and hearing acuity and perceptual organization become capable of assuming many of the visual properties associated with depth, distance, and other spatial factors. Hence, in the blind, hearing is developed as though it were a radarlike mechanism to be used for localization and to determine the proximity of the identifiable environment. (Oral Physiol.)

functional Pertaining to the movements and actions of a part. (Oral Surg.)

— Of or pertaining to the functions of an organ, part, or prosthesis. (Remov. Part. Prosth.)

fungate (fŭn′gāt) To produce funguslike growths; to grow rapidly like a fungus. (Oral Path.)

fungus (fŭn′gŭs) A class of vegetable organisms of a low order of. development, including mushrooms, toadstools, and molds. Many are saprophytic and/or pathogenic for man, e.g., *Candida albicans, Histoplasma, Trichophyton, Actinomyces,* and *Blastomyces.* Oral and systemic moniliasis (thrush) is produced by overgrowth of *Candida albicans,* which is a saprophytic resident in the oral cavity. When physiologic processes are sufficiently impaired, the organism may gain a foothold and assume a pathogenic role. (Periodont.)

furcation (fer-kā′shŭn) All divisions of the root portion of a tooth. (Oper. Dent.)

   root f. The interradicular denudation that may occur in multirooted teeth due to periodontal disease. (Periodont.)

furnace An apparatus in which to generate heat. (Oper. Dent.)

   inlay f. A furnace used for eliminating the wax from an inlay mold and establishing the proper condition and temperature of the investment to receive the molten casting gold. (Oper. Dent.)

   porcelain f. A furnace used for fusing, firing, or glazing dental porcelain for inlays, crowns, and pontics. (Oper. Dent.)

fusion The uniting or joining together of two or more entities. The fusion temperature of an alloy lies just below the lower limit of its melting range, which is particularly important in soldering operations because temperatures near or above fusion temperature will decrease ductility. (D. Mat.) (see also **concrescence; range, melting**)

— The process of producing fused teeth. (Oral Diag.)

   f. of metal (see **metal, fusion of**)

   nuclear f. The union of atomic nuclei to form heavier nuclei, resulting in the release of enormous quantities of energy when certain light elements unite (as in the combining of heavy-hydrogen nuclei to form helium nuclei, which takes place in the activity of the sun or in the explosion of a hydrogen bomb). (Oral Radiol.)

Fusobacterium fusiforme (fū″zō-băk-tē′rē-ŭm) **(Vincent's bacillus)** A microorganism that, along with *Borrelia vincentii,* is implicated in the causation of necrotizing ulcerative gingivitis. Although both *Fusobacterium fusiforme* and *Borrelia vincentii* are inhabitants of the oral cavity, they may become pathogenic when tissue resistance is impaired. (Periodont.)

Fusobacterium nucleatum A genus of schizomycetes, an anaerobic gram-negative bacterium often seen in necrotic tissue and implicated, but not conclusively, with other organisms in the causation and perpetuation of periodontal disease. (Periodont.)

❧ G ❧

g (see **gram**)

gag A surgical device for holding the mouth open. (Anesth.)

gagging An involuntary retching reflex that may be stimulated by something touching the posterior palate or throat region. (Comp. Prosth.; Remov. Part. Prosth.)

gait Manner of walking; a cyclic loss and regaining of balance by a shift of the line of gravity in relationship to the center of gravity. A person's gait is as characteristic and as individual as his fingerprints. (Oral Med.; Oral Physiol.)

cerebellar g. An unsteady, irregular gait characterized by short steps and a lurching from one side to the other; most commonly seen in multiple sclerosis or other cerebellar diseases. (Oral Med.)

festinating g. A gait characterized by rigidity, shuffling, and involuntary hastening. The upper part of the body advances ahead of the lower part. It is associated with paralysis agitans and postencephalitic Parkinson's syndrome. (Oral Med.)

sensor ataxic g. An irregular, uncertain, stamping gait. The legs are kept far apart, and either the ground or the feet are watched, since there has been a loss of knowledge of the position of the lower limbs. This gait is caused by an interruption of the afferent nerve fibers and may be associated with tabes dorsalis and sometimes with multiple sclerosis and other lesions of the nervous system. (Oral Med.)

spastic g. (creeping palsy) A slow, scuffing gait in which the patient appears to be wading in water. There is restricted movement at the knee and hip. This gait may be associated with multiple sclerosis, syphilis, combined systemic disease, or other diseases affecting the spinal pyramidal tracts. (Oral Med.)

staggering g. A reeling, tottering, and tipping gait in which the individual appears as if he may fall backward or lose his balance. It is associated with alcoholic and barbiturate intoxication. (Oral Med.)

waddling g. Exaggerated alteration of lateral trunk movements, with an exaggerated elevation of the hip, suggesting the gait of a duck; characteristic of progressive muscular dystrophy. (Oral Med.)

galactin (gah-lăk'tĭn) (see **hormone, lactogenic**)

galvanic current (see **current, galvanic**)

galvanism The electric current generated between two metals of different electromotive potential in the presence of an electrolyte. With saliva as the electrolyte, adjacent restorations of different metals may generate an electric current that will stimulate the pulp and injure the mucosa. This usually occurs only when a fresh amalgam comes in contact with gold. (Oral Diag.)

galvanotherapy (see **ionization**)

gamma A microgram; the millionth part of a gram. (Oral Med.; Pharmacol.)

ganglion(ia) (găng'glē-on) Any collection or mass of nerve cells that serves as a center of nervous influence. (Anesth.)

basal g. A group of forebrain nuclei that, with the related structures of brain, play an important role in the regulation of muscle tone and motor control. The cell groups of these ganglia and their respective nerve tracts are classified as the extrapyramidal motor system to differentiate them from the pyramidal motor system, which goes directly from the cerebral cortex to the lower motor neuron. Disease associated with the basal ganglia is manifested by three principal motor abnormalities: disturbance of muscle tone, derangement of movement, and loss of associated or automatic movement. (Oral Physiol.)

ciliary g. A parasympathetic nerve ganglion in the posterior part of the orbit. It receives preganglionic fibers from the region of the oculomotor nucleus and sends postganglionic fibers via short ciliary nerves to (1) the constrictor muscle of the iris (constriction of pupil) and (2) circular fibers of the ciliary muscle (accommodation for vision). (Oral Physiol.)

otic g. A ganglion located medial to the mandibular nerve just below the foramen ovale in the infratemporal fossa. It supplies the sensory and secretory fibers for the parotid gland. Its sensory fibers arise from the facial and glossopharyngeal nerves. (Oral Physiol.)

sphenopalatine g. One of the four ganglia of the autonomic nervous system associated with the head and neck region. It is located deep in the pterygopalatine fossa and is intimately associated with the maxillary nerve. It lies distal and medial to the maxillary tuberosity. Its fibers supply the mucous membrane of the roof of the pharynx, the tonsils, the soft and hard palates, and the nasal cavity. The mucous and serous secretions of all the mucous membranes in the oropharynx are also mediated by this ganglion. (Oral Physiol.)

submaxillary g. A ganglion located on the medial side of the mandible between the lingual nerve and the submaxillary duct. It is distributed to the sublingual and submaxillary glands. The sensory fibers arise from the lingual branch of the trigeminal nerve, i.e., the chorda tympani of the facial nerve. (Oral Physiol.)

ganglionitis, acute posterior (găng″glē-ō-nī′tĭs) (see **herpes zoster**)

gangrene Death of tissue en masse; e.g., gangrene of the pulp is total death and necrosis of the pulp. (Oral Diag.)

gap, interocclusal (see **distance, interocclusal**)

gap arthroplasty Surgical correction of ankylosis by creation of a space between the ankylosed part and the portion in which movement is desired. (Oral Surg.)

gargoylism (see **syndrome, Hurler's**)

GAS (see **syndrome, general adaptation**)

gas Any elastic aeriform fluid in which the molecules are separated from one another and thus have free paths. (Anesth.)

laughing g. (see **nitrous oxide**)

noble g. A gas that will not oxidize; the inert gases; e.g., helium or neon. (D. Mat.)

olefiant g. (see **ethylene**)

suffocating g. A gas employed in warfare that causes intense irritation of the bronchial tubes and lungs, resulting in pulmonary edema; among gases so employed are phosgene and diphosgene-oxychlorcarbon. (Anesth.)

gasometer (găs-ahm′ĕ-ter) A calibrated instrument or vessel for measuring the volume of gases. Used in clinical and physiologic investigation for measuring respiratory volume. (Anesth.)

Gaucher's cell, disease (gō-shāz′) (see under appropriate nouns)

gauge An instrument used to determine the dimensions or caliber of an object. (Anesth.)

Boley g. A vernier type of instrument used for measuring in the metric system. It is accurate to tenths of millimeters. (Oper. Dent.)

undercut g. An attachment used in conjunction with a dental cast surveyor to measure the amount of infrabulge of a tooth in a horizontal plane. (Remov. Part. Prosth.)

gel (jĕl) A colloid in solid form, jellylike in character. Hydrocolloid impression materials are examples of gels. A gel has a brush-heap structure—the fibril-forming spaces, or micelles—that hold water. (D. Mat.)

g. strength (see **strength, gel**)

g. time (see **time, gel**)

gelation time (jĕ-lā′shŭn) (see **time, gel**)

gemination (jĕm″ĭ-nā′shŭn) Division of a tooth bud that results in the formation of double, or twin, crowns on a single root with a single pulp canal. (Oral Path.)

gene One of a paired unit of inheritance arranged linearly along chromosomes. (Oral Med.)

— Fundamental unit of inheritance located in the chromosome. It determines and controls hereditarily transmissible characteristics. (Oral Radiol.)

g. locus (see **locus, gene**)

sex-linked g. A gene located on a sex chromosome. (Oral Med.)

generated path (**chew-in**) A track made by repeated use by man or animals. The paths are generated without thought but by use. In creating occlusal paths of opposite protuberances, the patient is asked to move the mandible side to side horizontally and fore and aft. These movements will generate the paths in which the peaks, ridges, or crests of teeth will run and thus keep in contact with the wax. (Gnathol.)

g. occlusal p. (see **path, occlusal, generated**)

generator A device that converts mechanical energy into electrical energy. (Oral Radiol.)

x-ray g. A device that converts electrical energy into electromagnetic energy (photons). (Oral Radiol.)

genetic effects of radiation (jĕ-nĕt′ĭk) Those changes produced in the individual's genes and chromosomes of all nucleated body cells, both somatic and gonadal. The more common meaning relates to the effect produced in the reproductive cells. It is believed that any amount of radiation received by the gonads before the end of the reproductive period is likely to add to the number of undesirable genes present in the population. Such mutated genes may have no recognizable effect for a number of generations, but potentially, practically all will eventually result in untoward changes in the form of spontaneous genetic abnormalities. (Oral Radiol.)

genetics The science that deals with the origin

of the characteristics of an individual. (Orthodont.)

genial tubercle (see **tubercle, genial**)

genioplasty (jē′nē-ō-plăs″tē) A surgical procedure, performed either intraorally or extraorally, to correct deformities of the mandibular symphysis. (Oral Surg.)

genotype (jē′nō-tīp) The aggregate of ordered genes received by offspring from both parents; e.g., a person with blood group AB is of genotype AB. (Oral Med.)

gentian violet (jĕn′shŭn) (see **violet, gentian**)

geographic tongue (see **tongue, geographic**)

geometric unsharpness Impairment of image definition due to the geometric penumbra. (Oral Radiol.) (see also **penumbra, geometric; x-ray beam**)

geometry of x-ray beam The effect of various factors on the spatial distribution of radiation emerging from an x-ray generator or source. (Oral Radiol.) (see also **law, inverse-square; penumbra, geometric** and subentries; **x-ray beam** and subentries)

geriatrics (jĕr″ē-ăt′rĭks) The department of medicine or dentistry that treats all problems peculiar to advanced age and the aging, including the clinical problems of senescence and senility. (Comp. Prosth.; Remov. Part. Prosth.)

dental g. The part of dentistry that deals with the dental problems of patients of advanced age. (Comp. Prosth.; Remov. Part. Prosth.)

germicide A substance capable of killing a wide variety of microorganisms. More specifically, one capable of killing all microorganisms, except for spores, with which it is in contact for a standard period of time. (Oral Med.; Pharmacol.)

gerodontics (jĕr″ō-dahn′tĭks) **(gerodontology)** The branch of dentistry that deals with the diagnosis and treatment of the dental conditions of aging and aged persons. (Comp. Prosth.; Remov. Part. Prosth.)

gerodontology (jĕr″ō-dahn-tol′ō-jē) (see **gerodontics**)

giant follicular lymphoblastoma (see **lymphoblastoma, giant follicular**)

giantism (macrosomia) Marked overgrowth involving a single tooth or, as in hyperpituitarism, the entire body. (Oral Diag.)

— Excessive growth resulting in a stature larger than the range of normal for age and race. (Oral Med.)

infantile g. Excessive growth occurring before adolescence. (Oral Med.)

primary g. Excessive growth not attributable to a definite cause. (Oral Med.)

secondary g. Excessive growth secondary to a disorder of the adrenal, pineal, gonadal, or pituitary gland. (Oral Med.)

gift A transfer of personal property, made voluntarily and without consideration or qualification. (D. Juris.)

Gigli's wire saw (jēl′yēz) (see **saw, Gigli's wire**)

Gillies' operation (see **operation, Gillies'**)

Gillmore needle (see **needle, Gillmore**)

Gilson fixable-removable bar (see **connector, cross arch bar splint**)

gingiva(e) (jĭn′jĭ-vah) The fibrous tissue covered by mucous membrane that immediately surrounds a tooth and is continuous with its pericemental ligament (periodontal ligament). (Comp. Prosth.; Oper. Dent.; Orthodont.; Remov. Part. Prosth.)

— The mucous membrane that covers the alveolar processes of the maxillae and mandible and surrounds the necks of the teeth. (Periodont.)

g., abrasion The attrition (scraping or wearing away) of the gingival tissue by harsh irritants such as coarse foods or faulty toothbrushing. Atrophic or inflammatory changes may occur. (Periodont.)

g., anatomy The covering of the alveolar processes and the marginal parts of the teeth. It is characterized as either free or attached gingiva, the line of division between the two being an imaginary line between the bottom of the gingival sulcus and the gingival groove. The margin of the gingiva describes a wavy course around the four surfaces of the tooth, with the interproximal surfaces constituting the part of the gingiva nearest the occlusal surface of the teeth. (Periodont.)

g., architecture The structural arrangement of the various tissue components of the gingivae, consisting of a corium of connective tissue covered by stratified squamous epithelium. (Periodont.)

attached g. The portion of the gingivae extending from the free gingival groove, which demarcates it from the free or marginal gingivae, to the mucogingival junction, which separates it from the alveolar mucosa. This tissue is firm, dense, stippled, and tightly bound down to the underlying periosteum, tooth, and bone. (Periodont.)

a. g. extension (see **extension, gingiva, attached**)

g., blanching Lightening of gingival color due to stretching and diminution of blood supply; usually of a temporary nature. (Periodont.)

g., bleeding The flowing of blood from the marginal gingival area (particularly the sulcus), seen in such conditions as gingivitis, marginal periodontitis, injury, and ascorbic acid deficiency. Bleeding may be spontaneous or may result from the mild stimuli of a toothbrush, coarse food, etc. (Periodont.)

— A prominent symptom of periodontal disease produced by ulceration of the sulcular epithelium and an inflammatory process. (Periodont.)

blood supply to g. The vascular supply to the gingival mucous membrane. It arises from the vessels that pass on the gingival side of the outer periosteum of bone and anastomoses with blood vessels of the periodontal membrane and intra-alveolar blood vessels. (Periodont.)

cleft g. (see **cleft, gingival**)

g., color The color of the gingival tissues in health and in disease. It varies with the thickness and degree of keratinization of the epithelium, the blood supply, the pigmentation, and the alterations produced by diseased processes affecting the gingival tissues. In health, often described as coral pink. (Periodont.)

connective tissue of g. The binding and supportive element of the gingival tissue, lying subjacent to the epithelium. Healthy connective tissue is composed of an orderly arrangement of gingival fibers that attach the gingivae to the tooth structure, indifferent fibers, fibroblasts, blood and lymphatic vessels, nerve fibers, etc. The derangements produced in disease consist of structural alterations of the fiber apparatus of the gingivae, variations in size and number of blood vessels, and changes in both cellular arrangement and type. (Periodont.)

consistency of g. Visual and tactile characteristics of healthy gingival tissue. Visual consistency varies from a smooth velvet to an orange peel, either finely or coarsely grained. The tactile consistency of the gingival tissue should be firm and resilient. (Periodont.)

g., deformity (see **deformity, gingival**)

g., discoloration A change from the normal coloration of the gingivae; associated with inflammation, diminution of blood supply, abnormal pigmentation, etc. (Periodont.)

elephantiasis g. (see **fibromatosis gingivae**)

g., epithelial architecture The epithelial covering of gingivae, which consists of stratified squamous epithelium that possesses some degree of keratinization, and papillary projections into the connective tissue. In health the sulcular epithelium does not extend in rete pegs into the underlying corium. (Periodont.)

free g. The unattached coronal portion of the gingiva that encircles the tooth to form the gingival sulcus. (Periodont.)

g., hereditary enlargement Overgrowth of the gingivae as a result of some inherited tendency. (Oral Diag.)

g., hormonal enlargement Enlargement of the gingivae associated with hormonal imbalance during pregnancy. (Oral Diag.)

g. hyperplasia (see **hyperplasia, gingival, Dilantin**)

interdental g. (interproximal g.; interdental ligament) The soft supporting tissue, consisting of prominent horizontal collagen fibers, that normally fills the space between two contacting teeth. (Oper. Dent.; Periodont.)

interproximal g. (see **gingiva, interdental**)

lymphatic drainage of g. Lymphatic drainage that follows the course of the gingival blood supply, i.e., from the lymphatic vessels on the gingival side of the periosteum of the alveolar process to the lymphatic vessels in the periodontal membrane to vessels leading into the alveolar bone. (Periodont.)

marginal g. The part of the free gingiva that is localized at the labial, buccal, lingual, and palatal aspects of the teeth. (Periodont.)

microscopic appearance of g. Stratified squamous epithelium that varies in degree of keratinization and overlies a corium of connective tissue with interspersed blood vessels and nerves. Rete pegs of epithelium project downward into the connective tissue corium, except from the base of sulcular epithelium. The gingival fiber apparatus is readily discerned. (Periodont.)

normal g. Gingival tissues free of disease and of structural and topographic alterations. (Periodont.)

g., physiology The function of the gingival tissues. The gingivae encircle the teeth and serve as a mucosal covering for the underlying tissues; the gingival fiber apparatus serves as a barrier to apical migration of the epithelial attachment and serves to bind the gingival tissues to the teeth, thus contributing to tooth support. The normal topographic attributes of the gingivae permit the free flow of food away from the occlusal surfaces and from the cervical and interproximal areas of the teeth, promoting the self-cleansing ability of the tissues and providing protection to the gingivae and to the underlying tissues. (Periodont.)

g., pigmentation The deposition of coloring matter in the gingival tissue. Variations in gingival color may be correlated with the complexion of the individual (as in the Negro and in persons of Mediterranean origin) or may be a reflection of pathologic influences, as in the melanin pigmentation associated with hypoadrenocorticism (Addison's disease). Gingival pigmentation may be due to physiologic or pathologic factors. The physiologic factors include the melanin pigmentation of dark-complexioned individuals. The pathologic pigmentations result from nevi, depositions of heavy metals (e.g., lead and bismuth within areas of marginal inflammation), foreign bodies (amalgam), and systemic disorders (e.g., Addison's disease and Peutz-Jeghers syndrome). (Periodont.)

g., retraction (see **retraction, gingival**)

self-cleansing g. The topographic attributes of the gingival tissues that are conducive to the smooth and unimpeded passage of food over the surface of the tissues. These attributes include a thin gingival margin, interdental tissue sluiceways, semilunar mesiodistal curvature to the gingival margin, etc. (Periodont.)

g., shrinkage The lessening in size of gingival tissue, principally in the following circumstances: (1) the diminution of gingival enlargement to a more physiologic form by removal of the local irritant, control of contributing systemic etiologic factors (if present), surgical curetment of the edematous and hyperplastic tissues, and/or adequate home oral physiotherapy; (2) the elimination of a gingival or periodontal pocket by the therapeutic removal of accretions from the tooth surfaces and/or the degenerated and irreversibly diseased tissues lining the pocket; (3) the reduction of a gingival or periodontal pocket by diminution of edema, usually as a result of therapeutic elimination of subgingival deposits and curetment of the soft tissue wall of the pocket. (Periodont.)

g., stippling A series of small depressions or a network of low ridges characterizing the surface of the gingivae, varying in consistency from a smooth velvet to that of an orange peel, either finely or coarsely grained. (Periodont.)

g., surface texture The texture of the attached gingivae, which normally consists of a stippled surface and ranges from smooth velvet to a distinct orange peel. In gingival inflammatory conditions, the gingival fiber apparatus is destroyed; with the edema, cellular infiltration, and concomitant swelling, the surface stippling is lost and the gingiva takes on a smooth, shiny edematous appearance. In later states of inflammatory gingival involvement in which fibrosis has occurred, stippling returns. (Periodont.)

g., topography The form of the healthy gingival tissues. The marginal gingivae and the interdental papillae have a characteristic shape. (Periodont.)

transitional g. The gingiva adjacent to a residual ridge; with a modified form as related to its tooth. (Fixed Part. Prosth.)

gingival Pertaining to or in relation to the gingiva. (Oper. Dent.)

g. crater A concave depression in the gingival tissue. Especially seen in area of former apex of the interdental papilla as a result of the gingival destruction associated with necrotizing ulcerative gingivitis, or when food impaction occurs against the tissue subjacent to the contact points of adjacent teeth. (Periodont.)

　interdental g. c. A bony crater occurring at the crest of the interdental alveolar septum. (Periodont.) (see also **bony crater**)
　— A saucer-shaped depression in the interproximal gingival papilla. (Periodont.)

g. defense mechanisms Multifactional system that attempts to maintain gingival health and defense against exogenous attack; consists of structural mechanisms as well as mechanical, chemical, and cellular mechanisms. (Periodont.)

g. mat The gingival connective tissue composed of coarse, broad collagen fibers that serve to attach the gingivae to the teeth and to hold the free gingivae in close approximation to the teeth. (Periodont.)

g. position The level of the gingival margin in relation to the tooth. (Periodont.)

subg. At a level apical to the gingival extent of the preparation or restoration. (Oper. Dent.)

g. sulcus (preferred to gingival crevice) (see **sulcus**)

g. third Relating to the most apical one third

of a given clinical crown or of an axial surface cavity or preparation. (Oper. Dent.)

gingivectomy (jĭn″jĭ-věk′tō-mē) Surgical excision of unsupported gingival tissue to the level where it is attached, creating a new gingival margin apical in position to the old. An integral phase of gingivectomy is the concurrent surgical production of physiologic architectural form in the gingival tissues. A procedure designed to eliminate a gingival or periodontal pocket by removing its soft tissue mass and to provide an approach operation for more extensive surgical procedures. (Periodont.)

g. in edentulous area Elimination of periodontal pockets surrounding abutment teeth; requires the removal of gingival tissue on the adjacent edentulous area. (Periodont.)

gingivitis (jĭn″jĭ-vī′tĭs) Any inflammation of the gingival tissue. (Oral Diag.; Oral Path.; Periodont.)

— An inflamed condition of the gingiva; e.g., that is caused by pressure contact of a partial denture unit. (Remov. Part. Prosth.)

bacteria in g. The causative organisms in gingival inflammation. The common chronic forms of gingivitis, from a bacterial standpoint, are nonspecific, with the exception of acute necrotizing ulcerative gingivitis, in which there is an apparent specificity of the bacterial flora: the fusospirochetal organisms. (Periodont.)

bismuth g. Metallic poisoning caused by bismuth given for treatment of systemic disease; characterized by a dark, bluish line along the gingival margin. (Oral Diag.)

catarrhal g. (catarrhal stomatitis) A transitory inflammation of the gingival and/or oral mucous membranes accompanied by erythema, swelling, and occasional epithelial desquamation; usually a result of the change in the oral bacterial flora. (Periodont.)

chronic atrophic senile g. Gingival inflammation characterized by atrophy and areas of hyperkeratosis; found primarily in elderly women. (Oral Diag.)

desquamative g. An inflammation of the gingivae characterized by the tendency of the surface epithelium to desquamate. The disease is a clinical entity, not a pathologic entity. It is most frequently associated with the menopause but may be associated with any biologic stress. (Oral Diag.)

chronic d. g. The form of gingivitis accompanied by separation of epithelium from the underlying connective tissue, leaving a burning, raw, bleeding surface. Includes

gingivosis, a desquamative condition correctable by systemic therapy with nicotinamide and pyridoxine. Gingivosis is the desquamative gingivitis associated with either artificial or natural menopause, resulting from loss of estrogenic stimulation to mucous membranes. It may be a form of lichen planus. (Periodont.)

eruptive g. (ē-rŭp′tĭv) Gingival inflammation occurring at the time of eruption, particularly of the permanent teeth. It is associated with the lack of deflecting contours of the erupting crown, resultant food impaction, and accumulation of debris. (Periodont.)

faulty fillings in g. Faulty restorations which, by virtue of their irritant action and by serving as a nidus of food accumulation, are etiologic factors in the initiation and perpetuation of gingival disease. (Periodont.)

fusospirochetal g. (see **gingivitis, necrotizing ulcerative**)

g. gravidarum (see **gingivitis, pregnancy**)

hemorrhagic g. Gingivitis characterized by profuse bleeding, especially that associated with ascorbic acid deficiency. (Periodont.)

herpetic g. Inflammation of the gingivae caused by herpesvirus. (Periodont.) (see also **gingivostomatitis, herpetic**)

hormonal g. Gingivitis associated with endocrine imbalance, the endocrinopathy being modified, in most instances, by the influence of local environmental factors. (Periodont.)

hyperplastic g. Gingivitis characterized by proliferation of the various tissue elements, epithelium, and connective tissue. Rarely it is accompanied by dense infiltration of inflammatory cells. (Periodont.)

idiopathic g. Gingival inflammation of unknown causation. (Periodont.)

inflammatory cells in g. The types of cells present in inflammation of gingival tissue. Since the gingival inflammatory process is usually chronic and progressive in nature, the inflammatory cells are, for the most part, lymphocytes, plasma cells, and some histiocytes. With acute exacerbations, polymorphonuclear leukocytes are also present. (Periodont.)

g. and malposed teeth The role of the malposition of teeth in gingivitis in the dental arches. Malposition may predispose the gingivae to inflammation by permitting food impaction or impingement on the tissues, by providing irregular spaces in which calculus may be deposited, etc. (Periodont.)

marginal g. Inflammation of the gingivae limited to its margins. (Oral Diag.)

— Inflammation of the gingivae localized to the marginal gingivae and interdental papillae. (Periodont.)

necrotizing ulcerative g. (fusospirochetal g., NUG, trench mouth, ulcerative g., ulceromembranous g., Vincent's g., Vincent's infection) An inflammation of the gingivae characterized by necrosis of the interdental papillae, ulceration of the gingival margins, the appearance of a pseudomembrane, pain, and a fetid odor. (Oral Diag.)

— A clinically recognizable syndrome characterized by painful, hyperemic gingivae, absence of interdental papillae, ulceration of gingivae with pseudomembrane formation, and fetid mouth odor. The condition is not histologically specific. (Oral Path.)

— An acute, sometimes chronic, gingivitis characterized by ragged, iregular ulceration of the gingival margin and interdental papillae, progressive necrosis of the epithelium and/or gingival corium, an intense erythema of the gingival tissues, a fetid taste and odor, thick and ropy saliva, pain, etc. May also prevail as a form of stomatitis, pharyngitis, etc. Etiologic factors associated with this disease are emotional stress, debilitating illnesses, poor nutritional status, and the fusospirochetal organisms. (Periodont.)

epithelial changes in n. u. g. The characteristic changes in the marginal epithelium in necrotizing ulcerative gingivitis, which are ulceration, necrosis, and sloughing. Fusospirochetal organisms can be demonstrated both on and within the epithelium in histologic preparations. (Periodont.)

inflammatory cells in n. u. g. Prevalent cellular infiltrate in necrotizing ulcerative gingivitis, including polymorphonuclear leukoctyes, plasma cells, and lymphocytes. In the acute phase polymorphonuclear leukocytes predominate. (Periodont.)

nephritic g. (uremic g., uremic stomatitis) A membrane form of stomatitis and gingivitis associated with a failure of kidney function. It is accompanied by pain, ammoniacal odor, and increased salivation. (Periodont.)

pregnancy g. (g. gravidarum, hormonal g.) Enlargement or hyperplasia of the gingivae due to hormonal imbalance during pregnancy. (Oral Diag.; Oral Path.)

puberty g. An enlargement of the gingival tissues confined to the anterior segment and perhaps present in only one arch. The lingual tissue generally remains unaffected. (Pedodont.)

scorbutic g. Gingivitis associated with vitamin C (ascorbic acid) deficiency. (Periodont.)

streptococcal g. Inflammation of the gingivae caused by streptococci. (Oral Diag.)

ulcerative g. (see **gingivitis, necrotizing ulcerative**)

ulceromembranous g. (see **gingivitis, necrotizing ulcerative**)

uremic g. (see **gingivitis, nephritic**)

Vincent's g. (see **gingivitis, necrotizing ulcerative**)

gingivoplasty (jĭn"jĭ-vō-plăs'tē) The surgical contouring of the gingival tissues to secure the physiologic architectural form necessary for the maintenance of tissue health and integrity. (Periodont.)

gingivosis (jĭn"jĭ-vō'sĭs) A noninflammatory degenerative condition of the gingivae. The term is applied to desquamative gingivitis. (Oral Diag.; Oral Path.)

— An unusual, severe type of gingival disease seen in malnourished and chronically ill persons. The disease possesses three stages: low-grade edema of the interdental papillae progressing to marginal and attached gingivae; profuse and spontaneous bleeding of the gingivae, terminating in necrosis of the affected gingivae; and a chronic stage characterized by necrosis of gingivae with recession and denudation of roots. (Periodont.)

gingivostomatitis (jĭn"jĭ-vō-stō"mah-tī'tĭs) An inflammation that involves the gingivae and the oral mucosa. (Periodont.)

herpetic g. An inflammation of the gingivae and oral mucosa caused by primary invasion of herpesvirus. It occurs chiefly in childhood, one attack giving immunity to generalized stomatitis but not to isolated lesions (herpetic lesions). The gingivae are red and swollen, the mucosa is red and soon shows vesicles and ulcers, the mouth is painful, and the temperature is elevated. The course is about 14 days. (Oral Diag.)

— Infection of the gingivae and oral mucosa by herpesvirus; usually occurs in children. (Oral Path.)

— An acute viral infection of the oral mucosa due to herpes simplex virus; characterized by diffuse erythema, vesiculation, and ulceration of the mucosa. This painful disease lasts 10 to 14 days, is seen most commonly in children and adolescents, and terminates when effective antibody titer exists in the body to combat herpesvirus. (Periodont.)

acute h. g. (see **stomatitis, herpetic, acute**)

membranous g. A disease, or group of diseases, in which false membranes form on the gingivae and oral mucosa; the membranes have a grayish white coloration and are surrounded by a narrow red margin. Detachment of the membrane leaves a raw, bleeding surface. One cause is mixed pyogenic infection in which *Streptococcus viridans* and staphylococci predominate. (Periodont.)

white folded g. (see **nevus spongiosus albus mucosa**)

ginglymus (jĭng′glĭ-mŭs) (**hinge joint**) A joint that allows motion around an axis. (Comp. Prosth.; Remov. Part. Prosth.)

glabella (glah-bĕl′ah) The most anterior point on the frontal bone. (Orthodont.)

gland(s) An organ producing a specific product or secretion. (Oral Physiol.)

Blandin and Nuhn's g. Minor anterior lingual salivary glands, partly serous and partly mucous. The duct of each gland opens on the inferior surface of the tongue. (Oral Path.)

ectopic sebaceous g. (see **spots, Fordyce's**)

endocrine g. Any one of the glands of internal secretion; a hormone-secreting gland; e.g., the pituitary gland, thyroid gland, parathyroid glands, adrenal glands, ovaries, and testes. (Periodont.)

pituitary g. (hypophysis) An endocrine gland located at the base of the brain in the sella turcica. It is composed of two parts: the pars nervosa, which is an extension of the anterior part of the hypothalamus, and the pars intermedia, which is an epithelial evagination of secretory tissue from the stomodeum of the embryo. By its structural and functional relationships with the nervous system and with the endocrine glands, it acts as a mediator of both the nervous system and the endocrine system. (Oral Physiol.)

salivary g. Glands in the mouth that secrete saliva. Three major groups of salivary glands contribute their secretions to form the whole saliva; accessory mucous glands found within oral mucosa contribute also in small part. The prime glands are the parotid, submaxillary, and sublingual. (Periodont.)

accessory s. g. Glands located at the posterior aspect of the dorsum of the tongue behind the vallate papillae and along the margins of the tongue; also located in the pal-ate, labial mucosa, and buccal mucosa. The secretion is mucous. (Periodont.)

parotid s. g. The largest of the salivary glands; situated between the ramus of the mandible in front, the mastoid process and sternocleidomastoideus behind, and the zygomatic arch above; irregularly wedge shaped, with the lateral surface flattened and the medial aspect more or less pointed toward the pharyngeal wall. Its secretion, which is serous, traverses Stensen's duct to empty into the mouth at the ductal orifice on the buccal mucosa opposite the upper molar teeth. (Periodont.)

sublingual s. g. The smallest of the principal salivary glands. It lies below the mucous membranes of the floor of the mouth at the sides of the lingual frenum and is in contact with the sublingual depression on the inner side of the mandible. Its numerous ducts open directly into the mouth on the sides of the lingual frenum and/or join to form the duct of Bartholin (sublingual duct), which enters into the submaxillary duct (Wharton's duct). Its secretion is mucous in nature. (Periodont.)

submaxillary s. g. A gland that has an irregular form and is situated in the submaxillary triangle, bordered anteriorly by the anterior belly of the digastricus and posteriorly by the stylomandibular ligament. Its mucoserous section is carried by Wharton's duct, whose orifice lies at the summit of a small papilla (submaxillary caruncle) at the side of the lingual frenum. (Periodont.)

glass, lead Lead-impregnated glass used in windows of control booths and in protective shields to protect radiologists and their assistants from primary and scattered radiation. (Oral Radiol.)

glaze Ceramic veneer in dentistry, usually a transparent glass; applied to porcelain to provide a glossy and impermeable surface. (D. Mat.)

— A critical stage in the final firing of dental porcelain when complete fusion takes place, with the formation of a thin, vitreous, glossy surface (glaze). (Fixed Part. Prosth.)

glenoid The fossae in the temporal bone in which condyles of the mandible articulate with the skull. (Orthodont.)

glide(s) The passage of one object over another as guided by their contracting surfaces.

— The sounds "w" and "wh" and the sound

"y," which are voiced as bilabial and palatal glides, respectively. The rapid movement of the lips or tongue from a set position toward a neutral vowel ("u," as in up). (Cleft Palate)

mandibular g. Side-to-side, protrusive, and intermediate movement of the mandible, occurring when the teeth or other occluding surfaces are in contact. (Comp. Prosth.; Remov. Part. Prosth.)

occlusal g. Movement induced by deflective tooth contact that diverts the mandible from a normal path of closure to a centric jaw relation. (Remov. Part. Prosth.)

gliding occlusion (see **occlusion, gliding**)

globulin A class of proteins. (Oral Med.)

antihemophilic g. (see **factor VIII**)

antihemophilic A g. (see **factor VIII**)

antihemophilic B g. (see **factor IX**)

glossalgia (glah-săl'jē-ah) Painful sensations in the tongue. (Oral Diag.; Oral Path.)

glossectomy (glah-sĕk'tō-mē) Surgical removal of the tongue, a portion of the tongue, or a lesion of the tongue. (Oral Surg.)

glossitis (glah-sī'tĭs) Inflammation of the tongue. (Oral Diag.; Oral Med.; Oral Path.; Periodont.)

g. areata exfoliativa (see **tongue, geographic**)

atrophic g. (bald tongue, smooth tongue) Atrophy of the glossal papillae, resulting in a smooth tongue. The tongue may be pallid or erythematous and may appear small or enlarged. Atrophic glossitis may be associated with anemias, pellagra, vitamin B complex deficiencies, sprue, or other systemic diseases or may be local in origin. Because atrophy may be one phase, and circumscribed, painful, glossal excoriations may be another phase of one or more of the same systemic disease(s), much confusion in terminology has arisen; e.g., Moeller's glossitis; Hunter's glossitis; slick, glazed, varnished, glossy, or bald tongue; chronic superficial erythematous glossitis; glossodynia exfoliativa; beefy tongue; and pellagrous glossitis. (Oral Med.)

benign migratory g. (see **tongue, geographic**)

chronic superficial erythematous g. (see **glossitis, Moeller's**)

Clarke-Fournier g. (see **glossitis, interstitial sclerous**)

Hunter's g. (see **glossitis, Moeller's**)

interstitial sclerous g. (Clarke-Fournier g.) Nodular, lobulated, indurated tongue associated with terminal syphilis. (Oral Med.)

median rhomboid g. A developmental defect appearing as a red, slightly elevated area of the tongue just anterior to the foramen cecum. It is of no clinical significance and results from trapping of the median lobe of the tongue (tuberculum impar) at the surface during development. (Oral Diag.)

g. migrans (see **tongue, geographic**)

Moeller's g. (chronic superficial erythematous g., glossodynia exfoliativa, Hunter's g., pellagrous g.) Chronic, superficial, irregular atrophy of the mucosa of the tongue. It may be caused by allergy, neural disturbance, vitamin B complex deficiency, etc. A smooth, red, painful tongue associated with pernicious anemia. (Oral Diag.)

— Superficial, smooth, circumscribed, painful erythematous patches on the edges and dorsum of the tongue; associated initially with pernicious anemia but now known to be associated with many systemic diseases. It has also been described as pellagrous glossitis. (Oral Med.; Oral Path.)

pellagrous g. (see **glossitis, Moeller's**)

glossodynia (glos″ō-dĭn'ē-ah) Painful sensations in the tongue; a sensation of burning in the tongue; a sore tongue. (Oral Diag.; Oral Med.; Oral Path.; Oral Surg.)

g. exfoliativa (see **glossitis, Moeller's**)

glossoplasty (glos'ō-plas″tē) A surgical procedure performed on the tongue. (Oral Surg.)

glossoplegia (glos″ō-plē'jē-ah) Paralysis of the tongue; may be unilateral or bilateral. (Oral Diag.)

glossopyrosis (glos″ō-pī-rō'sĭs) Burning sensation of the tongue. (Oral Med.; Oral Surg.)

glossorraphy (glos″or'ah-fē) Suture of a wound of the tongue. (Oral Surg.)

glossotomy (glah-sot'ō-mē) Excision or incision of the tongue. (Orthodont.)

glottal (glot'tăl) Pertaining to, or produced in or by, the glottis. The sound of "h" is a voiceless glottal fricative. The airstream on the exhalation phase moves unimpeded through the larynx, pharynx, and oral cavities. (Cleft Palate)

glottidospasm (glot-tĭ'dō-spăzm) (see **laryngospasm**)

glottis (glot'ĭs) The vocal apparatus of the larynx, consisting of the true vocal cords (vocal folds) and the opening between them (rima glottidis). (Anesth.)

glucagon (gloo'kah-gahn) (**hyperglycemic factor, hyperglycemic-glycogenolytic factor, HGF**) A hormone of the pancreas that raises the blood sugar by increasing hepatic glycogenolysis. (Oral Med.)

glucocorticoids (gloo″kō-kor'tĭ-koidz) (**anti-in-**

flammatory hormone, 11-oxycorticoids) Adrenocortical steroid hormones that affect glycogenesis in the liver. They are anti-inflammatory, are active in protection against stress, and affect carbohydrate and protein metabolism. Typical of the group are cortisol and cortisone. (Oral Med.)

glucoside (gloo′kō-sīd) A glycoside in which the sugar component is glucose. (Oral Med.; Pharmacol.)

glyceride (glĭs′er-īd) An ester of glycerin with one or more aliphatic acids. (Oral Med.; Pharmacol.)

glycerite (glĭs′er-īt) A solution or suspension of a drug in glycerin. (Oral Med.; Pharmacol.)

glycogenolysis (glī″kō-jĕ-nol′ĭ-sĭs) The formation of blood glucose by hydrolysis of stored liver glycogen. (Oral Med.)

glyconeogenesis (glī″kō-nē″ō-jĕn′ĕ-sĭs) The formation of glucose by the liver from noncarbohydrate precursors (e.g., glycogenic amino acids) and the glycerol portion of fat molecules. (Oral Med.)

glycoside (glī′kō-sīd) A compound that contains a sugar as part of the molecule. (Oral Med.; Pharmacol.)

glycosuria (glī″kō-sū′rē-ah) Presence of sugar in the urine. It is due most commonly to diabetes mellitus but may occur from a lowered renal threshold (renal glycosuria) in pregnancy, in inorganic renal disease, and in patients taking adrenocorticosteroids. (Oral Med.)

Gm (see **gram**)

gnathic organ (năth′ĭk) A collective organ assembled about the upper and the lower dentolingual surface and used to pronounce the consonants: th, t, d, n, l, and r. (Gnathol.)

gnathion (năth′ē-ahn) The lowest point in the lower border of the mandible at the median plane. It is a point on the bony border palpated from below and naturally lies posterior to the tegumental border of the chin. (Comp. Prosth.; Orthodont.; Remov. Part. Prosth.)

gnathode (nă-thōd′) A gnathographically mounted dental cast. (Gnathol.)

gnathodynamometer (nă″thō-dī″nah-mom′ĕ-ter) An instrument used for measuring biting pressure. (Comp. Prosth.)

    Bimeter g. A gnathodynamometer equipped with a central bearing point of adjustable height. (Comp. Prosth.)

Gnathograph (năth′ō-grăf) An articulator designed by McCollum. It resembles the Hanau instrument but differs chiefly by having a provision for increasing the intercondylar distance,

an important determinant of groove directions in the occlusal surfaces of teeth. (Gnathol.)

Gnathokin (năth′ō-kĭn) An experimental instrument made to study how given cusps articulate in protrusive balance with various given slants and curvatures of the condyle paths. (Gnathol.)

Gnatholator An articulator by Granger that has since been succeeded by an improved instrument called the Simulator (or Gnathosimulator). (Gnathol.)

gnathologic instrument Term often used as a synonym for an articulator. Any dental instrument used for diagnosis and treatment, such as a probe for determining the depth of a periodontal pocket, is a gnathologic tool. (Gnathol.)

gnathology (nah-thol′ō-jē) The science of the masticatory system, including physiology, functional disturbances, and treatment. (Comp. Prosth.)

— A method for occlusal treatment utilizing a precision adjustable articulator and pantographic records of mandibular movements and jaw positions. (Fixed Part. Prosth.)

— A branch of biology devoted to learning how gnathic organs should grow and mature; how teeth are best related to the jaw joints for ingesting and digesting food; and how to treat growth failures, damaged teeth, periodontal ills, and tooth losses to recover as fully as possible the gnathic functions. (Gnathol.)

gnathoschisis (nah-thos′kĭ-sĭs) (see **jaw, cleft**)

Gnathoscope Name of an articulator designed by McCollum that had tiltable remnant hinge "axles" that were set in stirrup mounts that could be swiveled and turned so that the setting of each condylar element would provide an approximate path of travel for the condyles of the patient. (Gnathol.)

gnathostatics (năth″ō-stăt′ĭks) A technique of orthodontic diagnosis based on relationships between the teeth and certain landmarks on the skull. (Oral Diag.) (see also **cast, gnathostatic**)

goiter (goi′ter) Enlargement of the thyroid gland. (Oral Diag.)

    colloid g. (endemic g., iodine deficiency g., simple g.) Visible enlargement of the thyroid gland without obvious signs of hypofunction or hyperfunction of the gland; due to inadequate intake or to an increased demand for iodine. (Oral Med.)

    endemic g. (see **goiter, colloid**)

    exophthalmic g. A disease of the thyroid gland consisting of hyperthyroidism, exophthalmos, and goiterous enlargement of the thyroid gland. A diffuse primary hyperplasia of the thyroid gland of obscure origin; may occur at any age. It produces nervousness, muscular weakness, heat intolerance, tremor, loss of weight, lid lag, and absence of winking and may lead to thyrotoxic heart disease and thyroid crisis. (Oral Med.)

iodine deficiency g. (see **goiter, colloid**)

nodular g., nontoxic Recurrent episodes of hyperplasia and involution of colloid goiter, resulting in a multinodular goiter. Symptoms are related to pressure. (Oral Med.)

simple g. (see **goiter, colloid**)

goitrogens (goi′trō-jĕnz) Agents such as thiouracil and related antithyroid compounds that are capable of producing goiter. Included are such agents as soybeans, cabbage, and thiocyanate, which produce goiter not treatable by the administration of iodine. (Oral Med.)

gold A precious or noble metal; yellow, malleable, ductible, nonrusting; much used in dentistry in pure and alloyed forms. (Oper. Dent.)

crystal g. (see **gold, mat**)

fibrous g. (see **foil, gold**)

g. file (see **file, gold**)

g. foil (see **foil, gold**)

g. f. cylinder (see **foil cylinder**)

g. f. pellet (see **pellet, foil**)

inlay g. An alloy, principally gold, used for cast restorations. Desired physical properties may be obtained by selecting those with varying ingredients and/or proportions. Acceptable alloys are classified by A.D.A. specifications according to Brinell hardness: Type A—soft, Brinell 40 to 75; Type B—medium, Brinell 70 to 100; Type C—hard, Brinell 90 to 140. (D. Mat.)

g. inlay A cast restoration of gold alloy fabricated outside the mouth and cemented into the prepared cavity; usually refers to the intracoronal type of restoration. (Oper. Dent.)

g. knife (see **knife, gold**)

mat g. (**crystal g., sponge g.**) A noncohesive form of pure gold prepared by electrodeposition. Sometimes used in the base of restorations and then veneered or overlaid with cohesive foil. (D. Mat.)

powdered g. Fine granules of pure gold, formed by atomizing the molten metal or by chemical precipitation. For clinical use it is available either as clusters of the granules, or as pellets of the powder contained in an envelope of gold foil; the pellets range in diameter from 1 to 3 mm. (Oper. Dent.)

— A form of pure gold; very thin, flakelike crystals formed by electrodeposition. Used in combination with cohesive gold foil in gingival-third foil restorations. (Oper. Dent.)

g. saw (see **saw, gold**)

sponge g. (see **gold, mat**)

g., wedging principle The fundamental tenet or rule in the compaction of gold foil. The rule is to pack the foil tightly between the confirming peripheral walls of a cavity preparation, utilizing controlled compaction force to wedge the parallel walls apart or to compress the dentin by lateral pressure. It is accomplished by stepping the condenser from the central area of the mass of gold toward the walls. (Oper. Dent.)

white g. A gold alloy with a high palladium content. It has a higher fusion range, lower ductility, and greater hardness than a yellow gold alloy. (D. Mat.)

Goldent Proprietary name for a direct gold restorative material. It consists basically of varying amounts of powdered gold contained in a wrapping or envelope of gold foil. (Oper. Dent.)

Goldman-Fox knife (see **knife, Goldman-Fox**)

Golgi's corpuscles (gol′jēz) (see **corpuscle, Golgi's**)

gomphosis (gahm-fō′sĭs) A form of joint in which a conical body is fastened into a socket, as a tooth is fastened into the jaw. (Oral Surg.)

gonad (gō′năd, gon′ăd) An ovary or testis, the site of origin of eggs or spermatozoa. (Oral Radiol.)

gonadotrophin (gō-năd″ō-trōf′ĭn) (see **gonadotropin**)

gonadotropin (gō-năd″ō-trōp′ĭn) (**gonadotropic hormone**) A gonad-stimulating hormone derived either from the pituitary gland (e.g., follicle-stimulating hormone [FSH] and a luteinizing hormone [LH], which is also an interstitial cell–stimulating hormone [ICSH]) or from the chorion (e.g., chorionic gonadotropin, which is found in the urine of pregnant women). (Oral Med.)

chorionic g. (see **hormone, pregnancy**)

gonion (gō′nē-on) The lowest, posterior, and most outward point of the mandibular angle. (In the location of the point, the patient is cautioned not to turn his head but to look straight ahead.) (Orthodont.)

good faith Honesty of intention. Generally, not a sufficient defense in a dental malpractice lawsuit. (D. Juris.)

Good Samaritan legislation Statutes enacted in some states providing that physicians and dentists who render aid in an emergency situation are not liable to the injured party for alleged malpractice unless there is a showing of willful wrong. (D. Juris.)

good will The custom or patronage of any established trade, business, or professional practice. (D. Juris.)

Gothic arch tracer (see **tracer, needle point**)

Gothic arch tracing (see **tracing, needle point**)

gr (see **grain**)

graft A slip or portion of tissue used for implantation. (Oral Implant.; Oral Surg.) (see also **donor site; recipient site**)

    allograft A graft between genetically dissimilar members of the same species. (Oral Surg.)

    alloplast g. A graft of an inert metal or plastic material. (Oral Surg.)

    autogenous g. A graft taken from one portion of an individual's body and implanted into another portion of the same individual's body. (Oral Implant.)

        a. bone g. A bone graft taken from one part of a patient's body and transplanted to another part of the same patient's body; e.g., the transfer of a portion of the iliac crest to the mandible. (Oral Surg.)

        — The implantation of living bone tissue from the same individual into another part of the body. This tissue becomes incorporated into the healing process and survives afterward as a functioning part of the periodontium. (Periodont.)

    auto-g. A graft taken from one part of the body and transplanted to another part. (M.F.P.)

    — The transfer of tissue—e.g., mucous membrane, teeth, skin, or bone—from one site to another on the same patient. (Oral Surg.)

    — A graft transferred from one position to another within the same individual. (Oral Surg.)

    g. donor site The site from which bone graft material is taken and implanted into the periodontal defect. (Periodont.)

    filler g. A graft used for the filling of defects, such as bone chips used to fill a cyst. (Oral Surg.)

    free g. A portion of the masticatory mucosa that is completely detached from its original site and transferred to another site. (Periodont.)

    — A graft of tissue completely detached from its original site and blood supply. (Oral Surg.)

    full-thickness g. A skin graft consisting of the full thickness of the skin with none of the subcutaneous tissues. (Oral Surg.)

heterogenous g. A graft implanted from one species to another. (Oral Implant.)

heterograft A graft of tissue taken from a donor of one species to be grafted into a recipient of another species. (M.F.P.; Oral Surg.)

homogenous g. A graft taken from a member of a species and implanted into the body of a member of the same species. (Oral Implant.)

homograft A graft of tissue taken from a donor of the same species as the recipient. (M.F.P.)

— A graft between genetically similar individuals of the same species. (Oral Surg.)

iliac g. A bone graft whose donor site is the crest of the ilium. Various locations of the iliac crest duplicate areas of the mandible and curvatures of the midfacial skeleton. (Oral Surg.)

isograft A graft between individuals with identical or histocompatible antigens. (Oral Surg.)

kiel g. Denatured calf bone used to fill defects or restore facial contour. Often used for chin and nasal augmentation. (Oral Surg.)

mucosal g. A split-thickness graft involving the mucosa. (Oral Surg.)

onlay bone g. A graft in which the grafted bone is applied laterally to the cortical bone of the recipient site, frequently to improve the contours of the chin or the malar eminence of the zygomatic bone. (Oral Surg.)

pedicle g. A stem or tube of tissue that remains attached near the donor site to nourish the graft during advancement of a skin graft. (Oral Surg.)

split-thickness g. A graft that varies in thickness and contains only mucosal elements and no subcutaneous tissue. (Oral Surg.)

swaging g. A procedure analogous to bone grafting. Also referred to as a contiguous transplant that involves a greenstick fracture of bone bordering on an infrabony defect and the displacement of bone to eliminate the osseous defect. (Periodont.)

Thiersch's skin g. A split-thickness skin graft containing cutaneous and some subcutaneous tissues, the line of cleavage being through the rete peg layer. (Oral Surg.)

grain (gr) A unit of weight equal to 0.0648 g.

— A crystal of an alloy. (D. Mat.)

    g. boundary The junction of two grains growing from different nuclei, impinging on each other and causing discontinuity of the lattice structure. Important in corrosion and brittleness of metals. (D. Mat.)

g. growth (see **growth, grain**)

gram (Gm, g) The basic unit of mass of the metric system. Equivalent of 15.432 gr. (D. Mat.)

Gram's stain (see **stain, Gram's**)

granules, sulfur (see **actinomycosis**)

granulocytopenia (grăn″u-lo-sĭ″to-pē′nē-ah) A deficiency in the number of granulocytic cells in the bloodstream. (Oral Diag.)

granuloma (grăn″u-lo′mah) A localized mass of granulation tissue. (Oral Diag.)

    chronic g. (chronic apical periodontitis) Chronic inflammatory tissue surrounding the apical foramina as a result of irritation from within the root canal system. (Endodont.)

    dental g. A mass of granulation tissue surrounded by a fibrous capsule attached at the apex of a pulp-involved tooth. It produces a fairly well demarcated radiolucency. (Oral Diag.; Oral Path.)

    eosinophilic g. (ē″o-sĭn″o-fĭl′ĭk) Chronic localized histoplasmosis X. A disease characterized by radiolucent areas in the bones, including the skull and jaws. Histiocytes and eosinophils characterize the lesions microscopically. Faulty lipid metabolism appears to be its cause. (Oral Diag.)

    — A granulomatous inflammatory disease of unknown etiology, usually monofocal in bone but sometimes affecting soft tissues. Sheets of histiocytes and masses of eosinophils characterize the lesion histologically. (Oral Path.)

    giant cell reparative g. An abnormal reparative reaction to an injury, characterized by fibroblastic proliferation with numerous giant cells. It may be peripheral (i.e., on the gingiva, as in giant cell epulis) or central (i.e., within the bone, producing a radiolucency). Most giant cell lesions of the jaws are reparative granulomas rather than neoplasms. (Oral Diag.)

    — A benign tumorlike growth composed of highly cellular fibrous connective tissue in which are located numerous vascular channels, multinucleated giant cells, and foci of hemosiderin. The lesion may be within the bone (central) or on the gingiva (peripheral). (Oral Path.)

    peripheral g. c. r. g. (giant cell epulis, osteoclastoma) A tumorlike pedunculated or sessile lesion believed to represent an exuberant repair phenomenon. It is composed of a matrix of young fibrous connective tissue that contains numerous multinucleated giant cells. (Oral Path.) (see also **granuloma, giant cell reparative**)

    pyrogenic g. A tumorlike mass of granulation tissue produced in response to minor trauma in some individuals. It is highly vascular and bleeds readily. (Oral Diag.)

    — A tumorlike growth occurring on the gingivae, lips, or tongue as a result of an exuberant repair phenomenon. (Oral Path.)

    reticuloendothelial g. (see **disease, lipoid storage**)

grasp The manner in which an instrument is held.

    finger g. A modification of the palm and thumb grasp; it is more useful with modern, smaller-handled instruments. The handle is held by the four flexed fingers rather than allowed to rest in the palm, and the thumb is used to secure a rest. Used when working indirectly on the upper arch. (Oper. Dent.)

    instrument g. Manner of holding a dental instrument in operative dentistry; classified as pen, inverted-pen, palm-and-thumb, and finger grasps. (Pen and finger grasps are the most useful.) (Oper. Dent.)

    — A method of holding the instrument with the fingers in such a manner that freedom of action, control, tactile sensitivity, and maneuverability are secured. The most common grasp is the pen grasp. (Periodont.)

    palm-and-thumb g. A grasp that is similar to the hold on a knife when one is whittling wood; the handle rests in the palm and is grasped by the four fingers, while the thumb rests on an adjoining object. (Oper. Dent.)

    pen g. A grasp in which the instrument is held somewhat as a pen is held, with the handle in contact with the bulbous portion of the thumb and index finger and the shank in contact with the radial side of the bulbous portion of the middle finger (not crossing the nail) while the handle rests against the phalanx of the index finger. (Oper. Dent.)

    — A preferred method of holding periodontal and other operative instruments. The tips of the thumb, forefinger, and middle finger are all in direct contact with the shank of the instrument. This grasp offers the tactile sensitivity so vital to instrumentation. (Periodont.)

        inverted p. g. A grasp that is similar to the pen grasp, except that the wrist is flexed so that the working part of the instrument points toward rather than away from the operator. (Oper. Dent.)

gratis Free, without reward or consideration. (D. Juris.)

Graves' disease (see **goiter, exophthalmic**)

gravity, specific The weight of 1 ml of a liquid material or 1 cc of a solid material. (D. Mat.)
— A number indicating the ratio of the weight of a substance to that of an equal volume of water. (Remov. Part. Prosth.)

grid A device used to prevent as much scattered radiation as possible from reaching an x-ray film during the making of a radiograph. It consists essentially of a series of narrow lead strips closely spaced on their edges and separated by spacers of low density material. (Oral Radiol.)

crossed g. An arrangement of two parallel grids rotated in position at right angles to each other. (Oral Radiol.) (see also **grid, parallel**)

focused g. A grid in which the lead foils are placed at an angle so that they all point toward a focus at a specified distance. (Oral Radiol.)

moving g. A grid that is moved continuously or oscillated throughout the making of a radiograph. (Oral Radiol.)

parallel g. A grid in which the lead strips are oriented parallel to each other. (Oral Radiol.)

Potter-Bucky g. A grid utilizing the principle of the moving grid, with an oscillating movement. (Oral Radiol.)

stationary g. A nonoscillating or nonmoving grid; the image of its strips will be visible on the radiograph for which it is used. (Oral Radiol.)

grinding, selective Modification of the occlusal forms of teeth by grinding at selected places marked by spots made by articulating paper or marked by parts of the teeth as they cut through a thin layer of wax placed over the teeth. (Comp. Prosth.; Remov. Part. Prosth.)

grinding-in The process of correcting errors in the centric and eccentric occlusions of natural or artificial teeth. (Comp. Prosth.; Remov. Part. Prosth.)

groove A linear channel or sulcus, especially on the surface of a tooth. (Oper. Dent.)

abutment g. A transverse groove that may be cut in the bone across the alveolar ridge to furnish positive seating for the implant framework and to prevent tension of the tissue. (Oral Implant.)

developmental g. A fine depressed line in the enamel of a tooth that marks the union of the lobes of the crown in its development. (Oper. Dent.)

gingival g., free The shallow line or depression on the surface of the gingiva between the free and the attached gingivae. It denotes the junction of the free and the attached gingivae. (Periodont.)

interdental g. A linear, vertical depression on the surface of the interdental papillae; functions as a sluiceway for the egress of food from the interproximal areas. (Periodont.)

retention g. A groove formed by opposing vertical constrictions in the tooth that provide a horseshoelike grip on the tooth. (Fixed Part. Prosth.)

ground, electrical Electrical connection with the earth (or other ground); also, a large conducting body (e.g., automobile chassis, airplane fuselage, or the earth itself) used as a common return for the electrical circuit, and as an arbitrary zero of potential. (Oral Radiol.)

g. state The state of a nucleus, an atom, or a molecule when it has its lowest energy. All other states are termed excited. (Oral Radiol.)

grounded Pertaining to an arrangement whereby an electrical circuit or equipment (e.g., x-ray generator) is connected by an electrical conductor with the earth or some similarly conducting body. (Oral Radiol.)

group, blood (see **blood groups**)

group function (see **function, group**)

group practice (see **practice, group**)

group purchase The purchase of dental services, either by postpayment or prepayment, by a large group of people. (Pract. Man.)

growth Increase in size. (Orthodont.)

grain g. A phenomenon resulting from heat treatment of alloys. In excessive amounts this growth produces undesirable physical properties. (D. Mat.)

GTT (see **test, glucose tolerance**)

guaranty A contract that some certain and designated thing shall be done exactly as it is agreed to be done. (D. Juris.)

guard, bite An acrylic resin appliance designed to cover the occlusal and incisal surfaces of the teeth of a dental arch so as to stabilize the teeth and/or provide a flat platform for the unobstructed excursive glides of the mandible. (Periodont.) (see also **plane, bite**)

guard, mouth A resilient intraoral device worn during participation in contact sports to reduce the potential for injury to the teeth and associated tissue. (Orthodont.)

guard, night An acrylic resin device used to stabilize the teeth and to minimize the effects of traumatic occlusal habits. (Periodont.) (see also **plane, bite**)

guardian A person appointed to take care of the person or property of another; one who legally has the care and management of the person, or the property, or both, of a child until the child attains his or her majority. (D. Juris.)

Guérin's fracture (gā-rănz') (see **fracture, Guérin's**)

guidance A mechanical or other means for controlling the direction of movement of an object.

condylar g. (see **guide, condylar**)

c. g. inclination (see **guide, condylar, inclination**)

incisal g. The influence on mandibular movements by the contacting surfaces of the mandibular and maxillary anterior teeth. (Comp. Prosth.; Fixed Part. Prosth.; Remov. Part. Prosth.)

i. g. angle (see **angle, incisal guidance**)

guide A device for directing the motion of something.

anterior g. The part of an articulator contacted by the incisal guide pin to maintain the selected separation of the upper and lower members of the articulator. The guide influences the changing relationships of mounted casts in eccentric movements. (Comp. Prosth.; Remov. Part. Prosth.) (see also **guide, incisal**)

adjustable a. g. An anterior guide, the superior surface of which may be varied to provide desired separation of the casts in various eccentric relationships. (Comp. Prosth.; Remov. Part. Prosth.)

condylar g. (condylar guidance) The mechanical device on an articulator; intended to produce guidance in articulator movement similar to that produced by the paths of the condyles in the temporomandibular joints. (Comp. Prosth.; Fixed Part. Prosth.; Remov. Part. Prosth.)

c. g. inclination (c. guidance inclination) The angle of inclination of the condylar guide mechanism of an articulator in relation to the horizontal plane of the instrument. (Comp. Prosth.; Fixed Part. Prosth.; Remov. Part. Prosth.)

incisal g. (anterior guide) The part of an articulator that maintains the incisal guide angle. (Comp. Prosth.; Remov. Part. Prosth.)

i. g., adjustment Occlusal adjustment that produces a minimum of overbite (vertical overlap) and a maximum of overjet (horizontal overlap), eliminates fremitus and racking effects on the anterior segment of teeth in the protrusive glide, and attains maximal incisive group function. (Periodont.)

i. g. angle (see **angle, incisal guide**)

g. plane (see **plane, guide**)

guideline, Cummer's Term suggested by W. E. Cummer to indicate the line of greatest convexity of an abutment tooth surface at a chosen inclination, as determined by a selected path of placement and removal of a removable prosthesis; more commonly known by the term applied by Edward Kennedy: the "surveyed height of contour." (Remov. Part. Prosth.)

gum(s) The fibrous and mucosal covering of the alveolar process or ridges. (Comp. Prosth.; Remov. Part. Prosth.) (see also **gingiva**)

g. contour (see **contour, gingival**)

g. cuff, implant (see **epithelial cuff, implant**)

g. pads Edentulous segments of the maxillae and mandible that correspond to the underlying primary teeth. (Pedodont.)

gumma (gŭm'ah) A granulomatous, gummy lesion of tertiary syphilis. The palate and tongue are sites of predilection in the oral region. A similar lesion occurring with tuberculosis is designated a tuberculous gumma. (Oral Diag.; Periodont.)

— A granulomatous, destructive lesion of tertiary syphilis. (Oral Med.)

— A rubbery, gray-white, tumorlike mass commonly found on mucocutaneous surfaces in tertiary syphilis. Also seen in liver, bone, and testes. (Oral Path.)

Gunning's splint (see **splint, Gunning's**)

Gunn's syndrome (see **syndrome, Gunn's**)

gutta-percha (gŭt"ah-per'chah) The coagulated juice of various tropical trees that has certain rubberlike properties. Used for temporary sealing of dressings in cavities; also used in the form of cones for filling root canals and in the form of sticks for sealing cavities over treatment. (Endodont.)

— The sap of the sapotaceous order of trees. Coagulated by boiling; hardens on exposure to air. (Oper. Dent.)

baseplate g.-p. Gutta-percha combined with fillers and coloring materials, and rolled into sheets. Used for making temporary restorations, filling root canals, separating teeth, and retracting gingival tissue. (Oper. Dent.)

g.-p. points Fine, tapered cylinders of gutta-percha used, because of their radiopacity, for radiographic ascertainment of pocket depth and topography; used also as a root canal filling material. (Periodont.)

g.-p., temporary stopping Gutta-percha mixed with zinc oxide and white wax. Used for temporary sealing of dressings in cavities. (Oper. Dent.)

gypsum (jĭp'sŭm) The dihydrate of calcium sulfate ($CaSO_4 \cdot 2H_2O$). Alpha-hemihydrate and beta-hemihydrate are derived from gypsum. (D. Mat.)

H

h II (see **hemophilia B**)

habit A frequently repeated practice that may produce injury to the teeth, their attachment apparatus, the oral mucous membranes, the mandibular musculature, the temporomandibular articulation, etc. Oral habits include bruxism, clenching, clamping, tongue thrusting, lip biting, cheek biting, etc. (Periodont.)

bruxism h. (see **bruxism**)

clamping h. The prolonged or sustained application of the mandibular teeth to the maxillary teeth, a practice that may produce injury to the various elements of the stomatologic system. (Periodont.)

clenching h. (see **clenching**)

occupational h. A habit that is associated with a vocation and that is formed and performed either by necessity or for convenience; e.g., the holding of nails between the teeth by shoemakers or the biting of thread by seamstresses and tailors. (Periodont.)

oral h. A habit that causes changes in occlusal relationships; e.g., thumb and finger habits, tongue habits, reverse swallowing, and lip sucking. Any one of the repeated acts of indefinite motivation performed by structures of the stomatologic system that may be detrimental to the integrity of the teeth, their attaching and supporting structures, the tongue, mucous membranes, temporomandibular articulation, etc. (Pedodont.)

h. reminder Any effective appliance for breaking pernicious oral habits. (Pedodont.)

tongue h. Afunctional movements of the tongue, repeated either consciously or unconsciously, that may produce deviations of tooth position or damage to the tissues of the tongue and the attachment apparatus of teeth. (Periodont.)

habituation A state in which an individual involuntarily tends to continue the use of a drug. Generally refers to the state in which an individual continues self-administration of a drug because of psychologic dependence without physical dependence. (Oral Med.; Pharmacol.)

Hageman trait (hahg'măn) (see **factor XII**)

half-life The time in which a radioactive substance will lose half of its activity through disintegration. (Oral Radiol.)

biologic h.-l. The time in which a living tissue, organ, or individual eliminates, through biologic processes, half of a given amount of a substance that has been introduced into it. (Oral Radiol.)

effective h.-l. Half-life of a radioactive isotope in a biologic organism, resulting from the combination of radioactive decay and biologic elimination.

$$\text{Effective half-life} = \frac{\text{Biologic half-life} \times \text{Radioactive half-life}}{\text{Biologic half-life} + \text{Radioactive half-life}}$$

(Oral Radiol.)

physical h.-l. The average time (t½) required for the decay of half the atoms in a given amount of a radioactive substance. Each radionuclide (radioactive isotope or radioisotope) has a specific half-life. (Oral Radiol.)

half-value layer (HVL) The thickness of a specified material (usually aluminum, copper, or lead) required to decrease the dosage rate of a beam of x rays at a point of interest to half its initial value. A determination of the half-value layer of a given x-ray beam is used to denote the quality of the x-ray beam. The half-value layer will vary depending on kilovolt peak and the amount of filtration at the source. (Oral Radiol.)

h.-v. l., half thickness The thickness or surface density, of a layer of a specified material that attenuates the beam to such an extent that the exposure rate is reduced to one half, under narrow beam conditions. (Oral Radiol.)

halisteresis (hah-lĭs″ter-ē′sĭs) A theory of the method of bone resorption according to which bone salts can be removed by a humoral mechanism and returned to the tissue fluids, leaving behind a decalcified bone matrix; osteolysis. This is not considered to be the mechanism under which resorption occurs in periodontal disease. (Periodont.)

halitosis (hăl″ĭ-tō′sĭs) **(bad breath, bromopnea, fetor ex ore, offensive breath)** Offensive odor of the breath due to local and metabolic conditions; e.g., poor oral hygiene, periodontal disease, sinusitis, tonsillitis, suppurative bronchopulmonary disease, acidosis, and uremia. (Oper. Dent.; Oral Diag.; Oral Med.)

Haller's plexus (see **plexus, Haller's**)

halogen (hăl′ō-jĕn) An element of a closely related group of elements consisting of fluorine, chlorine, bromine, and iodine. (Oral Med.; Pharmacol.)

halothane (hăl′ō-thān) A potent anesthetic agent synthesized by Suckling. (Anesth.)

hamartoma A localized error in the composition of the tissue elements of an organ. May be anatomically manifested in three ways, either singly or in combination: by abnormal quantity, by abnormal structure, or by degree of maturation of the tissue components. (Oral Path.)

Hamberger's schema (see **schema, Hamberger's**)

Hamburger's phenomenon (see **phenomenon, Hamburger's**)

hamular notch (see **notch, pterygomaxillary**)

hamular process (see **process, hamular**)

hand air syringe (see **syringe, hand air**)

hand condenser (see **condenser, hand**)

hand pressure (see **pressure, hand**)

handpiece An instrument used to hold rotary instruments in the dental engine or condensing points in mechanical condensing units. It is connected by an arm, cable, belt, or tube to the source of power (motor, air, or water). (Oper. Dent.)

   air turbine h. A handpiece with a turbine powered by compressed air. (Oper. Dent.)

   cervix h. The constricted, highly polished portion that connects the base of the insert to the head. (Oper. Dent.)

   contra-angle h. A binangled instrument for use with the dental engine; permits access to areas difficult or impossible to reach with a straight handpiece. (Oper. Dent.)

   high-speed h. A type of rotary or vibratory cutting tool that operates at speeds above 12,000 rpm. It is propelled by gears, belt, or turbine or is operated by ultrasonic mechanical vibrations with an abrasive powder/water slurry. Generally classified as an air turbine, a hydraulic turbine, a high-speed handpiece on a conventional dental engine, or an ultrasonic handpiece. (Oper. Dent.)

      ultra h.-s. h. A handpiece designed to permit rotational speeds of 100,000 to 300,000 rpm. (Oper. Dent.)

   right-angle h. A monangled instrument used with mechanical condensers to reach some operating areas. (Oper. Dent.)

   straight h. A handpiece whose axis is in line with the rotary instrument. The simplest handpiece for a direct approach. (Oper. Dent.)

   ultrasonic h. A type of tooth-cutting device; cutting is produced by aluminum oxide slur-

ry directed on the instrument tip, which vibrates at a frequency of 29,000 cycles/sec, which is above audible range. (Oper. Dent.)

   water-turbine h. A handpiece with a turbine powered by water under pressure. (Oper. Dent.)

Hand-Schüller-Christian disease (hănd-shĭl′er-krĭs′chăn) (see **disease, Hand-Schüller-Christian**)

Hansen's disease (see **leprosy**)

hard of hearing Term applied to persons whose hearing is impaired but who have enough hearing left for practical use. (Cleft Palate)

hardener An ingredient (potassium alum) of the photographic and radiographic fixing solution that serves to harden the gelatin of the film to prevent softening and swelling of the gelatin. (Oral Radiol.)

hardening The process of setting or becoming firm.

   age h. The precipitation of intermetallic compounds that alters certain physical properties in alloys; usually brought about through heat treatment. (D. Mat.)

   precipitation h. (see **tempering**)

   h. solution (see **solution, hardening**)

   strain h. An increase in proportional limit due to distortion of the space lattice and fracture of grain boundaries through cold work. Ductility is markedly reduced. (D. Mat.)

   — An increase in hardness or strength caused by plastic deformation at temperatures lower than the recrystallization range. (Oper. Dent.)

   work h. The hardening of a metal by cold work, such as repeated flexing. (Remov. Part. Prosth.)

hardness (of a substance) The ability of a material to resist an indenting type of load. Usually considered to be somewhat indicative of the ability of a material to withstand abrasion or attrition. (D. Mat.)

   — Resistance to indentation measured by any one of the following tests: Brinell, Mohs, Rockwell, Vickers, or Knoop. (Oper. Dent.)

   — Resistance of a metal to permanent deformation; usually an indentation or scratching test is used to test hardness. (Remov. Part. Prosth.)

hardness, Mohs Relative scratch resistance of minerals based on an arbitrary scale: 10, diamond; 9, corundum; 8, topaz; 7, quartz; 6, orthoclase; 5, apatite; 4, fluorite; 3, calcite; 2, gypsum; and 1, talc. (Mineralogy)

hardness (of x rays) Term used to indicate in a general way the quality of x radiation, "hardness" being a function of wavelength; the shorter the wavelength, the "harder" the x radiation. (Oral Radiol.)

harelip (cheiloschisis, left lip, congenital cleft lip) Congenital nonunion or inadequacy of soft and hard tissues related to the lip. The deformity may be extensive enough to involve the nose, alveolar process, hard palate, and velum. The extent of deformity varies among individuals. Various classifications have been established to identify the extent of a cleft. (Cleft Palate)

— A cleft of the upper lip, either unilateral or bilateral, at the embryonal junction of the median nasal process and the maxillary process. A rare midline cleft may occur in the lower lip at the embryonal junction of the two mandibular processes. (Oral Diag.)

— A congenital defect or cleft in the upper lip. (Oral Path.)

— A deformity of the lip resulting from improper union or lack of union of the maxillary process with the nasomedial process during the second month of intrauterine development. (Orthodont.)

harmony, occlusal The nondisruptive relationship of an occlusion to all its factors, e.g., the neuromuscular mechanism, the temporomandibular joints, the teeth and their supporting structures. (Comp. Prosth.; Remov. Part. Prosth.)

functional o. h. An occlusal relationship of opposing teeth in all functional ranges and movements that will provide the greatest masticatory efficiency without causing undue strain or trauma on the supporting tissues. (Comp. Prosth.; Fixed Part. Prosth.; Remov. Part. Prosth.)

Hatch clamp (see **clamp, gingival, Hatch**)

hatchet An angled cutting hand instrument in which the broad side of the blade is parallel with the angle(s) of the shank. Used to develop internal cavity form. May be bibeveled or single beveled like a chisel, in which case the instrument is paired with another. (Oper. Dent.)

enamel h. An angled cutting hand instrument in which the broad side of the blade is parallel with the angle(s) of the shank. May be bibeveled or single beveled like a chisel, in which case the instrument is paired with another. Used primarily with a chipping or a lateral scraping stroke to develop internal cavity form. (Oper. Dent.)

haversian system (see **osteon**)

Hawley appliance, chart, retainer (see under appropriate noun)

hay rake (see **appliance, hay rake**)

hazard, radiation The hazard that exists in any area to which a person has access while radiation equipment is in operation and the dosage rate is greater than the permissible dosage rate. (Oral Radiol.)

head, steeple (see **oxycephalia**)

headache Pain in the cranial vault due to intracranial, extracranial, or psychogenic causes: intracranial vascular dilation, space-occupying lesions, diseases of the eyes, ears, and sinuses, extracranial vascular dilation, sustained muscular contraction, and hysteria. (Oral Med.)

cluster h. (see **neuralgia, facial, atypical**)

lower-half h. (see **neuralgia, facial, atypical**)

migraine h. A severe type of headache (often unilateral) associated with nausea, vomiting, and other sensory disturbances, such as blurring of vision. It usually occurs periodically. (Oral Diag.)

—A paroxysmal pain, usually initially unilateral in the temporal, frontal, and retroorbital area; may become steady and generalized and may persist for hours or days and recur periodically. Visual disturbances, scotomas, or hallucinations may precede or accompany the headache. (Oral Med.)

headcap The part of an extraoral orthodontic appliance that engages the back of the head, incorporating the skull as a source of resistance for tooth movement, and gives attachment to the intraoral element of the appliance. (Orthodont.)

plaster h. A cap, constructed of plaster-of-paris gauze, that embodies points for applying fixation and traction appliances in the treatment of mandibular and maxillofacial injuries. (Oral Surg.)

headdress Protective covering for the patient's head. (Oper. Dent.)

headgear The apparatus encircling the head or neck and providing attachment for an intraoral appliance in use of extraoral anchorage. (Orthodont.)

radiologic h. A device used to protect the head from injury by radiation. (Oral Radiol.)

health A bodily state in which all parts are functioning properly. Also refers to the normal functioning of a part of the body. A state of normal functional equilibrium; homeostasis. (Periodont.)

patient h. The state of bodily soundness of the patient; his absolute or relative freedom from physical and/or mental disease. The state of health of the patient is an important consideration affecting the etiology, diagnosis, prognosis, and treatment of oral disease. (Periodont.)

hearsay The testimony given by a witness who relates not what he knows personally but what others have told him or what he has heard said by others. (D. Juris.)

heart block The condition in which the muscular interconnection between the auricle and ventricle is interrupted so that the auricle and ventricle beat independently of each other. (Anesth.)

heart failure A sudden, sometimes fatal cessation of the heart's action. (Oral Surg.)

acute h. f. A rapid and marked impairment of the cardiac output. (Oral Med.)

backward h. f. Congestive heart failure in which the initiating factor is increased venous pressure resulting from ventricular failure to empty the atria. (Oral Med.)

congestive h. f. A clinical syndrome resulting from chronic cardiac decompensation associated with left-sided and/or right-sided heart failure. Left-sided failure may be due to rheumatic mitral valvular disease, aortic valvular disease, systemic hypertension, or arteriosclerotic disease. Manifestations include orthopnea, paroxysmal dyspnea, pulmonary edema, cough, and cardiac asthma. Right-sided failure results most commonly from pulmonary congestion and hypertension associated with left-sided failure but may be due to anemia, myocarditis, beriberi, or dysrhythmia. Manifestations include peripheral pitting edema, ascites, cyanosis, oliguria, and hydrothorax. (Oral Med.)

forward h. f. Heart failure initiated by decreased cardiac output that leads to decreased blood supply to tissues, decreased excretion of salt (Na^+) and salt retention, elevated venous pressure, and edema. (Oral Med.)

heat The state of a body or of matter that is perceived as opposed to cold and is characterized by elevation of temperature.

applied h. Therapeutic application of wet or dry heat to increase circulation and produce hyperemia, to accelerate dissolution of infection and inflammation, to increase absorption from tissue spaces, to relieve pain, to relieve muscle spasm and associated pain, and to increase metabolism. (Oral Physiol.)

a. h., contraindications Conditions that preclude the use of heat application: peripheral neuropathy, conditions in which maximum vasodilation and inflammation are already present, acute inflammatory conditions in which more swelling will cause exquisite (acute) pain and pulpitis, septicemia, and malignancies. (Oral Physiol.)

a. h., general physiologic effects The physiologic effects of generally applied wet or dry heat: increase in body temperature, generalized vasodilation, rise in metabolism, decrease in blood pressure, increase in pulse rate and circulation, and increase in depth and rate of respiration. (Oral Physiol.)

a. h., local physiologic effects The physiologic effects of locally applied wet or dry heat to the intraoral and/or extraoral tissues: increase in caliber and number of capillaries, increased absorption due to capillary dilation, increased lymph formation and flow, relief of pain, relief of spasm, increase of phagocytes, and a rise in local metabolism. (Oral Physiol.)

h. and cold, applied The most commonly employed physical agents in dental practice; they modify the physiologic processes and have both a systemic and a local effect. The principal effect on the tissues is mediated by the alteration in the circulatory mechanisms. Properly used, heat and cold have a salutary therapeutic result; improperly used, they may produce serious pathologic consequences. (Oral Physiol.)

h. loss, metabolic causes Biologic factors that influence heat loss: redistribution of blood vasodilation and vasoconstriction, variations in blood volume, tendency of fat to insulate the body, and evaporation. (Oral Physiol.)

h. loss, physical causes Physical factors that influence heat loss: radiation, convection, and conduction; evaporation from the lungs, skin, and mucous membranes; the raising of inspired air to body temperatures; and the production of urine and feces. (Oral Physiol.)

h. production, metabolic causes Chemical factors of the body that cause heat production: specific dynamic action of food, especially protein, that results in a rise of metabolism; a high environmental temperature that, by raising temperatures of the tissues, increases the velocity of reactions and thus increases heat production; and stimulation of the adrenal cortex and thyroid glands by the hormones of the pituitary glands. (Oral Physiol.)

h. treatment (see **treatment, heat**)

heavy function (see **function, heavy**)

hebephrenia (hĕb″ĕ-frē′nē-ah) A form of schizophrenia in which the individual behaves like a child; e.g., giggling and acting silly. (Oral Med.)

heel effect (see **effect, heel**)

Heerfordt's syndrome (see **fever, uveoparotid**)

height of contour (see **contour, height of**)

helium (hē′lē-ŭm) A colorless, odorless, tasteless gas; one of the inert gaseous elements that was first detected in the sun and is now obtained from natural gas. Symbol, He; atomic number, 2; atomic weight, 4.003. Used in medicine as a diluent for other gases. (Anesth.)

hemangioameloblastoma (hē-măn″jē-ō-ah-mēl″ō-blăs-tō′mah) A neoplasm in the jaw that has characteristics of ameloblastoma and hemangioma. (Oral Diag.)

hemangioendothelioma (hē-măn″jē-ō-ĕn″dō-thē″lē-ō′mah) A neoplasm characterized by overgrowth of endothelial cells. It may have malignant properties and may invade locally or metastasize. (Oral Diag.)

— A malignant tumor formed by proliferation of endothelium of the capillary vessels. (Oral Path.)

hemangiofibroma (hē-măn″jē-ō-fī-brō′mah) A benign neoplasm characterized by proliferation of blood channels in a dense mass of fibroblasts. (Oral Diag.)

hemangioma (hē-măn″jē-ō′mah) A benign neoplasm characterized by blood vascular channels. A cavernous hemangioma consists of large vascular spaces. A capillary hemangioma consists of many small blood vessels. (Oral Diag.)

— A benign tumor composed of newly formed blood vessels. (Oral Path.)

hemangiopericytoma (hē-măn″jē-ō-pĕr″ĭ-sī-tō′mah) A vascular tumor composed of pericytes. (Oral Path.)

hemataerometer (hĕm″ăt-ā″er-om′ĕ-ter) A device for determining the pressure of the gases in the blood. (Anesth.)

hematemesis (hĕm″ah-tĕm′ĕ-sĭs) Vomiting of blood. (Oral Diag.)

hematocrit (hē-măt′ō-crĭt) **(packed-cell volume)** The percentage of the total blood volume composed of red blood cells (erythrocytes). Normal values are 42% to 45%. (Oral Diag.)

— The percentage of the total volume of a blood sample that is taken up by the red blood cells. Normal values: children 32% to 65%; adult men, 42% to 53%; adult women, 38% to 46%. (Oral Med.)

hematoma (hē″mah-tō′mah) A mass of blood in the tissue as a result of trauma or other factors that cause the rupture of blood vessels. (Oral Diag.)

— A tumefaction produced by extensive local hemorrhage into tissue or body space. They vary in color according to the state of blood deterioration. (Oral Diag.)

hematosis (hĕm″ah-tō′sĭs) Oxygenation or aeration of the venous blood in the lungs. (Anesth.)

hematuria (hĕm″ah-tū′rē-ah) Blood in the urine. (Oral Diag.)

— Presence of an abnormal number of red blood cells in the urine. (Oral Med.)

    gross h. Visible evidence of blood in the urine. It may occur from neoplasms of the kidney and bladder, hemorrhagic diathesis, hypertension with renal epistaxis, or acute glomerular nephritis. (Oral Med.)

    microscopic h. Demonstration of hematuria during the microscopic examination of centrifuged urine. It may be due to the same causes as gross hematuria or to toxicity of drugs, embolic glomerulitis, vascular diseases, or chronic glomerular nephritis. (Oral Med.)

hemianesthesia (hĕm″ē-ăn″ĕs-thē′zē-ah) Anesthesia or loss of tactile sensibility on one side of the body. (Anesth.; Oral Diag.)

hemiatrophy (hĕm″ē-ăt′rō-fē) Atrophy of one half of the body, an organ, or a part; e.g., facial hemiatrophy. (Oral Diag.)

hemiglossectomy (hĕm″ē-glŏ-sĕk′tō-mē) Surgical removal of half of the tongue. (Oral Surg.)

hemihypertrophy (hĕm″ē-hī-per′trō-fē) Excessive growth of half of the body, an organ, or a part; e.g., facial hemihypertrophy. (Oral Diag.)

hemiplegia (hĕm″ē-plē′jē-ah) In medical jurisprudence, paralysis of one side of the body. (D. Juris.)

hemisection The complete sectioning through the crown of a tooth into the furcation region to remove the involved portion of the crown and root. (Endodont.)

    h. for interradicular involvement Removal of one or two roots, leaving the other in situ; may be indicated treatment when furcations can be probed from one aspect to the other. (Periodont.)

hemoglobin (hē″mō-glō′bĭn) The oxygen-carrying red pigment of the red blood corpuscles. It is a reddish, crystallizable conjugated protein consisting of the protein globulin combined with the prosthetic group, heme. (Anesth.)

    h. estimation Determination of the hemoglobin content of the blood. By the Sahli method,

14 to 17 g/100 ml of blood is normal, and 15.1 Sahli units are taken as 100% for estimation of hemoglobin percentages. (Oral Diag.)

hemoglobinopathy (hē″mō-glō″bǐ-nop′ah-thē) Any one of a group of genetically determined diseases involving abnormal hemoglobin; e.g., sickle cell disease, in which hemoglobin S occurs, and hemoglobin C disease. (Oral Med.)

paroxysmal nocturnal h. An acquired hemolytic anemia of unknown cause characterized by increased hemolysis during sleep, resulting in the presence of hemoglobin in the urine on awakening. (Oral Med.)

hemolysin (hē-mol′ĭ-sĭn) An antibody that causes hemolysis of red blood cells in vitro. (Oral Med.)

hemophilia (hē″mō-fĭl′ē-ah) **(bleeder's disease)** A sex-linked genetic disease manifested in males and characterized by severe hemorrhage. (Oral Diag.)

— A hereditary hypoprothrombinemia characterized by a delayed clotting time of the blood. It is inherited by males through the mother as a sex-linked characteristic. (Oral Path.)

h. A (classic h.) A hemorrhagic diathesis due to a deficiency of antihemophilic globulin (AHG); inherited as a recessive sex-linked characteristic and characterized by recurrent bouts of bleeding from even trivial injury. The coagulation time is prolonged, but the bleeding time is normal. (Oral Med.)

h. B (Christmas disease, h. II, hemophilioid state C) A hemorrhagic diathesis due to a deficiency of plasma thromboplastin component (PTC); transmitted as a sex-linked recessive characteristic and characterized clinically by the same manifestations as classic hemophilia. There is a delay in the generation of thromboplastin. The platelet count, bleeding time, tourniquet test, and thrombin and prothrombin times are normal. (Oral Med.)

h. C (plasma thromboplastin antecedent [PTA] deficiency, Rosenthal's syndrome) A hemophilia-like condition thought to be due to a deficiency of plasma thromboplastin antecedent (PTA), transmitted as a simple autosomal dominant, and characterized by a moderate bleeding tendency after extraction of teeth or after tonsillectomy. Prothrombin consumption and thromboplastin generation are abnormal. (Oral Med.) (see also **factor XI**)

classic h. (see **hemophilia A**)

vascular h. A hereditary hemorrhagic disorder affecting both sexes and associated with a deficiency of antihemophilic globulin and vascular abnormalities characteristic of pseudohemophilia (von Willebrand's disease). The bleeding time is prolonged, and severity of bleeding varies considerably from one person to another. (Oral Med.)

hemophilioid state A (hē″mō-fĭl′ē-oid) (see **parahemophilia**)

hemophilioid state C (see **hemophilia B**)

hemoptysis (hē-mop′tĭ-sĭs) Expectoration of blood, by coughing, from the larynx or lower respiratory tract. (Oral Diag.)

hemorrhage (hĕm′or-ĭj) Escape of blood from the blood vessels; bleeding. (Oral Diag.)

hemorrhagic bone cyst (see **cyst, hemorrhagic**)

hemosiderin (hē″mō-sĭd′er-ĭn) A dark yellow-brown pigment that contains iron. (Oral Path.)

hemostasis (hē″mō-stā′sĭs) The arrest of an escape of blood. (Oral Surg.)

hemostatic (hē″mō-stăt-ĭk) An agent used to reduce bleeding from minute vessels by hastening the clotting of blood or by the formation of an artificial clot. (Oral Med.; Pharmacol.)

Henderson's test (see **test, Henderson's**)

hepatitis (hĕp″ah-tī′tĭs) Inflammation of the liver. (Oral Med.)

homologous serum h. (homologous serum jaundice, serum h., syringe jaundice, type B h.) A viral hepatitis clinically difficult to distinguish from epidemic infectious hepatitis. It is transmitted by human serum (parenteral injection, transfusions, lacerations). The incubation period is 40 to 90 days or longer. Principal manifestations are jaundice, gastrointestinal symptoms, anorexia, and malaise. (Oral Med.)

infectious h. (IH, type A h.) A viral hepatitis that is frequently epidemic in nature and that has an incubation period of 1 to 4 or even 7 weeks. It is usually transmitted by the virus in fecal matter but may be transmitted by human serum (transfusions, lacerations, needle puncture). (Oral Med.)

serum h. (see **hepatitis, homologous serum**)

hereditary benign intraepithelial dyskeratosis A hereditary disease seen in triracial isolates (white, Indian, Negro). It involves the oral mucosa and periodic seasonal keratoconjunctivitis. (Oral Diag.)

heredity The inheritance of resemblance, physical qualities, or disease from a familial predecessor; the passage of characteristics from one generation to its progeny by genetic linkage. (Periodont.)

Hering-Breuer reflex (hĕr'ĭng-broi'er) (see **reflex, Hering-Breuer**)

hermetic seal (see **seal, hermetic**)

herpangina (her"păn-jī-nah) **(Coxsackie A disease)** A disease of children caused by Coxsackie virus and characterized by ulcers at the posterior region of the soft palate. (Oral Diag.)

— A viral disease of children occurring usually in summer and characterized by sudden onset, fever (100° to 105° F), sore throat, and oropharyngeal vesicles. It is due to Coxsackie A viruses and is self-limiting. (Oral Med.)

herpes labialis (her'pēz lā"bē-ăl'ĭs) **(cold sore)** A disease of the lips caused by herpesvirus and characterized by vesicles that rupture, leaving ulcers. The local lesions are often called fever blisters or cold sores. Herpes simplex of the lips. (Oral Diag.; Oral Path.)

herpes simplex (hĕr'pēz sĭm'plĕx) Infection caused by the herpes simplex virus. Primary infection, occurring most often in children between 2 and 5 years of age, may result in apparent clinical disease or such manifestations as acute herpetic gingivostomatitis, keratoconjunctivitis, vulvovaginitis, or encephalitis. Recurrent manifestations include herpes labialis (fever blisters or cold sores), dendritic corneal ulcers, or genital herpes simplex. (Oral Med.)

— An acute viral disease characterized by the formation of groups of vesicles on the skin and mucous membranes, such as the borders of the lips. (Oral Path.) (see also **herpes labialis**)

— The virus or the acute viral disease affecting the skin and mucous membranes. The disease is characterized by erythema, vesicles, ulceration, and pain. (Periodont.)

herpes zoster (her'pēz zahs'ter) **(acute posterior ganglionitis, shingles)** An inflammatory disease caused by a virus and affecting the cerebral ganglia and the ganglia of the posterior nerve roots. The lesions are vesicles that rupture and ulcerate and that are present on the skin over the distribution of the nerves from the affected ganglia. (Oral Diag.)

— An acute viral disease with lesions involving the dorsal spinal root or cranial nerve and producing vesicular eruption in areas of the skin corresponding to the involved sensory nerve. Pain is a prominent feature and may persist, although skin lesions subside in 1 to 2 weeks. (Oral Med.)

— An acute viral disease caused by *Herpesvirus varicellae* and characterized by the formation of vesicles having reddish peripheries in the cutaneous areas supplied by certain nerve trunks. (Oral Path.)

— Acute inflammatory disease of the cerebral ganglia and the ganglia of the posterior nerve roots, characterized by the appearance of the small vesicles on erythematous bases over the line of distribution of the nerve trunks. Oral lesions occur on the anterior portion of the tongue, the soft palate, the cheek, and occasionally, the gingivae. (Periodont.)

herpetic lesion (see **lesion, herpetic**)

herpetic ulcer (see **ulcer, herpetic**)

heteresthesia (hĕt"er-ĕs-thē'zē-ah) Variation in the degree of cutaneous sensibility on adjoining areas of the body surface. (Anesth.)

heterograft (see **graft**)

heterozygous (hĕt"er-ō-zī'gŭs) Term indicating that genes lying at equivalent loci on chromosome pairs are different. (Oral Med.)

HGF (see **glucagon**)

hiccup An involuntary spasmodic contraction of the diaphragm that causes a beginning inspiration that is suddenly checked by closure of the glottis, thus producing a characteristic sound. (Anesth.)

hidrosis (hī-drō'sĭs) The secretion of sweat. (Oral Diag.)

high labial arch (see **arch, high labial**)

high lip line (see **lip line, high**)

high speed (see **speed, high**)

high-pressuring The forcing of extensive dental treatment on a patient who is not completely convinced of its necessity. (Pract. Man.)

high-pull headgear Apparatus designed to give an upward pull on the face-bow. (Orthodont.)

high-speed handpiece (see **handpiece, high-speed**)

hinchazon (hĭnch"ah-zon') (see **beriberi**)

hinge axis (see **axis, hinge**)

hinge axis determination (see **axis, hinge, determination**)

hinge axis–orbital plane (see **axis, hinge, orbital plane**)

hinge axis point (see **point, hinge axis**)

hinge-bow The kinematic face-bow used to determine the location of the hinge axis when it is rearmost is a three-piece instrument with independently adjustable arms controlled by slow screws that lengthen or shorten them. Other slow screws raise or lower the caliper points to find the spots in or on the skin near the tragi where only rotary movements occur when the jaw is opened and closed at the rearmost point. (Gnathol.) (see also **face-bow, kinematic**)

hinge movement (see **movement, hinge**)

hinge position (see **position, hinge**)

Hinton's test (see **test, Hinton's**)

hippus, respiratory (hĭp'ŭs) Dilation of the pupils occurring during inspiration, and contraction of the pupils occurring during expiration; often associated with pulsus paradoxus. (Anesth.)

Hirschfeld-Dunlop file (see **file, Hirschfeld-Dunlop**)

Hirschfeld's method; point, Hirschfeld's silver (see under appropriate noun)

hirsutism (her'sūt-ĭzm) Increased body or facial hair, which is especially noted in the female. (Oral Diag.)

histiocyte (hĭs'tē-ō-sīt") A large phagocytic cell found in the interstices of the tissues; of reticuloendothelial origin. (Periodont.)

histiocytosis, nonlipid (hĭs"tē-ō-sī-tō'sĭs) (see **disease, Letterer-Siwe**)

histiocytosis X A group of diseases characterized by abnormal histiocytic activity. Includes a chronic disseminated type (Hand-Schüller-Christian disease) and a chronic localized type (eosinophilic granuloma). (Oral Diag.)

acute disseminated h. X (see **disease, Letterer-Siwe**)

chronic disseminated h. X (see **disease, Hand-Schüller-Christian**)

histoclasia, implant (hĭs"tō-klā'zē-ah) A condition of the tissues existing in the presence of an implant in which the implant is not directly involved. It is a condition of the oral mucosal tissues in which the pathology is due to some external cause, e.g., salivary calculus or attached prosthetic appliances. (Oral Implant.)

histoplasmosis (hĭs"tō-plăz-mō'sĭs) A disease caused by the fungus *Histoplasma capsulatum* and affecting the reticuloendothelial system. Ulceration of the oral mucosa may occur. (Oral Diag.)

— A systemic mycotic infection caused by *Histoplasma capsulatum*. (Oral Path.)

history, case The events associated with a disease condition that may aid in its diagnosis. Family, medical, dental, nutritional, personal, and social histories may be included. (Oral Diag.)

— A record of the facts obtained from the patient that will assist in arriving at a diagnosis. (Oral Surg.)

— A detailed and concise compilation of all physical, dental, social, and mental factors relative and necessary to diagnosis, prognosis, and treatment. (Periodont.; Pract. Man.)

dental c. h. An investigation into experiences, attitudes, and treatment and conditions present at the time of examination. (Pract. Man.; Periodont.)

histotoxic (hĭs-tō-tahk'sĭk) Relating to poisoning

of the respiratory enzyme system of the tissues. (Anesth.)

hives (see **urticaria**)

Hodgkin's disease (see **disease, Hodgkin's**)

hoe An angled instrument with the broad dimension of its blade perpendicular to the axis of the shank of the shaft; used to develop internal form of cavity preparations, as compared with a chisel, which is intended to cut enamel. Used with a push, pull, or scraping stroke. (Oper. Dent.)

— An instrument designed for the removal of calcareous deposits from the teeth. Its working blade is bent to a right angle, thus permitting a pull stroke when the edge of the angled blade is applied so as to engage the apical edge of the calculus. (Periodont.)

hold To possess by reason of a lawful title. (D. Juris.)

holder An apparatus or instrument that is used to hold something. (Oper. Dent.)

broach h. (see **broach holder**)

clamp h. (see **holder, rubber dam clamp**)

matrix h. (see **retainer, matrix**)

rubber dam h. An apparatus used to hold a rubber dam in place on the face and to secure the edges of the dam clear of the field of operation; usually metal clips, which are connected by adjustable tapes or elastic placed around the back of the head, grip each side of the dam. (Endodont.; Oper. Dent.)

rubber dam clamp h. (clamp h.) An instrument used to engage the holes or notches of the flanges of a rubber dam clamp, so that the clamp can be placed on a tooth, adjusted, or removed. (Oper. Dent.)

Hollenback condenser (see **condenser, pneumatic**)

hollow bulb That portion of a prosthesis made hollow to minimize weight. (M.F.P.)

home care The physiotherapeutic measures employed by the patient for the maintenance of dental and periodontal health. Includes proper toothbrushing, stimulation of gingival tissues, etc. (Periodont.)

homeostasis (hō"mē-ō-stā'sĭs) Term used to describe the tendency toward physiologic equilibration; e.g., acid-base balance, pH level of blood, or blood sugar level. (Oral Med.)

— A concept that is basic to the comprehension of cell and tissue behavior. When applied to cellular behavior, the term homeostasis means a tendency of cells, tissues, and organisms to maintain the consistency of the internal environment. This simple principle also applies when the organism must adjust to external stimuli that arise from complex social situations. Responses to these motivations are considered adjustments in behavior and express the external relationships between the person and his social environment. (Oral Physiol.)

cell h. The tendency of biologic tissues and processes to maintain a constancy of environment consistent with their vitality and well-being. For cells to maintain their stability or equilibrium, the cell membranes must be in continuous interaction with both the internal (intracellular) environment and the external (extracellular) environment. When the equilibrium of any component is disturbed, the interaction permits automatic readjustment by giving rise to stimuli that result in restoration of the equilibrium. (Oral Physiol.)

homograft (see **graft**)

homozygous (hō-mō-zī′gŭs) Term indicating that genes lying at equivalent loci on chromosome pairs are the same. (Oral Med.)

hook, skin A metallic instrument ending in a fine, sharp hook for handling soft tissues during surgery. (Oral Surg.)

Hoover's sign (see **sign, Hoover's**)

HOP Abbreviation for high oxygen pressure. (Anesth.)

horizontal overlap (see **overlap, horizontal**)

horizontal plane (see **plane, horizontal**)

hormone(s) Biochemical secretions of the endocrine glands that, in relatively small quantities, partially regulate the physiologic activity of the tissues, organs, organ systems, and other endocrine glands, and of the nervous system itself. The hormonal secretions are conducted and distributed throughout the body by the circulation of the bloodstream and tissue fluids. (Oral Physiol.)

adenohypophyseal h. Hormones secreted by the adenohypophysis. Includes seven distinct hormones: somatotropin (STH), thyrotropin (TSH), prolactin, follicle-stimulating hormone (FSH), luteinizing hormone (LH), melanocyte-stimulating hormone (MSH), and adrenocorticotropic hormone (ACTH). (Oral Med.)

adrenal medullary h. Hormones secreted by adrenal medulla, including two catechol-amines: epinephrine and norepinephrine. (Oral Med.)

adrenocortical h. Steroid hormones secreted by the adrenal cortex that are biologically active in one or more of the following states: stress, inflammation, metabolism of carbohydrates, proteins, electrolytes, and water.

(Oral Med.) (see also **steroid, adrenocortical**)

— A hormone produced by the adrenal cortex, the principal constituent of which is hydrocortisone, a 17-OH ketosteroid. (Periodont.)

adrenocorticotropic h. (see **ACTH**)

adrenotropic h. (see **ACTH**)

androgenic h. (see **hormones, sex, male**)

anterior pituitary-like h. (see **hormone, pregnancy**)

antidiabetic h. (see **insulin**)

antidiuretic h. (ADH, vasopressin) A hormone of the posterior pituitary gland that encourages reabsorption of water by acting on the epithelial cells of the distal portion of the renal tubule. The pressor-antidiuretic principle of the neurohypophysis. It raises blood pressure by its effect on the peripheral blood vessels and exerts an antidiuretic effect (antifacultative resorption of water in the renal tubules). An absence of ADH causes diabetes insipidus. (Oral Med.)

anti-inflammatory h. (see **glucocorticoids**)

corticosteroid h. (see **steroid, adrenocortical**)

corticotropic h. (see **ACTH**)

diabetogenic h. Principally, the pituitary growth hormone, which tends to elevate the blood sugar by acting as an antagonist to insulin. It is probably not a distinct entity, and its effects are probably related to those of known pituitary hormones. (Oral Med.)

estrogenic h. (follicular h.) Substances capable of producing estrus in lower animals. In women they prepare the uterus for the action of progestational hormones, suppress the follicle-stimulating hormones, and are active in maintaining secondary female sex characteristics. Include estradiol, estrone, and estriol. (Oral Med.)

— Any one of the ovarian or adrenal hormones (e.g., estradiol, estrone, and estriol) that is capable of stimulating changes of a cyclic nature in the genital system. One of the ovarian or adrenal hormones capable of affecting the cyclic changes of the female genital system. (Periodont.)

follicle-stimulating h. A pituitary tropic hormone that promotes the growth and maturation of the ovarian follicle and, with other gonadotropins, induces secretion of estrogens, and possibly spermatogenesis. (Oral Med.)

follicular h. (see **hormones, estrogenic**)

gastrointestinal h. Hormones that regulate motor and secretory activity of the digestive organs, i.e., gastrin, secretin, and cholecystokinin. (Oral Med.)

gonadotropic h. (see **gonadotropin**)

 chorionic g. h. A glycoprotein secreted by placental tissue early in normal pregnancy but also found in the urine or blood in association with chorioepitheliomas and some neoplastic diseases of the testis. (Oral Med.)

growth h. (somatotropic h., somatotropin) A pituitary hormone that stimulates growth of soft tissues and long bones at the epiphyses. It also has a diabetogenic effect. (Oral Med.)

— A growth, or somatotropic, hormone that is secreted by the anterior lobe of the pituitary gland and that exerts an influence on skeletal growth. As long as the growth apparatus is functional, it is responsive to the effects of the hormone. (Oral Physiol.)

ketogenic h. Term used to describe a factor of the anterior pituitary hormone responsible for ketogenic effect. It is probably not an entity differing from known pituitary hormones. (Oral Med.)

lactogenic h. (galactin, mammotropin, prolactin) A pituitary hormone that stimulates lactation. (Oral Med.)

luteal h. (see **hormones, progestational**)

luteinizing h. A pituitary hormone that causes ovulation and development of the corpus luteum from the mature graafian follicle. It is called an interstitial cell–stimulating hormone because of its action on the testis in maintaining spermatogenesis and because of its role in the development of accessory sex organs. (Oral Med.)

melanocyte-stimulating h. (intermedin, MSH) A hormone of the middle lobe of the pituitary gland that increases melanin deposition by the melanocytes of the skin. (Oral Med.)

N h. (see **hormone, nitrogen; steroid, C-19 cortico-**)

neurohypophyseal h. Octapeptides of the neural lobe: oxytocin and vasopressin. (Oral Med.)

nitrogen h. (N h.) C-19 corticosteroids that have androgenic and protein anabolic effects. (Oral Med.)

parathyroid h. Hormones of the parathyroid gland that have a profound effect on calcium and phosphorus metabolism. There is increasing evidence that there are probably two such hormones: a calcium-mobilizing principle and a substance that produces phosphaturia. Abnormalities of parathyroid function include hyperparathyroidism and hypoparathyroidism. (Oral Med.)

— The secretory product of the parathyroid glands that controls the renal excretion of phosphorus and consequently calcium. Excessive secretion of the parathyroid hormone, by lowering the renal threshold for phosphorus, produces generalized bone resorption, formation of fibrous marrow in the spongiosa, and, in young individuals, hypocalcification of the teeth. (Periodont.)

pituitary h. Hormones of the anterior lobe of the pituitary gland, including the growth hormones (somatotropin 1, lactogenic hormone, prolactin, galactin, mammotropin) and pituitary tropins (gonadotropins, thyrotropic hormone, and ACTH). Whether or not a true diabetogenic pituitary hormone exists is a question. The melanocyte-stimulating hormone is secreted by the middle lobe of the pituitary gland, and vasopressin and oxytocin are secreted by the posterior lobe of the pituitary gland. (Oral Med.)

pregnancy h. (anterior pituitary-like h., antuitrin S, chorionic gonadotropin) A gonadotropic hormone found in the urine during pregnancy; it is a product of the very early placenta. (Oral Med.)

progestational h. (luteal h.) Hormones produced during the phase of the menstrual cycle just preceding menstruation. Includes progesterone, pregnanediol, and pregneninolone. (Oral Med.)

proinflammatory h. (see **mineralocorticoids**)

"S" h. (glucocorticoid factor, sugar h.) A factor in the secretions of the adrenal cortex related to the regulation of carbohydrate metabolism. (Oral Med.)

sex h. Steroid hormones that are produced by the testes and ovaries and that control secondary sex characteristics, the reproductive cycle, development of the accessory reproductive cycle, and development of the accessory reproductive organs. Also included are the gonadotropins produced by the pituitary gland. (Oral Med.)

 female sex h. Hormones secreted by the ovary. They include two main types: the follicular, or estrogenic, hormones produced by the graafian follicle, and the progestational hormones from the corpus luteum. (Oral Med.)

 male sex h. (androgenic h., C-19 steroids) Hormones found in the testes, the urine, or the blood. Included are testosterone found in the testes, andosterone excreted into the urine, and dehydro-3-epiandrosterone found in the blood. (Oral Med.)

somatotropic h. (see **hormone, growth**)

steroid h. A group of biologically active organic compounds that are secreted by the adrenal cortex, testis, ovary, and placenta, and that have in common a cyclopentanoperhydrophenanthrene nucleus. (Oral Med.)

sugar h. (see **hormone, "S"; steroid, C-21 cortico-**)

testicular h. Hormones elaborated by the testis (chiefly testosterone) that promote the growth and function of the male genitalia and secondary sex characteristics and that have potent protein anabolic effects. (Oral Med.)

thyroid h. Hormonal variants, including thyroxin and triiodothyronine, derived from the thyroid gland. Thyroid hormone acts as a catalyst for oxidative processes of the body cell and thus regulates the rates of body metabolism and stimulates body growth and maturation. (Oral Med.)

thyroid-stimulating h. (see **hormone, thyrotropic**)

thyrotropic h. (thyroid-stimulating h., TSH) A pituitary hormone that regulates the growth and activity of the thyroid gland. (Oral Med.)

horn, pulp A small projection of vital pulp tissue directly under a cusp or developmental lobe. (Oper. Dent.)

p. h., recessional lines The lines along which the pulp has receded during the growth of the dentin. They lead from the axio-occlusal margin or crest of pulp on one of its angles toward the point of each of the cusps of a tooth and constitute an important factor in the design of cavity preparations because accidental pulp exposure may occur through cutting across such a line. (Oper. Dent.)

hospital An institution for the care of sick, wounded, infirm, or aged persons; generally incorporated as a nonprofit organization. (D. Juris.)

host site An anatomic area surgically prepared to receive an implant or graft. (Oral Implant.)

Howard's method (see **method, Howard's**)

Howe's silver nitrate (see **silver nitrate, ammoniacal**)

Howe's silver precipitation method (see **method, Howe's silver precipitation**)

h.s. Abbreviation for *hora somni,* a Latin phrase meaning at bedtime. (Oral Med.; Pharmacol.)

humectant (hū-měk'tănt) A substance that prevents loss of moisture. (Oral Med.; Pharmacol.)

Hunter's glossitis (see **glossitis, Moeller's**)

Hunt's syndrome (see **syndrome, Hunt's**)

hurt To molest or restrain; not restricted to physical injuries; also includes mental pain, discomfort, or annoyance. (D. Juris.)

husband A man who has a wife. (D. Juris.)

Hutchinson-Gilford syndrome (see **syndrome, Hutchinson-Gilford**)

Hutchinson's incisors (see **incisors, Hutchinson's**)

Hutchinson triad (see **triad, Hutchinson**)

HVL (see **half-value layer**)

hyalinization (hī"ah-lǐn"ǐ-zā'shŭn) The appearance of an acellular, avascular, homogeneous area in the periodontal ligament where compression of the ligament between bone and tooth occurs as a result of orthodontic forces. (Orthodont.)

h. of periodontal ligament A degenerative process due to long-continued occlusal trauma in which the fibers become hyalinized into a homogeneous mass. (Periodont.)

hyaluronidase (hī"ah-lū-ron'ǐ-dās) An enzyme that produces hydrolysis of hyaluronic acid, the cementing substance of the tissues. Produced by certain pathogenic bacteria formed in testes. (Periodont.)

hydraulicity (hī"draw-lǐ'sǐ-tē) The ability of a material (cement) to set while in contact with moisture. (Oper. Dent.)

hydraulic pressure (see **pressure, hydraulic**)

hydremia (hī"drē'mē-ah) Increase in blood volume caused by an increase in serum volume. This may result from cardiac failure, renal insufficiency, pregnancy, or the intravenous administration of fluids. (Oral Physiol.)

hydroalcoholic (hī"drō-ăl-kō-hol'ĭk) Containing both water and alcohol. (Oral Med.; Pharmacol.) (see also **solution**)

Hydrocal (hī'drō-kăl) Trade name for a gypsum product, alpha-hemihydrate, known as artificial stone. It is used for making casts. (Comp. Prosth.; D. Mat.; Oper. Dent.; Remov. Part. Prosth.)

hydrocephalus (hī"drō-sěf'ah-lŭs) Abnormal accumulation of fluid in the cranial vault, resulting in a disproportionately large cranium. (Oral Diag.)

hydrocolloid (hī"drō-kol'oid) The materials listed as colloid sols with water; used in dentistry as elastic impression materials. Hydrocolloids can be reversible or irreversible. (Comp. Prosth.; Oper. Dent.; Periodont.; Remov. Part. Prosth.)

—An agar-base impression material. (D. Mat.)

irreversible h. (alginate) A hydrocolloid whose physical condition is changed by a chemical action that is not reversible. It is an impression material that is elastic when set. (Comp. Prosth.; Remov. Part. Prosth.) (see also **alginate**)

—Gel formed by precipitation of insoluble calcium alginate—an irreversible chemical reaction. A material employed in making diagnostic casts and partial denture impressions. (D. Mat.)

reversible h. (agar-agar type) A hydrocolloid whose physical condition is changed by temperature. The material is made fluid by heat and becomes an elastic solid on cooling. (Comp. Prosth.; Remov. Part. Prosth.)

— A hydrocolloid that changes from the sol to the gel state or from the gel to the sol state with temperature change—purely a physical phenomenon. Materials used for inlay, crown, and other indirect restorative procedures. (D. Mat.)

hydrocortisone (hī″drō-kor′tē-sōn) **(cortisol)** A glucocorticosteroid secreted by the adrenal cortex in response to stimulation by ACTH. It is antianabolic, stimulates gluconeogenesis, and probably acts on some cellular system in response to a need for adaptation to change (stress). (Oral Med.)

hydrolysis (hī-drol′ĭ-sĭs) Reaction between the ions of salt and those of water to form an acid and a base, one or both of which is only slightly dissociated. A process whereby a large molecule is split by the addition of water. The end products divide the water, the hydroxyl group being attached to one and the hydrogen ion to the other. (Anesth.)

— The splitting of a compound into two parts, with the addition of the elements of water. (Oral Med.; Pharmacol.)

hydrophilic (hī″drō-fĭl′ĭk) Having an affinity for water. Opposite of lipophilic. (Oral Med.; Pharmacol.) (see also **ointment, hydrophilic**)

hydroquinone (hī-drō-kwĭn′ōn) A reducing agent used as an inhibitor in resin monomers to prevent polymerization during storage. (D. Mat.)

— One of the two chemicals used as reducing agents in film-developing solutions. It is made from benzene (paradihydroxy-benzene) and is sensitive to thermal changes. Above 70° F its action is rapid; below 60° F it becomes inactive. Its action is to control the contrast of the film. (Oral Radiol.)

hydrostatic pressure (hī″drō-stăt′ĭk) (see **pressure, hydrostatic**)

hydrotherapy (hī″drō-thĕr′ah-pē) An empirical adjunct to oral physiotherapy where forced water irrigation is used to cleanse subgingival spaces, remove debris from interproximal spaces, and cleanse pockets. (Periodont.)

hydroxyapatite (hī-drok″sē-ăp′ah-tīt) A mineral compound of the general formula $3Ca_3(PO_4)_2 \cdot Ca(OH)_2$, which is the principal inorganic component of bone, teeth, and dental calculus. (Periodont.)

hygiene (hī′jēn) The science of health and its preservation.

oral h. (mouth h.) The practice of personal oral physiotherapy; the maintenance of a state of oral cleanliness and improved tissue tone by toothbrushing, tissue stimulation and massage, hydrotherapy, etc., for the prevention of disease and the preservation of oral health. (Periodont.)

— The general care given by the patient to the teeth, oral structures, and oral prosthesis, if any. (Remov. Part. Prosth.)

radiation h. The art and science of protecting human beings from injury by radiation. Since any amount of radiation is harmful in some degree, the ideal objective is to prevent the exposure of any person without a definite medical purpose. (Oral Radiol.)

hygienist, dental A person trained in an accredited school or dental college and licensed by the state in which she resides to practice the art of dental prophylaxis under the direction of a licensed dentist. (Pract. Man.)

— One trained and utilized to perform initial scaling for new patients, teach oral physiotherapy, and maintain recall patients, among many other duties necessary for a well-functioning office. (Periodont.)

hygroma (hī-grō′mah) A sac or cyst swollen with fluid.

h. colli cysticum (cystic h., cystic lymphangioma) A cavernous lymphangioma involving the neck. It may be of large size, impairing breathing and swallowing. (Oral Diag.)

hygroscopic (hī″grō-skop′ĭk) Having the property of absorbing moisture. When applied to gypsum products in contact with free water during their set, the resultant expansion is implied. (Oper. Dent.) (see also **expansion, hygroscopic**)

— Having such a strong affinity for water that it tends to absorb moisture from the air to an unusual degree. (Pharmacol.)

h. investment (see **investment, hygroscopic**)

hypacusis (hī″pah-kū′sĭs) A hearing disorder associated with diminished hearing function. (Oral Physiol.)

hypalgesia (hī″păl-jē′zē-ah) Diminished sensitiveness to pain that results from a raised pain threshold. (Anesth.)

hyper- (hī′per) A prefix signifying above, beyond, or excessive. (Anesth.)

hyperadrenocorticism (hī″per-ah-drē″nō-kor′tĭ-sĭzm) Adrenocortical hyperfunction due to neoplasia of the cortex, hyperplasia of the cortex secondary to an increase in ACTH, or prolonged administration of steroid hormones of ACTH. Manifestations include hyperglycemia, edema, hypertension, glycosuria, negative nitrogen balance, acne, and hirsutism. (Oral Med.) (see also **syndrome, adrenogenital; syndrome, Cushing's**)

hyperalgesia (hī″per-ăl-jē′zē-ah) A greater-than-normal sensitivity to pain that may be due to a painful stimulus or a lowered pain threshold. (Anesth.)

— An altered pain threshold, resulting in a superficial, poorly localized burning sensation to stimuli that are not normally painful. (Oral Med.)

hyperalgia (hī-per-ăl′jē-ah) Abnormal sensitivity to pain. (Anesth.)

hypercalcemia (hī″per-kăl-sē′mē-ah) **(hypercalcinemia)** Elevated blood calcium level. (Oral Diag.)

— Abnormal elevation of calcium in the blood. Causes include primary hyperparathyroidism, sarcoidosis, multiple myeloma, malignant neoplasms, prolonged androgen therapy, massive doses of vitamin D, etc. Symptoms suggestive of hypercalcemia are nausea, vomiting, constipation, polyuria, weight loss, muscular weakness, and polydipsia. The normal level of total serum calcium is 8.5 to 10.5 mg/100 ml. (Oral Med.)

hypercalcinemia (see **hypercalcemia**)

hypercalcinuria (see **hypercalciuria**)

hypercalciuria (hī″per-kăl″sē-ū′rē-ah) **(hypercalcinuria)** Excessive urinary excretion of calcium. (Oral Diag.)

— A condition in which there is an excessive increase in urinary calcium excretion. Major causes include primary hyperparathyroidism, hypervitaminosis D, excessive milk intake, metastatic malignancy, immobilization, and renal tubular acidosis. (Oral Med.) (see also **hypercalcemia** for normal values)

hypercapnia (hī″per-kăp′nē-ah) Presence of more than the normal amount of carbon dioxide in the blood tissues due to either an increase of carbon dioxide in the inspired air or a decrease in elimination. (Anesth.)

hypercementosis (hī″per-sē″měn-tō′sĭs) Excessive formation of cementum on the roots of one or more teeth. (Oral Diag.)

— Excessive production of the cementum of a tooth. (Oral Path.)

— Formation of excessive secondary cementum, especially about the root apices; primarily, a proliferative cementoblastic action to maintain biologic width of the periodontal membrane. (Periodont.)

hypercenesthesia (hī″per-sěn″ěs-thē′zē-ah) A feeling of exaggerated well-being such as is seen in general paralysis and sometimes in mania. (Anesth.)

hyperchloremia (hī″per-klō-rē′mē-ah) Excessive concentration of chloride in the plasma. Normal range is 98 to 106 mEq/L. It may occur in water depletion, dehydration, decreased bicarbonate concentration, or metabolic acidosis. (Oral Med.)

hyperemia (hī″per-ē′mē-ah) **(congestion)** Excessive amount of blood in the vessels in any part of the body. (Anesth.; Oral Diag.)

— An increased and excessive amount of blood in a tissue. The hyperemia may be active or passive. (Oral Physiol.)

— Increased accumulation and flow of blood through a tissue or part of the body. (Periodont.)

active h. Hyperemia caused by an increased flow of blood to an area by active dilation of both the arterioles and capillaries. It is associated with neurogenic, hormonal, and metabolic function. (Oral Physiol.)

passive h. Hyperemia caused by a decreased outflow of blood from an area. It may be generalized, resulting from cardiac, renal, or pulmonary disorders, or it may be localized, as in the oral cavity, and caused by pressure from mechanical or physical obstruction or by pressure from a tumor, denture, filling, or salivary calculus. (Oral Physiol.)

hyperesthesia (hī″per-ěs-thē′zē-ah) Excessive sensitivity of the skin or of a special sense. (Anesth.)

— Excessive sensitivity of a part or region. (Oper. Dent.; Oral Diag.)

hyperesthetic (hī″per-ěs-thět′ĭk) Pertaining to or affected with hyperesthesia. (Anesth.)

hyperfunction Increase in activity of a part or in the stresses applied to a part; particularly, the adaptive changes occurring in the attachment apparatus of a tooth incident to increased or heavy function. (Periodont.)

hypergammaglobulinemia (hī″per-găm″ah-glob″ū-lĭn-ē′mē-ah) An excess of gamma globulin in the blood. It occurs in chronic granulomatous inflammations, chronic bacterial infections, liver disease, multiple myeloma, lymphomas, and dysproteinemias. (Oral Med.)

hyperglobulinemia (hī″per-glob″u-lĭn-ē′mē-ah) Abnormally high concentration of globulins in the blood. (Oral Med.)

hyperglycemia (hī″per-glī-sē′mē-ah) Increase in the concentration of sugar in the blood. It is a feature of diabetes mellitus. (Oral Med.)

hypergonadism (hī″per-gō′năd-ĭzm) Excessive secretion of hormonal agents by the testes or ovaries. Gingival changes induced by the administration of estrogens and androgens include an increase in keratinization and hyperplasia of epithelial and connective tissue. (Periodont.)

hyperhidrosis (hī″per-hī-drō′sĭs) Excessive sweating, which may be generalized or localized. (Oral Diag.; Oral Med.)

    gustatory h. Increased sweating in the preauricular region, forehead, or face associated with eating. (Oral Diag.; Oral Surg.) (see also **syndrome, auriculotemporal**)

    masticatory h. Excessive sweating associated with chewing. The cause is traumatic injury producing anastomosis of the facial nerve with a sympathetic branch. (Oral Diag.)

hyperkalemia (hī″per-kah-lē′mē-ah) Abnormally elevated concentration of serum potassium. It may occur in renal failure, shock, and advanced dehydration, and in association with high intracellular potassium in Addison's disease. Normal adult range of serum potassium is 4.0 to 5.5 mEq/L. (Oral Med.)

hyperkeratosis (hī″per-ker″ah-tō′sĭs) Excessive formation of keratin; e.g., in leukoplakia. (Oral Diag.)

— Overproduction or retention of keratin on a skin or mucosal surface. (Oral Path.)

— Excessive deposition of keratin on the superficial layers of the eptihelium or the conversion of a superficial layer of the epithelium into keratin. Excessive production of keratin in any portion of the oral mucosa is considered to be a pathologic state. Some of the causes are vitamin A deficiency, mechanical or chemical irritation to the tissue, excessive androgenic and estrogenic stimulation, and neoplastic changes. (Periodont.)

hypermagnesemia (hī″per-măg″nĕ-sē′mē-ah) Excess of magnesium in the blood serum. Normal range is 1.5 to 2.5 mEq/L. It may result in respiratory failure and coma and may occur in untreated diabetic acidosis, renal failure, and severe dehydration. (Oral Med.)

hypernasality (hī″per-nāz-ăl′ĭ-tē) Excessive nasal resonance usually accompanied by emission of air through the nasal passageways. (Cleft Palate)

hypernatremia (hī″per-nā-trē′mē-ah) Abnormally elevated concentration of serum sodium. It may occur rarely in nephrosis, congestive heart failure, and Cushing's disease and after administration of ACTH, cortisone, or deoxycorticosterone. Normal adult range of serum sodium is 135 to 145 mEq/L. (Oral Med.)

hyperocclusion (traumatic) Premature tooth contact during mouth closure. (Endodont.)

hyperostosis (hī″per-os-tō′sĭs) Excessive growth of bone, as in infantile cortical hyperostosis. (Oral Diag.)

— Hypertrophy of bone. (Oral Path.) (see also **exostosis**)

    infantile cortical h. (Caffey's disease; Smyth's syndrome) Disturbance in bone development most often observed between the third and sixth month of life and characterized by sudden, localized swellings of the face and extremities and by new subperiosteal bone formation. (Oral Diag.)

    — A disease of infants of unknown etiology and characterized by tender soft tissue swelling that is followed by hyperostosis of the cortex of the underlying bone. The mandible, clavicle, and ulna are most frequently affected. (Oral Path.)

hyperoxia (hī″per-ok′sē-ah) An excess of oxygen in the system. (Anesth.)

hyperparathyroidism (hī″per-păr″ah-thī′roid-ĭzm) **(generalized osteitis fibrosa cystica, von Recklinghausen's disease of bone)** Excessive secretion of parathyroid hormone leading to osteitis fibrosa cystica. (Oral Diag.)

— Increased parathyroid function due to primary hyperplasia, to a functioning neoplasm of the parathyroid glands, or to secondary hyperplasia related most often to chronic renal insufficiency. Manifestations are related to abnormalities of the bones, kidneys, and blood vessels. Skeletal changes are referred to as generalized osteitis fibrosa cystica or von Recklinghausen's disease. Brown tumors, which are essentially giant cell tumors, may develop generally, as well as in the jaws. Kidney changes include renal stones and nephrocalcinosis. Calcification of muscles in arteries occurs. Renal rickets is associated with secondary hyperparathyroidism in children with chronic renal disease. Laboratory findings include high serum calcium, low phosphorus, and a normal or high alkaline phosphatase. Renal impairment, such as occurs in secondary hyperparathyroidism, tends to nullify hypercalcemia because of an increased loss of calcium in the urine. (Oral Med.)

— Abnormally increased activity of the parathyroid glands causing loss of calcium from the bones and resulting in tenderness in bones, spontaneous fractures, muscular weakness, and osteitis fibrosa. (Oral Path.)

— Excessive production of parathormone by the parathyroid gland (as in parathyroid hyperplasia and/or adenoma), resulting in increased renal excretion of phosphorus by lowering of the renal threshold for this substance. The pathologic changes produced are osteoporotic or osteodystrophic in nature as a consequence of withdrawal of calcium and phosphorus from osseous tissues. (Periodont.)

h., brown node of (see **node, brown, of hyperparathyroidism**)

hyperphosphatemia (hī″per-fos″fah-tē′mē-ah) Elevated blood phosphate level. (Oral Diag.)

— Abnormal elevation of phosphatase in the blood. An increase in alkaline phosphatase may occur in metabolic bone disease, liver disease, Paget's disease, osteogenic sarcoma, metastatic carcinoma from the prostate to bone, and local bone disease. Acid phosphatase is elevated in carcinoma of the bone that has metastasized from the prostate gland. Normal range of alkaline phosphatase in adults is 2 to 5 Bodansky units; in children, it is 5 to 15 units. Normal range of acid phosphatase is 0.1 to 0.8 unit. (Oral Med.)

— Increased concentration of inorganic phosphates in the blood serum. May occur in childhood and also in acromegaly, renal failure, and vitamin D intoxication. Normal adult range of serum inorganic phosphorus is 2.5 to 4.2 mg/100 ml. (Oral Med.)

hyperphosphaturia (hī″per-fos″fah-tū′rē-ah) Excessive excretion of phosphate in the urine. (Oral Diag.)

hyperpituitarism (hī″per-pĭ-tū′ĭ-tăr-ĭzm″) A condition caused by excessive production of the hormones secreted by the pituitary gland. An excess of the growth hormone results in giantism or acromegaly; an excess of ACTH produces Cushing's syndrome. (Oral Med.)

hyperplasia (hī″per-plā′zē-ah) Abnormal multiplication or increase in the number of normal cells in normal arrangement in a tissue, resulting in a thickening or enlargement of the tissue. (Comp. Prosth.; Oral Path.; Remov. Part. Prosth.)

— Increased growth of a tissue by increase in the number of cells. (Oral Diag.)

denture h. (denture hypertrophy) Enlargement of tissue beneath a denture that is traumatizing the soft tissue. If it occurs in the mucobuccal fold, it may be called epulis fissuratum. (Oral Diag.)

gingival h. Enlargement of the gingival tissue due to proliferation of its cellular elements. Hereditary or inflammatory etiology may be involved. (Periodont.)

—Proliferation of gingival epithelium to form elongated rete pegs and proliferation of fibroblasts with increased collagen formation in the underlying connective tissue; leads to nodular enlargement of the gingiva in diphenylhydantoin sodium therapy. (Oral Path.)

— A more or less bulbous gingival enlargement, primarily produced by proliferation of connective tissue elements; often accompanied by gingival inflammation as a result of trauma to the hyperplastic tissues and coincidental with or following the ingestion of diphenylhydantoin sodium. (Periodont.)

Dilantin g. h. (dī-lăn′tĭn) **(Dilantin enlargement)** Enlargement of the gingivae caused by the use of diphenylhydantoin sodium (Dilantin sodium) in the treatment of epilepsy. (Oral Diag.)

idiopathic g. h. (see **fibromatosis gingivae**)

inflammatory fibrous h. (see **epulis fissuratum**)

papillary h. A growth in the midline of the hard palate, usually in the relief area of a denture; characterized by a papillary, or raspberry, appearance. (Oral Diag.)

inflammatory p. h. (inflammatory papillomatosis, multiple papillomatosis, papillary hyperplasia) A condition of unknown etiology but associated with the presence of maxillary dentures. Characterized by numerous red papillary projections on the hard palate. (Oral Path.)

hyperplastic tissue (see **tissue, hyperplastic**)

hyperpnea (hī″perp-nē′ah) Abnormal increase in respiratory volume; an abnormal increase in the rate and depth of breathing. (Anesth.)

hyperpotassemia (hī″per-pot″ah-sē′mē-ah) (see **hyperkalemia**)

hyperproteinemia (hī″per-prō″tē-ĭ-nē′mē-ah) Abnormal increase in serum and plasma proteins. (Oral Med.)

hyperproteinuria (hī″per-prō″tē-ĭ-nū′rē-ah) (see **albuminuria**)

hypersalivation (see **sialorrhea**)

hypersensitive Abnormally sensitive. (Anesth.)

hypersensitiveness A state of altered reactivity in which the body reacts more strongly than normal to a foreign agent. (Anesth.)

hypersensitivity Adverse reaction to contact with specific substances in quantities that usually produce no reaction in normal individuals. (Oral Diag.)
— Usually, an allergic tendency. In general, a tendency to react with unusual violence to stimuli. (Oper. Dent.; Oral Med.; Pharmacol.)
— A common complaint after periodontal therapy in which dentin may be exposed, resulting in pain in the teeth or sensitivity to heat, cold, and sweet substances. (Periodont.)
   atopic h. (see **atopy**)
   bacterial h. Delayed inflammatory reaction due to previous sensitization of the host by an antigen. (Periodont.)
hypersensitization The process of rendering abnormally sensitive or the condition of being abnormally sensitive. (Anesth.)
hypersthenuria (hī″per-sthĕ-nū′rē-ah) Urine with an abnormally high specific gravity. It is seen in uncontrolled diabetes mellitus and in severe dehydration. (Oral Med.)
hypersusceptibility (hī″per-sŭh-sĕp″tĭ-bĭl′ĭ-tē) A condition of abnormal susceptibility to poisons, infective agents, or agents that are entirely innocuous in the normal individual. (Anesth.)
hypersympathicotonus (hī″per-sĭm-păth″ē-kō-tō′nŭs) Increased tonicity of the sympathetic nervous system. (Anesth.)
hypersystolic (hī″per-sĭs-tol′ĭk) Characterized by hypersystole; having heartbeats of excessive force. (Anesth.)
hypertarachia (hī″per-ta-răk′ē-ah) Extreme irritability of the nervous system. (Anesth.)
hypertelorism (hī″per-tē′lō-rĭzm) Excessive distance between paired organs. (Oral Med.) (see also **syndrome, Greig's** for ocular hypertelorism)
— Abnormal width between two organs or parts. Ocular hypertelorism is a feature of craniofacial deformity associated with defective development of the sphenoid bone. (Oral Diag.)
hypertension (hī″per-tĕn′shŭn) High blood pressure. (Oral Diag.)
— Abnormal elevation of systolic and/or diastolic arterial pressure. Systolic hypertension is generally related to emotional stress, sclerosis of the aorta and large arteries, or aortic insufficiency. Diastolic hypertension may be due to obscure causes (essential), renal disease, or endocrine disorders. (Oral Med.)
   essential h. Elevated blood pressure of unknown etiology. (Oral Med.)
   malignant h. Elevated blood pressure characterized by a progressive course uncontrollable by medication. (Oral Med.)

hyperthyroidism (Parry's disease) Excessive production of thyroid hormones, resulting in increased metabolism, exophthalmos, and other symptoms. (Oral Diag.)
— Abnormalities of calorigenic mechanisms, body tissues, blood, and body fluids and of the circulatory, muscular, and nervous systems due to an excessive elaboration of thyroid hormone. Manifestations include increased sweating, increased appetite, intolerance to heat, weight loss, increased protein-bound iodine (PBI), early shedding of primary teeth and early eruption of permanent teeth, tachycardia, palpitation, tremors, nervousness, muscular weakness, diarrhea, increased excretion of calcium and phosphorus, hypocholesterolemia, creatinuria, and osteoporosis. May occur as the result of primary hyperplasia, hyperfunctioning nodular goiters, functional benign tumor, or adenoma of the thyroid gland. (Oral Med.) (see also **goiter, exophthalmic**)
— Excessive secretion of the thyroid hormone, leading to weight loss, excitability, generalized osteoporosis, and increased basal metabolism. (Oral Path.)
— Excessive production of thyroxin by the thyroid gland or increased or excessive functional activity of the thyroid gland, resulting in increased metabolic rate, exophthalmos, tachycardia, excessive perspiration, nervousness, osteoporosis, and periodontal lesions resembling those seen in periodontosis. (Periodont.)
hypertonic (hī″per-ton′ĭk) Having an osmotic pressure greater than that of the solution with which it is compared. (Anesth.)
hypertrichosis (hī″per-trĭ-kō′sĭs) Excessive growth of hair on the body, possibly as a result of endocrine dysfunction, as in the hirsutism accompanying excessive adrenocortical function. (Periodont.)
hypertrophy Morbid enlargement or overgrowth of an organ or part due to an increase in size of its constituent cells. (Comp. Prosth.; Orthodont.; Remov. Part. Prosth.)
— Enlargement or overgrowth of an organ or part due to an increase in the size of its constituent cells. (Oral Diag.; Oral Path.)
   denture h. (see **hyperplasia, denture**)
   muscle h. Hypertrophy denotes an increase in the size or number of constituent fibers of a muscle. Any other condition (e.g., inflammation, tumor, or fatty infiltration) that increases the size of a muscle is called pseudohypertrophy. True or physiologic hypertrophy results from excessive activity of muscle. Genetic and hormonal factors play

a role in determining the size of muscles; e.g., muscles in the male tend to be larger than in the female in the temporal and facial regions. The histologic characteristics of hypertrophied muscle are normal. The fibrils are slightly wider in diameter than is normal, and the only change might be a slight increase in vascularity. (Oral Physiol.)

hyperventilation Abnormally prolonged, rapid, and deep breathing; also the condition produced by overbreathing of oxygen at high pressures. It is marked by confusion, dizziness, numbness, and muscular cramps brought on by such breathing. (Anesth.)
— Rapid, deep, forced breathing frequently resulting from anxiety. It results in a transient loss of carbon dioxide and respiratory alkalosis. Symptoms include anxiety, circumoral numbness, tingling sensation, faintness, and occasionally, carpopedal spasms, tetany, and syncope. (Oral Med.)

hypervitaminosis A (hī″per-vī″tah-mǐ-nō′sǐs) The effects of toxic doses of vitamin A. Manifestations include bone fragility, xeroderma, nausea, headache, and loss of hair. (Oral Med.)

hypervitaminosis D The toxic effects of ingesting large amounts of vitamin D. Manifestations include symptoms due to hypercalcemia, impairment of renal function, and metastatic calcification. (Oral Med.)

hypervolemia Increased blood volume. (Oral Med.)

hypnalgia (hǐp-nǎl′jē-ah) Pain that recurs during sleep. (Anesth.)

hypnesthesia (hǐp″nĕs-thē′zē′ah) Sleepiness. (Anesth.)

hypnic (hǐp′nǐk) Inducing or pertaining to sleep. (Anesth.)

hypno- (hǐp′nō) Combining form denoting a relationship to sleep. (Anesth.)

hypnosis (hǐp-nō′sǐs) A condition of artificially induced sleep or of a trance resembling sleep. (Anesth.)
— Sleep or a state closely resembling sleep, induced by drugs, psychologic means, or both. A trancelike state induced by psychologic means. (Oral Med.; Pharmacol.)

hypnotic (hǐp-not′ǐk) A drug that induces sleep or depresses the central nervous system at a cortical level. (Anesth.)
— Causing sleep or a trance. (Oral Med.; Pharmacol.) (see also **sedative**)

hypnotism The method or practice of inducing sleep. (Anesth.)
— In medical jurisprudence, a mental state rendering the patient susceptible to suggestion at the will and inducement of another. (D. Juris.)

hypnotize (hǐp′nō-tīz) To put into a state of hypnosis. (Anesth.)
— To introduce a trance by means of the power of suggestion. Utilized to secure the cooperation of patients by the alleviation of fears. (Pract. Man.)

hypo (hī′pō) An abbreviated form of the term hyposulfite, which is a synonym of sodium thiosulfate ($Na_2S_2O_3$), a solution used in photography and radiography to fix and harden the manifest image. (Oral Radiol.) (see also **fixation**)

hypo- (hī′po) A prefix signifying beneath, under, or deficient. (Anesth.)

hypoadrenocorticalism (hī″pō-ǎd-rē″nō-kor′tǐ-kǎl-ǐzm) **(adrenocortical insufficiency, hypoadrenocorticism)** Acute or chronic adrenocortical hypofunction, as in Waterhouse-Friderichsen syndrome or Addison's disease. (Oral Med.)

hypoadrenocorticism (hī″pō-ah-drē-nō-kor′tǐ-sǐzm) (see **hypoadrenocorticalism**)

hypoalgesia (hī″pō-ǎl-jē′zē-ah) Diminished sensation of pain resulting from a raised pain threshold. (Anesth.)

hypocalcemia (hī″pō-kǎl-sē′mē-ah) Lowered blood calcium level. (Oral Diag.)
— Abnormally low concentration of calcium in the blood; may be associated with hypoparathyroidism, rickets, osteomalacia, renal rickets, pancreatic disease, sprue, obstructive jaundice, or tetany. (Oral Med.)

hypocalcification (hī″pō-kǎl-si-fi-kā′shǔn) Reduced calcification, especially of enamel. It produces opaque white spots that may be discolored later. (Oral Diag.) (see also **fluorosis**)
   hereditary enamel h. A hereditary anomaly of enamel formation affecting the primary and permanent dentition in which the enamel peels off after tooth eruption and exposes dentin, giving the teeth a yellow appearance. (Periodont.)

hypocalciuria (hī″pō-kǎl′sē-ū′rē-ah) Decrease in urinary calcium. Normal values vary considerably but are roughly related to calcium intake. Various values are given; e.g., 100 to 200 mg/day on a normal diet, or 350 to 400 mg/day for calcium intake of 10 mg/kg of body weight in children. It may occur in hypoparathyroidism, rickets, osteomalacia, metastatic carcinoma of the prostate, and renal failure. (Oral Med.) (see also **test, Sulkowitch's**)

hypocapnia (hī″pō-kǎp′nē-ah) **(hypocarbia)** A

deficiency of carbon dioxide in the blood. (Anesth.)

hypocarbia (see **hypocapnia**)

hypocenesthesia (hī″pō-sĕn″ĕs-thē′zē-ah) Lack of the normal sense of well-being. (Anesth.)

hypochloremia (hī″pō-klō-rē′mē-ah) Decrease below normal of chloride concentration in the plasma. Normal range is 98 to 106 mEq/L. It may occur in adrenal insufficiency, persistent vomiting, renal failure, acute infections, and dehydration with sodium depletion. (Oral Med.)

hypochondria hī″pō-kon′drē-ah) **(hypochondriasis)** Anxiety about disease; a type of neurosis characterized by fear of disease or by simulated disease. (Oral Diag.)
— A neurosis characterized by an abnormal concern about body functions and health even though no organic disease is present. (Oral Med.)

hypochondriasis (hī″pō-kon-drī′ah-sĭs) (see **hypochondria**)

hypochromia (hī-pō-krō′mē-ah) **(hypochromasia)** Reduced staining quality of cells, particularly pale-staining red blood cells associated with hemoglobin deficiency. (Oral Diag.)

hypodermoclysis (hī″pō-der-mok′lĭ-sĭs) Subcutaneous injection of fluid in large volume. (Oral Med.; Pharmacol.)

hypodontia Fewer teeth than normal. (Orthodont.)

hypoesthesia Decreased sensitivity to touch or pressure. (Oral Diag.)

hypoestrogenism Diminished production of estrogenic substances by the ovaries, such as that which occurs during menopause. Lesions on the oral mucous membranes are of a desquamative nature. (Periodont.) (see also **gingivitis, desquamative**)

hypofibrinogenemia (hī″pō-fī-brĭn″ō-jĕ-nē′mē-ah) Reduction of fibrinogen in the blood. Excessive bleeding may occur following trauma. The deficiency of fibrinogen may be congenital or may be due to faulty synthesis associated with liver disease and defibrinogenation resulting from disorders of pregnancy involving the placenta and amniotic fluid. The normal range is 200 to 600 mg/100 ml of plasma. Clotting deficiencies do not occur until the concentration falls below 75 mg/100 ml. (Oral Med.)

hypogammaglobulinemia (hī″pō-găm″ah-glahb′ū-lĭ-nē′mē-ah) Deficiency of gamma globulin. It is usually manifested by recurrent bacterial infections. (Oral Med.)

hypogeusia (hī″pō-gū′zē-ah) Decreased sense of taste. (Oral Med.)

hypoglycemia (hī″pō-glī-sē′mē-ah) A condition existing when the concentration of blood sugar (true blood sugar) is 40 mg/100 ml or less. Symptoms may not occur even when the concentration is considerably less. Symptoms include nervousness, hunger, weakness, vertigo, and faintness. Hypoglycemia may occur in the fasting state and/or following the injection of insulin. (Oral Med.)

fasting h. Hypoglycemia occurring in the postabsorptive state; occurs in renal glycosuria, lactation, hepatic disease, or central nervous system lesions. (Oral Med.)

insulin h. Hypoglycemia due to improper administration of insulin. If hypoglycemia is severe, convulsions, coma, and death may occur. (Oral Med.) (see also **shock, insulin**)

mixed h. Hypoglycemia occurring during the fasting state and after the ingestion of carbohydrate; occurs in idiopathic spontaneous hypoglycemia of infancy, in anterior pituitary and adrenocortical insufficiency, and with tumors of the islet cells of the pancreas. (Oral Med.)

reactive h. Hypoglycemia occurring after the ingestion of carbohydrate with an excessive release of insulin, as in functional hyperinsulinism. (Oral Med.)

spontaneous h. Hypoglycemia that is functional (i.e., due to renal glycosuria, lactation, severe muscular exertion, etc.) or due to organic disease (i.e., due to hepatic disease, adrenocortical insufficiency, etc.). (Oral Med.)

hypogonadism (hī″pō-gō′năd-ĭzm) Gonadal deficiency due to abnormalities of the testes and ovaries or to pituitary insufficiency. Manifestations include eunuchism, eunuchoidism, Fröhlich's syndrome, amenorrhea, and incomplete development or maintenance of secondary sex characteristics. (Oral Med.)
— Diminished internal secretion of the testes or ovaries that may result in retarded eruption of teeth, marked bone loss, and widening of the periodontal ligament spaces. (Periodont.)

hypohidrotic ectodermal dysplasia (hī″pō-hī-drŏt′ĭk ĕk-tō-dĕr′mal dĭs-plā′zē-ah) Syndrome consisting of hypodontia, hypotrichosis, hypohidrosis, and other defects related to the development of ectodermal structures. (Oral Med.)

hypokalemia (hypopotassemia) Abnormally low serum potassium. It may occur in metabolic alkalosis, chronic diarrhea, Cushing's syndrome, primary aldosteronism, and excessive use of deoxycorticosterone, cortisone, or ACTH. (Oral Med.)

hypolarynx (hī″pō-lăr′ĭnks) The infraglottic compartment of the larynx that extends from the true vocal cords to the first tracheal ring. (Anesth.)

hypolethal (hī″pō-lē′thal) Not quite lethal; said of dosage. (Anesth.)

hypomagnesemia (hī″pō-măg″nĕ-sē′mē-ah) Deficiency of magnesium in the blood serum (normal values range from 1.5 to 2.5 mEq/L). It may be associated with chronic alcoholism, starvation, and prolonged diuresis in congestive heart failure. Manifestations include muscular twitching, convulsions, and coma. (Oral Med.)

hyponasality (hī″pō-nā-zăl′ĭt-ē) Lack of nasal resonance necessary to produce acceptable voice quality. The type of voice quality heard when the speaker's nose is occluded or he is suffering from a severe cold. (Cleft Palate)

hyponatremia (hī″pō-nah-trē′mē-ah) Abnormally low concentration of sodium in the blood serum. It may develop in adrenocortical insufficiency and chronic renal disease or with extreme sweating. (Oral Med.)

hypoparathyroidism (hī″pō-păr″ah-thī′roid-ĭzm) Decrease in parathyroid function, usually the result of surgical removal. Symptoms include tetany, irritability, and muscle weakness. The serum calcium is low, the blood phosphorus elevated, the blood magnesium reduced, and the alkaline phosphatase normal. (Oral Med.)

hypopharyngoscope (hī″pō-fah-rĭng′gō-skōp) An apparatus devised for bringing the lower part of the pharynx or hypopharynx into view. (Anesth.)

hypopharynx (hī″pō-făr′ĭnks) The division of the pharynx that lies below the upper edge of the epiglottis and opens into the larynx and esophagus. (Anesth.)

hypophosphatasia (hī″pō-fos″fah-tā′zē-ah) Deficiency of alkaline phosphatase resulting in deficient calcification of bone, excess osteoid tissue, irregular endochondral ossification, premature and early exfoliation of the teeth, and increased phosphoethanolamine in the urine. (Oral Med.)

— A familial disease in which the children may have very low serum alkaline phosphatase levels, total or partial aplasia of the cementum, and an abnormal periodontal ligament in the deciduous teeth. A decreased phosphatase level that has been linked to a premature loss of deciduous teeth in children. Examination reveals absence, hypoplasia, or dysplasia of cementum. (Periodont.)

hypophosphatemia (hī″pō-fos″fah-tē′mē-ah) Abnormally low concentration of serum phosphates. Blood phosphorus levels are low in sprue, celiac disease, and hyperparathyroidism and in association with an elevated alkaline phosphatase in vitamin D–resistant rickets and other diseases involving a renal tubular defect in resorption of phosphate. (Oral Diag.; Oral Med.)

hypophysis (see **gland, pituitary**)

hypopituitarism (hī″pō-pĭ-tū′ĭ-tăr-ĭzm) Decrease in the hormonal secretions of the pituitary gland. (Periodont.)

hypoplasia (hī″pō-plā′zē-ah) Defective or incomplete development of any tissue or structure. (Comp. Prosth.; Oper. Dent.; Oral Path.; Remov. Part. Prosth.)

    enamel h., chronologic A prenatal or postnatal systemic hypoplasia affecting amelogenesis occurring at the time of the systemic disorder. (Pedodont.)

    enamel h., hereditary (hereditary brown tooth) A hereditary anomaly of the enamel affecting the primary and permanent dentition in which a thin layer of hard enamel covering the yellow dentin gives the tooth a brown appearance. (Pedodont.)

    mandibular h. Abnormally small mandibular development; e.g., in micrognathia or brachygnathia. (Oral Diag.)

hypopnea (hī-pop′nē-ah) Abnormally shallow and rapid respirations. (Anesth.)

hypopotassemia (hī″pō-pot″ah-sē′mē-ah) (see **hypokalemia**)

hypoproteinemia (hī″pō-prō″tē-ĭ-nē′mē-ah) A decrease in serum and plasma proteins. (Oral Med.)

hypoprothrombinemia (hī″pō-prō-throm″bĭ-nē′mē-ah) A deficiency of prothrombin in the blood. It may be congenital or may be associated with vitamin K deficiency, large doses of salicylates, liver disease, or excessive anticoagulants. The normal level ranges from 70% to 120% plasma prothrombin concentration. There is little danger of hemorrhage if the prothrombin concentration is greater than 20% of normal. (Oral Med.)

hyposalivation (xerostomia) A decreased flow of saliva. It may be associated with dehydration, radiation therapy of the salivary gland regions, anxiety, the use of drugs such as atropine and antihistamines, vitamin deficiency, various forms of parotitis, and various syndromes (Sjögren's, Riley-Day, Plummer-Vinson, and Heerfordt's). (Oral Med.) (see also **asialorrhea**)

hyposensitive Less sensitive. (Anesth.)

hyposthenuria (hī″pōs-thĕ-nū′rē-ah) A condition in which the urine has an abnormally low specific gravity. It may occur in cases in which renal damage impairs concentrating power or when the kidneys are normal but lack hormonal stimulus for concentrations, as in diabetes insipidus. (Oral Med.)

hypotension (hī″pō-tĕn′shŭn) Abnormally low tension, especially low blood pressure. (Anesth.)

hypothalamus (hī″pō-thăl′ah-mŭs) A small extension of the brain that lies in the sella turcica in the cranium. It lies just at the superior level of the body of the sphenoid bone. It is intimately related structurally and functionally with the pituitary gland, and it is important in the central regulation of the endocrine glands, including the thyroid gland, pancreas, adrenal glands, and gonads. The most important visceral functions are under control of the hypothalamus because it functions in such close coordination with the endocrine glands. The control is mediated through its structural communication with the pituitary gland. (Oral Physiol.)

hypothetical question Assumed or proved facts and circumstances, stated so as to constitute a specific situation or state of facts, on which the opinion of an expert is asked, in producing evidence at a trial. (D. Juris.)

hypothyroidism (hī″pō-thī′roid-ĭzm) Deficiency of the thyroid hormone resulting in lowered basal metabolism and retarded growth. The condition is called cretinism in children and myxedema in adults. (Oral Diag.; Oral Path.)
— Diminished activity of the thyroid gland with decreased secretion of thyroxin, resulting in lowered basal metabolic rate, lethargy, sleepiness, dysmenorrhea in females, and a tendency toward obesity. Occasionally there is accompanying gingival hyperplasia. (Periodont.)
  congenital h. (see **cretinism**)

hypoxemia Deficient oxygenation of the blood. (Anesth.)

hypoxia Low oxygen content or tension. (Anesth.)
  anemic h. Hypoxia brought about by a reduction of the oxygen-carrying capacity of the blood due to a decrease in the complete blood counts or an alteration of the hemoglobin constituents. (Anesth.)
  anoxic h. Hypoxia due to inadequate oxygen in inspired air or interference with gaseous exchange in the lungs. (Anesth.)
  histotoxic h. Hypoxia that is the result of the inability of the tissue cells to use the oxygen that may be present in normal amount and tension. (Anesth.)
  metabolic h. Hypoxia due to an increased tissue demand for oxygen. (Anesth.)
  stagnant h. Hypoxia due to decreased circulation in an area. (Anesth.)

hysteresis (hĭs-tĕ-rē′sĭs) A physical phenomenon whereby a material such as a reversible hydrocolloid passes from a sol to a gel state at one temperature and a gel to a sol state at another. (D. Mat.)

hysteria (hĭs-tĕr′ē-ah) A disease or disorder of the nervous system, more common in females than males, not originating in lesions and due to psychic rather than physical causes. (D. Juris.)
— A psychoneurosis characterized by lack of control over emotions or acts, exaggeration of sensory impression, and simulation of disease or pain associated with disease. In some patients trismus, neuralgia, and temporomandibular joint disturbance may be hysterical in origin. (Oral Diag.)

I

I and D (surgical fistulation) Incision and drainage; the procedure of incising a fluctuant mucosal lesion to allow for the release of pressure and drainage of fluid exudate. (Endodont.)

-ia Latin suffix that indicates a condition (e.g., a disease) or a science, practice, or treatment. (Orthodont.)

iatrogenic (ī-ăt″rō-jĕn′ĭk) Originating as a result of professional care; e.g., an iatrogenic dermatitis. (Oral Med.)

— Pertaining to a disease process adventitiously caused by therapy undertaken by the dentist or other therapist during the course of treatment. (Oral Physiol.)

-ics Indicative of a science, practice, or treatment. In dentistry the trend is from the use of -ia to the use of -ics; e.g., about 1937 the term orthodontics began to replace the term orthodontia. In ancient Greek times the adjectival ending -ikos was used without a following noun to indicate a practice; e.g., ethics. The ending -ics, unlike -ia, can indicate only a practice, not a condition. To be preferred to -ia. (Comp. Prosth.; Remov. Part. Prosth.)

icterus (ĭk′ter-ŭs) (see **jaundice**)

  acholuric i. (see **jaundice, hemolytic, congenital**)

-id reaction (see **reaction, -id**)

identity Sameness; the fact that a subject, person, or thing before a court is the same as it is claimed to be. (D. Juris.)

idiopathic disease (see **disease, idiopathic**)

idiopathic enlargement (ĭd″ē-ō-păth′ĭk) (see **enlargement, idiopathic**)

idiosyncrasy (ĭd″ē-ō-sĭng′krah-sē) Abnormal or unusual response to a drug when an extremely small dose has been given. The reaction may be similar to that of toxic overdose. (Anesth.)

— Tendency to react atypically or with unusual violence to a food, drug, or cosmetic. Also, any characteristic peculiar to an individual. (Oral Med.; Pharmacol.)

ignorance of law (see **law, ignorance of**)

illegal Not authorized by law; illicit. (D. Juris.)

illuminator (light box) A source of light with uniform intensity for viewing radiographs. The ideal illuminator should be of such a size or be adaptable to such a size as to permit only that light passing through the films to reach the eye. A small, intense spot illuminator is used for interpretation of the areas of increased radiographic density. (Oral Radiol.)

illusion (ĭ-lū′zhŭn) In medical jurisprudence, an image or impression in the mind created by some external object which, instead of denoting reality, is distorted or mistaken, the error being caused by the imagination of the observer, not by any defect in the organs of sense. Seen in certain reactions in general anesthesia or intoxication. (D. Juris.)

illustration A drawing or photograph used to help clarify the patient's concept of proposed treatment and conditions present. (Pract. Man.)

image, latent The invisible image produced on photographic or radiographic film by the action of light or radiation before development. (Oral Radiol.)

imbalance, occlusal An inharmonious relationship between the maxillary and mandibular teeth during closure or functional jaw movements. (Orthodont.)

imbedded (see **embedded**)

imbibition (ĭm″bĭ-bĭsh′ŭn) Absorption of liquid. Gel structures are particularly susceptible to imbibition. (D. Mat.)

— Absorption of a fluid, which is accompanied by a swelling of the gel; e.g., when a hydrocolloid is immersed for long periods, its water content is increased by the process of imbibition. This process occurs to a lesser degree in an alginate than in an agar hydrocolloid. (Remov. Part. Prosth.)

immediate denture (see **denture, immediate**)

immune reaction (see **reaction, immune**)

immunity Exemption from service or from duties that the law ordinarily requires other citizens to perform (e.g., jury duty). (D. Juris.)

— Condition of an organism whereby it successfully resists or is not susceptible to injury or infection. (Oper. Dent.)

immunization with silver nitrate (ĭm″ū-nĭ-zā′shŭn) The process of rendering enamel and dentin immune from caries by impregnating the surface of the tooth with silver precipitated from silver nitrate solution by means of formalin or eugenol. (Oper. Dent.)

immunoglobulins (ĭm″ū-nō-glŏb′ū-lĭnz) **(Ig)** Serum proteins (gamma globulins) synthesized by plasma cells that act as antibodies and are important in the body's defense mechanisms against infection. Main classes are designated as IgG, IgA, and IgM. (Oral Med.)

impact strength (see **strength, impact**)

impacted tooth (see **tooth, impacted**)

impaction (ĭm-păk′shŭn) Situation in which an unerupted tooth is wedged against another tooth or teeth or otherwise located so that it cannot erupt normally. (Oral Surg.)

　food i. Abnormal lodging of food against the gingival margin, producing an irritational effect with subsequent gingival inflammation. Impaction may also occur within a gingival or periodontal pocket with similar consequences. Horizontal and vertical impaction may occur. (Periodont.)

impaired function (see **function, impaired**)

impeachment of witness The questioning of the veracity of a witness by means of evidence obtained for that purpose. (D. Juris.)

impetigo (ĭm″pĕ-tī′gō) An inflammatory disease of the skin characterized by pustules. (Oral Diag.)

impingement (ĭm-pĭnj′mĕnt) An area of over-compaction, displacement, or compression of a tissue by some unit of a removable prosthesis. Also, an area of traumatization of the periodontal membrane caused by an occlusal force on a tooth that produces a laterally directed stress. (Remov. Part. Prosth.)

implant A graft or insert set firmly onto or deeply into the alveolar process prepared for its insertion. It may support a crown or crowns, a partial denture, or a complete denture. (Comp. Prosth.; Oral Implant.; Remov. Part. Prosth.)

— A device, usually alloplastic, surgically inserted into or onto the jawbone. To be used as a prosthodontic abutment, it should remain quiescent and purely incidental to local tissue physiology. (Oral Implant.)

　abutment of i. The portion of an implant that protrudes through the gingival tissues and that is designed to support a prosthodontic appliance. (Oral Implant.)

　arthroplastic i. A cast chrome-alloy glenoid fossa prosthesis available in right and left models in fifty shapes for each side. (Oral Implant.)

　bone i. (see **graft, autogenous, bone; graft, iliac; graft, kiel; graft, onlay bone; graft, swaging**)

　cervix of i. That portion of an implant which connects the infrastructure with the abutment as it passes through the mucoperiosteum. (Oral Implant.)

　endosseous i. (see **implant, endosteal**)

　endosteal i. An appliance that is placed into the alveolar and/or basal bone and that protrudes through the mucoperiosteum, thus serving as a prosthodontic abutment (such implants are occasionally used for fracture fixation devices or as sources for orthodontic anchorage). (Oral Implant.)

　anchor e. i. An implant with a narrow buccolingual wedge-shaped infrastructure that is designed to be placed deep into the bone. The outline of the implant appears similar to a nautical anchor, and there are a variety of sizes and shapes to satisfy many anatomic and prosthodontic needs. They are cast of chromium-cobalt surgical alloy and annealed. (Oral Implant.)

　　arms of a. e. i. The major portion of the implant infrastructure. These extensions leave the shank at its deepest point and curve anteriorly and posteriorly. (Oral Implant.)

　　crown of a. e. i. The abutment part of an anchor implant. (Oral Implant.)

　　flukes of a. e. i. The end portions of the arms that rise to the most superficial portion within the bone.

　　seating instrument of a. e. i., arm type A bayonet-shaped device designed to assist in seating an anchor implant by straddling its arms over a specially designed "seating notch." (Oral Implant.)

　　seating instrument of a. e. i., crown type A bayonet-shaped, double-ended device designed to assist in seating an anchor implant by cupping its crown or abutment. (Oral Implant.)

　　shaft of a. e. i. The cervix of an anchor implant. (Oral Implant.)

　blade e. i. An implant with a narrow (buccolingually) wedge-shaped infrastructure bearing openings or vents through which tissue grows to obtain retention. These implants may have one or more cervices on each. They are supplied in a variety of sizes, shapes, and configurations to fulfill many anatomic and prosthodontic requirements, and may be constructed of cast chromium-cobalt alloy or machined of titanium. (Oral Implant.)

　　complete-arch b. e. i. A blade type of implant, designed either with or without direct bone impression, to be inserted into a completely edentulous ridge as a single appliance bearing multiple abutments. (Oral Implant.)

　　leading edge of b. e. i. The part of the

wedge-shaped infrastructure that is narrowest and deepest within the bone. It is straight and unbroken in conformation. (Oral Implant.)

fenestrated l. e. of b. e. i. A scalloped or broken leading edge that enters the bone more easily and with less trauma to the host site. (Oral Implant.) (see also **host site**)

shoulder of b. e. i. That unbroken surface of the wedge-shaped infrastructure which is widest and most superficial. It is this part which is tapped during the seating of the implant. (Oral Implant.)

ceramic e. i. An endosteal implant of a variety of designs constructed of silicate or porcelain. (Oral Implant.)

endodontic e. i. An implant with a threaded or nonthreaded pin that fits into a root canal and extends beyond the dental apex into the adjacent bone, thereby lengthening the clinical root. (Oral Implant.)

oblique e. e. i. An implant passing obliquely through a dental root and into the bone beyond. It is used in this manner in instances when direct extensions from the canal would cause the implant to be located outside the bone. (Oral Implant.)

helicoid e. i. A two-piece endosteal implant consisting of a helical steel spring that is inserted into bone as a female, and a male that may be placed postoperatively and serves as the abutment. (Oral Implant.)

needle e. i. (pin e. i.) A smooth, thin shaft (self-perforating) that serves as an implant usually in conjunction with two others, the three being placed in bone in tripodal conformity. (Oral Implant.)

mandrel of n. e. i. A hollow device available in full, half, and shallow depths into which needle implants fit. The mandrel, in turn, is used in the contraangle to drive the needle implant into place. (Oral Implant.)

ramus e. i. A blade type of implant designed for the anterior part of the ramus. Its abutments are found at the anterior end and emerge in the retromolar area. (Oral Implant.) (see also **implant, endosteal, blade**)

frame type of r. e. i. A prefabricated mandibular full-arch implant consisting of two posterior ramus implants: an anterior (symphyseal) endosteal compo-

nent and a conjunction bar. (Oral Implant.)

seating instrument of e. i. A device designed to be placed on a portion of an implant so that malleting on it will seat the implant into the bone. It usually has an angled or bayoneted shaft to enable it to protrude from the mouth in a more or less vertical direction. The blade end has a specialized shape to grip, grasp, or fit over a portion of the shoulder, abutment, arm, or crown of the implant so that it will be seated. (Oral Implant.)

spiral e. i. A screw type of implant, either hollow or solid, usually consisting of abutment, cervix, and infrastructure. (Oral Implant.)

C. M. (crête manche) s. e. i. A narrow-diameter screw implant designed for thin ridges. (Oral Implant.)

fabricated i. A custom-designed implant constructed for a specific operative site. (Oral Implant.)

gingival cuff i. The cicatricial epithelium that surrounds the implant cervix at its point of emergence. (Oral Implant.)

infrastructure of i. The part of an implant that is designed to give it retention (e.g., the mesh frame of a subperiosteal implant, the flutes of a spiral endosteal implant, or the shoulder portion of a blade implant). (Oral Implant.)

intraosseous i. A bone fixation tube used to obtain a canal traversed by the metal tube serving as a denture support. (Oral Implant.)

intraperiosteal i. An artificial appliance made to conform to the shape of a bone and placed beneath the outer, or fibrous, layer of the periosteum. (Oral Implant.)

magnetic i. A tissue-tolerated, magnetized metal placed within the bone to aid denture retention. It is composed of two parts: the implant magnet, the part that is placed within the bone; and the denture magnet, the part that is placed within the denture. (Oral Implant.)

mesostructure i. An intermediate superstructure. A series of splinted copings, each of which fits over an implant abutment or natural tooth and over which fits the completed prosthodontic appliance. (Oral Implant.)

oral i. A device or substance, biologic or alloplastic, that is surgically inserted into the soft or hard oral structures, to be used for functional or cosmetic purposes. (Oral Implant.)

polymer tooth replica i. An acrylic resin implant, shaped like the tooth recently extracted, that is placed into the tooth's alveolus. Its surface has a series of porosities designed to attract ingrowth of surrounding tissues. (Oral Implant.)

stock i. An implant, usually endosteal, that is available in manufactured form in uniform sizes and shapes. (Oral Implant.)

subperiosteal i. An appliance consisting of an open-mesh frame designed to fit over the surface of the bone beneath the periosteum. Attached to this frame are one or more mucoperiosteal piercing posts, which serve as prosthodontic abutments. These implants are usually cast of a surgical chromium-cobalt alloy. (Oral Implant.)

anterior s. i. An implant placed in the anterior part of an edentulous mandible and designed to supply abutments in the two cuspid regions. It may or may not have posterior subperiosteal extensions. (Oral Implant.)

complete s. i. An implant used for an entire edentulous jaw. (Oral Implant.)

fixation screw of s. i. Screws, 5 to 7 mm long, that are made of the same surgical alloy as the implant and that are used to to affix the implant to the underlying bone. (Oral Implant.)

screw hole of s. i. An opening made in a strut to permit the placement of a screw for purposes of fixation. The complete subperiosteal implant has three screws, each of which is countersunk to allow for level seating of the screw head. (Oral Implant.)

single-tooth s. i. An implant designed to replace a single missing tooth; usually unsupported by adjacent natural teeth. (Oral Implant.)

strut of s. i. A thin, striplike component of an infrastructure. (Oral Implant.)

peripheral s. of s. i. The part of the infrastructure that makes up its most remote outlines. (Oral Implant.)

primary s. of s. i. The portion of the infrastructure, usually connected to the periphery, that crosses the crest of the bony ridge and to which the abutment devices are attached. (Oral Implant.)

secondary s. of s. i. Other infrastructure connectors generally used to supply rigidity to the frame. (Oral Implant.)

unilateral s. i. An implant that is used in a single quadrant only. It is usually intended to serve as an abutment for a free-end denture base. (Oral Implant.)

universal s. i. A subperiosteal implant that is used for an entire jaw in which some teeth are present. The infrastructure circumvents these existing teeth, with its periphery passing buccally, labially, palatally, or lingually to them. (Oral Implant.)

superstructure of i. A completed prosthesis that is supported entirely or in part by an implant. It may be a removable or fixed prosthesis and may be a single crown or a complete arch splint. (Oral Implant.)

transosteal i. An implant that is designed for the anterior mandible and that passes through both inferior and superior (alveolar) cortices. It is usually inserted via a submental skin incision. (Oral Implant.)

two-piece i. An implant, either endosteal or subperiosteal, having its infrastructure and abutment in separate parts. Generally, the abutment, which is threaded, is screwed to the infrastructure some weeks after its incision, so that healing has taken place. (Oral Implant.)

implantation, tooth A procedure used in the treatment of periodontosis; the first molar is extracted, and the tooth germ of the third molar is transplanted to the extraction site. (Periodont.)

implantodontics (ĭm-plăn″tō-don′tĭks) The division of dentistry that deals with the science of implanting foreign materials into or onto the jawbones. (Oral Implant.)

implantodontist (ĭm-plăn″tō-don′tĭst) A dentist who is engaged in and proficient in the art and practice of implantodontics. (Oral Implant.)

implantodontology (ĭm-plăn″tō-don-tŏl′ō-je) The study of the placement of a foreign material into or onto the jawbones to replace or support artificial dentition. (Oral Implant.)

implantologist, oral (ĭm-plăn-tol′ō-jĭst) A dentist who practices the art and science of oral implantology. (Oral Implant.) (see also **implantology, oral**)

implantology, oral (ĭm-plăn-tol′ō-je) The art and science of dentistry that concerns itself with the surgical insertion of materials and devices into, onto, and about the jaws and oral cavity for purposes of oral maxillofacial, or occlusal rehabilitation and/or cosmetic correction. (Oral Implant.)

implied Inferred; conceded. (D. Juris.)

impression An imprint, or negative form, of the teeth and/or other tissues of the oral cavity made in a plastic material that becomes relatively hard, or set, while in contact with these tissues. An impression is made in order to produce a positive form, or cast, of the recorded tissues. Impressions are classified according to the materials of which they are made (e.g., reversible or irreversible hydrocolloid impression, modeling compound impression, modeling plastic impression, plaster impression, or wax impression), according to the structures included or recorded in the impression material (e.g., edentulous impression or dentulous impression), and according to its purpose (e.g., complete denture impression, partial denture impression, or inlay impression). (Comp. Prosth.; Fixed Part. Prosth.; Oper. Dent.; Orthodont.)

— An imprint or negative likeness of an object from which a positive reproduction may be made. (Remov. Part. Prosth.)

anatomic i. An imprint or negative record of the form of a dental arch or portion thereof that records the shape of the structures in a passive or unstrained form, making possible a static relationship of a prosthesis produced from such an impression. (Remov. Part. Prosth.)

i. area (see **area, impression**)

boxing of an i. (see **boxing of an impression**)

bridge i. An impression made for the purpose of constructing or assembling a fixed restoration, fixed partial denture, or bridge. (Fixed Part. Prosth.)

cleft palate i. An impression of the upper jaw of a patient with a cleft (incomplete closure, or union) in the palate. (Comp. Prosth.)

closed mouth i. An impression made while the mouth is closed and with the patient's muscular activity molding the borders. (Comp. Prosth.)

complete denture i. An impression (negative record) of an edentulous arch made for the purpose of constructing a complete denture. It includes the entire area of the basal seat and the limiting structures around the borders of the basal seat area. (Comp. Prosth.)

composite i. An impression consisting of two or more parts. (M.F.P.)

correctable i. An impression whose surface is capable of alteration by the removal from or addition to some area of its surface or border. (Remov. Part. Prosth.)

dual i. (see **technique, impression, dual**)

duplicating i. (see **duplication**)

elastic i. An impression made in a material that will permit registration of undercut areas by springing over projecting areas and then returning to its original position. (Oper. Dent.)

final i. (secondary i.) An impression used for making the master cast. (Comp. Prosth.; Fixed Part. Prosth.; Remov. Part. Prosth.)

fluid wax i. An impression of the functional form of subjacent structures made with selected waxes that are applied (brushed on) to the impression surface in fluid form. (Comp. Prosth.; Remov. Part. Prosth.)

functional i. An impression of the supporting structures in their functional form. (Remov. Part. Prosth.) (see also **structure, supporting, functional form of**)

hydrocolloid i. An impression made of a hydrocolloid material. (Comp. Prosth.; Fixed Part. Prosth.; Remov. Part. Prosth.)

lower i. (see **impression, mandibular**)

mandibular i. (lower i.) An impression of the mandibular jaw and related tissues and dental structures. (Comp. Prosth.; Fixed Part. Prosth.; Remov. Part. Prosth.)

i. material (see **material, impression**)

maxillary i. (upper i.) An impression of the maxillary jaw and related tissues and dental structures. (Comp. Prosth.; Fixed Part. Prosth.; Remov. Part. Prosth.)

mercaptan i. An impression made of mercaptan (polysulfide), a rubber base elastic material. (Remov. Part. Prosth.)

partial denture i. An impression of part or all of a partially edentulous arch made for the purpose of designing or constructing a partial denture. (Remov. Part. Prosth.)

pickup i. An impression made with the superstructure frame in place on the abutments in the mouth after the implant has been surgically inserted and the mouth has healed. The superstructure frame is picked up by the impression material, and an accurate impression of the oral mucosal tissue over the implant is obtained. (Oral Implant.)

preliminary i. (primary i.) An impression made for the purpose of diagnosis or the construction of a tray for making a final impression. (Comp. Prosth.; Fixed Part. Prosth.; Remov. Part. Prosth.)

primary i. (see **impression, preliminary**)

secondary i. (see **impression, final**)

sectional i. An impression that is made in sections. (Comp. Prosth.)

snap i. (see **impression, preliminary**)

i. surface (see **denture foundation area; surface, basal**) surgical bone i. A negative likeness of the exposed bony surfaces necessary to support the implant substructure. (Oral Implant.)

i. technique (see **technique, impression**)

i. tray (see **tray, impression**)

upper i. (see **impression, maxillary**)

welded inlay i. A method of procuring a negative likeness of an inlay preparation by incremental welding of the impression compound by heat and impression into an immobilized matrix. (Oper. Dent.)

impulse An uncontrollable wave of excitation transmitted along a nerve fiber due to a stimulus. (Anesth.)

— A surge of electric current for a short time span; e.g., in a 60-cycle AC current, there are 120 impulses per second. (Oral Radiol.)

— An excitation wave. (Oral Physiol.)

muscle i. A wave of excitation along a muscle fiber initiated at the neuromuscular endplate; accompanied by chemical and electrical changes at the surface of the muscle fiber and by activation of the contractile elements of the muscle fiber; detectable electronically (electromyographically); and followed by a transient refractory period. (Oral Physiol.)

nerve i. A wave of excitation along a nerve fiber initiated by a stimulus; accompanied by chemical and electrical changes at the surface of the nerve fiber; propagated at speeds of 1 to 100 meters per second; detectable electronically; and followed by a transient refractory period during which further stimulation has no effect. (Oral Physiol.)

in chief Principal; directly obtained. Evidence obtained from a witness on his examination in court by the party producing him. (D. Juris.)

in pais (ĭn pā') A legal transaction that has been accomplished without legal proceedings. (D. Juris.)

in potestate parentis (ĭn pō-těst'ăt pah-rěn'tĭs) Under the authority of the parent. (D. Juris.)

inacidity Absence of acidity. (Anesth.)

inactivate To render inactive; to destroy the activity of. (Anesth.)

inactivator A substance added to a culture medium to prevent the activity of an inoculant. Penicillinase is added to the culture medium to prevent the activity of penicillin that might be carried over from a root canal treatment. (Endodont.)

inadequacy, velopharyngeal (věl"ō-făh-rĭn'jē-ăl) A lack of functional closure of the velum to the postpharyngeal wall, allowing air and sound to enter the nasopharynx and nasal cavities, thus producing a hypernasal voice quality. (Cleft Palate)

inadmissible That which cannot be admitted under the established rules of law. (D. Juris.)

inchacao (ĭn-chah-kah'ō) (see **beriberi**)

incipient (ĭn-sĭp'ē-ěnt) Beginning, initial, commencing. (Oper. Dent.)

incisal (ĭn-sī'zăl) Relating to the cutting edge of the anterior teeth, the incisors or cuspids. (Oper. Dent.)

i. angle (see **angle, incisal**)

i. guidance angle (see **angle, incisal guidance**)

i. guide (see **guide, incisal**)

i. guide pin (see **pin, incisal guide**)

i. rest (see **rest, incisal**)

incision (ĭn-sĭzh'ŭn) The act of cutting or biting.

i. and drainage (see **I and D**)

i. of food The phase of the masticatory cycle, performed by utilization of the incisor teeth, that cuts or separates the bolus of food. As food is placed between the anterior teeth, the mandible is elevated in a pattern of closure to incise the bolus. (Periodont.)

preauricular i. The incision of the soft tissue anterior to the external ear that permits access to the temporomandibular joint. (Oral Surg.)

relieving i. A cut into the soft tissues adjacent to a wound to permit a tension-free closure. (Oral Implant.)

Risdon's i. The incision of the soft tissues in the area of the mandibular angle that permits access to the lateral surface of the mandibular ramus, the subcondylar neck, and the condylar area. (Oral Surg.)

incisive foramen (see **foramen, incisive**)

incisive papilla (see **papilla, incisive**)

incisor(s) (ĭn-sī'zor) A cutting tooth. One of the four anterior teeth of either jaw. (Oper. Dent.)

— The anterior teeth; the upper and lower central and lateral incisors. The teeth performing the initial act of the masticatory cycle—incision of a food bolus. (Periodont.)

central i. The first incisor. (Comp. Prosth.)

Hutchinson's i. Malformed teeth caused by the presence of congenital syphilis during tooth development. The incisors usually are shorter than normal, show a single permanent notch on each incisal edge, and are screwdriver shaped. (Oral Diag.)

lateral i. The second incisor. (Comp. Prosth.; Orthodont.; Remov. Part. Prosth.)

i. point (see **point, incisor**)

inclination (ĭn"klĭ-nā'shŭn) The angle of slope from a particular item of reference.

axial i. The alignment of a tooth in a vertical plane in relationship to its basal bone structure. (Periodont.)

lateral condylar i. The direction of the lateral condyle path. (Comp. Prosth.; Remov. Part. Prosth.)

i. of tooth (see **tooth, inclination of**)

income The return in money from one's business, practice, or capital invested; gains, profit. (D. Juris.)

incompatibility (ĭn"kom-păt"ĭ-bĭl'ĭ-tē) Term that refers to a disharmonious relationship among the ingredients of prescriptions and other drug mixtures. (Oral Med.; Pharmacol.)

chemical i. A situation in which two or more of the ingredients of a drug interact chemically, with resulting deterioration of the mixture. (Oral Med.; Pharmacol.)

incontinentia pigmenti (see **syndrome, Bloch-Sulzberger**

incubator (ĭn'kū-bā-tor) A laboratory container with controlled temperature for the cultivation of bacteria. (Endodont.)

index The ratio of a measurable value to another value desired but less easily measured. (Anesth.)

— Information used for the measurement of a disease on an epidemiologic basis. (Periodont.)

— A core or mold used to record or maintain the relative position of a tooth or teeth to one another and/or to a cast. A guide, usually made of plaster of paris, used to reposition teeth, casts, or parts in order to reproduce their original positions. (Comp. Prosth.) (see also **splint**)

Broders' i. (**Broders' classification**) A system of grading of epidermoid carcinoma suggested by Broders. Tumors are graded from I to IV on the basis of cell differentiation. Grade I tumors are highly differentiated (there is much keratin production); Grade IV tumors are poorly differentiated (cells are highly anaplastic, with almost no keratin formation). (Oral Path.)

— Classification and grading of malignant neoplasms according to the proportion of malignant cells to normal cells in the lesion. (Oral Surg.)

cardiac i. The minute volume of blood per square meter of body surface. (Anesth.)

carpal i. The degree of ossification of the carpal bones noted in radiographs of the wrist; a method of determining the state of skeletal maturation. (Orthodont.)

cephalic i. Head shape and size. (Orthodont.)

DEF i. A dental caries index applied to the primary dentition in somewhat the same manner as the DMF index is used for classifying permanent teeth. The letter D stands for decayed; E for extraction indicated because of caries; and F for filled. Missing primary teeth are ignored in this index because of the uncertainty in determining whether they were extracted because of advanced caries or exfoliated normally. (Pedodont.)

DMF i. A dental caries index based on the number of persons, number of teeth, or number of tooth surfaces showing evidence of caries attack. These basic signs for permanent teeth are a demonstrable lesion of caries, a filling or other restoration, or a missing permanent tooth. These categories are indicated by D (for decayed), M (for missing or indicated for extraction), and F (for filled), usually written as DMF. Analysis may be based on the average number of DMF teeth (sometimes called DMFT) per person or the average number of DMF tooth surfaces (DMFS). (Pedodont.)

gingiva–bone count i. (**Dunning-Leach i.**) An index that permits differential recording of both gingival and bone conditions to determine gingivitis and bone loss. (Periodont.)

gnathic i. Relationship of jaw size to head size. (Orthodont.)

icterus i. (see **test, Meulengracht's**)

malocclusion i. A measure of the severity of a malocclusion, obtained by assigning values to a series of defined observations. (Orthodont.)

measuring i. An expression of relationship of one measurable value to another, or a formula based on measurable values. Indices of great value in the evolution of the degree and incidence of periodontal disease are the PMA index and the periodontal disease index (Russell index). (Periodont.)

oral hygiene i., simplified (**Greene-Vermillion i.**) An index made up of two components: the debris index and the calculus index, which are based on numerical determination representing the amount of debris or calculus found on six preselected tooth surfaces. (Periodont.)

periodontal disease i. (**Russell i.**) An index that measures the condition of both the gingiva and the bone individually for each tooth and arrives at the average status for periodontal disease in a given mouth without reference to type or etiology of disease. (Periodont.)

periodontal i. (**Ramfjord i.**) A thorough clinical examination of the periodontal status of six teeth: $\dfrac{6}{41}\;\;\dfrac{14}{6}$, with an evaluation of the gingival condition, pocket depth, calculus and plaque deposits, attrition, mobility, and lack of contact. (Periodont.)

PMA i. (Schour-Massler i.) An index used for recording the prevalence and severity of gingivitis in schoolchildren by noting and scoring three areas: the gingival papillae (P), the buccal or labial gingival margin (M), and the attached gingiva (A). (Periodont.)

Pont's i. The relation of the width of the four incisors to the width between the first premolars and the width between the first molars. (Orthodont.)

Russell i. (see **index, periodontal disease**)

salivary lactobacillus i. A count of the lactobacilli per milliliter of saliva; used as an indicator of present dental caries activity. The test is of questionable value in individual patients, although its use in large groups led to valuable information on caries activity. (Oral Diag.)

saturation i. A number indicating the hemoglobin content of a person's red blood cells as compared with the normal content. (Anesth.)

therapeutic i. The ratio of toxic dose to effective dose. (Oral Med.; Pharmacol.)

ventilation i. The index obtained by dividing the ventilation test by the vital capacity. (Anesth.)

indication That which serves as a guide or warning. (Anesth.)

indirect method (see **method, indirect**)

indirect pulp capping (see **capping, pulp, indirect**)

indirect retention (see **retention, indirect**)

induced Produced artificially. (Anesth.)

induction The act or process of inducing or causing to occur. (Anesth.)

inertia (ĭn-er′shuh) According to Newton's law of inertia, the tendency of a body that is at rest to remain at rest, and a body that is in motion to continue in motion with constant speed in the same straight line unless acted on by an outside force. The force needed to overcome the inertia of the body depends on the weight of the body and the rate at which it is moving. More effort is required per unit of work accomplished to start the incision of food than to complete the incision because of the difference in the inertia of the mandible at the two moments of time. At the first moment of incision, the mandible is stationary;

during the incisive movement, the mandible is in motion. (Oral Physiol.)

infantilism (ĭn-făn′tĭ-lĭzm) A disturbance marked by retention of childhood characteristics into adult life. Tooth eruption may be delayed or absent. (Oral Diag.)

— Arrested or retarded growth and arrest of primary and secondary sexual characteristics. (Oral Med.)

infarct (ĭn′farkt) Death of a tissue due to partial occlusion of a vessel or vessels supplying the area. (Oral Path.)

infection (ĭn-fĕk′shŭn) Invasion of the tissues of the body by disease-producing microorganisms and the reaction of these tissues to the microorganisms and/or their toxins. The mere presence of microorganisms without reaction is not evidence of infection. (Oral Diag.; Oral Path.; Periodont.)

focal i. The process in which microorganisms located at a certain site (focus) in the body are disseminated throughout the body to set up secondary sites (foci) of infection in other tissues. (Oral Diag.)

hemolytic streptococcal i. Infection usually caused by Group A hemolytic streptococci. Such infections include scarlet fever, streptococcal sore throat, cellulitis, and osteomyelitis. (Oral Med.)

— An infection caused by streptococci that produce a toxic substance (hemolysin) that will lyse the erythrocytes and liberate hemoglobin from red blood cells. (Periodont.)

i., resistance The ability of an individual to fight off the detrimental effects of microorganisms and their toxic products. A complexity involving individual and interacting factors; e.g., antibody formation, adequate nutrition, tissue tone, circulation, and emotional stability. (Periodont.)

i., susceptibility The degree of capability of being influenced by or involved in the pathologic processes produced by microorganisms and/or their toxins. (Periodont.)

Vincent's i. (see **gingivitis, necrotizing ulcerative**)

infiltrate (ĭn-fĭl′trāt) Material deposited by infiltration. (Anesth.)

infiltration (ĭn″fĭl-trā′shŭn) Accumulation in a tissue of a substance not normal to it. (Anesth.)

inflammatory i. Influx or accumulation of inflammatory elements (cellular and exudative) in the interstices of the tissues as a result of tissue injury by physical, chemical, microbiologic, and other irritants. Cellular elements include lymphocytes, plasma cells, polymorphonuclear leukocytes, and/or the macrophages of reticuloendothelial origin. (Periodont.)

local i. The prevention of excitation of the free nerve endings by literally flooding the immediate area with a local anesthetic solution. (Anesth.)

inflammation (ĭn″flah-mā′shŭn) The cellular and vascular response or reaction to injury. It is characterized by pain, redness, swelling, heat, and disturbance of function. It may be acute or chronic. The term is not synonymous with infection, which implies an inflammatory reaction initiated by invasion of living organisms. (Oral Diag.; Oral Path.)

gingival i. The alterations occurring in the gingivae as a result of irritation by physical, chemical, microbiologic, and other agents. Generalized characteristics include enlargement due to edema and tissue hyperplasia, loss of stippling due to the breakdown of members of the gingival fiber apparatus and to tissue edema, gingival retraction due to loss of gingival fiber support, redness due to engorgement of the capillaries with blood, bleeding through an area of ulceration of the pocket epithelium, variable degrees of pain, etc. (Periodont.)

granulomatous i. Chronic inflammation in which there is formation of granulation tissue. (Oral Path.)

periodontal i. (see **periodontitis**)

inflation (ĭn-flā′shŭn) The act of distending with air or with a gas. (Anesth.)

influences, local environmental Factors or agents within the oral cavity that are responsible for the initiation, perpetuation, or modification of a pathologic state within the stomatognathic system. (Periodont.)

influences, systemic environmental Systemic factors that may initiate, perpetuate, or modify disease processes within the stomatognathic system. Generally, the oral manifestations of systemic disease are modified by the influence of local environmental factors. (Periodont.)

infrabony pocket (ĭn′frah-bō-nē) (see **pocket, infrabony**)

infrabulge (ĭn′frăh-bulj) The surface of the crown of a tooth cervical to the clasp guide line, survey line, or surveyed height of contour. (Remov. Part. Prosth.)

infraclusion (ĭn″frah-kloo′zhŭn) (**infraversion**) The position occupied by a tooth when it has failed to erupt sufficiently to the line of oc-

clusion, which is higher in the maxillae and lower in the mandible. (Orthodont.)

infracrestal pocket (ĭn″frah-krĕs′tal) (see **pocket, infrabony**)

infradentale (ĭn″frah-dĕn-tă′lē) The most anterior point of the alveolar process of the mandible. (Orthodont.)

infrastructure, resection The act of removing a strut or more usually a shoulder portion of an implant without removing the implant. (Oral Implant.)

infraversion (ĭn″frah-ver′zhŭn) (see **infraclusion**)

infusion Therapeutic introduction of a fluid, e.g., saline solution, into a vein. In contrast to injection, infusion suggests the introduction of a larger volume of a less concentrated solution over a more protracted period. (Anesth.; Pharmacol.)

— A term used in pharmacy for a liquid extract prepared by steeping a plant substance in water. (Oral Med.; Pharmacol.)

ingate (see **sprue**)

inhalant (ĭn-hā′lănt) A medicine to be inhaled. (Anesth.)

inhalation (ĭn-hah-lā′shŭn) The drawing of air or other vapor into the lungs. (Anesth.)

endotracheal i. Inhalation of an anesthetic mixture into the lungs through an endotracheal catheter at low or atmospheric pressure. (Anesth.)

inhaler, nasal A device that is placed over the nose to permit inhalation of anesthetic agents. (Anesth.)

inhibition (ĭn″hĭ-bĭsh′ŭn) A neurologic phenomenon associated with the transmission of an impulse across a synapse. An impulse can be blocked from passing a synapse in a reflex situation by the firing of another, more dominant nerve. Inhibition can be achieved directly by preventing the passage of an impulse along an axon, or it can be achieved by liberation of a chemical substance at the nerve ending. This chemical inhibition is demonstrated by the sympathetic-parasympathetic control over smooth muscle activity in a blood vessel. Inhibition is the restraining of a function of a tissue or organ by some nervous or hormonic control. It is the opposite of excitation. (Oral Physiol.)

inhibitor of cholinesterase (ĭn-hĭb′ĭ-tor, kō″lĭn-ĕs′ter-ās) A chemical that interferes with the activity of the enzyme cholinesterase. (Anesth.)

inion (ĭn′ē-on) The most elevated point on the external occipital protuberance in the midsagittal plane. (Orthodont.)

initiator (ĭ-nĭsh′ē-ā″tor) A chemical agent added

to a resin to initiate polymerization. (D. Mat.)

injection (ĭn-jĕk′shŭn) The act of introducing a liquid into a part such as the bloodstream or tissue. (Anesth.)

— A liquid preparation designed for parenteral administration. (Oral Med.; Pharmacol.)

i. molding (see **molding, injection**)

injury The insult, harm, or hurt applied to tissues; may evoke dystrophic and/or inflammatory response from the affected part. (Periodont.)

frequency of i. Repetitious infliction of injury within a time period. The greater the frequency of insult to a tissue, the greater the likelihood of damage to its components. (Periodont.)

root i. Damage to the root, especially to the cementum, when an excessive force is placed on the tooth. (Periodont.)

toothbrush i. Insult or damage to the teeth and their investing structures produced by faulty toothbrushing. Lesions include tooth and gingival abrasion, with inflammatory or atrophic changes occurring in the gingivae. (Periodont.)

inlay (ĭn′lā) A restoration of metal, fired porcelain, or plastic made to fit a tapered cavity preparation and fastened to or luted into it with a cementing medium. (Oper. Dent.)

i. furnace (see **furnace, inlay**)

setting i. The procedure of fitting a casting to a preparation; adjusting the occlusal function and contact areas; securing the proper, clean dry field; cementing the cleaned, polished casting in aseptic, dry prepared cavity; and completing the final finishing and polishing of the restoration. (Oper. Dent.)

i. wax (see **wax, inlay**)

innervation (ĭn″er-vā′shŭn) Distribution or supply of nerves to a part. (Anesth.)

arterial i. The supply of nerves to the muscles of the arterial vessels. There are two mechanisms that control the muscular action of the blood vessels from the largest artery to the smallest arteriole: the nervous system and the chemical agents in the blood and tissues. The arterial vessels are supplied by two sets of nerves—the vasoconstrictors of the sympathetic system and the vasodilators of the parasympathetic system. These nerves, with the associated biochemical factors, keep the muscles of the arterial system in a state of continuous and partial contraction, a state of tonus. In tonus, the muscles of the arterial system are in constant readiness to adjust to the circulatory needs. (Oral Physiol.)

reciprocal i. The simultaneous stimulation or activation of a flexor pattern when the extensor musculature is inhibited; rhythmic chewing is achieved efficiently when the masticatory muscles are reciprocally innervated. This permits alternate elevation and depression of the mandible in a smooth, coordinated sequence of actions. (Oral Physiol.)

input, sensory The summation of all the stimuli that flow into the nervous system to the cortex, the subcortical brain, and other integrating nerve structures. Collectively, the stimuli are the exteroceptors, the proprioceptors, the chemoreceptors, the special senses, and the psychic phenomena associated with memory and recall. These stimuli are correlated, organized, and integrated in the brain. The stimuli for motor activity flow out to stimulate secretion with muscle contraction. Information about this activity feeds back into the pool of sensory information. There is thus a continuous cycle of sensation, organization, motor activity, and feedback for as long as activity persists in life. (Oral Physiol.)

insert, intramucosal (ĭn″trah-mū-kō′săl) (**mucosal insert, implant button**) A nonreactive metal appliance that is affixed to the tissue-borne surface of a denture and that offers added retentive qualities to the denture. An intramucosal insert consists of a base, a cervix, and a head. (Oral Implant.)

base of i. i. The round, two-tiered discoid structure that affords solid anchorage of the device in the denture when it is embedded into and covered with self-curing acrylic resin. (Oral Implant.)

base-preparing bur of i. i. A specially designed bur constructed to cut a seat in the denture base of the proper size to permit precise placement of either the intramucosal insert or the surgical indicator stylus. It is used in a dental handpiece. (Oral Implant.)

cervix of i. i. The constricted, highly polished portion of the intramucosal insert that connects the base of the insert to the head. (Oral Implant.)

head of i. i. The elliptical-shaped portion of an insert that is designed to obtain retention about itself when placed into the mucosal tissues. (Oral Implant.)

insert, mucosal (see **insert, intramucosal**)

insertion (ĭn-ser′shŭn) The act of implanting or, as it refers to regional analgesia, the act of introducing the needle into the tissues. (Anesth.)

— The placing of a dental prosthesis in the

mouth. (Comp. Prosth.; Fixed Part. Prosth.; Remov. Part. Prosth.)

path of i. The direction in which a prosthesis is inserted and removed. (Comp. Prosth.)
— The direction of movement of an appliance or prosthesis from the point of initial contact of its rigid parts with the supporting teeth to the place of final rest. (Comp. Prosth.; Remov. Part. Prosth.)

choice of p. of i. The varying of the direction of insertion and removal of a partial denture by alteration of the plane to which the guiding abutment surfaces are made parallel. The choice is a compromise to best fulfill four demands: to encounter the least interference, to provide needed retention, to establish adequate guiding-plane surfaces, and to provide acceptable esthetics. (Remov. Part. Prosth.)

insidious (ĭn-sĭd′ē-ŭs) Coming on in a stealthy manner. (Anesth.)

insoluble Not susceptible to being dissolved. (Anesth.)

inspection Visual examination of the body or portions thereof, which is an integral phase of the physical or dental examination procedure. (Periodont.)

inspiration The act of drawing air into the lungs. (Anesth.)

inspirator (ĭn′spĭ-rā″tor) A form of inhaler or respirator. (Anesth.)

inspirometer (ĭn-spĭ-rom′ĕ-ter) An instrument for measuring the force, frequency, or volume of the inspirations. (Anesth.)

instruction of partial denture patient (see **denture, partial, instruction of patient**)

instrument(s) A tool or implement, especially one used for delicate or scientific work. (Oper. Dent.)

amalgam condenser i. (amalgam plugger) An instrument used to compact plastic amalgam. (Oper. Dent.)

carving i. (see **carver**)

classification of i. names Classification of instruments by name to denote purpose (e.g., excavator), to denote position or manner of use (e.g., hand condenser), to describe the form of the point (e.g., hatchet), or to describe the angle of the blade in relation to the handle. (Oper. Dent.)

cutting i. An instrument used to cut, cleave, or plane the walls of a cavity preparation; the blade ends in a sharp, beveled edge. Unless otherwise specified, it refers to a hand instrument rather than to a rotary type. May

be a direct or lateral cutting instrument. (Oper. Dent.)

bibeveled c. i. (bī′bĕv-ĕld) An instrument in which both sides of the end of the blade are beveled to form the cutting edge, as in a hatchet. (Oper. Dent.)

rotary c. i. A power-activated instrument used in a dental handpiece; e.g., a bur, mounted diamond point, mounted carborundum point, wheel stone, or disk. (Oper. Dent.)

single-beveled c. i. An instrument in which one side of the end of the blade is beveled to form the cutting edge, as in a wood chisel. (Oper. Dent.)

diamond i. A rotary abrasive instrument, wheel, or mounted point. Made of fine diamond chips bonded into a desired form; used to reduce tooth structure. (Oper. Dent.)

double-plane i. An instrument with the curve of the blade in a plane perpendicular to that of the angles of the shank. (Oper. Dent.)

formula name of i. Method of naming and describing dental hand instruments. Measurements are in the metric system. The working point is described first, and then the formula is given in three (or sometimes four) units. The first figure denotes the width of the blade in tenths of millimeters, the second shows the length of the blade in millimeters, and the third indicates the angle of the blade in relation to the shaft in centigrades or hundredths of a circle. Whenever it is necessary to describe the angle of the cutting edge of a blade with its shaft, the number is entered in brackets as the second number of the formula. Paired instruments are also designated as *right* or *left;* in lateral cutting instruments the one used to cut from right to left is termed *right;* in direct cutting instruments with right and left bevels, the one having the bevel on the right side of the blade as it is held with the cutting edge down and pointing away from the observer is termed *right.* (Oper. Dent.)

i. grasp (see **grasp, instrument**)

hand i. An instrument used principally with hand force. (Oper. Dent.)

holding i. An instrument used to support gold foil while a foil restoration is inserted. (Oper. Dent.)

McCall's i. Periodontal instruments of various sizes and shapes designed by John Oppie McCall; used for gingival curettage and for dislodging accretions from the tooth surfaces. (Periodont.)

i. parts Handle or shaft, blade or nib, and shank. (Oper. Dent.)

blade The part bearing a cutting edge; it begins at the terminal angle of the shank and ends at the cutting edge. (Oper. Dent.)

nib The counterpart of the blade in the condensing instrument; the end of the nib is the face. (Oper. Dent.)

shaft or handle The part that is grasped by the operator's hand while he is using the instrument. (Oper. Dent.)

shank The part that connects the shaft and the blade or nib. (Oper. Dent.)

plastic i. An instrument used to manipulate a plastic restorative material. (Oper. Dent.)

screwdriver i. An instrument made of surgical alloy; it may have a screw holder at its tip designed to drive screws into the bone. (Oral Implant.)

i. sharpening (see **sharpening, instrument**)

single-plane i. An instrument with all its angles and curves in one plane; when the instrument lies on a flat surface, the cutting edge and the blade will parallel the surface. (Oper. Dent.)

i. stop A device, usually metal, that can be placed on a reamer or file to mark the exact measurement of the root. This prevents the instrument from going beyond the apex since it strikes the incisal, or occlusal, part of the tooth. (Endodont.)

instrumentation (ĭn″stroo-měn-ta′shŭn) The use of, or work done by, instruments in the treatment of a patient. (Oper. Dent.)

— The proper utilization of instruments in the performance of an operation. (Periodont.)

insufficiency, adrenocortical (ah-drē″nō-kor′tĭ-kăl) (see **hypoadrenocorticalism**)

insufficiency, functional Inadequacy of usage of, stimulation to, a part of the body, often resulting in atrophic tissue changes. (Periodont.)

insufflation (ĭn″sŭ-flā′shŭn) The act of blowing a powder, vapor, gas, or air into a cavity; e.g., into the lungs. (Anesth.)

endotracheal i. The forcing of an anesthetic mixture into the lungs through an endotracheal catheter under pressure. (Anesth.)

mouth-to-mouth i. The oldest recorded procedure for artificially ventilating the lungs. The lungs are inflated by blowing into the mouth, and expiration either is passive or is assisted by compressing the thorax. Adequate ventilation is produced, and the procedure should be utilized when other techniques are not applicable; e.g., in thoracic injury.

Auxiliary airway tubes are available for use when mouth-to-mouth insufflation is required. Such tubes maintain the airway and prevent the tongue from obstructing the glottis. (Oral Physiol.)

insufflator (ĭn′suh-flā″tor) An instrument used in insufflation. (Anesth.)

insulator, thermal A material having a low thermal conductivity. (D. Mat.)

insulin (antidiabetic hormone) A hormone produced by the beta cells of the islets of Langerhans in the pancreas. It promotes a decrease in blood sugar. Its action may be influenced by the pituitary growth hormone, ACTH, "S" hormones of the adrenal cortex, epinephrine, glucagon, and thyroid hormone. (Oral Med.)

i. shock (see **shock, insulin**)

insurance Protection against damage, loss, etc.

health i. Insurance that provides financial return when the dentist is unable to practice his profession due to prolonged illness. (Pract. Man.)

liability i. Insurance protecting the dentist from financial loss due to liability suits. (Pract. Man.)

life i. A protective contract providing for compensation to the beneficiaries of the insured. (Pract. Man.)

malpractice i. In dentistry, insurance covering accidents or catastrophes that may occur during the performance of professional duties. (Pract. Man.)

retirement i. Life insurance that carries, as an additional benefit, payments to the insured when he or she reaches a specific age. (Pract. Man.)

insurer The company accepting premiums in return for specific or speculative benefits. The insurance company issuing the policy. (D. Juris.)

intake The substance or quantities thereof taken in and utilized by the body. (Anesth.)

integration, neurologic The factors in the production of speech (i.e., respiration, phonation, resonance, and articulation), which are highly coordinated (some sequentially and some simultaneously) by the central nervous system. Speech is a learned function, and adequate hearing and vision and a normal nervous system are required for its full development. When the speech function comes into conflict with the other vital functions of the maxillofacial structures, it is speech that suffers. This is particularly true when the conflict is with the important reflex actions of coughing, sneezing, hiccuping, and regurgitating. (Oral Physiol.)

intelligence The basic mental potential or the native intellectual ability of a person, in contradistinction to learning. It represents the innate ability to make adaptations to new situations. (Oral Physiol.)

i. quotient (IQ) An estimate of the intellectual status of a child in terms of an index determined by dividing the mental age in months by the actual age in months and reducing the results to a percentage. Hence, the IQ of a child of 100 months with a mental age of 80 months would be 80. (Oral Physiol.)

dental i. q. An estimated appraisal of a patient's appreciation for dental services. (Pract. Man.)

intensifying screen (see **screen, intensifying**)

intensity of an x-ray beam The amount of energy in an x-ray beam per unit volume or area. (Oral Radiol.)

radiation i. Energy flowing through a unit area perpendicular to the beam per unit of time. It is expressed in ergs per square centimeter or in watts per square centimeter. This is not synonymous with dose rate in air. (Oral Radiol.)

interaction According to Newton's law of interaction, the phenomenon in which every force is accompanied by an equal and opposite force. For every force there are two bodies—one to exert the force and one to receive it. Furthermore, whenever there is one force, another force must also be involved. If there is force to the right on one body, there is force to the left on another. Since the one force acts as long as the other, the impulses are equal. The total momentum of the two interacting bodies cannot change. Continuous interaction is demonstrated between the food that is masticated and the force applied to the food. (Oral Physiol.)

interalveolar space (ĭn″ter-ăl-vē′ō-lar) (see **distance, interarch**)

interarch distance (see **distance, interarch**)

interceptive occlusal contact (see **contact, interceptive occlusal**)

interceptive orthodontics (see **orthodontics, interceptive**)

intercondylar distance (ĭn″ter-kon′dĭ-lar) The distance between the vertical axes of a pair of condyles. (Comp. Prosth.; Fixed Part. Prosth.; Remov. Part. Prosth.)

intercuspation (ĭn″ter-kŭs-pā′shŭn) The cusp-to-fossa relationship of the upper and lower posterior teeth to each other. The meshing of cusps of opposing teeth. (Comp. Prosth.; Fixed Part. Prosth.; Remov. Part. Prosth.)

interdental (ĭn″ter-děn′tal) Situated between the proximal surfaces of the teeth of the same arch or between any two teeth in the same arch. (Comp. Prosth.; Remov. Part. Prosth.)

i. canal (see **canal, interdental**)

i. embrasure (see **embrasure, interdental**)

i. septum (see **septum, interdental**)

i. splint (see **splint, interdental**)

interdigitation (ĭn″ter-dĭj″ĭ-tā′shŭn) (see **intercuspation**)

interface (ĭn′ter-fās) The surface, such as a plane surface, formed between the walls of a prepared cavity or extracoronal preparation and a restoration. It forms a common boundary between the tooth structure and the restorative material. (Oper. Dent.)

interfacial surface tension (see **tension, interfacial surface**)

interference, cuspal (see **contact, deflective occlusal**)

interference, occlusal Any tooth-to-tooth contact that interferes with jaw movement—e.g., if during working movement the lingual cusp of an upper tooth is contacting a buccal cusp of a lower tooth on the opposite side, a nonworking or balancing interference is present. (Periodont.)

interference, slip Irregularities at grain boundaries that prevent or interfere with the slippage of one grain on another. (D. Mat.)

interim denture (see **denture, interim**)

intermaxillary Between the two maxillae. (Often incorrectly used to mean between the upper and lower jaws.) (Comp. Prosth.)

— Between the maxillae and mandible. (Orthodont.)

i. anchorage (see **anchorage, maxillomandibular**)

i. elastic (see **elastic, maxillomandibular**)

i. fixation (see **fixation, maxillomandibular**)

i. relation (see **relation, maxillomandibular**)

i. traction (see **traction, maxillomandibular**)

intermedin (ĭn-ter-mē′dĭn) (see **hormone, melanocyte-stimulating**)

intern A dental or medical college graduate serving and residing for twelve months in a hospital, usually during the first year after receiving his D.D.S., D.M.D., or M.D. degree. (Oral Surg.)

interocclusal (ĭn″ter-ŏ-kloo′sal) Between the occlusal surfaces of the maxillary and mandibular teeth. (Comp. Prosth.; Orthodont.; Remov. Part. Prosth.)

i. clearance (see **clearance, interocclusal**)

i. distance (see **distance, interocclusal**)

i. gap (see **distance, interocclusal**)

i. record (see **record, interocclusal**)

i. rest space (see **distance, interocclusal**)

interoceptors (ĭn″ter-ō-sĕp′torz) Those sensory nerve end receptors lining the mucous membrane of the respiratory and digestive tracts which, although not in direct contact with the outer environment, respond to stimuli ultimately received from it. They are similar to exteroceptors but differ from them essentially in their location, which is in the viscera. (Oral Physiol.)

interpolate (ĭn-ter′pō-lāt) To insert intermediate terms in a series according to the trend of the series; to calculate intermediate values according to observed values. (Oral Radiol.)

interposition arthroplasty (ăr′thrō-plăs″tē) The surgical correction of ankylosis by the separating of the immobile fragment from the mobilized fragment and the interpositioning of a substance—such as fascia, cartilage, metal, or plastic—between them. (Oral Surg.) (see also **ankylosis**)

interpretation Evaluation of the morphologic and topographic attributes of the tissues as seen on a radiograph as an aid to diagnosis. The evaluation of variations in opacity as registered on a radiograph; the assessment of normal and pathologic conditions as an aid to diagnosis. (Periodont.)

— Translation of radiographic changes seen by the dentist into real variations in the object radiographed for diagnostic purposes. (Oral Radiol.)

radiographic i. (radiologic i., roentgenographic i.) An opinion formed from the study of a radiograph. (Comp. Prosth.; Remov. Part. Prosth.)

— An impression held by a radiologist resulting from his study of radiographic findings. (Oral Radiol.)

radiologic i. (see **interpretation, radiographic**)

interproximal Between the proximal surfaces of adjoining teeth. (Oper. Dent.)

interradicular alveoloplasty (ĭn″ter-rah-dĭk′ū-lar ăl-vē′ō-lō-plăs″tē) **(intraseptal alveoloplasty)** Removal of the interradicular bone and the collapsing of the cortical plates to a more normal alveolar contour. (Oral Surg.) (see also **alveolectomy**)

interridge distance (see **distance, interarch**)

interview A question-and-answer conference, at which time the parties concerned state the principles and facts regarding their relationship. In dental practice, this usually refers to the relationship between dentist and employee, and between dentist and patient. (Pract. Man.)

intolerance Inability to endure or withstand. (Anesth.)

intra-arterial Situated within an artery or arteries. (Anesth.)

intracellular (ĭn″trah-sĕl′ū-lar) Situated or occurring within a cell or cells. (Anesth.)

intracoronal (ĭn″trah-kō-rō′nal) Pertaining to the inside of the coronal portion of a natural tooth; usually refers to the form of both the tooth preparation and the subsequent restoration; e.g., intracoronal preparation or intracoronal restoration (inlay). (Fixed Part. Prosth.)

i. attachment (see **attachment, intracoronal**)

i. retainer (see **retainer, intracoronal**)

intramaxillary anchorage (see **anchorage, intramaxillary**)

intramaxillary elastic (see **elastic, intramaxillary**)

intramucosal insert (see **insert, intramucosal**)

intramuscular (ĭn″trah-mŭs′kū-lar) Situated in the substance of a muscle. (Anesth.)

intraoral (ĭn″trah-or′al) Within the mouth. (Comp. Prosth.; Fixed Part. Prosth.)

i. tracing (see **tracing, intraoral**)

intraosseous fixation (ĭn″trah-os′ē-ŭs) (see **fixation, intraosseous**)

intrapulmonary (ĭn″trah-pul′mō-ner″ē) Situated in the substance of a lung. (Anesth.)

intrapulmonic (ĭn″trah-pul-mon′ĭk) Occurring in the substance of the lungs. (Anesth.)

intravenation (ĭn″trah-vē-nā′shŭn) The act of injecting anything into a vein. (Anesth.)

intravenous (ĭn″trah-vē′nŭs) In, into, or from within a vein or veins. (Anesth.)

intraversion Indicating teeth or other maxillary structures that are too near the medial plane. (Orthodont.)

intrinsic coloring Coloring from within. The incorporation of pigment within the material of a prosthesis. (M.F.P.)

intrude To move a tooth apically. (Orthodont.)

intrusion A depression; an inward projection. (Orthodont.)

intubate (ĭn′tū-bāt) To treat by intubation. (Anesth.)

intubation (ĭn″tū-bā′shŭn) Insertion of a tube; especially the introduction of a tube into the larynx through the glottis for the introduction of air, etc. (Anesth.)

intubator (ĭn′tū-bāt-or) An instrument used in intubation. (Anesth.)

inunction (ĭn-ŭngk′shŭn) Local application of a drug in an oily or semisolid vehicle such as an ointment, or the preparation that is thus applied. (Oral Med.; Pharmacol.)

invagination of enamel (see **dens in dente**)

epithelial i. Downgrowth of epithelium along

the cervical tract of an implant. (Oral Implant.)

inventory An itemized compilation of materials on hand. (Pract. Man.)

    equipment i. A detailed listing of all the non-expendable items owned by the dentist and used in the practice of his profession. (Pract. Man.)

    materials i. A detailed listing of expendable supplies that are on hand in the practice. This is a constantly fluctuating list, depending on the quantity of the various materials presently on hand. (Pract. Man.)

inverse-square law (see **law, inverse-square**)

inversion The state of being upside down. (Orthodont.)

invest (ĭn-vĕst′) To surround, envelop, or embed in an investment material, e.g., a gypsum product. (Comp. Prosth.; Fixed Part. Prosth.; Oper. Dent.; Remov. Part. Prosth.)

investing (ĭn-vĕst′ĭng) The process of covering or enveloping wholly or in part an object such as a trial denture, tooth, wax form, or crown with a refractory investment material before curing, soldering, or casting. (Comp. Prosth.; Fixed Part. Prosth.; Remov. Part. Prosth.)

    vacuum i. The investing of a pattern within a vacuum to form a mold. (Comp. Prosth.; Fixed Part. Prosth.; Remov. Part. Prosth.)

investment (ĭn-vĕst′mĕnt) Any material used in dentistry to invest an object. The material used to enclose or surround a pattern of a dental restoration for casting or molding or to maintain the relations of metal parts during soldering. (Comp. Prosth.; Fixed Part. Prosth.; Oper. Dent.; Remov. Part. Prosth.)

    casting i. Material from which the mold is made in fabrication of gold or cobalt-chromium castings. (Comp. Prosth.; Remov. Part. Prosth.)

        gypsum-bonded c. i. Casting investment that can be bonded by alpha-hemihydrate, a derivative of gypsum, because the fusion temperatures of the metal alloys to be cast in it are relatively low. All gold alloy investments and some low-fusing cobalt-chromium alloy investments are gypsum bonded. (D. Mat.)

        phosphate-bonded c. i. Casting investment that is bonded by a phosphate and a metallic oxide that react to form a hard mass; generally used for high-fusing alloys. (D. Mat.)

        silica-bonded c. i. Casting investment that is bonded by a silica gel that reverts to

cristobalite in heating and that is generally used for high-fusing alloys. (D. Mat.)

    hygroscopic i. An investment specially designed for use with the hygroscopic investing techniques. (D. Mat.)

    refractory i. An investment material that can withstand the high temperatures used in soldering or casting. (Comp. Prosth.; Remov. Part. Prosth.)

    sectional i. A mold made in sections. (Comp. Prosth.; Remov. Part. Prosth.)

    soldering i. A quartz investment, preferably one with a very low thermal expansion, used for the investment of appliances during the soldering procedure. (D. Mat.)

invisible foil (see **foil, lingual approach**)

involucrum (ĭn″vō-lū′krŭm) A covering; usually a covering of new bone around a sequestrum. (Oral Path.; Oral Surg.)

involuntary Performed independently of the will. (Anesth.)

involute (ĭn′vō-loot) To decrease normally, in size and functional activity, an organ whose role in the body economy is temporary or confined to certain periods of life. Involute should be distinguished from atrophy, which means to waste away from abnormal causes. (Oral Physiol.)

involvement The state of becoming involved.

    bifurcation i. (bī″fŭr-kā′shŭn) The extension of pocket formation into the interradicular area of multirooted teeth in periodontitis. (Periodont.)

    interradicular i. The extension of periodontal pocket formation into the interradicular area of multirooted teeth. (Periodont.) (see also **involvement, bifurcation; involvement, trifurcation**)

    pulp i. A condition wherein consideration of the vitality or health of the dental pulp is a factor. (Oper. Dent.)

    trifurcation i. A condition in which periodontal disease has so destroyed the marginal tissue of the maxillary molars that the interradicular area is exposed. (Periodont.)

iodine A halogen element that is nonmetallic in nature; atomic weight, 126.91. Essential as a nutritional element because it is vital to the production of thyroxin by the thyroid gland. In radioactive form, it is used as a diagnostic substance to determine the ability of the thyroid gland to take up iodine. In tincture form it is used as a locally applied antiseptic, germicide, and disclosing solution. (Periodont.)

    protein-bound i. (PBI) Iodine bound to protein, mainly thyroxin in the plasma. The thyroid hormone is precipitated by protein-denaturing agents, and, in general, the amount of iodine in a protein precipitate indicates the amount of thyroid hormone present and is thus an index of thyroid activity. Various values are given for thyroid function: hypothyroidism, 0 to 3.5 μg/ml of protein-bound iodine; euthyroidism, 3.5 to 8 μg/ml; hyperthyroidism, values higher than 8 μg/ml. (Oral Med.)

iodism (iodine poisoning, iodine stomatitis) Acute or chronic intoxication due to the ingestion or absorption of iodides. Manifestations of acute poisoning include abdominal pain, nausea, vomiting, hypersalivation, conjunctivitis, and collapse. Chronic manifestations include hypersalivation, fever, coryza, swelling and tenderness of the salivary glands, and dermatitis and stomatitis in hypersensitive individuals. It is a toxic condition that sometimes follows the use of preparations containing iodine. (Oral Med.; Pharmacol.)

iodophor (ī-ō′dō-for) A loose chemical compound of iodine with certain organic compounds; e.g., polyvinylpyrrolidone. (Oral Med.; Pharmacol.)

ion (ī′on) An atomic particle, atom, or chemical radical bearing an electric charge, either negative or positive. (Oral Radiol.)

i. pair Two particles of opposite charge, usually the electron and the positive atomic residue resulting after the interaction of ionizing radiation with the orbital electrons of atoms. The average energy required to produce an ion pair is approximately 33 (or 34) electron volts. (Oral Radiol.)

ionic medication (see **ionization**)

ionization (ī″on-ĭ-zā′shŭn) The process or the result of a process by which a neutral atom or molecule acquires either a positive or a negative charge. (Oral Radiol.)

avalanche i. (Townsend i.) The multiplicative process in which a single charged particle accelerated by a strong electric field produces additional charged particles through collision with neutral gas molecules. (Oral Radiol.)

i. chamber (see **chamber, ionization**)

air-equivalent i. c. (see **chamber, ionization, air-equivalent**)

i. density The number of ion pairs per unit volume. (Oral Radiol.)

i. path (ionization track) The trail of ion pairs produced by ionizing radiation in its passage through matter. (Oral Radiol.)

i. potential The potential necessary to separate

one electron from an atom, resulting in the formation of an ion pair. (Oral Radiol.)

ionizer (see **electrolyzer**)

iontophoresis (ī-on″tō-fō-rē′sĭs) Application, by means of an appropriate electrode, of a galvanic current to an ionizable agent in contact with a surface in order to hasten the movement into the tissue of the ion of opposite charge to that of the electrode. Usually a cumbersome and uncertain procedure. (Pharmacol.) (see also **ionization**)

IQ (see **intelligence quotient**)

irradiation (ĭ-rā″dē-ā′shŭn) The exposure of material to roentgen or other radiation. (One speaks of radiation therapy but of irradiation of the patient.) (Oral Radiol.)

— Exposure to radiation. (Oral Radiol.)

irresuscitable (ĭr″rē-sŭs′ĭ-tah-bl) Beyond the possibility of being revived. (Anesth.)

irreversibility (ĭr″rē-ver″sĭ-bĭl′ĭ-tē) The quality of being incapable of being revived. (Anesth.)

irreversible (ĭr″rē-ver′sĭ-bl) Incapable of being reversed or returned to the original state. (Oral Radiol.)

i. hydrocolloid (see **hydrocolloid, irreversible**)

irrigation (ĭr″ĭ-gā′shŭn) The technique of using a solution to wash or flush debris from the root canal of a tooth. (Endodont.)

irritability The quality of being irritable or of responding to a stimulus. (Anesth.)

irritant An agent that causes an irritation or stimulation. (Anesth.)

— An agent (toxic, bacterial, physical, chemical, etc.) that is capable of inducing functional derangements or organic lesions of the tissues. (Periodont.)

chemical i. A chemical agent that causes irritation. The primary agents that have an etiologic relationship to periodontal disease are plaque and calculus. Other agents that serve as a medium for the growth of microorganisms include food debris, sloughed cells, and necrotic material. (Periodont.)

irritation The act of stimulating. Any condition of functional derangement and nervous irritability. (Anesth.)

i. of gingival tissues (see **impingement**)

mechanical i. Tissue damage, injury, or insult by physical forces directed against the tissue; e.g., the tissue irritation produced by faulty toothbrushing. (Periodont.)

i. from overstimulation (see **impingement**)

ischemia (ĭs-kē′mē-ah) Local and temporary deficiency of blood. (Anesth.; Remov. Part. Prosth.)

— A focal deficiency of blood to a part of the

body or simply a local anemia. It results from encroachment on the lumen of an artery or the capillaries supplying the affected area. The reduction in the lumen may be caused by allergic hypersensitivity, degeneration of the tunica intima (atherosclerosis), inflammation, physical pressure, pharmacologic and toxic agents, and/or neurogenic disorders. (Oral Physiol.)

isobar (ĭ'sō-bahr) In radiochemistry, one of two or more different nuclides having the same mass number. (Oral Radiol.)

isomers (ĭ'sō-merz) Organic compounds having the same empirical formula, i.e., the same number of the same atoms, but different structural formulas and therefore different physical and chemical properties. (Oral Med.; Pharmacol.)

— One of several nuclides having the same number of neutrons and protons but capable of existing, for a measurable time, in different quantum states with different energies and radioactive properties. The isomer of higher energy commonly decays to one with lower energy by a process known as isomeric transition. (Oral Radiol.)

optical i. Two isomers whose structures, dextro- and levo-, differ only in a spatial arrangement that makes them mirror images. This occurs only when there is an asymmetric carbon atom, i.e., one attached to four different substituents. The pharmacologic activity often resides very largely in one of the two forms. (Oral Med.; Pharmacol.)

stereo-i. Molecules that differ only in the spatial arrangement of the atoms. This term

includes optical isomers. (Oral Med.; Pharmacol.)

isometric muscle contraction (ĭ''sō-mĕt'rĭk) (see **contraction, muscle, isometric**)

isosthenuria (i''sos-thĕ-nū're-ah) Excretion of urine with fixed specific gravity. It may occur in terminal renal disease when the specific gravity reaches that of the glomerular filtrate, 1.010. (Oral Med.)

isotone (ĭ'sō-tōn) One of several different nuclides having the same number of neutrons in their nuclei, but different mass numbers. (Oral Radiol.)

isotonic (ĭ''sō-ton'ĭk) Having a uniform toxicity or tension. (Anesth.)

— Equivalent in osmotic pressure. Specifically used in reference to a solution whose osmotic pressure is equal to that of a body fluid, such as blood plasma or tears, to which it is compared. (Anesth.; Oral Med.; Pharmacol.)

i. muscle contraction (see **contraction, muscle, isotonic**)

isotope (ĭ'sō-tōp) One of several nuclides having the same number of protons in their nuclei, and hence having the same atomic number but differing in the number of neutrons, and therefore in the mass number. The isotopes of a particular element have virtually identical chemical properties. (Oral Radiol.)

stable i. A nonradioactive isotope of an element. (Oral Radiol.)

itching (see **tickling and itching**)

Ivalon sponge Polyvinyl alcohol sponge.

Ivy loop wiring (see **wiring, Ivy loop**)

Ivy's test (see **test, Ivy's**)

❧ J ❧

jacket (see **crown, complete, veneer, acrylic resin; crown, complete, veneer, porcelain**)

jackscrew A threaded device used in appliances for separation or approximation of teeth or jaw segments. (Oral Surg.)

Jackson's sign (see **sign, Jackson's**)

Janet's test (see **test, Janet's**)

jaundice (jawn′dĭs) A condition characterized by an abnormal accumulation of bilirubin (red bile pigment) in the blood and manifested by a yellowish discoloration of the skin, mucous membranes, and cornea. Seen in hemolytic anemias, biliary obstruction, hepatitis, cholangiolitis, cirrhosis of the liver, etc. Oral mucous membranes may be pigmented. (Oral Diag.; Oral Med.; Periodont.)

acholuric j. Jaundice without bile in the urine. (Oral Med.)

epidemic j. (see **disease, Weil's**)

hemolytic j. (prehepatic j.) Excess bile pigments in the blood due to increased destruction of erythrocytes. (Oral Med.)

congenital h. j. (acholuric icterus, spherocytic anemia, hereditary spherocytosis) A familial hemolytic anemia transmitted as a mendelian dominant. The intrinsic defects of the red blood cells include a spheroidal shape (which allows them to be trapped by the spleen) and increased mechanical fragility. (Oral Med.)

hepatic j. (see **jaundice, hepatocellular**)

hepatocellular j. (hepatic j., infective j., medical j., toxic j.) Jaundice resulting from disease of liver cells by infectious agents or toxins, decreasing the ability of the liver to handle the bile pigments that are continually produced by the destruction of red blood cells. (Oral Med.)

homologous serum j. (see **hepatitis, homologus serum**)

infective j. (see **jaundice, hepatocellular**)

latent j. Increased bilirubin in the blood without clinical signs of jaundice. (Oral Med.)

medical j. (see **jaundice, hepatocellular**)

obstructive j. (posthepatic j.) Extrahepatic and intrahepatic obstruction of the biliary tract resulting in retrograde retention of bile pigments and jaundice. (Oral Med.)

posthepatic j. (see **jaundice, obstructive**)

prehepatic j. (see **jaundice, hemolytic**)

regurgitating j. Jaundice resulting from re-entry of conjugated bilirubin into the blood as a result of obstruction of the biliary tract or hepatocellular damage and failure to excrete conjugated bilirubin from liver cells. (Oral Med.)

retention j. An increase in bilirubin in the blood from hemolysis; failure of the liver cells to conjugate bilirubin or remove free bilirubin. (Oral Med.)

surgical j. Extrahepatic obstruction of the biliary tract. (Oral Med.)

syringe j. (see **hepatitis, homologous serum**)

toxic j. (see **jaundice, hepatocellular**)

jaw A common name for either the maxillae or the mandible; the meaning is usually extended to include their soft tissue covering. (Comp. Prosth.; Remov. Part. Prosth.)

cleft j. (gnathoschisis) A unilateral or bilateral failure of union of the median nasal and maxillary processes in the anterior palatal region, leaving a cleft or clefts through the alveolus. (Oral Diag.)

lumpy j. (see **actinomycosis**)

j. movement (see **movement, jaw**)

phossy j. (see **poisoning, phosphorus**)

j. reflex (see **reflex, jaw**)

j. relation (see **relation, jaw**)

jaw-to-jaw relationship The muscular and TMJ positioning of the mandible in relation to the maxillae with regard to tooth positioning, or intercuspation. (Periodont.)

jelly, petroleum (see **petrolatum**)

Johnston's method (see **method, chloropercha**)

joint(s) The junctions between bones and cartilages. Connective tissue that is usually free from cells and fibers generally covers bones and cartilages where they come together. The remaining ground substance is a tissue fluid, the synovial fluid, which has a high component of hyaluronic acid. In the cranial skeleton one bone butts directly against another, and there is little movement of the bones except during growth. Such a rigid union in the adult skull is termed a synarthrodial joint. A synarthrosis may be formed by thin, intervening layers of cartilage, by connective tissue, or by direct contact of bone to bone. The suture lines may be obliterated in adults with a synarthrodial joint when the bones joined together become fused as one bone. When bones move freely in contact, they have a diarthrodial joint

219

mechanism. The adjacent bone surfaces are typically covered by a film of cartilage and are bound by stout connective tissues, frequently enclosing a liquid-filled joint cavity. (Oral Physiol.)

Charcot's j. (shar-cōz') A manifestation of late syphilis in which there are degeneration, hypertrophy, hypermobility, and loss of contour of a joint, usually a weight-bearing joint. It is most common in tabes dorsalis. (Oral Med.)

hinge j. (see **ginglymus**)

j. mice Cartilaginous material present in the synovial spaces of a joint. (Oral Med.)

j. pathology Disorders of the joints. Joint activity is affected by diseases of metabolism such as arthritis, which affects the fluid, the membrane, and the subchondral bone; by neuromuscular disorders that restrict the motion in a joint or traumatize the joint structure by excessive force; by surgery associated with tumor; and by direct trauma from physical injury. The simplest trauma results from a single injury to the joint structures. It may be slight, causing only a strain on the ligaments or capsule of the joint. The response may be edema, restricted motion, and/or pain. Healing and repair are rapid, complete, and uneventful because of the rich vascular supply to the region of the joints. When the injury is severe enough to injure the synovial membrane, the dynamics and metabolism of the joint are affected and synovitis may ensue. The responses to such injury range from a short period during which the joint is painful and tender because of intra-articular pressures to a chronic alteration of the subchondral bone that results in osteoarthritis. (Oral Physiol.)

temporomandibular j. (see **articulation, temporomandibular**)

Jones protein (see **protein, Bence Jones**)

junction (jŭngk'shŭn) A place of coming together or union.

cementoenamel j. (**cervical line**) The junction of the enamel of the crown and the cementum of the root of a tooth. The area above the junction corresponds to the anatomic crown of the tooth; the area apical to the junction constitutes the anatomic root of the tooth. (Oper. Dent.; Periodont.)

dentinocemental j. The line of union or apposition of the cementum and dentin of a tooth. (Oper. Dent.; Periodont.)

dentinoenamel j. (**dentoenamel j.**) The linear area of juxtaposition of the enamel and dentin of the tooth crown, generally conforming to the shape of the crown. (Periodont.)

dentoenamel j. (see **junction, dentinoenamel**)

dentogingival j. The junction or contact relationship created between the gingival margin, a nonkeratinized epithelium, and the tooth surface. (Periodont.)

mucogingival j. The scalloped linear area denoting the approximation or separation of the gingivae and the alveolar mucosa. (Periodont.)

jurisprudence A body of law.

dental j. (**forensic dentistry**) The science that teaches the application of every branch of dental knowledge to the purposes of the law, including the elucidation of doubtful legal questions. (D. Juris.)

— The state laws and codes covering the legal limitations of the practice of the profession of dentistry. (Pract. Man.)

medical j. The science that applies the principles and practice of the different branches of medicine in the elucidation of doubtful questions in a court of justice. Also called forensic medicine. (D. Juris.)

jury A certain number of men and/or women selected according to law and sworn to inquire of certain matters of fact and to declare the truth on evidence submitted to them. (D. Juris.)

just Right; according to law and justice. (D. Juris.)

justice The constant and perpetual disposition to render every man his due. Also, the conformity of one's actions and will to the law. (D. Juris.)

juxtaposition Adjacent situation; apposition or contact. (Oral Surg.)

❧ K ❧

Kahn's test (see **test, Kahn's**)
kakke (kahk′kā) (see **beriberi**)
kaolin (kā′ō-lĭn) A fine, pure-white clay (hydrated aluminum silicate) used in porcelain teeth to add strength to the molded tooth prior to firing, and toughness and opacity to the fused porcelain product. (D. Mat.; Fixed Part. Prosth.)
Kaposi's sarcoma (see **sarcoma, Kaposi's**)
Kazanjian's operation (kah-zăn′jē-ŭnz) (see **operation, Kazanjian's**)
Kazanjian's procedure (see **operation, Kazanjian's**)
keloid (kē′loid) A dense, proliferative growth on the skin (hypertrophy of scar tissue) that appears to be an abnormal reaction to trauma, especially burns. Keloids tend to recur after excision and occur more frequently in Negroes than in Caucasians. (Oral Diag.; Oral Surg.)
keloplasty (kē′lō-plăs″tē) Excision of scar tissue in the skin. (Oral Surg.)
Kendall's compound B (see **corticosterone**)
Kendall's compound E (see **cortisone**)
Kennedy bar (see **connector, minor, secondary lingual bar**)
Kennedy classification A method of classifying partially edentulous conditions and partial dentures; based on the location of the edentulous spaces in relation to the remaining teeth. (Remov. Part. Prosth.)
keratin (ker′ah-tĭn) An insoluble sulfur-containing protein, composed primarily of the amino acids tyrosine and leucine; the main component of epidermis, hair, nails, keratinized epithelium, etc. (Periodont.)
keratinization (ker″ah-tin″ĭ-zā′shŭn) Term reserved for substances showing the characteristic x-ray diffraction pattern of keratin; e.g., the attached gingiva. (Periodont.)
keratoacanthoma (ker″ah-tō-ăk″ăn-thō′mah) A rapidly growing papular lesion with a superficial crater filled with keratin. (Oral Path.)
keratoconjunctivitis sicca (kĕr″ah-tō-kon-jŭnk″tĭ-vī-tĭs sĭk′ah) (see **syndrome, Sjögren's**)
keratocyst (ker-ah′tō-sĭst) A hornified cyst. (Oral Diag.)
keratohyalin granules (kĕr″ah-to-hī′ah-lĭn) Granules found in the granular layer that may quantitatively influence both its size and the development of the stratum. (Periodont.)

keratosis (ker″ah-tō′sĭs) A horny or cornified growth; e.g., a wart or callosity. (Oral Diag.; Oral Path.)
— A condition characterized by cornification, or hyperkeratinization, of the tissues. (Periodont.)
  focal k. Localized areas of increased cornification (hyperkeratinization). Such lesions are seen particularly on the lips. (Oral Diag.)
  k. follicularis (see **disease, Darier's**)
  seborrheic k. (**basal cell papilloma, verruca senilis**) Benign, pigmented, superficial epithelial tumors that clinically appear to be pasted on the skin of the trunk, arms, or face. Characterized histologically by marked hyperkeratosis, with keratin cyst formation, acanthosis of basal cells, and melanin pigmentation, all above the level of the adjacent epidermis. (Oral Path.)
  senile k. Leukoplakia of a dry surface. (Oral Path.) (see also **leukoplakia**)
    chronic s. k. Keratosis of the lips in elderly individuals. These lesions usually should be considered as precancerous. (Oral Diag.)
ketoacidosis (kē″tō-ăs″ĭ-dō′sĭs) A form of acidosis characterized by an increased accumulation of ketone bodies in the blood; e.g., the acidosis of uncontrolled diabetes mellitus. (Oral Med.)
ketone body (see **body, ketone**)
ketosis (see **ketoacidosis**)
kev Abbreviation for 1000 electron volts. (Oral Radiol.)
keyway The slot into which the male portion of precision attachments fits. (Oper. Dent.)
kg (see **kilogram**)
K.H.N. Abbreviation for Knoop hardness number. (D. Mat.) (see also **test, Knoop hardness**)
kilo- (kĭl′ō) Prefix meaning 1000. (Anesth.)
kilogram (kĭl′ō-grăm) (**kg**) 1000 g; or equivalent to about 2.2 lb avoirdupois. (Anesth.)
kilovolt (kĭl′ō-vōlt) (**kv**) Unit of electrical potential equal to 1000 volts. (Oral Radiol.)
  constant potential k. (**kvcp**) The potential in kilovolts of a constant voltage generator. (Oral Radiol.)
  k. peak (**kvp**) The crest value of the potential wave in kilovolts in an alternating current cycle. When only half of the wave is used,

the value refers to that of the useful half of the wave. (Oral Radiol.)

kilovoltage (kĭl′ō-vōl″tĭj) The potential difference between the anode and cathode of an x-ray tube. (Oral Radiol.)

constant potential k. The potential of a constant voltage generator, in constant potential kilovolts (kvcp). (Oral Radiol.)

equivalent kilovoltage (effective k.) The kilovoltage of monoenergetic radiation having the same half-value layer (HVL) as the heterogeneous beam produced by a peak kilovoltage in question. (Oral Radiol.)

peak k. The crest value of the potential wave, in peak kilovolts (kvp). (Oral Radiol.)

kinanesthesia (kĭn″ăn-ĕs-thē′zē-ah) Loss of the power to perceive the sensation of movement due to derangement of deep sensibility. (Anesth.)

kinematic face-bow (kĭn-ē-măt′ĭk) (see **face-bow, kinematic**)

kinesiology (kĭ-nē″sē-ol′ō-jē) The study of human motion that attempts to explain the manner in which movements of the body occur by considering collectively the information from the areas of anatomy, physiology, and mechanics. It does not profess to give the descriptive minutiae of anatomy or the complete picture of the biochemistry of muscle contraction, nor does it employ the mathematical precision of physics and its applied engineering. Kinesiology is essentially an applied science and is basically descriptive in nature. The principles of kinesiology may be used to describe the laws of articulation and the several theories of mandibular movement. (Oral Physiol.)

kink A bend or twist. (Anesth.)

Kirkland cement dressing, knife (see under appropriate noun)

Kirschner wire (see **wire, Kirschner**)

Kirstein's method (see **method, Kirstein's**)
Kline's test (see **test, Kline's**)
knife An instrument used for cutting that consists of a sharp-edged blade provided with a handle.

buck k. A periodontal knife possessing spear-shaped cutting points; used for interdental incision during gingivectomy. (Periodont.)

electronic k. An electrosurgical scalpel used to incise or shave tissue. If properly and judiciously used, it is a valuable aid for the contouring of gingival tissues to physiologic architectural form. (Periodont.)

gold k. An instrument, usually contra-angled, with a blade of knife form; used to trim excess metal and develop contour in foil restorations. (Oper. Dent.)

Goldman-Fox k. Any of a group of surgical instruments designed for the incision and contouring of gingival tissue. The No. 7 knife is heart shaped and is intended for the primary gingivectomy incision. The No. 11 knife is designed for interproximal incisions. (Periodont.)

Kirkland k. A heart-shaped knife, sharp on all edges, used for the primary gingivectomy incision. (Periodont.)

Merrifield's k. A knife that has a long, narrow, triangular blade in a shank; used for gingivectomy incisions. (Periodont.)

Knoop hardness test (see **test, Knoop hardness**)
Koeber's saw (see **saw, Koeber's**)
Koplik's spots (see **spots, Koplik's**)
Krause's corpuscles (see **corpuscle, Krause's**)
Kryptex (see **cement, silicophosphate**)
Küstner's test (kĭst′nerz) (see **test, skin, indirect**)
kv (see **kilovolt**)
kvcp (see **kilovolt, constant potential**)
kvp (see **kilovolt peak**)
kyphosis (kī-fō′sĭs) (**humpback**) An abnormal curvature of the spine with the convexity backward. (Oral Diag.)

L

label (lā'bĕl) Information placed on a package. The portion of the prescription in which the directions for use are stated. (Oral Med.; Pharmacol.) (see also **signa**)

labial (lā'bē-ăl) Of or pertaining to a lip. Toward a lip. (Comp. Prosth.; Oper. Dent.; Oral Surg.; Orthodont.; Remov. Part. Prosth.)
l. notch (see **notch, labial**)

labile (lā'bĭl) Unstable, as labile fever. (Oral Surg.)

labioversion (lā"bē-ō-ver'zhŭn) Any deviation of a tooth toward the lips from the line of occlusion or from a harmonious relationship to the dental arch. (Orthodont.; Periodont.)

labium superius oris (lā'bē-ŭm sū-pē're-ŭs ō'rĭs) Point of the upper lip lying in the midsagittal plane and a line drawn across the boundary of the mucous surface tangent to the curves. (Orthodont.)

laboratory The room in which the dentist or his auxiliaries perform professional services related to dental treatment but not done directly in the patient's mouth. (Pract. Man.)

laceration A wound produced by tearing; the process of tearing. (Oral Diag.; Oral Surg.)

laches (lătch'ĭz) Negligence; inexcusable delay; a failure to claim or enforce a claim or right at a proper time. (D. Juris.)

lacrimation, gustatory (see **syndrome, auriculotemporal**)

lactoflavin (lăk'tō-flā-vĭn) (see **vitamin B₂**)

lacuna (lah-kū'nah) A gap or space within bone. Within the bone are seen lacunae, containing osteocytes, from which canaliculi, containing protoplasmic processes of the osteocytes, radiate. Other lacunae are found primarily on the periphery of the bone surface and represent areas of bone resorption; they are of an irregular nature and often contain osteoclasts (Howship's lacunae; absorption lacunae). (Periodont.)

lambda (lăm'dah) The point in the skull at which the sagittal and lambdoid sutures meet. The strap of a rubber dam holder placed at this level will hold its position without slipping up or down. (Oper. Dent.; Orthodont.)

lamella, cemental (lah-mĕl'ah) The arrangement and deposition of cementum in incremental layers more or less parallel to the root configuration. (Periodont.)

lamina (lăm'ĭ-nah) A flat, thin plate.
l. dura Radiographic term denoting the plate of compact bone (alveolar bone) that lies adjacent to the periodontal membrane. It appears as a dense radiopaque line when the alveolar bone is in a state of health. When resorption of the alveolar bone occurs, the lamina dura appears radiographically to have lost its continuity, its thickness, and varying degrees of its radiopacity. (Oper. Dent.; Periodont.)
l. propria The zone of connective tissue subjacent to the epithelium of a mucous membrane. The lamina propria of the gingivae may be divided into two portions: that which is immediately subjacent to the epithelium, which interdigitates with the epithelial rete pegs, and an underlying layer of dense connective tissue that is contiguous with the submucosa. The gingival fibers enter into the lamina propria, attaching the gingivae to the tooth surface. (Periodont.)

laminagraphy (lăm'ĭ-năg'rah-fē) Body section radiography; used in dentistry in temporomandibular joint projections. (Oral Surg.)

lamp, mouth A device to produce light or illumination directly in the oral cavity and to transilluminate the dental tissues. (Oper. Dent.)

lance To cut open with a lancet; to incise. (Oral Surg.)

lancinating Pertaining to a stabbing pain; e.g., the pain occurring in tic douloureux. (Oral Surg.)

landmark An anatomic structure used as a guide for anatomic relationships; used in conductive anesthesia procedures, surgical dissections, radiologic examination, etc. (Oral Radiol.; Oral Surg.)
cephalometric l. (sĕf"ah-lō-mĕt'rĭk) One of the points located on oriented head radiographs from which lines, planes, and angles may be constructed in order to analyze the configuration and relationship of elements of the craniofacial skeleton. (Orthodont.)

laryngismus (lar"ĭn-jĭz'mŭs) Spasm of the larynx. (Anesth.)

laryngopharyngeal (lah-rĭng"gō-fah-rĭn'jē-al) Related jointly to the larynx and the pharynx. (Anesth.)

223

laryngopharynx (lah-rĭng″gō-făr′ĭngks) The lower portion of the pharynx, which extends from the corner of the hyoid bone or the vestibule of the larynx to the lower border of the cricoid cartilage. (Anesth.)

laryngoscope (lah-rĭng′gō-skōp) An instrument for examining the larynx. (Anesth.)

laryngospasm (lah-rĭng′gō-spăzm) Spasmodic closure of the larynx, sometimes noted during the induction phase of general anesthesia or during the recovery period. (Anesth.; Oral Surg.)

last will and testament The legal document describing the desires of a person for the distribution of his worldly goods after his death. (Pract. Man.)

latent image (see **image, latent**)

latent period (see **period, latent**)

lateral (lăt′ĕr-ăl) A position either to the right or the left of the midsagittal plane. (Comp. Prosth.; Orthodont.; Remov. Part. Prosth.)

  l. checkbite (see **record, interocclusal**)

  l. condylar inclination (see **inclination, lateral condylar**)

  l. condyle path (see **path, lateral condyle**)

  l. excursion (see **excursion, lateral**)

  l. movement (see **movement, lateral**)

  l. protrusion (see **protrusion, lateral**)

laterodetrusion (lăt″ĕr-ō-dē-tru′zhŭn) Noun that describes precisely the directions in which the muscles thrust a condyle outward and downward in the side shift preparatory to handling a large bolus of food. (Gnathol.)

lateroprotrusive (lăt″er-ō-prō-tru′sĭv) Pertaining to a movement direction of the jaw that has both sideward and forward components of movement. (Gnathol.)

lateroretrusive (lăt″er-ō-rē-tru′sĭv) Pertaining to a movement direction in cusp or condyle thrusts that has both lateral and backward components of movement. (Gnathol.)

laterotrusion (lăt″ĕr-ō-tru′zhŭn) The outward thrust given by the muscles to the rotating condyle or the condyle on the bolus side. When the jaw is thrown laterally, it seldom is from a pure rotation of the working condyle, because in most persons, the working side condyle moves as it rotates, or it moves outward and then is rotated. (Gnathol.)

  precurrent l. Laterotrusion in which the working side condyle is rotated as it is thrust laterally. (Gnathol.)

latex (lā′tĕks) Natural rubber. (Orthodont.)

latitude (lăt′ĭ-tūd″) The range between the minimum and maximum film exposures to radiation that yield images of structures whose photographic density differences are discernible under normal viewing conditions. Latitude chiefly varies directly with kilovoltage and inversely with contrast. (Oral Radiol.) (see also **contrast**)

lattice, space (lăt′ĭs) An arrangement of atoms in a definite relationship to each other, forming a lattice. (Oper. Dent.)

lavage (lah-vahzh′) Irrigation, or washing out, as in oral lavage. (Oral Surg.)

law(s) That which is laid down or established. An enforceable rule of conduct. (D. Juris.)

  Charles' l. The principle which states that all gases on heating expand equally and on cooling contract equally. (Anesth.)

  Dalton's l. The principle which states that the pressure of a mixture of gases equals the sum of the partial pressures of the constituent gases. So long as no chemical change occurs, each gas in a mixture of gases is absorbed by a given volume of solvent in proportion not to the total pressure of the mixture but to the partial pressure of the gas. (Anesth.)

  ignorance of l. Want of knowledge or acquaintance with the laws of the land insofar as they apply to the act, relation, duty, or matter under consideration. (D. Juris.)

  inverse-square l. The principle which states that the strength of x radiation from a point source varies inversely as the square of the distance; thus, as the distance is doubled, the intensity of the beam will be quartered. This does not apply in theory to scatter radiation from a broader source, although it may be used in a practical sense. (Oral Radiol.)

  moral l. The aggregate of those rules and principles of ethics that relate to right and wrong conduct and prescribe the standards to which the actions of persons should conform in their dealings with each other. (D. Juris.)

  neurologic l. (see **law of specific energy**)

  Newton's l., clinical application Clinical procedures and recommendations based on the laws of inertia, momentum, and interaction. For example, patients should have small occlusal tables for mastication; the widest possible bearing area for denture bases should be created; patients should introduce small quantities of food into the mouth for mastication; and food should be placed on the occlusal table in the first molar region to increase the efficiency of the lever system. (Oral Physiol.)

  Pascal's l. The principle which states that pressure applied to a liquid at any point is transmitted equally in all directions. (Remov. Part. Prosth.)

l. of specific energy (neurologic l.) The principle which states, in essence, that sensory quality is perceived according to the nerve that is excited, not according to the object that excites. If pressure placed on the eyeballs stimulates the retina, light is perceived, not pressure; similarly, electrical stimulation will produce sensations of smell, taste, touch, or pain in accordance with the nerve stimulated but not a sensation of electricity as such. The special, as well as the general, senses maintain this principle. (Oral Physiol.)

Wolff's l. The principle which states that all changes in the function of bone are attended by definite alterations in its internal structure. (Oral Surg.)

written l. Law or laws created by express legislation or enactment, as distinguished from unwritten or common law, which includes all law or laws from any other legal source. (D. Juris.)

lay Nonprofessional. (D. Juris.)

layer, Beilby's (bīl'bēz) An amorphous layer formed on the surface of metals by a disorientation of the crystalline structure during polishing. (D. Mat.)

LD₅₀ (see **dose, lethal, median**)

LD₅₀ time (see **time, median lethal**)

lead apron (see **apron, lead**)

lead glass (see **glass, lead**)

lead poisoning (see **plumbism**)

lease A conveyance of lands or tenements to a person for life, for a stated number of years, or at will, in consideration of rent or some other recompense. (D. Juris.)

lecithin (lĕs'ĭ-thĭn) A monoaminomonophosphatide found in nerve tissue, bile, blood, semen, egg yolk, etc.; usually occurs within all cells as lecithoprotein. (Periodont.)

ledger sheet An accounting form for keeping track of debits, expenditures, credits, and charges. (Pract. Man.)

Leede's test (see **test, capillary resistance**)

LeFort fracture (see **fracture, LeFort**)

legal In compliance with law. (D. Juris.)

leiomyoma (lī"ō-mī-ō'mah) A benign tumor derived from smooth muscle. (Oral Path.)

length The longest measure of an object, or the measurement between the two ends. A factor in the flexibility of major connectors and clasps and in the degree of efficiency of indirect retainers. (Remov. Part. Prosth.)

muscle l. The variable end-to-end measurement of a muscle. The physical changes in muscle observed in the isotonic and isometric states of contraction are related to the alteration in the striated bands of muscle. Many forms of activity of striated, or skeletal, muscle are associated with lever mechanisms. During the course of contraction, a muscle may be required to shorten, to maintain its length, or even to be lengthened. These states of active contraction are part of a highly coordinated synchronous and reciprocal relationship with other muscles. (Oral Physiol.)

tooth l. The distance along the long axis of the tooth from the apex of the root to the tip, or incisal edge, of the tooth. (Orthodont.)

lentula (lĕn-too'lah) A flexible spiral-wire instrument used in a handpiece to apply paste filling materials in root canals. (Endodont.)

leontiasis ossea (lē"on-tī'ah-sĭs os'ē-ah) An enlargement of the bones of the face leading to a lionlike appearance. It is recognized by some as a disease entity, but the name simply describes an appearance that may result from any of a number of diseases causing enlargement of the facial bones. (Oral Diag.)

— A clinical term applied to a slowly progressive disease that occurs in children and is characterized by hyperkeratosis of the facial bones, jaws, and skull, which results in a leonine appearance. Osseous encroachment may cause obliteration of sinuses, blindness, and malocclusion. (Oral Path.)

leproma Nodular lesion of leprosy seen on the skin, mucous membranes (including those of the eyes), upper respiratory tract, tongue, and palate. (Oral Med.)

leprosy (lĕp'rō-sē) (**Hansen's disease**) A chronic granulomatous infection caused by *Mycobacterium leprae*. It may exist in lepromatous (contagious), tuberculoid (noncontagious), and intermediate forms. (Oral Med.; Oral Path.)

leptocytosis, hereditary (lĕp"tō-sī-tō'sĭs) (see **thalassemia**)

Leptothrix (lĕp'tō-thrĭks) A filamentous microorganism, apparently not directly capable of pathogenicity, that may act as a nidus for the formation of dental calculus and its attachment to the tooth structure. Some investigators have associated this organism with the presence of periodontitis in human beings. (Periodont.)

lesion (lē'zhŭn) Any pathologic disturbance of a

tissue, with loss of continuity, enlargement, function, etc. (Oral Diag.)

cheek-chewing l. A lesion of the buccal mucosa caused by the patient's chewing his own cheek. (Oral Diag.)

extravasation l. (see **cyst, traumatic**)

herpetic l. A vesicle and/or ulceration of the mucosa caused by the herpes virus. (Oral Diag.)

herpetiform l. A painful ulceration of the oral mucosa with a red center and yellow border; occurs as a solitary lesion or in groups and appears similar to those lesions caused by herpesvirus. The term herpetiform is used as a clinical designation unless the viral cause has actually been demonstrated. (Oral Diag.)

indefinite bone l. (see **cyst, extravasation**)

traumatic bone l. (see **cyst, traumatic**)

Lesser's triangle (see **triangle, Lesser's**)

L.E.T. (see **transfer, linear energy**)

Letterer-Siwe disease (see **disease, Letterer-Siwe**)

leukemia (lū-kē′mē-ăh) A usually fatal disease of the blood-forming tissues characterized by a great increase in the white blood cell count (except in aleukemic leukemia). Oral lesions include gingival enlargement, severe gingivitis, and necrosis. Myeloid, lymphoid, and monocytic leukemias are the chief types. (Oral Diag.)

— An acute, subacute, or chronic disease of the white blood cell–forming tissue characterized by an unregulated, independent, profitless proliferation of leukocytes and precursors. It is usually manifested by the presence of large numbers of immature, abnormal white blood cells in the circulating blood. (Oral Med.)

— A malignant neoplasm characterized by an overproduction of white blood cells that appear in the circulating blood, most often in an immature form. (Oral Path.)

— A disease affecting the blood-forming tissues; characterized by abnormal proliferation of leukocytes and their precursors and attended by fatigue, weakness, fever, lymphadenopathy, splenomegaly, a tendency toward profuse tissue hemorrhage, ulceronecrotic lesions of the oral mucous membranes, diminished resistance to infection, etc. (Periodont.)

aleukemic l. A variety of leukemia marked by the proliferation of leukocytes within the blood-forming tissues, but without an increase in the white blood cell count; relatively few precursor cells are found in the blood smear. Although the finding of ab-

normal forms in the bloodstream is characteristic, the abnormal cells fail to appear in the blood in increased numbers. Oral lesions, when present, are ulceronecrotic and hypertrophic. (Oral Diag.; Periodont.)

lymphatic l. (lymphoid l.) An abnormal increase in white blood cells characterized by disturbance in the lymphocyte-producing tissues and abnormal numbers and types of lymphocytes. (Oral Diag.)

— A hyperplasia, of undetermined origin, affecting lymphoid tissue. Predominating cells are lymphocytes and lymphoblasts. Generally assumes a more chronic course than other forms of leukemia but may be acute. Oral lesions include swollen and hyperplastic gingivae, ulceronecrotic lesions, a marked tendency to gingival hemorrhage, etc. (Oral Path.; Periodont.)

lymphoid l. (see **leukemia, lymphatic**)

monocytic l. A malignant disease of the blood-forming cells characterized by excessive numbers of monocytes in the bloodstream. Oral manifestations include gingival enlargement and necrosis. (Oral Diag.; Oral Path.)

— A form of leukemia characterized by an abnormal increase in the number of monocytes. Manifestations include progressive weakness, anorexia, lymphadenopathy, hepatomegaly, splenomegaly, secondary anemia, etc. Oral lesions may be ulceronecrotic and hemorrhagic. (Periodont.)

myelogenous l. A malignant disease of the blood-forming apparatus characterized by excessive production of white blood cells (granulocytes) in the bone marrow. Oral manifestations may include gingival enlargement and necrosis. (Oral Diag.)

— Leukemia in which the leukocytes are of bone marrow origin; e.g., polymorphonuclear leukoctyes, myelocytes, and myeloblasts. (Oral Path.)

leukocyte (loo′kō-sīt) A white blood cell. (Oral Path.)

— White blood cell; a nucleated ameboid mass of protoplasm circulating in the blood. (Oral Physiol.) (see also **lymphocyte; monocyte**)

basophilic l. A basophil; a leukocyte that has coarse granules stainable with basic dyes and a bent lobed nucleus. (Oral Physiol.)

eosinophilic l. An eosinophil; a leukocyte that has coarse granules stainable with eosin and a bilobed nucleus. (Oral Physiol.)

immature l. One of several forms of leukocyte usually found in disease; e.g., myelocytes, myeloblasts, and lymphoblasts. (Oral Physiol.)

polymorphonuclear l. A neutrophil; a white blood cell with finely granular cytoplasm, an irregularly lobulated nucleus, and the appearance of a microphage. It is found in the tissues during acute inflammatory processes and in the superficial surface aspects of a lesion during subacute or chronic inflammation. The predominating leukocytes of the blood. Blood levels may be increased during acute inflammatory states, myelogenous leukemia, etc., and decreased in agranulocytosis (malignant neutropenia). (Periodont.)

— A neutrophil; a polymorph; a leukocyte that has fine granules stainable with neutral dyes and an irregularly lobed nucleus. (Oral Physiol.)

leukocytosis (loo″kō-sī-tō′sĭs) An increase in the leukocytes in the blood; may be a defensive reaction, as in inflammation, or may be due to a disturbance in white blood cell formation, as in leukemia. (Oral Diag.)

— An increase in the normal number of white blood cells. Various limits are given; e.g., leukocytosis in the adult is indicated when there are more than 10,000 white blood cells per cubic millimeter. (Oral Med.) (see also **eosinophilia; lymphocytosis; neutrophilia**)

leukoedema (loo″kō-ĕ-dē′mah) An innocuous oral condition characterized by a filmy, opalescent, white covering of the buccal mucosa consisting of a thickened layer of parakeratotic cells. It is most commonly associated with mechanical and chemical irritation. (Oral Diag.)

leukopenia (loo″kō-pē′nē-ah) A decrease in the normal number of white blood cells in the circulating blood. Various lower limits are given; e.g., leukopenia signifies less than 4000 white blood cells per cubic millimeter. (Oral Diag.; Oral Med.) (see also **lymphocytopenia; neutropenia**)

leukoplakia (loo″kō-plā′kē-ah) A white plaque formed on the oral mucous membrane from surface epithelial cells. It is leathery, opaque, and somewhat thickened. Excluded from this are the white lesions of lichen planus, white sponge nevus, burns, thrush, and other clinically recognizable entities. Leukoplakia, as used in this sense, is a clinical term in accordance with its classical meaning of a white plaque. (Oral Diag.)

— A premalignant surface lesion of the mucous membrane characterized by hyperkeratosis and dyskeratosis of the stratified squamous epithe-

lium. (Oral Path.) (see also **dyskeratosis; hyperkeratosis**)

— The development of white or off-white thickened patches of hyperkeratonic epithelium on mucosal surfaces. Histologically, hyperkeratosis, acanthosis, subepithelial and perivascular infiltrate of round cells, etc. may be seen. Dyskeratosis may be present. Leukoplakia lesions may progress to malignancy, with cellular atypicism, dyskeratosis, epithelial pearl formation, infiltration of malignant cells into connective tissue corium, etc. (Periodont.)

leukotaxine (loo″kō-tăk′sĭn) A substance that appears when tissue is injured and that can be recovered from inflammatory exudates. Increases capillary permeability and the diapedesis of leukocytes. (Oral Path.)

lev- (see **levo-**)

levarterenol The official (U.S.P.) drug name for norepinephrine. The British (B.P.) name is noradrenaline. In contrast to epinephrine, levarterenol produces its pressor effect primarily through vasoconstriction in certain areas rather than by cardiac excitatory action. (Anesth.; Pharmacol.) (see also **norepinephrine**)

level (lĕv′ĕl) To reduce the curve of Spee by intrusion and/or extrusion of the teeth in an arch. (Orthodont.)

leveling arch wire Arch wire used to align teeth in the same plane. (Orthodont.)

lever (lĕv′er) A bar or rigid body that is capable of turning about one joint or axis and in which are two or more other points where forces are applied. Egyptians understood, classified, and used levers 3000 years B.C. There are three classes of levers, and each has its own most effective use. (Gnathol.)

first-class l. A lever in which the fulcrum lies between the power source and the work produced. Its purpose is to lift great loads efficiently. A typical example of such a load in the human body is the head as it rests on the vertebral column. The fulcrum is at the axis of the cervical spine. The power for maintaining the head posture erect is provided by the powerful postcervical neck musculature, and the work performed is that energy necessary to overcome the force of gravity that could tend to cause the head and face structures to drop forward. The first-class lever, in such an instance, is a very efficient system for the production of considerable power. In the first-class lever the relationship between the length of the force arm and the length of the work-producing arm may vary; i.e., they may be equal, or either one may be longer than the other, with consequent alterations in efficiency. (Oral Physiol.)

second-class l. A lever in which the force arm is longer than the work-producing arm; thus the work produced is always greater than the energy used, with a resultant high efficiency. An example of a second-class lever in the body is seen in the action that takes place when a person stands on his toes. The fulcrum lies at the toes, the power arm is at the heel where the gastrocnemius muscle is inserted, and the work performed is represented by the elevation of the body weight, which rests on the bones of the metatarsal arch. Potentially the second-class lever is more efficient than the first-class lever, and it is considerably more efficient than the third-class lever. (Oral Physiol.)

third-class l. A lever in which the axis is at one end, the load at the other end, and the effort is exerted at a direction in between, as in a treadle. Its purpose is to speed the movement of the load. An example of the third-class lever in the body is the flexion of the elbow in the act of picking up a small weight. The fulcrum is at the elbow, the source of force (the biceps muscle) is attached close to the fulcrum in the forearm, and the work done is the elevation of a ball in the palm of the hand. The essential characteristic of this action is that, by a slight contraction of the muscle, the arm, which moves only a slight distance close to the fulcrum where the muscle is attached, moves a considerable distance at the work position, the hand. Thus rapid and extensive movement of a part of the body is effected by a combination of third-class levers. The third-class lever is the least efficient of the levers. It is not a strong, power-producing system like the second-class lever, but it does produce movement of a structure with a small expenditure of energy in a very short time. Thus the main contribution of the third-class lever in musculoskeletal activity is maneuverability of the tissues, as in the mechanical action of the mandible, rather than power production. It moves the tissues and elements into favorable positions so that the first-class and second-class levers can function more efficiently without dissipating their energies for changes in body position. (Oral Physiol.)

leverage (lĕv'er-ĭj) The mechanical advantage gained by the use of a lever. A factor in the magnification of stresses generated by an extension-base partial denture, etc. (Remov. Part. Prosth.)

levo- (**lēv-**) Prefix applied to the name of optical isomers that rotate the plane of polarized light to the left. (Oral Med.; Pharmacol.)

liability (lī″ah-bĭl'ĭ-tē) The state of being bound by law or justice to do something or to make something good; legal responsibility. (D. Juris.)

libel (lī'bĕl) That which is written and published, calculated to injure the character of another by bringing him into ridicule or contempt. (D. Juris.)

license Permission, accorded by a competent authority, granting the right to perform some act or acts that without such authorization would be contrary to law. (D. Juris.)

lichen planus (lī'kĕn plā'nŭs) A disease of unknown etiology affecting the skin and oral mucous membranes, either alone or concomitantly. The oral lesions are most common on the buccal mucous membrane, where they present a lacy pattern or bilateral network of raised white or bluish white, porcelain-like fine lines or a series of small, similarly appearing dots. The lesions are painless. On the tongue the lesions may appear as flat white plaques resembling leukoplakia. (Oral Diag.; Oral Path.)
— A dermatologic disease affecting the skin and mucous membranes; of unknown etiology but often associated with nervousness, fatigue, emotional depression, and allergy and considered to be a manifestation of quinacrine (Atabrine) therapy. Oral lesions often appear as white or blue-white striae forming an interweaving lacelike network of lines of epithelial thickening. Associated with the striated network; bullous or erosive lesions may be found. Histologically, varying degrees of hyperkeratosis and epithelial acanthosis may be found, with formation of sawtooth-shaped rete pegs of epithelium projecting into connective tissue corium. Subjacent to the epithelium is a band-like infiltrate of round cells with perivascular accumulation of leukocytes. Treatment is symptomatic. (Periodont.)

lien (lēn) A qualified right of property that a creditor has in specific property of his debtor as security for the debt or for performance of some act. (D. Juris.)

life, radioactive (see **half-life**)
   effective half-l. (see **half-life, effective**)

ligament (lĭg'ah-mĕnt) Any tough, fibrous connective tissue band that connects bones or supports viscera. Some of the ligaments are distinct fibrous structures; others are folds of fascia or of indurated peritoneum; still others are the relics of unused fetal organs. (Oral Surg.)

periodontal l. (PDL) The mode of attachment of the tooth to the alveolus. The ligament consists of numerous bundles of collagenous tissue (principal fibers) arranged in groups, between which is loose connective tissue, together with blood vessels, lymph vessels, and nerves. It functions as the investing and supportive mechanism for the tooth. (Periodont.)

  biologic width of p. l. The width of the periodontal ligament in normal, functioning teeth. It varies with the age of the individual and the functional demands made on the tooth, and in normalcy it is about 0.25 and 0.1 mm in width, narrowest at the center of the alveolus and widest at the margin and apex. (Periodont.)

sphenomandibular l. The ligament extending from the spine of the sphenoid bone to the mandibular lingula. (Oral Surg.)

stylohyoid l. A fibroelastic cord attached superior to the styloid process of the sphenoid bone. (Oral Surg.)

stylomandibular l. A ligament extending from the styloid process of the temporal bone and attached to the mandibular gonial angle. (Oral Surg.)

temporomandibular l. A triangular-shaped fibrous band extending from the lateral aspects of the root of the zygomatic process of the temporal bone to the mandibular subcondylar neck. (Oral Surg.)

ligate (lĭ′gāt) To tie or bind with a ligature or suture. (Oral Surg.)

ligation (lĭ-gā′shŭn) The operation of tying teeth with some form of knotted ligature. (Endodont.)

— The binding together of teeth with wire, string, thread, etc. for stabilization and immobilization during periodontal therapy; the application of a ligature to a tooth (teeth) as a phase of tooth movement in orthodontics; the occlusion of a blood vessel by applying a ligature circumferentially. (Periodont.)

surgical l. Exposure of an unerupted tooth with placement of a metal ligature around its cervix. The free ends of the ligature are fixed to a fine, precious-metal chain, which in turn is fixed to an orthodontic appliance for the purpose of placing traction on the unerupted tooth to cause its eruption. (Orthodont.)

ligature (lĭg′ah-tūr) A cord, thread, or fine wire tied around teeth for the purpose of holding a rubber dam in place on retained teeth with fractured roots or split crowns or on teeth that have been replanted. (Endodont.)

— Cord, thread, or wire used in tying off or binding. Sometimes used as a synonym for dental floss. (Oper. Dent.)

— A wire or threadlike substance used to tie a tooth to an orthodontic appliance or to another tooth. (Orthodont.)

  grass-line l. A ligature composed of the fibers of a grass-cloth plant (ramie); utilized for minor tooth movement. It depends for its activation in movement on the property of shrinkage of the ligature when it is wetted by the saliva of the patient. (Periodont.)

  steel l. A form of ligature, available as steel filaments in several useful diameters, used to bind teeth together to secure their stabilization and immobilization or, when properly applied, to produce desirable minor tooth movement. (Periodont.)

light box (see **illuminator**)

light, operating A light with a strong beam that may be directed for concentrated illumination of a part being operated on. (Oper. Dent.)

light touch (see **touch, light**)

limit Restriction.

  elastic l. (proportional l.) The greatest stress to which a material may be subjected and still be capable of returning to its original dimensions when the forces are released. (Comp. Prosth.; D. Mat.)

  proportional l. (see **limit, elastic**)

line Boundary; demarcation.

  l. angle (see **angle, line**)

  l. balancing A tracing of a gnathic projection plane that starts from the point of centricity and on the horizontal plane of projection runs forward and medially but on the vertical plane runs downward and forward. Line balancing is an orbital path of the opposite condyle that is moving outward in other component directions and turning about on its traveling axis. (Gnathol.)

  basophilic l. A group of microscopic sections of bone that stains darkly with hematoxylin. Represents periods of bone inactivity. (Oral Path.)

  Camper's l. The line running from the inferior border of the ala of the nose to the superior border of the tragus of the ear. (Comp. Prosth.; Remov. Part. Prosth.)

  cement l. The line of cement exposed at the margin of an inlay or crown.

  cemental l. (cementing l.) Basophilic line

distinguishing adjacent lamallae of bone; represents periods of inactivity of bone formation and resorption. (Periodont.)

cementing l. (see **line, cemental**)

cervical l. (see **junction, cementoenamel**)

cross arch fulcrum l. (see **line, fulcrum, cross arch**)

l. of draw The direction or plane of withdrawal or seating of a removable or cemented restoration. (Oper. Dent.)

external oblique l. A ridge of osseous structure on the body of the mandible extending from the anterolateral border to the mandibular ramus, passing downward and forward, after covering the buccocervical portion of the third molar, and ending by blending into the body of the mandible, lateral to the molar teeth. (Periodont.)

finish l. In cavity preparations, a minimal line of demarcation of the wall of the preparation at the cavosurface angle; usually results from a slice made by an abrasive disk. (Oper. Dent.)

l. focus A principle employed in the design of x-ray tubes, by which the effective focal spot is sharply reduced relative to the actual (larger) focal spot desirable to deal with the heat generated. It involves focusing the cathode stream, in the pattern of a thin rectangle, onto an anode truncated at about 20° to the transverse axis of the tube. (Oral Radiol.) (see also **spot, focal, effective**)

l. of force (see **force, line of**)

fulcrum l. Any imaginary line around which a removable partial denture tends to rotate. (Remov. Part. Prosth.)

　anteroposterior f. l. An imaginary line of rotation extending from a point in the rest area of the most distal abutment along the crest of the ridge of a distal extension partial denture to a point in the retromolar region. An imaginary line of rotation extending from the distal point of the fulcrum on an abutment rest area to the anterior point on the residual ridge in the anterior segment of the dental arch. An imaginary line of rotation between a point in the rest area of an abutment located posterior to a point similarly located farther anterior but on the same side of the arch. (Remov. Part. Prosth.)

　cross arch f. l. An imaginary line extending from the most distal rest area of a distal extension removable partial denture on one side to the most distal rest area on the opposite side, about which the denture will

tend to rotate when subjected to forces that tend to displace the denture base away from its basal seat; e.g., the denture will tend to rotate occlusally around an imaginary line connecting the two most anterior rest areas (one on either side of the arch), until the direct retainers are activated to resist such movement. (Remov. Part. Prosth.)

　vertical f. l. An imaginary vertical axis or line around which a removable partial denture rotates in the horizontal plane. (Remov. Part. Prosth.)

lead l. A bluish black patch on the gingival tissues, usually about 1 mm from the gingival crest. Caused by the deposition of fine granules of lead sulfide in the tissues. A sign of lead absorption in lead poisoning (plumbism). Bluish black specks may also be seen on the mucous membranes of the lips and cheeks. (Periodont.)

median l. The intersection of the midsagittal plane with the maxillary and mandibular dental arches. The center line divides the central body surface into right and left. (Comp. Prosth.; Orthodont.; Remov. Part. Prosth.)

mercurial l. A linear area of abnormal pigmentation of the gingival tissues associated with mercury poisoning. Seen along the gingival margin, it has been variously described as bluish, brownish, dirty reddish, or purplish in coloration. (Periodont.)

l. of occlusion The alignment of the occluding surfaces of the teeth in the horizontal plane. (Comp. Prosth.) (see also **plane, occlusal**)

— The line of greatest normal occlusal contact; the line with which, in form and position according to type, the teeth must be in harmony if they are in normal occlusion. (Orthodont.)

protrusive l. One of the three tracings made on each of the six projection planes of a jaw motion data recorder. It proceeds from the point of centricity forward when the stylus is on the mandibular bow of the apparatus, and the plane of projection is on the maxillary bow of the recording apparatus. If the stylus is held by the maxillary frame and the plane is held by the mandibular frame, the point of centricity marked on the plane is moved forward and the projected "protrusive" line is drawn reversely as are all other tracings of the "Gothic arch" traced lines. (Gnathol.) (see also **centricity, point of**)

survey l. A line produced on the various portions of a dental cast by a surveyor scriber or marker. It designates the greatest height of contour in relation to the orientation of the cast to the vertical scriber. (Remov. Part. Prosth.)

vibrating l. The imaginary line across the posterior part of the palate marking the division between the movable and relatively immovable tissues of the palate. (Comp. Prosth.; Remov. Part. Prosth.)

working l. The tracing of a gnathic projection plane that starts from the point of centricity and runs laterally. It is called a working line, in keeping with traditional language of dentists. More precisely, it records a "datum symptom" of a condyle motion direction made when the jaw is moved laterally in order to tumble the bolus and to get set for another chewing stroke. (Gnathol.)

linear energy transfer (L.E.T.) The linear rate of loss of energy by an ionizing particle traversing a material medium. (Oral Radiol.)

linen strip (see **strip, abrasive**)

liner, cavity (see **varnish, cavity**)

lines Elongated marks traced by a stylus on a gnathic projection plane, indicating direction of movement related variously to condyle movements. (Gnathol.)

lingua alba (see **tongue, white hairy**)

lingua nigra (see **tongue, black hairy**)

lingua villosa alba (see **tongue, white hairy**)

lingual (lĭng′gwahl) Next to, or toward, the tongue. (Comp. Prosth.; Oper. Dent.; Remov. Part. Prosth.)

— Pertaining to the tongue. (Orthodont.)

l. bar, major connector (see **connector, major, lingual bar**)

l. button Attachment welded to the lingual side of the cuspid, bicuspid, or molar bands. (Orthodont.)

l. peak, gingival A lingual peak that characterizes the normal interproximal tissue, which is composed of a lingual papilla and a buccal papilla connected interdentally in a triangular ridge depression termed a col. (Periodont.)

l. plate (see **connector, major, linguoplate**)

lingula (lĭng′gū-lah) A small, tonguelike projection of bone forming the anterior border of the mandibular foramen. (Periodont.)

linguoclusion (lĭng-gwō-klū′zhŭn) An occlusion in which the dental arch or group of teeth is lingual to normal. (Orthodont.)

linguoplate (see **connector, major, linguoplate**)

linguoversion The state of being displaced toward the tongue. (Oral Surg.)

— Term indicating any deviation from the normal line of occlusion toward the tongue. (Orthodont.)

— A position assumed by a tooth, as a result of displacing forces, that is lingual or medial to the line of occlusion or to a harmonious position in the dental arch. (Periodont.)

linkage (lĭngk′ĭj) The connection between two or more objects. Tendency of a group of genes to remain in continuous association from generation to generation. (Oral Physiol.)

cross l. (see **polymerization, cross**)

sex l. Inheritance of certain characteristics that are determined by genes located in the sex chromosomes. (Oral Radiol.)

lip biting An oral habit in which either lip is placed between the maxillary and mandibular teeth with more or less forcible application of the teeth to the lips, often resulting in displacement of the teeth, alterations of their attachment apparatus, and/or traumatic lesions of the dermal or mucosal surfaces of the lips. May be considered as one of the etiologic factors in occlusal traumatism. (Periodont.)

lip, cleft (see **harelip**)

congenital c. l. (see **harelip**)

lip, double A redundant fold of tissue on the mucosal side of the upper lip that gives the appearance of a second lip and that may become accentuated by habitually being sucked between the teeth. (Oral Diag.; Oral Path.)

lipid (lĭp′ĭd) Any one of a group of substances that includes the fats and esters having analogous properties. Lipids are organic substances, insoluble in water but soluble in alcohol, ether, and other fat solvents. (Anesth.)

plasma l. Lipid containing fatty acids esterified with glycerol to form neutral fat, cholesterol esters of the fatty acids, free cholesterol, and phospholipids such as lecithins, cephalins, and sphingomyelins. (Oral Med.)

Lipiodal (lĭp-ē′ō-dahl) Proprietary name for an iodized oil used as an opaque contrast medium in radiography. When it is placed within periodontal pockets and radiographs are made, the depth and topography of periodontal pockets may be ascertained. (Periodont.)

lip line, high The greatest height to which the lip is raised in normal function or during the act of smiling broadly. (Comp. Prosth.; Remov. Part. Prosth.)

lip line, low The lowest position of the lower lip during the act of smiling or voluntary retraction. The lowest position of the upper lip at rest. (Comp. Prosth.; Remov. Part. Prosth.)

lipoidosis (lĭp″oi-dō′sĭs) (see **disease, lipoid storage**)

lipoids (lĭp′oidz) Substances composed of long chains of fatty acids. They are stable and, when appropriately oxidized, are a great source of energy. They are stored intracellularly in globules and in specialized cells. They not only store energy but also relate to body contour and affect weight distribution and energy requirements. Fat is not soluble in water, but some fatty acids associated with the phosphates (the phospholipoids) are partially soluble. Other lipoids (the steroids) are essential to growth and to sexual and adrenocortical function. (Oral Physiol.)

lipoma (lĭ-pō′mah) A benign tumor characterized by fat cells. (Oral Diag.; Oral Path.)

lipophilic (lĭp-ō-fĭl′ĭk) Showing a marked attraction to, or solubility in, lipids. (Anesth.)
— Having an affinity for oil or fat. (Oral Med.; Pharmacol.)

lip pits (congenital lip fistulas) Congenital depressions, usually bilateral and symmetrically placed, on the vermilion portion of the lower lip. These pits may be circular or may be present as a transverse slit. The depression represents a blind fistula that penetrates downward into the lower lip to a depth of 0.5 to 2.5 cm. They often exude viscid saliva on pressure. (Cleft Palate)
— Bilateral pits that occur at the commissures of the lips. Other pits may occur at lines of embryonic fusion. (Oral Diag.)

lip retractors Apparatus to retract the lips when taking intraoral photographs. (Orthodont.)

Lipschütz body (lĭp′shĭtz) (see **body, Lipschütz**)

load An external force applied to an object. (D. Mat.)
  occlusal l. The stresses generated by functional and habitual contacting and rubbing of the occlusal surfaces of the upper and lower teeth. There are two components of such stress loads—the vertically directed components and those components that tend to move a tooth or denture laterally. (Comp. Prosth.; Remov. Part. Prosth.) (see also **force, occlusal**)

lobectomy (lō-bĕk′tō-mē) Excision of a lobe of an organ such as the submandibular gland or the lung. (Oral Surg.)

Lobstein's disease (lōb′stīnz) (see **osteogenesis imperfecta**)

local analgesia Loss of pain sensation over a specific area, caused by local administration of a drug that blocks nerve conduction. (Anesth.)

localization A direct, exact site or restriction to a limited area, such as localization of abscess. (Oral Surg.)
  radiographic l. Determination, by means of radiographs, of the location of an object or structure in the body or head. Usually accomplished by obtaining radiographs made from different angulations to the part in question. (Oral Radiol.)
  tactile l. The property of localization associated with the sense of touch. Perception of the location of a stimulus is more precise in the regions of the lips and the fingertips than elsewhere. This more precise perception results from a greater density of special touch receptors in a given area. (Oral Physiol.)

location The geographic spot in which the equipment is set up to practice dentistry. (Pract. Man.)

locator, abutment (see **abutment locator**)

locking gate A portion of the peripheral frame of a maxillary subperiosteal implant; attached by a hinge. This device permits the implant to be placed into an area of undercut. After the implant is seated, the gate is closed and locked, and wire is wrapped about two locking buttons. (Oral Implant.)

lockpin A soft metal pin used to attach an archwire to an orthodontic bracket. (Orthodont.)

locomotor ataxia (see **tabes dorsalis**)

locus, gene The position of a gene on the chromosome. (Oral Med.)

locus minoris resistentiae (lō′kŭs mī-nor′ĭs rē-sĭs-tĕn′chē-ē″) An area offering little resistance to invasion by microorganisms and/or their toxins. The junction between reduced enamel epithelium and oral epithelium within the epithelial wall of the gingival sulcus has been described as a weak link, providing a portal of entry for microorganisms and their toxins with initiation of pocket formation. (Periodont.)

loempe (lĕm′pē) (see **beriberi**)

logopedics (log″ō-pē′dĭks) The study and treatment of speech defects in children, involving habilitation or rehabilitation of speech. (Oral Physiol.)

loop, vertical A U-shaped bend in the archwire, which aids in the opening or closing of spaces in the arch. (Orthodont.)

loose premaxilla (see **premaxilla, loose**)

lordosis (lor-dō′sĭs) An anteroposterior curvature of the spine with the convexity facing forward. (Oral Diag.)

loss of bone (see **resorption of bone**)

loupe, binocular (loop) A magnifier that consists of lenses in an optical frame; it is worn like spectacles and is used with both eyes. (Oper. Dent.)

low lip line (see **lip line, low**)

lower ridge slope (see **slope, lower ridge**)

lozenge (lahz'ĕnj) (**troche**) A medicated, disk-shaped tablet designed to dissolve slowly in the mouth. (Oral Med.; Pharmacol.)

Ludwig's angina (lood'vĭgz) (see **angina, Ludwig's**)

lues (lū'ēz) (see **syphilis**)

luetic (loo-ĕt'ĭk) Pertaining to or affected by syphilis. (Oral Surg.)

lug (lŭg) The part of a casting that projects.

occlusal l. (see **rest, occlusal**)

retention l. A piece of metal that is soldered to either an orthodontic band or an artificial crown to create greater undercut for retention of the prosthesis. (Cleft Palate)

upright l. (see **connector, minor**)

vertical l. (see **connector, minor**)

lumen (loo'mĕn) The space within a tube structure, such as a blood vessel, tube, or duct. (Anesth.; Oral Surg.)

lupus (loo'pŭs) A disease of the skin and mucous membrane.

l. erythematosus A disease of unknown cause that occurs in two forms: disseminated lupus erythematosus is a fatal disease with fibrinoid lesions of the skin and mucosa; discoid (localized) lupus erythematosus may produce similar but less active lesions. The oral lesions in either type begin as areas of redness with radiating lines, suggesting lichen planus. A butterfly pattern of skin lesions over the nose and face is characteristic. (Oral Diag.)

— A superficial inflammation of the skin marked by disklike patches with raised red edges and covered with scales or crusts. (Oral Path.)

l. vulgaris Primary tuberculosis of the skin. (Oral Path.)

luxation (lŭk-sā'shŭn) Partial or complete detachment of a tooth from its socket resulting from trauma or a pathologic process. (Endodont.)

— Dislocation or displacement of a tooth or of the temporomandibular articulation. (Oral Surg.)

lymphadenitis (lĭm-făd"ĕ-nī'tĭs) Inflammation of the lymph glands, characterized chiefly by swelling, pain, and redness. (Oral Diag.; Oral Med.; Oral Path.)

lymphadenopathy (lĭm-făd"ĕ-nahp'ah-thē) A disease of the lymph nodes, which become enlarged. (Oral Med.)

— Enlarged, palpable lymph nodes, which are often symptomatic in periodontal states such as acute necrotizing ulcerative gingivitis. (Periodont.)

generalized l. Involvement of all or several regionally separated groups of lymph nodes by a systemic disorder. (Oral Med.)

regional l. Involvement of nodes draining a specific region; e.g., submental nodes draining the middle of the lower lip, floor of the mouth, or skin of the chin. (Oral Med.)

lymphadenosis, acute benign (lĭm-făd"ĕ-nō'sĭs) (see **mononucleosis, infectious**)

lymphangioma (lĭm-făn-jē-ō'mah) A benign neoplasm characterized by lymph vessel proliferation. A benign tumor of the lymph vessels. (Oral Diag.; Oral Path.)

cystic l. (see **hygroma, cystic**)

lymphoblastoma, giant follicular (**Brill-Symmers disease**) A malignant disease characterized by enlargement of the spleen and lymph nodes throughout the body. Lymphoblasts and reticular cells proliferate within lymphoid follicles, producing an increase in both the number and size of germinal follicles. (Oral Diag.; Oral Path.)

lymphocyte (lĭm'fō-sīt) A nongranular white blood corpuscle that arises from lymphatic tissue. (Oral Path.)

— A form of white blood cell originating in lymphoid tissues; possesses a single spherical nucleus and a nongranular cytoplasm. The lymphocytes comprise 25% of the white blood cells. Some lymphocytes, along with plasma cells and histiocytes, are found in clinically normal gingivae. Their numbers within the gingival connective tissue are increased in gingivitis and periodontitis. With progress of gingival inflammation to the underlying bone, lymphocytes are found within the marrow spaces of the supporting bone. (Periodont.)

— A mononucleated leukocyte with a nongranular protoplasm. (Oral Physiol.)

lymphocytopenia (lĭm"fō-sī"tō-pē'nē-ah) A decrease in the normal number of lymphocytes in the circulating blood. Various limits are given: e.g., a total number less than 600/mm³. It may be associated with agranulocytosis, hyperadrenocorticism, leukemia, advanced Hodgkin's disease, irradiation, and acute infections with neutrophilia. (Oral Med.)

lymphocytosis (lĭm"fō-sī-tō'sĭs) An absolute or relative increase in the normal number of lymphocytes in the circulating blood. Various limits are given; e.g., *absolute* lymphocytosis is said to be present if the total number of cells exceeds 4500/mm³, whereas *relative* lymphocytosis is said to be present if the percentage of lymphocytes is greater than 45% and the total number of cells is less than 4500/mm³. Lymphocytosis may be associated with infancy, exophthalmic goiter, mumps, rubella, infectious mononucleosis, sunburn, lymphatic leukemia, pertussis, and pyogenic infections in childhood. (Oral Diag.; Oral Med.)

lymphoepithelial lesion, benign (lĭm″fō-ĕp″ĭ-thē′lē-al) (see **disease, Mikulicz'**)

lymphoepithelioma (lĭm″fō-ĕp″ĭ-thē″lē-ō′mah) A malignant neoplasm arising from the epithelium and lymphoid tissue of the nasopharynx and characterized by cells of both tissues. May occur in the palate. (Oral Diag.; Oral Path.)

lymphoma (lĭm-fō′mah) Any neoplasm made up of lymphoid tissue. The term is a broad one, the malignant lymphomas including lymphosarcoma, Hodgkin's disease, reticulum cell sarcoma, and giant follicular lymphoblastoma. (Oral Diag.; Oral Path.)

lymphoreticulosis, benign inoculation (lĭm″fō-rĕ-tĭk″ū-lō′sĭs) (see **fever, cat-scratch**)

lymphosarcoma (lĭm″fō-sar-kō′mah) A malignant disease of the lymphoid tissues characterized by proliferation of atypical lymphocytes and their localization in various parts of the body. The jaws may be the sites of lymphosarcomas. (Oral Diag.; Oral Path.)

lysin (lī′sĭn) (see **plasmin**)

lysing effect (see **effect, lysing**)

lysis (lī′sĭs) Gradual abatement of the symptoms of a disease. Disintegration or dissolution of cells by a lysin. (Oral Surg.)

lysokinase (lī″sō-kī′nās) (see **fibrinokinase**)

lysozyme (lī′sō-zīm) An enzyme in major salivary secretions that may rupture bacterial cell walls and may regulate the oral flora. (Periodont.)

M

ma Abbreviation for milliampere.

macrocheilia (măk″rō-kī′lē-ah) Abnormally large lip. (Oral Diag.)

macrodontia (măk-rō-don′shē-ah) (**megadontismus**) Abnormally large teeth. One, several, or all teeth in a given individual may be involved. (Oral Diag.; Oral Path.; Orthodont.)

macrogingivae (măk″rō-jĭn′jĭ-vē) Abnormally large gingivae due to inflammation, heredity, scurvy, leukemia, neoplasia, diphenylhydantoin (Dilantin) therapy (in epilepsy), or hormonal stimulation of puberty or pregnancy. (Oral Diag.)

macroglobulinemia, essential (**macroglobulinemia of Waldenström**) Disturbance of the reticuloendothelial system characterized by increased numbers of macroglobulins in the serum, normochromic anemia, hemorrhagic diathesis, and lymphadenopathy. (Oral Med.)

macroglossia (măk″rō-glahs′ē-ah) An enlarged tongue due to muscle hypertrophy, vascular or neurogenic tumor, or endocrine disturbance. (Oral Diag.; Orthodont.)

amyloid m. (see **tongue, amyloid**)

macroglossic Descriptive of macroglossia. (Orthodont.)

macrognathia (măk″rō-năth′ē-ah) A definite overgrowth of the maxillae and mandible. (Orthodont.)

macrognathic (măk-rō-năth′ĭk) Descriptive of macrognathia. (Orthodont.)

macrophage (măk′rō-fāj) (see **histiocyte**)

macrosomia (see **giantism**)

macrostomia An abnormally large oral opening. (Oral Diag.; Orthodont.)

macule A lesion of the mucous membrane or cutaneous tissue that is not elevated above the surface. (Oral Surg.)

magistral prescription (see **prescription, extemporaneous**)

magnesium An elemental metal; atomic weight, 24.32. An essential nutritional substance. Deficiency produces irritability of the nervous system, trophic disturbances, etc. Experimental periodontal effects in rats include calculus formation, tooth mobility, and gingival hyperplasia. (Periodont.)

maintenance of denture (see **denture, maintenance of**)

maintenance, space (see **space maintainer**)

major connector (see **connector, major**)

making the turn The step in the procedure of inserting and condensing foil in a Class 3 cavity preparation at which the line of force is changed from an incisogingival direction to a gingivoincisal direction. (Oper. Dent.)

mal- (măl) Prefix meaning bad or fraudulent; e.g., maladministration, malpractice. (D. Juris.)

malalignment (măl″ah-līn′měnt) Out of normal alignment. (Orthodont.)

— Displacement of a tooth from its normal position in the dental arch. (Periodont.) (see also **buccoversion, buckling, crowding of teeth, distoversion, labioversion, linguoversion, mesioversion, torsiversion**)

malar (mā′lar) Pertaining to the cheek or the zygomatic bone. (Oral Surg.)

m. bone (see **bone, malar**)

malare Midpoint of intersection between the projection of the coronoid process and the lower contour of the malar bone. (Orthodont.)

Malassez, debris of (see **debris of Malassez**)

Malassez, rests of (see **debris of Malassez**)

maldevelopment Abnormal, imperfect, or deficient formation or development. (Orthodont.)

malfeasance (măl-fē′zěns) The wrongful doing of some act that the doer has not the right to perform. (D. Juris.)

malfunction (see **dysfunction**)

dental m. The incorrect action of opposing teeth in the process of mastication; sometimes referred to as malocclusion. (Orthodont.)

malice A wrongful act done intentionally, without legal justification or excuse, predicated on ill will toward some person. (D. Juris.)

m. in the law of libel and slander An evil intent arising from spite or ill will; willful and wanton disregard of the rights of the person defamed. (D. Juris.)

malignant (mah-lĭg′nănt) A term that, when used to describe a neoplasm, signifies that lesion's ability to metastasize and kill the host. (Oral Path.)

malingering Feigning of illness. (Oral Surg.)

malleability (măl″ē-ah-bĭl′ĭ-tē) Ability of a material to withstand permanent deformation under compressive forces without rupture. A malleable material may be hammered or rolled into the desired shape. (D. Mat.)

mallet A hammer instrument. (Oral Surg.)

  automatic m. (see **condenser, mechanical**)

  hard m. A small hammer with a leather-, rubber-, fiber-, or metal-faced head; used to supply force or to supplement hand force for the compaction of foil or amalgam and to seat cast restorations. (Oper. Dent.)

malocclusion Any deviation from a physiologically acceptable contact of opposing teeth or dentitions. (Comp. Prosth.; Remov. Part. Prosth.)

— An abnormal relation of the opposing teeth when brought into habitual opposition. The teeth in one arch come in abnormal contact with those in the other arch. (Oral Diag.; Orthodont.)

— Any deviation from normal occlusion of the teeth, usually associated with abnormal developmental growth of the jaws. (Periodont.)

  deflective m. A type of malocclusion occurring in persons who cannot close all their teeth while holding their condyles in the rearmost position. Instead, in closure they first contact one or two pairs of poorly coupled teeth. To gain occlusal contacts of the other teeth, they must move the jaw anteriorly, laterally, or anterolaterally, as the deflectors demand in their guidance. The fact that such deflectors are faceted as a result of wear would indicate that, perhaps, the temporal muscles attempt to close in a more rearward position than is allowed by the malocclusion. (Gnathol.)

malposed (măl-pōzd') In an abnormal position. (Oral Surg.)

malposition Abnormal position.

  m. of jaw Any abnormal position of the mandible. (Comp. Prosth.; Remov. Part. Prosth.)

  m. of teeth Improper position of teeth in relationship to the basal bone of the alveolar process, to adjacent teeth, and/or to opposing teeth. (Orthodont.; Periodont.)

malpractice The act or failure to act by a professional person that was the proximate cause of the injury to another, when said act was below the standard of care required of a reasonable person. (D. Juris.)

malrelationship Disturbance or disruption of the normal relation of conjoining structures. (Orthodont.)

mammotropin (măm″ō-trō'pĭn) (see **hormone, lactogenic**)

manage To conduct; to direct the concerns of a business, establishment, or practice. (D. Juris.)

management The art of administering all phases of a business or a profession. (Pract. Man.)

mandible Lower jawbone. (Comp. Prosth.; Remov. Part. Prosth.)

  architecture of m. Structural pattern of the various tissues comprising the mandible, the arrangement governed to a large degree by functional stimulation to the tissues. A change in function will result in a change in architecture; thus, in functional insufficiency, the supporting cancellous bone of the alveolar process undergoes disuse atrophy, and the periodontal membrane is thin, its principal fibers being replaced by indifferent fibers. Conversely, functional increase will result in increased density of periodontal fibers and reinforcement of the supporting bone. Inflammatory and neoplastic disease will also alter the structure of the mandible. (Periodont.)

  gliding movements of m. The nonmasticatory excursive movements of the mandible. The protrusive, right and left lateral, and lateral protrusive movements made with the teeth in contact. These movements are, in the main, nonfunctional excursions of the mandible. (Periodont.)

  inferior border of m. Lower edge of the mandible. Begins anterior to the insertion of the masseter muscle at the inferior surface of the angles of the mandible and is continuous anteriorly with the incisor region. (Periodont.)

  movements of m. (see **movement, mandibular**)

  posture of m. The physiologic rest position or the rest vertical relation of the mandible. (Periodont.)

  unlocking of m. The use of selective grinding to secure a free, unrestrained gliding and chewing movement of the mandible by reducing interference in the chewing cycle and in the various glide movements. One of the basic objectives of occlusal adjustment. (Periodont.)

mandibular (măn-dĭb'ū-lar) Pertaining to the inferior jaw. (Orthodont.)

  m. angle (see **angle of the mandible**)

  m. axis (see **axis, mandibular**)

  m. border (see **border, mandibular**)

  m. canal (see **canal, mandibular**)

  m. centric relation The closing relation of the mandible with the fixed craniofacial complex as determined clinically by jaw motion writing instruments. Such instruments carry six styluses that scribe on sleek tablets placed in reference relation to the two most convenient planes of projection. On each tablet are written arcs about both the near and the far condyle so that their point of union represents a point of centricity. After these arcs are written, the styluses are raised, the patient is encouraged to reach his jaw in the rearmost position, the styluses are dropped into writing contacts, and the patient is encouraged to start his protrusive records from the angle of union between the arcs. If he does so, it is assumed that centric relation has been determined. Because some persons have much precurrent laterotrusion and thus transtrude their condyles without causing any orbiting movements of the mandible, the rear styluses are placed near the posterior terminal position of the hinge axis to make the midmost condylar determinations more accurate. (Gnathol.) (see also **projection, planes of**)

m. condyle (see **condyle, mandibular**)

m. foramen (see **foramen, mandibular**)

m. glide (see **glide, mandibular**)

m. guide prosthesis A prosthesis with an extension designed to direct a resected mandible into a functional relation with the maxillae. (M.F.P.)

m. hinge position (see **position, hinge, mandibular**)

m. movement (see **movement, mandibular**)

m. notch (see **notch, mandibular**)

m. rest position (see **position, rest, mandibular**)

m. retraction (see **retraction, mandibular**)

mandibulofacial dysostosis (măn-dĭb″ū-lō-fā′shŭl) (see **syndrome, Treacher-Collins**)

mandrel (măn′drĕl) A shaft that supports or holds any object to be rotated. An instrument, held in a handpiece, that holds a disk, stone, or cup used for grinding, smoothing, or polishing. (Oper. Dent.)

— A shaft in which a tool is held. This term is sometimes used to mean a tool holder in the sense of an arbor or a chuck. (Remov. Part. Prosth.)

disk m. A mandrel designed to hold a polishing disk by means of a slip-on or split head so that the disk may be rotated forward or backward in the handpiece. (Oper. Dent.)

miniature d. m. A small-headed mandrel, useful with disks ⅜ and ½ inch in diameter. (Oper. Dent.)

Morgan's m. A disk mandrel with a split head; disks for such mandrels have a metal core that is held on the mandrel by frictional contact. (Oper. Dent.)

Snap-On m. Proprietary name for a mandrel with a split end to receive and hold a rubber polishing cup. (Oper. Dent.)

Mantoux test (mahn-too′) (see **test, Mantoux**)

manual Performed by the hand; used in the hand. (D. Juris.)

manudynamometer (măn″ū-dī-nah-mom′ĕ-ter) A device that measures the force exerted by the thrust of an instrument. (Oper. Dent.)

marble bone (see **osteopetrosis**)

margin An edge; a boundary line of a surface. In a restoration it is the counterpart of the cavosurface angle of the cavity prepared for that restoration. (Oper. Dent.)

bone m. The peripheral edge of a bone. (Periodont.)

thickened b. m. (see **bone, thickened margin of**)

enamel m. The part of the margin of a preparation that is laid in enamel. (Oper. Dent.)

free gum m. (see **margin, gingival, free**)

gingival m. The cavosurface angle of the wall of a cavity preparation closest to the apex of the root. (Oper. Dent.)

— The edge or the periphery of a restoration that approximates the gingival cavosurface angle of the prepared cavity. (Oper. Dent.)

— The crest or tip of the gingival tissues. (Periodont.)

free g. m. (**free gum m.**) The edge or summit of the gingival tissue immediately adjacent to the cervical portion of the crown of a natural tooth. The tissue is normally unattached to a depth of 2 to 2.5 mm. (Fixed Part. Prosth.; Remov. Part. Prosth.)

m. of safety The margin between lethal and toxic doses. (Anesth.)

marginal ridge (see **ridge, marginal**)

marginal spinning The burnishing of the margins of a casting during the initial setting of the cement to close the space between the margin and the preparation, resulting from the slight lifting of the marginal gold from its seat by the interposition of the cement. The rounded edge of the spinning tool must always be drawn along the margin and not across it. (Oper. Dent.)

margination Adhesion of the leukocytes to the luminal surface of blood vessel walls in the early stages of inflammation. (Oral Path.)

Marie's disease (see **acromegaly**)

marking medium (see **medium, marking**)

marsupialization (măr-su″pē-ah-lĭ-zā′shŭn) The opening of a cyst to establish communication with the external environment. (Oral Surg.) (see also **operation, Partsch's**)

MAS (**Ma.S., mas, milliampere-second**) The product of the milliamperes and the exposure time in seconds; e.g., 10 ma × ½ sec = 5 MAS. (Oral Radiol.)

mask Artificial covering.

　　full-face m. A device used in anesthesia to confine the gas that is delivered through the mask into the respiratory tract by way of the nose or mouth. (Anesth.)

　　rubber dam m. (see **pad, rubber dam**)

　　Wanscher's m. A mask for ether anesthesia. (Anesth.)

　　Yankauer's m. An open type of mask for administering ether. (Anesth.)

masking An opaque covering used to camouflage the metal or other parts of a prosthesis. (Comp. Prosth.)

mass number (symbol A) The number of nucleons (protons and neutrons) in the nucleus of an atom. (Oral Radiol.)

massage The systematic application of frictional rubbing and stroking to the gingival tissues for cleansing purposes, for increasing tissue tone, for increasing the circulation of blood through the tissues, and for increasing the keratinization of the surface epithelium. (Periodont.)

　　cardiac m. A systematic, rhythmic application of pressure to the heart to cause a significant blood flow in the treatment of a cardiac arrest; may be an open or closed chest procedure. (Oral Surg.)

master One having authority; one who directs, instructs, or superintends; an employer. (D. Juris.)

　　m. and servant relationship A relationship in which one person, for pay or other valuable consideration, enters into service of another for an agreed period; e.g., the relationship between a dentist and his assistant. (D. Juris.)

masticating apparatus (see **apparatus, masticating**)

masticating cycle (see **cycle, masticating**)

mastication The process of chewing food in preparation for swallowing and digestion. (Comp. Prosth.; Remov. Part. Prosth.)

— The act of chewing accomplished by the coordinated activity of the tongue, mandible, mandibular masculature, structural components of the temporomandibular joints, etc. and controlled by the neuromuscular mechanism. (Periodont.)

　　components of m. The various jaw movements made during the act of mastication as deter-

mined by the neuromuscular system, the temporomandibular articulations, the teeth, and the food being chewed. For purposes of analysis or description, the components of mastication may be categorized as opening, closing, left lateral, right lateral, or antero-posterior jaw movements. (Comp. Prosth.)

forces of m. (see **force, masticatory**)

insufficiency of m. Inefficiency or inadequacy of the chewing act, resulting in decreased functional stimulation to the investing and supporting structures of the teeth. Atrophic tissue changes and an increased suscepti-bility to infection in the tissues, which have a lowered resistance because of subnormal function, ensue. (Periodont.)

occlusal trauma in m. Injury or damage to the teeth that theoretically could occur as a re-sult of the contact between surfaces of the upper and lower teeth during mastication. However, because the forces applied to the teeth are relatively small, the time element of mastication is short, and the teeth touch only minimally during mastication, mastica-tion cannot account for the production of occlusal trauma. (Periodont.)

organ of m. (see **system, stomatognathic**)

physiology of m. The movements of the man-dible during the chewing cycle, which are controlled by neuromuscular action and cor-related to the structural attributes of the temporomandibular joints and the proprio-ceptive sense of the periodontal membranes. There are three phases in the physiology of mastication: the incision of food, mastica-tion of the bolus, and the act of swallowing. Accessory activity by the tongue and facial musculature facilitates the masticatory ac-tions. (Periodont.)

saliva in m. Increased in salivation, which serves to wet and lubricate the food to facilitate deglutition. (Periodont.)

second-class lever system in m. The function-ing of the masticatory tissues regarded as operating under the principle of the second-class lever. When the opposite, or contra-lateral, temporomandibular joint is regarded as the fulcrum, the work load is seen to be placed on the occlusal surfaces of the teeth, and the applied force is considered to be supplied by the masseter muscle on the side opposite the fulcrum, the system may be regarded as a second-class lever system. Out of these relationships there is a high level of efficiency, and the apparently small bulk of masseter muscle may produce a considerable amount of energy for mastication. During normal masticatory function, the masticatory tissues create work within both a second-class and a third-class lever relationship. (Oral Physiol.) (see also **lever, second-class**)

third-class lever system in m. The functioning of the masticatory tissues regarded as operating under the principle of the third-class lever. Traditionally, the masticatory levers have been classified essentially as third-class levers. The fulcrum is considered to be at the center of action of the masseter muscle and the work arm located more anteriorly in relation to the opposing occlusal forces. In this description, the fulcrum, the force, and the work positions are all on the same side of the mandible. This lever system is relatively inefficient. When the bolus of food is placed more distally or posteriorly, the efficiency of the lever increases as the distance of the work arm decreases. The masseter muscles have their mean position distal to the second and third molars, which means that when food is in the first molar, bicuspid, and anterior tooth positions, the lever system is progressively less efficient. (Oral Physiol.) (see also **lever, third-class**)

tongue in m. The muscular organ in the floor of the mouth whose function in the masticatory process consists in crushing some food by pressing it against the hard palate, forming it into a compact bolus, and assisting in placing it on the occlusal platform for tooth action. (Periodont.)

masticatory force (see **force, masticatory**)

masticatory movements (măs'tĭ-kah-tor"ē) (see **movements, mandibular, masticatory**)

mastoidale Lowest point on the contour of the mastoid process. (Orthodont.)

mat, gingival (see **gingival mat**)

mat gold (see **gold, mat**)

materia alba A soft white deposit around the necks of the teeth usually associated with poor oral hygiene; composed of food debris, dead tissue elements, and purulent matter; serves as a medium for bacterial growth. (Oral Diag.; Periodont.)

materia medica The study of drugs and their use. (Oral Med.; Pharmacol.)

material(s) Substance(s).

dental m. All the substances used to assist in rendering dental service. (Pract. Man.)

duplicating m. Materials used to copy casts, models, etc.; usually hydrocolloids. (D. Mat.)

filling m. Gutta-percha, silver cones, paste mixtures, or other substances used to fill root canals. (Endodont.)

impression m. Any substance or combination of substances used for making a negative reproduction or impression. (Comp. Prosth.; Remov. Part. Prosth.)

silicone rubber i. m. A dimethyl polysiloxane material whose polymerization is affected by an organ-metal compound and some type of alkyl silicate. (D. Mat.)

matrix (mā'trĭks) An intergranular substance that acts somewhat as a cementing material for other particles; e.g., zinc phosphate cement is made of undissolved zinc oxide particles, surrounded and held or cemented together by phosphate compounds. The phosphate compounds comprise the matrix. (D. Mat.) (see also **bone; splint**)

— A mechanical or artificial wall to complete the mold into which plastic material may be inserted. Also a mold into which something is formed. (Oper. Dent.)

amalgam m. A metal form, usually of stainless steel, about 0.0015 to 0.002 inch thick, adapted to a prepared cavity to supply the missing wall so that the plastic amalgam will be confined when it is condensed into the cavity. (Oper. Dent.)

bone m. The intercellular substance of bone. The organic fraction of compact bone makes up as much as 35% of the dry, fat-free weight of bone. Only a small part of this percentage is contributed by the cells; the remainder is the bone matrix. The matrix, which is impregnated with bone salts, has two chief components. The most prominent component is fibrillar in nature and is chemically a collagen. The other is the amorphous ground substance, whose most important compound is a mucopolysaccharide, chondroitin sulfate, and which is in intimate relationship with the intercellular tissue fluid. Dyes and radioactive isotopes introduced into the circulation diffuse in the bones so rapidly that the tissue fluid, which is small in amount, and the ground substance are considered to be coextensive, homogeneous, and interconnected. However, free fluid may be entirely absent from considerable areas of compact bone, especially in the adult. The presence or absence of tissue fluid has an important bearing on the freedom of exchange of ions between the bone and the blood and on the possibility of necrosis in bone injury. (Oral Physiol.)

Celluloid m. A strip of Celluloid used to mold cement into the desired shape. (Oper. Dent.) (see also **strip, plastic**)

custom m. A matrix made especially for a given location, tooth, or preparation. (Oper. Dent.)

direct porcelain m. A platinum-foil matrix adapted directly to the tooth preparation for the direct technique. (Oper. Dent.)

m. holder (see **retainer, matrix**)

mechanical m. (proprietary m.) A patented or manufactured type of matrix. (Oper. Dent.)

plastic m. A matrix of resin or plastic for use with cold-curing resin or cement. (Oper. Dent.)

platinum m. A matrix of wrought platinum foil, usually 0.001 inch or thinner, adapted to a die of a preparation for a fired porcelain restoration; serves as a vehicle to carry and maintain the applications of porcelain when they are placed in a furnace for firing. (Oper. Dent.)

proprietary m. (see **matrix, mechanical**)

m. retainer (see **retainer, matrix**)

T-band m. Matrix material cut with a T-shaped projection at one end; the lugs are bent over to engage the band as it encircles the tooth. (Oper. Dent.)

maxilla (măk-sĭl'ah) The irregularly shaped bone forming half of the upper jaw. The upper jaw is made up of the two maxillae. (Comp. Prosth.)

architecture of m. The structural pattern of the maxilla, modified by the functional stimulation afforded it. Since the mandible is a force transmitter because it is a moving and projecting bone, and the maxilla is stationary and receptive, the maxillae and mandible have different structural arrangements. (Periodont.)

maxillary (măk″sĭ-lĕr'ē) Pertaining to the superior jaw. (Orthodont.)

m. retrusion (see **retrusion, maxillary**)

m. sinus (see **sinus, maxillary**)

m. tuberosity (see **tuberosity, maxillary**)

maxillofacial (măk-sĭl″ō-fā'shŭl) Pertaining to the jaws and the face. (Comp. Prosth.; Orthodont.; Remov. Part. Prosth.)

m. prosthetics (see **prosthetics, maxillofacial**)

maxillomandibular relation (măk-sĭl″ō-măn-dĭb'ū-lar) (see **relation, maxillomandibular**)

maxillotomy (măk″sĭ-lot'ō-mē) Surgical sectioning of the maxilla to allow movement of all or a part of the maxilla into the desired portion. (Oral Surg.)

Mazzini's test (mah-zē'nēz) (see **test, Mazzini's**)

McCall's festoon, instrument (see under appropriate noun)

McShirley's electromallet (see **condenser, electromallet**)

MDR Minimum daily requirement, especially the Minimum Daily Requirements for Specific Nutrients compiled by the United States Food and Drug Administration. (Oral Med.; Pharmacol.)

mean foundation plane (see **plane, mean foundation**)

mean life (see **average life**)

measles An infectious disease caused by a virus. There are two types: rubeola and rubella (German measles). Both have oral manifestations. (Oral Diag.)

— An acute contagious disease caused by a virus and transmitted by direct contact and droplet infection. The incubation period is about 10 to 14 days. Onset is characterized by fever, malaise, coryza, conjunctivitis, and cough. Koplik's spots appear in 24 to 36 hours, and a characteristic morbilliform rash begins on the third or fourth day, spreads from the face to the whole body, and then declines after 4 or 5 days. (Oral Med.)

German m. (see **rubella**)

three-day m. (see **rubella**)

mechanically balanced occlusion (see **occlusion, balanced, mechanically**)

mechanism The manner of combination of parts that subserve a common function.

cough m. A short inspiration, closure of the glottis, forcible expiratory effort, and then release of the glottis, with a rush of air at a flow rate of 3000 to 4000 cc/sec. A cough is essentially used or regarded as a process for removing foreign material from the lungs. It involves two phases. In the first, the combined action of the cilia and bronchiolar peristalsis moves the material up to the main bronchi and the bifurcation of the trachea. Further movement out of the respiratory system depends on the cough mechanism. In all medical conditions in which this mechanism is abolished or reduced, secretions and foreign material accumulate in the alveoli, with a resultant reduction in the aerating surface and a predisposition to infection. Since ventilation of the lungs depends on a patent airway, the cough mechanism should always be utilized by patients whose inadequate ventilation of lungs may be related to obstruction of the airway. (Oral Physiol.)

guidance m. A natural process conceived as a machine or as functioning purely in accordance with mechanical laws. Most processes, either chemical or physical, are biologic mechanisms. Joints of the body are regarded as guidance mechanisms. (Gnathol.)

inhibitory-excitatory m. A mechanism that provides coordinated and continuous stimuli to the lower motor neuron for smooth, facile, and rapidly adjustable muscle contraction. This mechanism operates on every level of the central nervous system, from the final common pathway back up the spinal cord to the cerebrum. The excitatory phase of stimulation is transmitted directly to the nerve. Inhibiton, however, is effected not by stimulating the motor output directly, as is done in the parasympathetic nerves, but rather by the interaction of inhibitory mechanisms on the excitatory impulses. (Oral Physiol.)

investing m. The structures or tissues that surround the tooth, such as the periodontal membrane, cementum of the tooth, alveolar bone, and gingivae, and that provide retention and support for the tooth. (Periodont.)

respiratory control m. The mechanism by which the respiratory functions are controlled. There are three major factors in the control of respiration that concern the dentist: the neurogenic control of respiration, the chemical regulation of respiration, and the mechanical events leading to pulmonary ventilation. These three factors are significant in practice procedures because the dentist influences each of these factors in routine dental care; e.g., the patency of the airways is always subject to alteration by instrumentation, dental prostheses, and the use of pharmacologic agents, and the physically induced responses modify the rate and magnitude of the respiratory mechanism. (Oral Physiol.)

suspensory m. The hammocklike arrangement of the structures comprising the attachment apparatus (cementum, periodontal ligament, alveolar bone) that serve to support the tooth in the alveolus. The primarily oblique periodontal fibers are supported between the cementum and the alveolar bone into which they are attached, and thus a suspensory mechanism is formed. (Periodont.)

media (mē′dē-ah) The plural form of medium.

median (mē′dē-ăn) Pertaining to the middle.
  m. lethal dose (see **dose, lethal, median**)
  m. line (see **line, median**)
  m. mandibular point (see **point, median mandibular**)
  m. palatine suture (see **suture, intermaxillary**)
  m. retruded relation (see **relation, centric**)
  m. sagittal plane (see **plane, median sagittal**)

mediation Intervention; the act of a third person who interferes between two contending parties to reconcile them or to persuade them to adjust or settle their differences. (D. Juris.)

medication Impregnation with a medicine; a remedy.
— A drug. The administration of drugs. (Pharmacol.)

  ambulatory m. A single drug or a combination of drugs used to allay fear and reduce muscular tension in difficult children requiring dental procedures. The child remains conscious. (Pedodont.)

  complete m. Combination of synergistic drugs used in dental procedures for difficult children; the patient is in a state of sleep or light anesthesia. (Pedodont.)

  intracanal m. A drug used in the root canal system during the course of therapy. (Endodont.)

  official m. (see **drug, official**)

  officinal m. (see **drug, officinal**)

  repository m. Slowly soluble drug mixtures intended for parenteral injection and gradual absorption into the blood and hence into other tissues of the body. (Oral Med.; Pharmacol.)

  sustained release m. Oral dosage forms designed to be absorbed at various levels in the gastrointestinal tract, thus prolonging action. (Oral Med.; Pharmacol.)

medicine A remedy. Also, the art of healing.

  oral m. The discipline of dentistry that deals with the significance and relationship of oral and systemic disease. (Oral Med.)

  practice of m. A pursuit that includes the application and use of medicines and drugs for the purpose of curing or alleviating bodily diseases; surgery is usually limited to manual operations generally performed by means of surgical instruments or appliances. (D. Juris.)

mediotrusion A thrusting of the mandibular condyle inward (toward the median plane). When the right condyle is thrust outward (in laterotrusion) before it is rotated, the left condyle is thrust inward before it is orbited and is thus said to be in precurrent mediotrusion. If the left condyle is thrust outward before it is rotated, the right condyle is in precurrent mediotrusion. Each condyle will have an amplitude of transtrusion equal to the sum of the mediotrusion and the laterotrusion. However, if the right condyle is moved about its vertical axis just as soon as its laterotrusion is started, the left condyle will have its mediotrusion concurring with its orbiting, and vice versa. The transtrusion of each condyle will be so obscured in the elliptical tracing arcs that its amplitude is difficult to measure. (Gnathol.)

Mediterranean anemia (see **thalassemia major**)

Mediterranean disease (see **thalassemia major**)

medium(ia) An interposed agent or material; a carrier; a material serving as an environment for the growth of microorganisms. (Oral Path.)

    marking m. Any of several agents, such as carbon paper or inked ribbon, used to indicate an occlusal interference. Any of several agents, such as stencil correction fluid, rouge and alcohol, or pressure indicator paste, used to determine interference in the placement of a removable denture. (Remov. Part. Prosth.)

    radiopaque m. A substance that may be injected into a cavity or region to increase its density in x-ray examination and thereby aid in diagnosis. Lipiodol, Iodochloral, Parabodril, and Ioduron are examples of such materials. (Oral Diag.)

    Sabouraud's m. A nutrient agar used to grow fungi. It is especially useful for the growth and identification of *Candida albicans,* the causative agent of thrush. (Oral Med.)

    separating m. Materials used to prevent the attachment of one object or part to another. Any coating that is used on a surface and that serves to prevent another surface or material from adhering to the first; e.g., tinfoil, cellophane, or alginate, all of which are used to protect an acrylic resin from the moisture in the gypsum mold, and shellac, sandarac, liquid wax, or petrolatum, all of which are used to prevent two mixes of gypsum materials from adhering to each other. (Comp. Prosth.; Remov. Part. Prosth.)

medulla oblongata (mĕ-dul'ah ob-long-gah'tah) The direct upward extension of the spinal cord. It lies at the junction between the cerebrum and the spinal cord and is considered to be in a group with the pons and midbrain because the nuclei of all the cranial nerves except one are situated within this structural group. The medulla, which is the next immediate structure of the spinal cord, has several functions that are associated with the nuclei of the glossopharyngeal, vagus, spinal accessory, and hypoglossal nerves. These nuclei control the reflex actions of the pharynx, larynx, and tongue, which are related to deglutition, mastication, and the speech function. They are also concerned with the visceral reflexes of coughing, sneezing, sucking, vomiting, and salivation, as well as with other secretory functions. The small size and compact form of the medulla subject the body to serious disorganization of widely varying functions if disease or injury develops within its structure or if it is subject to unusual pharmacologic action. (Oral Physiol.)

megadontismus (mĕg-ah-don-tĭz'mŭs) (see **macrodontia**)

Meissner's corpuscles (mīs'nerz) (see **corpuscle, Meissner's**)

melanin (mĕl'ah-nĭn) The dark amorphous pigment of melanotic tumors, the skin, the hair, the choroid coat of the eye, and the substantia nigra of the brain. (Oral Path.)

melanocytes (mĕl'ah-nō-sīts") Dendritic cells of the gingival epithelium which, when functional, cause pigmentation regardless of race. (Periodont.)

melanoma (mĕl"ah-nō'mah) A malignant neoplasma characterized by pigment-producing cells. It usually is dark in color but may be amelanotic, i.e., free of pigment. (Oral Diag.)

— A malignant lesion of the melanin-producing cells. Rarely seen in the oral cavity. (Oral Path.)

melanosis (mĕl"ah-nō'sĭs) The condition in which melanin pigments appear in the tissues. Melanosis is normal in the gingivae of most dark-skinned individuals and occasionally in those with light skin. (Oral Diag.)

— A condition characterized by abnormal melanin pigment deposit or pigment metabolism. (Oral Path.)

melena (mĕ-lē'nah) The passage of dark or black stools; the color is produced by altered blood and blood pigments. (Oral Diag.)

melituria (mĕl"ĭ-tū'rĕ-ah) Presence of any sugar in the urine; e.g., glucose, lactose, pentose, fructose, maltose, galactose, or sucrose. (Oral Med.)

melting range (see **range, melting**)

membrane A thin layer of tissue that covers a surface or divides a space or organ. (Oral Physiol.)

    basement m. The delicate, PAS-positive, noncellular membrane on which the epithelium is seated. (Periodont.)

m. bone (see **bone, membrane**)

mucous m. (see **mucosa**)

Nasmyth's m. (see **cuticle, primary**)

periodontal m. A modified periosteum consisting of collagenous connective tissue fibers that connect the tooth to the alveolar bone. Its principal functions are to provide nutrition to the cementum and bone for metabolic needs, to provide support by organizing and distributing the stresses of occlusal function, to maintain and replace bone and cementum, and to provide proprioception and pain reception for adjustive mechanisms associated with occlusal function. (Oral Physiol.)

— The tissue that surrounds the root(s) of a tooth and attaches it to the bony alveolus. Basically composed of numerous white collagenous fibers extending from tooth to alveolar bone with an interposed area of intermediate plexus, numerous capillaries coursing between and perpendicular to the fiber bundles, fibroblasts generally oriented in the direction of the fibers, osteoblasts adjoining the alveolar bone, occasional cementoblasts approximating the cementum, nerve fibers, lymphatic vessels, etc. A part of the attachment apparatus. (Periodont.)

p. m. attachment Bundles of collagen in fibers of the periodontal membrane, together with an interposed intermediate plexus (Sharpey's fibers). These fibers form the attachment of the periodontal membrane to the root cementum on one side and to the alveolar bone on the other. (Periodont.)

biologic width of p. m. The width in millimeters of the periodontal membrane from the surface of the cementum to the surface of the alveolar bone, i.e., physiologic width. (Periodont.)

blood supply of p. m. Arises from the marrow of the supporting bone and passes through lateral perforations in the alveolar bone and also from the periapical blood vessels. (Periodont.)

blood vessels in p. m. The blood vessels found in the periodontal membrane arise mainly from the marrow of the supporting bone through the lateral perforations of the alveolar bone and, to some extent, from the periodontal vessels. They form an intricate and elaborate anastomosing network, the blood vessels appearing to course perpendicular to and between the principal fiber bundles. (Periodont.)

hyalinization of p. m. Conversion, by degeneration, of portions of the periodontal membrane into albuminoid or vitreous-like material. Seen in occlusal traumatism, experimental lathyrism, etc. (Periodont.)

p. m. in hyperthyroidism Effect of hyperthyroidism on the periodontal membrane. For example, in hyperthyroidism induced with thyroxin in experimental animals, the periodontal membrane will appear wider, with resorption of alveolar bone. There may be increased vascularity and degeneration of the alveolar group of periodontal membrane fibers. (Periodont.)

inflammation in p. m. The rare involvement of the periodontal membrane in inflammatory disease states. The periodontal membrane is almost always spared when inflammatory disease affects the periodontium. In a few instances an inflammatory cellular infiltrate may be seen in the marginal area of the periodontal membrane between the fiber groups around the periodontal membrane vessels. (Periodont.)

injuries to p. m. Hemorrhage, thrombosis, and necrosis of the periodontal membrane as a result of occlusal traumatism. In addition, hyalinization of the connective tissue and even cartilage formation have been noted. In acute occlusal traumatism, tearing of the periodontal fibers on the tension side, accompanied by crushing of the periodontal membrane on the pressure side, may be noted. (Periodont.)

p. m. in mastication The function of the periodontal membrane in the masticatory process. The periodontal membrane serves to transmit functional masticatory forces to the remaining portions of the attachment and supporting apparatus of the tooth. The fluids of the periodontal membrane are physiologically forced through the cribriform channels of the alveolar bone into the narrow spaces of the supporting bone, serving as a functional stimulus to bone formation. The direct pressure of these membrane fluids against the alveolar bone also serves as a stimulus for the preservation of its integrity. (Periodont.)

p. m. nerves The two varieties of nerves, myelinated and unmyelinated, that are present in the periodontal membrane. Their endings have been described as knoblike swellings, rings around fiber bundles, and free endings between periodontal membrane fibers. The nerves are primarily proprioceptive, and a sense of localization is imparted through them. (Periodont.)

physiologic width of p. m. The width of the periodontal membrane in normal, functioning teeth. (Periodont.)

p. m. in protein deficiency Degenerative changes in the periodontal membrane as a result of experimentally induced protein deficiency. There is widening of periodontal membrane space due to alveolar and supporting bone resorption, degeneration of the principal fibers (probably due to an adverse ratio of collagen formation to collagen destruction—turnover rate of collagen), and replacement of fibers by loose edematous connective tissue, with increased capillarity and some hyalinization of connective tissue fibers. (Periodont.)

p. m. space The radiolucent area (noted on radiographs as a dark line) occupied by the periodontal membrane and lying between the tooth cementum and the lamina dura. (Periodont.)

thrombosis of p. m. Thrombosis of the blood vessels of the periodontal membrane may be seen as a result of occlusal traumatism. (Periodont.)

traumatic injury to p. m. Injury manifested by blood vessel thrombosis, necrosis of the intermediate plexus area and subsequently of the areas occupied by cemental and alveolar fibers, hyalinization, etc. According to some authorities, the superimposition of injury by tension to the periodontal membrane can allow the spread of gingival inflammation directly into the periodontal membrane. (Periodont.)

p. m. in vitamin A deficiency Effect on the periodontal membrane when there is an insufficient supply of vitamin A. In acute vitamin A deficiency produced in experimental animals, the connective tissue of the periodontal membrane showed hyaline degeneration with loss of cellular detail. (Periodont.)

p. m. in vitamin B deficiency Effect on the periodontal membrane when there is an insufficient supply of vitamin B. In vita-min B deficiency the periodontal membrane space appears greatly enlarged on radiographs, and microscopic examination reveals an absence of the principal fibers. (Periodont.)

subimplant m. The fibrous connective tissue that regenerates from the periosteum and that forms between the inner surface of the implant framework and the bone surface. All vertical and lateral stresses applied to the implant abutments are borne by this membrane. (Oral Implant.)

memomotion A movie photographic technique used to assist in analysis of work procedures. (Pract. Man.)

menarche The beginning of the menstrual function. (Oral Diag.)

meniscectomy (měn″ĭ-sěk′tō-mē) Excision of an intra-articular meniscus. (Oral Surg.)

menopause Cessation of menstruation in the human female occurring variably from approximately 45 to 50 years of age. It is accompanied by diminution of estrogen formation, often with atrophic changes occurring in the oral mucous membranes and gingivae. (Periodont.)

oral symptoms of m. Burning sensation and dryness of the mouth; salty taste; edematous, reddened, atrophic-appearing, tender mucosa; glossitis; and often desquamative gingivitis. (Periodont.)

mental foramen (see **foramen, mental**)

mental retardate An individual who is intellectually inadequate in his society. (Pedodont.)

meperidine hydrochloride (mě-per′ĭ-dēn) Ethyl 1-methyl-4-phenyl 4-piperidine carboxylate hydrochloride; a narcotic employed for its analgesic, sedative, and spasmolytic effect. The usual dose for adults is 50 to 100 mg. (Periodont.)

mephenesin (mě-fěn′ĭ-sĭn) An antispasmodic drug, 3-ortho-toloxy-1,2-propanediol. Utilized for the preparation of apprehensive patients for dental and periodontal procedures because of its ability to produce muscular relaxation and euphoria. Usual dosage for an adult is 1 Gm, in either tablet or elixir form 20 minutes prior to the dental appointment. (Periodont.)

merbromin (mer-brō′mĭn) A mercury-bromine compound used as a germicide for disinfection of the skin, mucous membrane, and wounds. Used in 10% alcoholic solution (Scott-Wilson reagent) in the treatment of moniliasis. (Periodont.)

mercaptan (mer-kăp′tăn) The basic ingredient

of the polysulfide polymer employed in rubber base impression materials. (D. Mat.) (see also **Thiokol**)

mercurial (mer-kū'rē-ăl) A compound that owes its activity to the mercury it contains. (Oral Med.; Pharmacol.)

m. line (see **line, mercurial**)

mercurialism (mercury poisoning) Poisoning due to the ingestion of pure mercury, its salts, or its vapor. Manifestations of acute intoxication include nausea, vomiting, abdominal cramps, oral and pharyngeal pain, uremia, dehydration, diarrhea, and shock. Manifestations of chronic poisoning include hypersalivation, diarrhea, vertigo, depression, intention tremor, and stomatitis. (Oral Med.) (see also **acrodynia; stomatitis, mercurial**)

— Poisoning by ingestion or absorption of mercury compounds. (Periodont.) (see also **line, mercurial**)

Mercurochrome Proprietary brand of merbromin.

Merkel's corpuscles (see **corpuscle, Merkel's**)

Merkel's disks (see **corpuscle, Merkel's**)

Merrifield's knife (see **knife, Merrifield's**)

mesh, suspending Tantalum metal mesh extending approximately 2 mm beyond the margins of an implant magnet. The mesh is attached to the magnet to suspend it in a position level with the bony margins if the vault is prepared too deeply and to prevent it from rotating in the vault in the bone. (Oral Implant.)

mesial (mē'zē-ăl) Situated in the middle; median, toward the middle line of the body or toward the center line of the dental arch. (Comp. Prosth.; Oper. Dent.; Orthodont.; Remov. Part. Prosth.)

mesioclusion (mē"zē-ō-kloo'zhŭn) Anterior relationship of the lower jaw to the upper jaw. (Orthodont.)

bilateral m. Mesioclusion on both sides. (Orthodont.)

unilateral m. Mesioclusion on one side. (Orthodont.)

mesiodens (mē'zē-ō-dĕnz) A supernumerary tooth appearing in an erupted or unerupted state between the two maxillary central incisors. (Oral Diag.)

— An accessory tooth, usually peg shaped and usually occurring between the maxillary central incisors. (Oral Path.)

mesioversion (mē-zē-ō-ver'zhŭn) When applied to a tooth, a term indicating that the tooth is closer than normal to the median plane or midline. When applied to the maxillae or mandible, it means that the jaw is anterior to its normal position. (Orthodont.)

mesocephalic (mēz"ō-sĕ-fǎl'ĭk) Descriptive term applied to a head size between dolichocephalic and brachycephalic (76 to 81). (Orthodont.)

mesodontia (mēz-ō-don'shē-ah) Medium-sized teeth. (Orthodont.)

mesognathic (mē-sŏ-nǎth'ĭk) Having an average relationship of jaws to head. (Orthodont.)

mesostomia (mēz-ō-stō'mē-ah) An oral fissure of medium size. (Orthodont.)

mesostructure conjunction bar A connecting bar joining implant abutment copings together. Bar and copings together make up the mesostructure. (Oral Implant.)

metabolism (mē-tăb'ō-lĭzm) The sum of chemical changes involved in the function of nutrition. There are two phases: anabolism (constructive or assimilative changes) and catabolism (destructive or retrograde changes). (Anesth.)

— The phenomena of synthesizing foodstuffs into complex tissue elements (anabolism) and complex substances into simple ones in the production of energy (catabolism). (Periodont.)

basal m. (see **basal metabolic rate**)

bone m. The continual complex of anabolism and catabolism taking place in bone when it is in physiologic equilibrium. Bone is a highly labile substance that reflects the adequacy of general body metabolism. (Periodont.) (see also **bone, alveolar, metabolism**)

cell m. The complexity of anabolic and catabolic processes occurring within cellular structures. (Periodont.)

energy m. The transformation of energy in living tissues, consisting of anabolism (storage of energy) and catabolism (the dissipation of energy). (Oral Physiol.)

substance m. The sum of all the physical and chemical processes by which living organized tissues are produced and maintained. (Oral Physiol.)

metachysis (mē-tăk'ĭ-sĭs) Blood transfusion; the introduction of any substance directly into the bloodstream by mechanical means. (Anesth.)

metal An element possessing luster, malleability, ductility, and conductivity of electricity and heat. (D. Mat.)

base m. Archaic term referring to nonprecious metals or alloys; e.g., iron, lead, copper, nickel, chromium, and zinc. In dentistry, a term usually referring to the stainless steel and chrome-cobalt-nickel alloys. (D. Mat.)

fusion of m. Blending of metals by melting together. (Oper. Dent.)

m. insert teeth (see **tooth, metal insert**)

noble m. A precious metal, usually one that does not readily oxidize; e.g., gold or platinum. (D. Mat.)

solidification of m. The change of metal from the molten to the solid state. (Oper. Dent.)

wrought m. A cast metal that has been cold worked in any manner. (D. Mat.)

metalloid (mĕt′ăh-loid) A nonmetallic element that behaves as a metal under certain conditions. Carbon, silicon, and boron are three examples. These elements may be alloyed with metals. (D. Mat.)

Metaphen, tincture of (mĕt′ah-fĕn) Proprietary brand of tincture of nitromersol. (Pharmacol.)

metaphysis (mĕ-tăf′ĭ-sĭs) The line of junction of the epiphysis with the diaphysis of a long bone. (Oral Physiol.)

metaplasia (mĕt″ah-plā′zē-ah) Change in the type of adult cells in a tissue to a form that is not normal for that tissue. (Oral Path.)

metastasis (mĕ-tăs′tah-sĭs) The transfer of a disease by blood vessels, lymph vessels, or the respiratory tract (aspiration) from one organ or region to another not directly contiguous with it. Usually used in reference to malignant tumor cells, but bacteria can also metastasize (e.g., in focal infection). (Oral Diag.; Oral Path.)

meter, dose rate Any instrument that measures radiation dose rate. (Oral Radiol.)

integrating d. r. m. Ionization chamber and measuring system designed for determining the total accumulated radiation administered during an exposure. (Oral Radiol.)

meter, radiation An instrument for the measurement of exposure to radiation. (Oral Radiol.)

dosimeter r. m. An instrument used to detect and measure an accumulated exposure to radiation—commonly a pencil-sized ionization chamber with built-in self-reading electrometer used in personnel radiation monitoring. (Oral Radiol.)

integrating r. m. An instrument consisting in principle of an ionization chamber feeding responses to an integrating system, for the determination of the total accumulated radiation exposure. (Oral Radiol.)

methemoglobinemia (mĕt-hē″mō-glō″bĭ-nē′mē-ah) An abnormality of hemoglobin as a result of exposure to industrial substances or the ingestion of toxic agents such as phenacetin, sulfonamides, aniline nitrates, and nitrates. A rare congenital form is seen most commonly in Greeks. Symptoms include generalized cyanosis, headache, drowsiness, and confusion. (Oral Med.)

method A manner of performing an act or operation; a technique.

Bell m. A method of toothbrushing in which the bristles are guided upward over the maxillary teeth and gingivae and downward over the mandibular teeth and gingivae; sometimes referred to as the physiologic method. A soft multitufted toothbrush is used. (Periodont.)

Callahan's m. (see **method, chloropercha**)

Charters' m. A method of toothbrushing in which the brush is held horizontally, with the bristles lying against the teeth and gingivae and pointed in a coronal direction at 45° so that the bristles lie half on the teeth and half on the gingivae. A vibratory cycle of a very constricted diameter is negotiated so that the brush head moves in a circular movement but the brush bristles remain fairly stationary while being agitated. The circular vibration loosens debris and pumps the bristles into interproximal areas to massage the tissues. (Periodont.)

chloropercha m. (**Callahan's m., Johnston's m.**) The method of filling root canals in which gutta-percha cones are dissolved in a chloroform-rosin solution in the root canal. The canal is flooded with the chloroform solution. A preselected gutta-percha cone is then pumped carefully into and out of the canal. As the cone dissolves, the material is forced into the apex as a plastic mass. Other cones and ocasionally additional chloroform solution are added until the canal is sealed. (Endodont.)

filling m. The procedure used to fill a root canal of a tooth. (Endodont.)

Fones' m. (**Fones' technique**) A toothbrushing technique in which, with the teeth occluded and with the brush at more or less right angles to the teeth, large sweeping, scrubbing circles are described. With the jaws parted, the palatal and lingual surfaces of the teeth are scrubbed utilizing smaller circles. Occlusal surfaces are brushed in an anteroposterior direction. (Periodont.)

Hirschfeld's m. A toothbrushing method in which the bristles are placed against the axial surfaces of the teeth, with slight incisal or occlusal inclination from a right-angled application, in simultaneous contact with teeth and gingivae, and then rotated in a circle of exceedingly small diameter. Occlusal surfaces are brushed energetically. (Periodont.)

Howard's m. A method of artificial respiration. The patient is placed on his back, his hands are placed under his head, and a cushion is placed so that his head is lower than his abdomen. The physician applies rhythmical pressure upward and inward with his hands against the lower lateral parts of the patient's chest. (Anesth.)

Howe's silver precipitation m. A method of depositing silver in enamel and dentin by the application of ammoniacal silver nitrate solution and its reduction with formalin or eugenol. (Oper. Dent.)

indirect m. A procedure involving an intervening medium; e.g., the formation of a wax pattern on a die. Made from an impression of a prepared cavity, rather than fabricated directly on the tooth in the mouth. (Oper. Dent.)

— The technique of construction of a restoration on a cast or model of the original; e.g., the indirect method of inlay construction, in which a die of amalgam or other material is made from an impression of the prepared tooth, a wax pattern formed, and the cast inlay fitted and finished on the die. (Remov. Part. Prosth.)

Johnston's m. (see **method, chloropercha**)

Kirstein's m. A method of inspection of the larynx without a laryngoscope by inclining the head far back and depressing the tongue; autoscopy. (Anesth.)

lateral condensation m. The method in which a preselected gutta-percha cone is sealed into the apex of the root. The balance of space is filled with other gutta-percha cones forced laterally with a spreader. (Endodont.)

segmentation m. The method in which a preselected gutta-percha cone is cut into segments. The tip section is sealed into the apex of the root. The other segments are usually warmed and condensed against the first piece with a plugger. Additional pieces are then used until the space is obliterated. (Endodont.)

silver cone m. The method in which a prefitted silver cone is sealed into the apex of the root canal. If irregularities in canals occur, the space not sealed with the cone is obliterated with gutta-percha by lateral condensation or segmentation. (Endodont.)

split cast m. A procedure for checking the ability of an articulator to receive or be adjusted to a maxillomandibular relation record. (Comp. Prosth.)

— A procedure for indexing casts on an articulator to facilitate their removal and replacement on the instrument. (Comp. Prosth.; Remov. Part. Prosth.)

Stout's m. (see **wiring, continuous loop**)

methyl methacrylate (mĕth′ĭl mĕth-ak′rĭ-lāt) An acrylic resin, $CH_2=C(CH_3)COOCH_3$, derived from methyl acrylic acid. Monomer is the single molecule and polymer is the polymerization product. (D. Mat.)

Meticorten Proprietary form of prednisone.

Meulengracht's test (moi′lĕn-grăkts) (see **test, Meulengracht's**)

metric system (see **system, metric**)

mev One million electron volts. (Oral Radiol.)

micelle (mī-sĕl′) Any one of the spaces formed by the brush structure of fibrils in colloidal gels. The spaces are occupied by water in hydrocolloid impressions. (D. Mat.)

microcephalus (mī″krō-sĕf′ah-lŭs) An abnormally small head. (Oral Diag.)

Micrococcus gazogenes (mī″krō-kahk′ŭs gah′zō-jĕnz) (see **Veillonella alcalescens**)

microcurie One millionth of a curie. (Oral Radiol.)

microcytosis, hereditary (mī″krō-sī-tō′sĭs) (see **thalassemia; thalassemia major**)

microdontia (mī″krō-don′shē-ah) Abnormally small teeth. Term may apply to one, several, or all the teeth of a given individual. (Oral Diag.)

— Abnormally small tooth or teeth. (Oral Path.; Orthodont.)

microgenia (mī″krō-jē′nē-ah) Abnormal smallness of the chin. (Oral Surg.)

microglossia (mī″krō-glahs′ē-ah) An abnormally small tongue. (Oral Diag.; Orthodont.)

— An undersized tongue. (Oral Surg.)

microglossic Descriptive of microglossia. (Orthodont.)

micrognathia (mī″krō-năth′ē-ah) An abnormally small jaw; e.g., in brachygnathia. (Oral Diag.) (see also **brachygnathia**)

— A receding mandible; unusual smallness of the mandible, indicating a lack of normal development of the maxillae and the mandible. (Oral Surg.; Orthodont.) (see also **retrognathism**)

micrognathic Descriptive of micrognathia. (Orthodont.)

microleakage The seepage of fluids, debris, and microorganisms along the interface between a restoration and the walls of a cavity preparation. (Oper. Dent.)

micrometer (mī′krō-mē″ter) A millionth of a meter (10^{-6} meter). (D. Mat.)

micron (see **micrometer**)

microorganism A minute living organism, such as a bacterium, virus, rickettsia, yeast, or fungus. These organisms may exist as part of the normal flora of the oral cavity without producing disease; with disturbance of the more or less balanced interrelationship between the organisms or between the organisms and host resistance, individual forms of microorganisms may overgrow and induce disease in the host's tissues. Of course, organisms foreign to the individual may invade and produce pathologic processes. (Periodont.)

microradiography A process by which a radiograph of a small object is produced on fine-grained photographic film under conditions that permit subsequent microscopic examination or enlargement of the radiograph at linear magnifications of up to several hundred. (Oral Radiol.)

microstomia (mī″krō-stō′mē-ah) A small oral fissure. (Orthodont.)

microtia (mī-krō′shē-ah) Aplasia or hypoplasia of the pinna of the ear, with a closed or missing external auditory meatus. (M.F.P.)

midbrain The portion of the brain located superior to the pons and medulla and containing the motor nuclei of the ocular motor and trochlear nerves. It also contains the major pathways and decussations of fibers from the cerebrum and cerebellum. Disturbances in the midbrain, as a rule, do not prevent contraction of the muscle groups. Such disturbances merely effect an incoordination of the muscular activities. The major diseases associated with the midbrain generally involve pupillary and ocular motor dysfunctions. (Oral Physiol.)

midline The line equidistant from bilateral features of the head. (Orthodont.)

migraine (see **headache, migraine**)

migration, tooth (see **tooth, drifting**)

Mikulicz' aphtha, disease, syndrome (mĭk′ū-lĭch) (see under appropriate noun)

Mikulicz' ulcer (see **periadenitis mucosa necrotica recurrens**)

milled-in curve (see **path, milled-in**)

milled-in path (see **path, milled-in**)

Miller's organism (see **organism, Miller's**)

milliampere (mĭl″ē-ăm′pēr) In radiography, milliamperage signifies the amount of current flowing in the tube circuit. With time (seconds) it is an indication of roentgen ray quantity. (Oral Radiol.)

millicurie One thousandth of a curie. (Oral Radiol.)

milliliter (ml) (mĭl″ĭ-lē′ter) The preferred unit of volume used in prescription writing. It is based on the fundamental unit, the liter. One liter equals 1000 milliliters. In prescriptions the terms ml and cc are often used interchangeably because they are so nearly equal. (Oral Med.; Pharmacol.)

milling-in The procedure of refining or perfecting the occlusion of removable dentures by placing abrasives between their occluding surfaces while the dentures make contact in various excursions on the articulator. (Comp. Prosth.; Remov. Part. Prosth.)

milliroentgen (mĭl″ĭ-rĕnt′gĕn) A submultiple of the roentgen, equal to one thousandth of a roentgen. (Oral Radiol.)

mineralization Bioprecipitation of inorganic substance. (Oral Med.; Oral Physiol.)

mineral oil (see **oil, mineral**)

mineral salt (see **salt, mineral**)

mineralocorticoids (mĭn″er-ăl-ō-kor′tĭ-koidz) (**proinflammatory hormones**) Adrenal corticosteroids that are active in the retention of salt and in the maintenance of life of adrenalectomized animals. Typical are deoxycorticosterone and aldosterone. Aldosterone is a natural hormone for salt retention but also has some regulatory effect on carbohydrate metabolism. (Oral Med.)

minim (mĭn′ĭm) A unit of volume in the traditional apothecary system. It equals 0.0616 ml. A drop is sometimes used as a crude approximation of the minim. (Oral Med.; Pharmacol.)

minor A person of either sex under the age of majority; i.e., one who has not attained the age at which full civil rights are granted; an infant. (D. Juris.)

m. connector (see **connector, minor**)

miotic (mī-ah′tĭk) A drug that constricts the pupil. (Anesth.)

misconduct A deviation from duty, injurious to another, by one employed in a professional capacity. (D. Juris.)

misfeasance (mĭs-fē′zĕns) The improper performance of some act that one may lawfully do. (D. Juris.)

misrepresentation An intentionally false statement regarding a matter of fact. (D. Juris.)

mistake Some unintentional act, omission, or

error due to ignorance, surprise, or misplaced confidence. (D. Juris.)

mithridatism (mĭth′rĭ-dā″tĭzm) (see **tolerance, acquired**)

mitigation (mĭt″ĭ-gā′shŭn) Alleviation; abatement or diminution of a penalty imposed by law. (D. Juris.)

m. of damages A reduction of damages based on facts that show the plaintiff's course of action does not entitle him to as large an amount as the evidence on his side would otherwise justify the jury in allowing him. (D. Juris.)

mix To form by combining ingredients. (Oper. Dent.)

mixed dentition (see **dentition, mixed**)

mixing, vacuum A method of mixing materials, such as gypsum products and water, in a vacuum. (Comp. Prosth.; Fixed Part. Prosth.; Remov. Part. Prosth.)

MLD (see **dose, lethal, minimum**)

MLT (see **time, median lethal**)

MO (see **cavity, MO**)

mobility Loosening of a tooth or teeth, an important diagnostic sign that may result not only from a decrease in root attachment or changes in the periodontal ligament but also from destruction of the gingival fiber apparatus and transseptal fibers. (Periodont.)

m. of tooth (see **tooth mobility**)

MOD (see **cavity, MOD**)

model A replica, usually in miniature. (Comp. Prosth.; Oper. Dent.; Remov. Part. Prosth.) (see **cast,** *n.*)

— An object (metal, plaster, etc.) formed or poured in a matrix or impression. A positive likeness of some desired form. A positive reproduction of the form of the tissues of the upper or lower jaw; made in an impression over which appliances may be fabricated. (Orthodont.)

— A positive replica of the dentition and surrounding or adjoining structures used as a diagnostic aid and/or base for construction of orthodontic and prosthetic appliances. (Periodont.)

— A reproduction of the oral cavity or parts of the oral cavity used to illustrate the existing conditions and proposed treatment to patients. (Pract. Man.)

casting m. (see **cast, refractory**)

implant m. (see **cast, implant**)

m. of prepared cavity (see **die**)

study m. (see **cast, diagnostic**)

modeling composition (see **plastic, modeling**)

modeling compound (see **compound, impression; plastic, modeling**)

modeling plastic (see **plastic, modeling**)

moderator A chairman; one who presides over an assembly, group, or panel. (D. Juris.)

modiolus (mō-dī′ō-lŭs) A point distal to the corner of the mouth where several muscles of facial expression converge. (Comp. Prosth.)

modulus A constant that numerically indicates the amount in which a certain property is possessed by any object. (D. Mat.)

m. of elasticity (see **elasticity, modulus of**)

m. of resilience (see **resilience, modulus of**)

m. of rigidity (see **rigidity**)

Young's m. (see **elasticity, modulus of**)

Moeller's disease (mĕ′lerz) (see **scurvy, infantile**)

Moeller's glossitis (mĕ′lerz) (see **glossitis, Moeller's**)

Mohs scale (see **hardness scale**)

molar A reference solution in which the concentration is stated with regard to the number of gram molecular weights per liter of solution. (D. Mat.)

— One of the twelve teeth in man located distal to the second bicuspid on each side of each arch. (Oper. Dent.)

bicuspidized m. The process of separating the roots of a lower molar and restoring the two endodontically treated roots coronally as bicuspids. (Endodont.)

mulberry m. A malformed first molar with a crown suggesting the appearance of a mulberry. It may be a manifestation of congenital syphilis, although other diseases affecting the enamel organ during morphodifferentiation may produce a similar lesion. (Oral Diag.)

— A molar characterized by dwarfing of the cusps and hypertrophy of the enamel around them. Seen in hereditary syphilis. (Oral Path.)

m. sheath A rectangular metallic tube soldered or welded to the molar bands. (Orthodont.)

mold (mould) A form in which an object is cast or shaped. The process of shaping a material into an object. The term used to specify the shape of an artificial tooth or teeth. (Comp. Prosth.; Oper. Dent.; Remov. Part. Prosth.)

molding Shaping.

border m. (see **border molding**)

compression m. The act of pressing or squeezing together to form a shape in a mold. The process of forming a denture base material into the shape of the base by pressing the material into a split mold (two or more parts contained in a flask). (Comp. Prosth.) (see also **molding, injection**)

—Adaptation by pressure of a plastic material to the negative form of a split mold. (Remov. Part. Prosth.)

injection m. Adaptation of a plastic material to the negative form of a closed mold by forcing the material into the mold through appropriate gateways. (Comp. Prosth.; Fixed Part. Prosth.; Remov. Part. Prosth.) (see also **molding, compression**)

tissue m. (see **border molding**)

mole A pigmented nevus. (Oral Path.)

molecular weight (see **weight, molecular**)

molecule A chemical composition of two or more atoms that forms a specific chemical substance. (Anesth.)

molimina, menstrual (mō-lĭm′ĭ-nah) Circulatory symptoms, psychic tension, irritable behavior, belligerence, and other personality alterations prior to or during menstruation. The cause is unknown. (Oral Med.)

molluscum fibrosum (see **neurofibromatosis**)

momentum Quantity of motion. Newton's law of momentum can be expressed as the product of mass and velocity. When a body is acted on by a force, the momentum of that body is changed in the direction of the force. Also, the momentum is proportionate to the amount of the force applied and to the duration of the force acting on the body. Momentum is thus directly associated with inertia. The greater the inertia of the body, the greater the force that must be applied to change the momentum. (Oral Physiol.)

money General term for the representation of value; currency; cash. (D. Juris.)

mongolism (mon′gō-lĭzm) (**Down's syndrome**) Extreme mental deficiency of a congenital type associated with features of the Mongolian race, such as slanted eyes. (Oral Diag.)

— Clinical syndrome (Down's) associated with the autosomal abnormalities trisomy-21 or translocations 13-15/21-22, or 21/22. Affected children have almond-shaped eyes, a rather roundish head, and increased susceptibility to infection. They are mentally retarded, commonly suffer from acute leukemia, and often have congenital heart disease, a heavily fissured and protruding tongue, delayed dentition, and underdeveloped nose, short fingers, and broad simian-like hands. (Oral Med.; Pedodont.)

Monilia albicans (mō-nĭl′ē-ah ăl′bĭ-kănz) (see **Candida albicans**)

moniliasis (mō″nĭ-lī′ah-sĭs) Surface fungous infection caused by *Candida albicans;* affects the mucous membrane of the oral cavity, gastrointestinal tract, and vagina. (Oral Diag.; Oral Path.) (see also **thrush**)

— Infection by a fungus of the genus *Candida,* usually *Candida albicans.* May involve the mouth (thrush), female genitalia, skin, hands, nails, and/or lungs. Oral moniliasis refers to thrush or to mycotic stomatitis. The latter term is sometimes applied to erythematous patches that are not typical of the usual white patches of thrush. (Oral Med.)

monitoring Periodic or continuous determination of the dose rate in an occupied area (area monitoring) or of the dose received by a person (personnel monitoring). (Oral Radiol.)

area m. Routine monitoring of the level of radiation of any particular area, building, room, equipment, or outdoor space. Some laboratories distinguish between routine monitoring and survey activities. (Oral Radiol.)

personal m. Monitoring of any part of an individual, his breath or excretions, or any part of his clothing. (Oral Radiol.)

personnel m. A systematic, periodic check of the radiation dose each person receives during his working hours. (Oral Radiol.)

monkey An animal often used for experimental purposes in medicine and stomatology. Its dental and oral structures are morphologically and functionally similar to those of human beings, permitting an associated correlation of experimental findings. (Periodont.)

Monobloc (see **activator**)

monocyte (mon′ō-sīt) A large nongranular leukocyte containing a single oval or indented nucleus and more protoplasm than a lymphocyte. (Oral Physiol.)

monocytosis (mon″ō-sī-tō′sĭs) Increase in the number of monocytes in the peripheral bloodstream. Various limits are given; e.g., a total number in excess of $800/mm^3$, regardless of the percentage, or a total greater than 8% with the total number less than 800; in both cases the presence of monocytosis is indicated. It may be associated with chronic pyogenic infections, subacute bacterial endocarditis, infectious hepatitis, monocytic leukemia, rickettsial disease, and protozoan infections. (Oral Diag.; Oral Med.)

monomer (mon′ō-mer) A single molecule. In commercial resin products, the term applies to the liquid, which is usually a mixture of monomers. (D. Mat.)

residual m. The unpolymerized monomer remaining in the appliance or restoration after processing. (D. Mat.)

mononucleosis, infectious (mon″ō-nū″klē-ō′sĭs) (**acute benign lymphadenosis, "kissing disease," "student's disease"**) An acute disease characterized by increased numbers of abnormal mononuclear cells in the blood, enlargement of lymph nodes, fever, malaise, and, often, pharyngitis and stomatitis. (Oral Diag.)

— An acute infectious disease of unknown cause most commonly affecting young adults and older children. Manifestations include fever, sore throat, cervical lymphadenopathy, petechial hemorrhages of the soft palate, and, at times, purpura with thrombocytopenia. Early leukopenia and relative lymphocytosis occur, with later increases in the number of large leukocytoid lymphocytes. The heterophil (usually sheep cell) antibody titer is significantly increased in most instances. (Oral Med.; Oral Path.)

— A disease of viral origin, characterized by influenza-like manifestations: malaise, fever, headache, myalgia, throat inflammation, lymphadenopathy, splenomegaly, presence of abnormal lymphocytes in the blood, petechial hemorrhages of the mucous membranes, and necrotizing ulcerative gingival lesions. The incidence and degree of severity of signs and symptoms are variable. Diagnosis lies in the establishment of an accurate differential diagnosis from influenza and necrotizing ulcerative gingivitis, demonstration of a large number of atypical lymphocytes in the blood, and correlative diagnosis by heterophil agglutination reaction for the determination of antibody titer to the virus. (Periodont.)

monostotic Affecting a single bone. (Oral Path.)

Monson curve (see **curve, Monson**)

moot Subject to argument; undecided. (D. Juris.)

moral Relating to the conscience or moral sense or to the general principles of correct conduct. (D. Juris.)

Morgan's mandrel (see **mandrel, Morgan's**)

moron A mentally defective individual with an IQ between 50 and 70. In the adult moron the mental age corresponds to that of a child of 8 to 12 years of age. (Oral Med.)

morphology The branch of biology that deals with the form and structure of an organism or part, without regard to function. (Oper. Dent.)

determinants of occlusal m. Variable factors that determine the forms given to the crowns of teeth restored in metals, such as mandibular centricity; the intercondylar distance; the distance of teeth from the sagittal plane; the character and steepness of the articulating eminences or the kinds of lateral and protrusive paths of the condylar axes; and the overlaps of the anterior teeth. (Gnathol.)

mortgage A right given to the creditor over the property of the debtor for the security of his debt; invests the creditor with the power of having the property seized and sold in default of payment. (D. Juris.)

chattel m. A mortgage of goods or personal property. (D. Juris.)

mortgagee The person who takes or receives a mortgage. (D. Juris.)

motion, envelope of The three-dimensional space circumscribed by border movements and by occlusal contacts of a given point of the mandible; also called movement space (Posselt). Each mandibular cusp tip and each mandibular fossa pit have spaces in which they are confined by the outlines of border movement. Often, cross sections of such envelopes at particularly assigned levels are projected on the horizontal plane. A point in the top of the condyle that could represent the vertical axis has a free but relatively limited area of movement along its cranial joint surface. The envelope of such a movement among patients varies in length from 10 to 12 mm and in width from 2 to 3 mm, and its shape depends on the shape of the lateral and medial condyle paths. (Gnathol.) (see also **movement, border, posterior**)

motivation The stimulus, incentive, or inducement to act or react in a certain way. Purposeful human behavior is motivated behavior, which means that either physiologic or social stimuli activate or motivate a person to do something. The simplest form of motivated behavior is the response to the simple reflex of pain. More complex motivations are thirst and hunger, which are sustained and do not abate until some adjusted action is taken. It is not to be inferred that a single stimulus motivates behavior. On the contrary, motivation at any one time is a function of a complex pattern of stimulations, some coming from the internal environment of the body itself and others from the external environment as one perceives it. Thus all the inner and outer stimuli that bear on a person at one time constitute his psychologic (motivating) environment and jointly determine his behavior. (Oral Physiol.)

— In dentistry, that force, drive, or reason that creates a desire on the part of the patient to receive dental services. (Pract. Man.)

poor m. Absence of sufficient positive motivation to act or react in a desired way. The unmotivated or poorly motivated patient can waste the professional skills of many treatment disciplines and the extensive physical resources of offices, clinics, and other institutions. The problem in managing unmotivated patients is to decide whether or not to provide treatment, and if it is provided, how extensive it should be and at what level or restored function it should be terminated. Motivation is poor when it is exclusively specific and is directed to only one aspect of treatment. The consequence of specific motivation is manifested in the patient's inability and unwillingness to learn the skills needed for successful wearing of dentures and to accept less functional activity than that provided by a normal dentition. (Oral Physiol.)

motor Pertaining to a muscle, nerve, or center that produces or effects movement.

m. output The activity that results from the integrative phenomena associated with brain activity. It is expressed in function as muscle contraction of the smooth and striated muscle and as secretion of the exocrine and endocrine glands, and, in effect, represents the total behavioral activity of human life. Whereas sensory phenomena have many avenues that feed into the brain, motor activity is expressed in terms of the simple, direct state of muscle contraction and glandular secretion. Thus muscle activity is expressed in terms of locomotion, hand-learned skills, speaking, mastication, and all forms of human activity that involve motion. (Oral Physiol.)

m. pathway All reflex actions of muscle are achieved by the passage of nerve impulses through the final common pathway—the muscle fibers. The lower motor neuron (the motor route of the cranial nerve) is the final pathway for the structures that are innervated by the cranial nerves. Impulses traverse these nerves to their respective muscles from every level of the spinal cord, the hindbrain, the midbrain, and the cerebral cortex. The cranial motor neurons collate these multiple stimuli and transmit sequences of stimuli to the motor end-plate, which in the normal muscle effects a smooth, continuous, controlled contraction. (Oral Physiol.)

m. unit The entity consisting of the lower motor neuron, the motor end-plate, and the muscle fibers supplied by the end-plate. The final motor activity resulting from a sequence of stimulations to the lower motor neuron is considered a function of the motor unit. The proportion of nerve fibers to the muscle fibers in motor units is designated as the innervation ratio. Motor units may have ratios ranging from 1:4 to 1:150. The closer the ratio approximates unity, the greater the finesse of specificity of the muscular action. The eye muscles have the highest ratio of striated muscles, and the tongue, facial, masticatory, and pharyngeal muscles succeed in that order. (Oral Physiol.)

mottled enamel (see **fluorosis, chronic endemic dental**)

moulage A model of a part or a lesion; e.g., a model of the face. It may be of wax or plaster and usually is colored by painting. (Oral Diag.)

mould (see **mold**)

mount, x-ray A windowed, stiff material on which radiographs are arranged in a specific order to correspond with the charts of the teeth. (Pract. Man.)

mounting The laboratory procedure of attaching the maxillary and/or mandibular cast to an articulator or similar instrument. (Comp. Prosth.; Remov. Part. Prosth.)

m. board A jig used in mounting the maxillary cast on the top articulator frame. The mounting board enables the dentist to determine the patient's axis so that the maxillary cast can be positioned accurately. The axis of the patient is represented by an imaginary line between the axis-orbital caliper points; the centrically related axis of the articulator is represented by two outjetting points located one on either side of the sagittal plane of the articulator and at an equal distance from the sagittal plane. The two outjetting points are positioned to align closely with the caliper points of the face-bow so that the following common errors can be avoided: (1) failing to make the midpoint of the axis space between the caliper points coincide with the articulator; (2) inadvertently increasing the angle between the plane of the arms and the plane of the bite fork as a result of the weight of the cast and the viscosity of the plaster while the upper member of the articulator is being closed down into the "mix"; and (3) failing to provide the same gravity freedom for the caliper arms that they had when they were astride the patient's face and the bite fork was between his teeth. (Gnathol.)

split cast m. A cast with the margins of its base or capital beveled or grooved to permit accurate remounting on an articulator. Split remounting metal plates may be used instead of beveling or grooving in the casts. (Comp. Prosth.; Remov. Part. Prosth.)

mouth breathing (see **breathing, mouth**)

mouth, denture-sore Traumatization and inflammation of the oral mucous membranes produced by ill-fitting dentures, hypersensitivity to the chemical components of the denture, and/or proliferation of *Candida albicans* with subsequent monilial infection. (Periodont.)

mouth guard (see **guard, mouth**)

mouth hygiene (see **hygiene, oral**)

mouth lamp (see **lamp, mouth**)

mouth preparation (see **preparation, mouth**)

mouth rehabilitation (see **rehabilitation, mouth**)

mouth-to-mouth insufflation (see **insufflation, mouth-to-mouth**)

mouth, trench (see **gingivitis, necrotizing ulcerative**)

mouthwash A mouth rinse possessing cleansing, germicidal, and/or palliative properties. (Periodont.)

movement(s) Any change of place or of position of a body. (Remov. Part. Prosth.)

Bennett m. The bodily lateral movement or lateral shift of the mandible resulting from the movements of the condyles along the lateral inclines of the mandibular fossae during lateral jaw movement. (Comp. Prosth.; Fixed Part. Prosth.; Remov. Part. Prosth.)

— Movement involving the cuspal relations of the teeth in both an anterior and a posterior direction, which enables the mandible to move freely to and from centric relation without restraint. (Periodont.)

— Movement in which the muscles of the mandibular condyles are thrust outward as well as forward, producing a "lateral thrust" of the condyle movement, which was named after Bennett. (Gnathol.)

bodily m. Movement of a tooth so that the crown and root apex move the same amount in the same direction, thus maintaining the same axial inclination; opposed to tipping movement. (Orthodont.)

border m. Any extreme muscular movement

limited by bone, ligaments, or other soft tissues. (Comp. Prosth.)

posterior b. m. Any movement of the mandible occurring while the mandible is its most posterior relation to the maxillae. This movement occurs in the vertical plane from the level of occlusal contact to the level of maximal opening of the jaws. (Comp. Prosth.)

hinge m. An opening or closing movement of the mandible on the hinge axis. A movement around a single axis. (Comp. Prosth.; Remov. Part. Prosth.)

intermediary m. (intermediate m.) All mandibular movements between the extremes of mandibular excursions. (Comp. Prosth.; Remov. Part. Prosth.)

intermediate m. (see **movement, intermediary**)

jaw m. All changes in position of which the mandible is capable. (Comp. Prosth.; Remov. Part. Prosth.)

labial m. The labial progression of a tooth, either by bodily movement or by tipping movement, occurring as a result of excessive tongue pressure against the lingual aspects of the teeth, disequilibrium between tongue and lip pressure against the teeth, diminution of periodontal support in combination with aforementioned factors, or a purposeful consequence of orthodontic therapy. (Periodont.)

lateral m. A movement of a body to one side of its established position. (Comp. Prosth.; Remov. Part. Prosth.)

l. m. of jaw Movement of the mandible sideways; usually considered as a relation of the mandible in a nearly horizontal plane around one condyle. (Comp. Prosth.; Remov. Part. Prosth.)

lingual m. Lingual progression of a tooth or teeth, either by bodily movement or by tipping movement, from the line of occlusion or from a harmonious position in the dental arch. Movement occurs as a result of disequilibrium between lip and tongue forces on the teeth, occlusal interferences producing lingual displacement, habits, etc. (Periodont.)

mandibular m. Any movement of the lower jaw. (Comp. Prosth.; Remov. Part. Prosth.)

— Activities of the mandibular chewing muscles: (1) ingesting, egesting, digesting, and swallowing food; (2) uttering language sounds ranging from whispers to shouts of joy or groans of great pain; (3) uttering wordless expressions of deep or insane emotions; (4) investigating oral and dental relations in an attempt to relearn the reoriented tools; and (5) equally contracting the front and back muscles of the head and neck to protect the neck joints in heavy lifting or in fierce athletics. (Gnathol.)

free m. m. Mandibular movement made without tooth interference. An uninhibited movement of the mandible. (Comp. Prosth.; Remov. Part. Prosth.)

functional m. m. All natural, proper, or characteristic movements of the mandible made during speaking, chewing, yawning, swallowing, and other associated movements. (Comp. Prosth.; Fixed Part. Prosth.; Remov. Part. Prosth.)

masticatory m. m. The translatory and rotary movements of the mandible that are used in the course of chewing food. (Comp. Prosth.; Remov. Part. Prosth.)

— Excursive actions of the mandible made during chewing, opening, closing, protruding, lateral, and lateral protrusive movements; governed by the size and consistency of the food bolus, the patient's pain threshold, the anatomic structure and functional attributes of the temporomandibular joints, the mandibular musculature, the restraining ligaments associated with the mandible, the presence or absence of disease, etc. (Periodont.)

opening m. m. The movement of the mandible executed during jaw separation. (Comp. Prosth.; Remov. Part. Prosth.)

perverted m. m. Movement of mandibular muscles for other than masticatory purposes. The secondary, or acquired, uses are sometimes called nonfunctional or parafunctional. If mandibular movements are overused for emotional purposes or misused to hold objects in either indulgent or work habits, the overlaps of the incisors are disturbed, the teeth are misplaced, their edges may be worn, and the postcanine teeth may wear off in latercursive motions. Such overuse is said to be due to unintended activity, which is called nonfunctional activity. (Gnathol.)

tipping m. The movement of a tooth in any direction while its apex remains in almost the original position. (Orthodont.)

tooth m. Temporary or permanent deviation of a tooth from its normally fixed position in the dental arch. Also, mobility of teeth.

When teeth exhibit mobility patterns, movement may be buccolingual, mesiodistal, occlusoapical, rotational, etc. Movement of teeth into different positions in the dental arch may be produced by repositioning them mesially, distally, buccally, lingually, occlusally, etc. (Periodont.)

— Slight movement of a tooth as a result of some altered environmental condition. Movement of a tooth with which contact is to be made may occur between the time of making the final impression of a partially edentulous dental arch and the time of placing the cast portion of the prosthesis. The immediate result is that the cast metal portion of the prosthesis cannot be perfectly seated. If the framework, with temporary bases, is worn for a short period of time (usually until the next day), the teeth will have returned to their former positions. At this time the correctable impression of the ridge areas may be accurately related to the remaining teeth. (Remov. Part. Prosth.)

distal t. m. Migration of a tooth in a distal direction as the result of traumatic occlusal forces, loss of support by removal of distally adjacent tooth, etc.; also the purposeful distal movement of teeth in orthodontic therapy. (Periodont.)

translatory m. Motion of a body at any instant when all points within the body are moving at the same velocity and in the same direction. (Comp. Prosth.; Fixed Part. Prosth.; Remov. Part. Prosth.)

MPD (see **dose, maximum permissible**)

MSH (see **hormone, melanocyte-stimulating**)

mucobuccal fold (see **fold, mucobuccal**)

mucobuccal reflection (see **fold, mucobuccal**)

mucocele (mu'kō-sēl) (see **cyst, mucous**)

mucolabial fold (see **fold, mucolabial**)

mucopolysaccharidosis (**MPS**) Genetic disorder involving mucopolysaccharide metabolism and leading to excess storage of the material in the tissues. Forms include MPS I, II, III, IV, V, and VI. Eponymic designations are Hurler, Hunter, Sanfilippo, Morquio, Scheie, and Maroteaux-Lamy syndromes. (Oral Med.)

mucosa (**mucous membrane**) (mū-kō'sah) A membrane, composed of epithelium and lamina propria, that lines the oral cavity and other canals and cavities of the body that communicate with external air. (Oral Diag.; Oral Path.)

— A lining tissue of a part of the body such as the gastrointestinal tract, the respiratory tract, or the genitourinary tract; it is composed of epithelium overlying a connective tissue corium. (Periodont.)

alveolar m. The covering on the alveolar process loosely attached to bone; extends from the mucogingival junction to the vestibular fornix and from the lower jaw to the sublingual sulcus. (Periodont.)

color of a. m. A deeper tone than the attached gingivae; usually dark pink to rose (with variations). (Periodont.)

texture of a. m. A smooth surface similar, in large measure, to that of the buccal mucosa. (Periodont.)

m. in menstruation Transitory changes—in gingivae, for example—resembling those seen in pregnancy, with hyperemia, swelling, and sometimes hemorrhage. Occasionally oral herpetic lesions are seen. (Periodont.)

oral m. Lining of the oral cavity; composed of the stratified squamous epithelium and the underlying lamina propria. (Oral Path.)

palatine m. The mucous membrane covering the palate. (Periodont.)

mucositis (mū″kō-sī′tĭs) Inflammation of the mucous membrane. (Comp. Prosth.; Oral Diag.; Remov. Part. Prosth.)

chronic atrophic senile m. Mucosal inflammation characterized by atrophy and found primarily in elderly women. (Oral Diag.)

fusospirochetal m. Mucosal inflammation associated with fusiform and spirochetal microorganisms. (Oral Diag.)

mucostatic Pertaining to the normal, relaxed condition of mucosal tissues covering the jaws. (Comp. Prosth.; Remov. Part. Prosth.)

— An agent that arrests the secretion of mucus. (Oral Med.; Pharmacol.)

mucous membrane (see **mucosa**)

mucous patch (see **patch, mucous**)

mucoviscidosis (mū″kō-vĭs″ĭ-dō′sĭs) (see **disease, fibrocystic**)

mulberry molars First permanent molars in which the occlusal surface is composed of an aggregate of enamel nodules. All four molars are involved, usually as the result of congenital syphilis. (Oral Diag.)

mulling (mŭh′lĭng) The final step of mixing dental amalgam; a kneading of the triturated mass to complete the amalgamation. (Oper. Dent.)

mumps (parotitis) An infectious disease of viral origin affecting the salivary glands (and other glands) with swelling and pain. (Oral Diag.)

— An acute infectious viral disease chiefly involving the parotid glands but, at times, the other salivary glands, testes, and ovaries. The incubation period is 12 to 26 days; transmission is by droplet spread and direct contact; communicability begins about 2 days prior to the appearance of symptoms and lasts until swelling of the glands has abated. Symptoms begin with vague pain in the parotid region, followed by headache, malaise, low-grade fever, and then swelling of the glands. Temperature may rise to 104° F and last 1 to 3 days. (Oral Med.)

— A contagious parotitis caused by the virus *Rabula inflans* and characterized by swelling of the parotid gland and sometimes of the pancreas, ovaries, and testicles. (Oral Path.) (see also **parotitis**)

iodide m. (iodine m.) Enlargement of the thyroid gland due to iodides. (Oral Med.)

iodine m. (see **mumps, iodide**)

murmur A humming or blowing sound heard on auscultation. (Oral Med.)

aortic m. A murmur resulting from insufficiency of the aortic valve secondary to involvement by rheumatic fever or tertiary syphilis. (Oral Med.)

apical diastolic m. A murmur heard over the apex of the heart and caused by mitral stenosis, relative mitral stenosis, or aortic insufficiency. (Oral Med.)

apical systolic m. A murmur heard at the apex of the heart in systole and caused by mitral insufficiency, which may result from rheumatic heart disease, or by relative mitral insufficiency, which may result from congestive heart failure associated with arteriosclerosis or hypertension. The murmur may also have a functional basis. (Oral Med.)

basal diastolic m. A murmur heard over the base of the heart and caused by aortic insufficiency resulting from rheumatic heart disease or syphilis, by relative aortic insufficiency associated with diastolic hypertension, or by a patent ductus arteriosus. (Oral Med.)

basal systolic m. A murmur heard over the base of the heart and caused by aortic stenosis resulting from rheumatic heart disease or by relative stenosis of the aortic valve resulting from aortic dilation secondary to arteriosclerosis or hypertension. The murmur may also be functional or may be due to congenital heart or vascular defects. (Oral Med.)

cardiac m. (heart m.) An abnormal sound heard in the region of the heart at any time during the heart's cycle. Murmurs may be named according to the area of generation (mitral, aortic, pulmonary, or tricuspid) and according to the period of the cycle (diastolic or systolic). (Oral Med.)

functional m. (innocent m., inorganic m.) A murmur resulting from the position of the body, severe anemia, or polycythemia. Not related to structural changes in the heart. (Oral Med.)

heart m. (see **murmur, cardiac**)

innocent m. (see **murmur, functional**)

inorganic m. (see **murmur, functional**)

mitral m. Heart murmur produced by a defect in the mitral valve. The most common form of murmur in rheumatic heart disease. (Oral Med.)

organic m. A murmur due to structural changes in the heart or in the great vessels of the heart. (Oral Med.)

muscle(s) An organ that, by cellular contraction, produces the movements of life. There are two varieties of muscle structure: striated, including all the muscles in which contraction is voluntary and the heart muscle (in which contraction is involuntary), and unstriated, smooth, or organic, including all the involuntary muscles (except the heart), such as the muscular layer of the intestines, bladder, and blood vessels. (Oral Physiol.)

ciliary m. Tiny smooth muscle at the junction of the cornea and sclera, consisting of two groups of fibers: circular fibers (which exert parasympathetic control through the oculomotor nerve and the ciliary ganglion) and radial fibers (which exert sympathetic control). Responsible for accommodation for far vision through flattening of lens. (Oral Physiol.)

m. contraction (see **contraction, muscle**)

concentric m. c. (see **contraction, muscle, concentric**)

eccentric m. c. (see **contraction, muscle, eccentric**)

isometric m. c. (see **contraction, muscle, isometric**)

isotonic m. c. (see **contraction, muscle, isotonic**)

elasticity of m., physical The physical quality of being elastic, of yielding to passive physical stretch. (Comp. Prosth.; Remov. Part. Prosth.)

elasticity of m., physiologic The biologic quality, unique for muscle, of being able to change and resume size under neuromuscu-

lar control. (Comp. Prosth.; Oper. Dent.; Remov. Part. Prosth.)

elasticity of m., total The combined effect of muscle. (Comp. Prosth.; Oper. Dent.; Remov. Part. Prosth.)

facial m. The muscles of expression, frequently called the mimetic muscles. They are quite variable in contour, are widely distributed over the scalp and face, and tend to be especially concentrated about the orbits, the outer ear, and the lips. It is the mobility of the lips, especially, which has extended the usefulness of the facial muscles in expressing motion, speech, and intelligence. The facial muscles, as a group, have only one bony origin in the facial skeleton. The muscles form a circular rim around the perimeter of the facial bones and extended anteriorly as a tube of tissue in which the lumen narrows and terminates in the orbicularis oris. The structure of the facial muscles may be regarded as a truncated cone in which the base rests on the skeleton (origin) in a fixed position, whereas the truncated top of the cone (insertion in the orbicularis oris) is variable in diameter and height. The lips are thus extensible and retractable and can constrict like a purse string. (Oral Physiol.)

functional changes of m. Asymmetric modifications in length, diameter, and bulk of muscle fibers as a result of variations in function. Muscle responds to normal function by maintenance of bulk. An increase in bulk is caused by an increase in the number of capillaries and in the mean diameter of individual muscle fibers. It is the response to function that accounts for the asymmetry of musculature, which is frequently found when the growth patterns have been influenced by a traumatogenic agent such as disease, injury, or surgery, and also by the functional processes of the body itself, such as posture and habit. Asymmetry is not necessarily pathologic; e.g., it may be the result of differences in habits of chewing, incision, speech sounds, and facial gestures. (Oral Physiol.)

m. hypertenseness Increased muscular tension that is not easily released but that does not prevent normal lengthening of the muscle. Hypertenseness is found in patients with general nervousness. (Comp. Prosth.)

innervation of m., reciprocal A phenomenon of antagonistic muscles demonstrated during a concentric contraction such as that of the temporal muscle. Innervation of the antagonist, the external pterygoid muscle, is partially inhibited, so that freedom of action in flexing the temporomandibular joint is possible. This phenomenon demonstrates inhibition of antagonistic skeletal muscles in a reflex arc brought about automatically by a reduction of the motor discharges from the central nervous system. One of the two muscles in the reflex arc is activated, and the activity of the other is depressed. (Oral Physiol.)

masticatory m. The powerful muscles that elevate and rotate the mandible so that the opposing teeth may occlude for mastication. Considerable pressure can be generated by these muscles when the teeth occlude; in some psychic and neurotic disorders the teeth and the investigating bone tissues may be destroyed as the result of pressure. On the other hand, these muscles can move the mandible with the extremely sensitive changes in position necessary for rapid, precise speech. Their general configuration and position are relatively constant and do not vary significantly from person to person. (Oral Physiol.)

mechanical energy of m. A phenomenon manifested as motion resulting from the shortening mechanisms of the muscle fiber, which converts chemical potential energy into mechanical energy. The dynamics of motion is based on increasing the magnitude of the mechanical energy inherent in the shortening of the muscle. The mechanism to achieve increments in energy is thus a schema of multiple arrangements of muscle fibers, a system of skeletal levers, and a system of reciprocal innervation and gradation of muscle responses. Ultimately, muscle tissue dynamics is based on the biochemical and biophysical mechanisms of contraction of the muscle fiber, which is responsible for the liberation of energy and the development of force for motion. (Oral Physiol.)

m. memory A kinesthetic phenomenon by which a muscle or set of muscles may involuntarily produce movement that follows a pattern that has become established by frequent repetition over a long period of time. (Remov. Part. Prosth.)

ocular m., function The action of the eye muscles in moving the eyeballs. The eyes are in a position of rest (their primary position) when their direction is maintained simply by the tone of the ocular muscles.

This condition prevails when the gaze is straight ahead into distance and not directed to any particular point in space. The visual axes are then parallel. When the eyes view some distant definite object, they are turned by contraction of the ocular muscles and converge so that the visual axes meet at the observed object, and an almost identical image of the object falls on a corresponding point on each fovea, the centralis of the retina. The adjustment of the eye movements for acute observation is called fixation, and the point where the visual axes meet is the fixation point. Thus the interplay of the ocular muscles permits rapid, reciprocally controlled movement of the eyeballs for fixation. (Oral Physiol.)

physical characteristics of m. Primarily, elasticity. A muscle is an elastic body. Its individual fibers follow Hooke's law of elastic bodies; i.e., the amount of elongation is proportional to the stretching force. The muscle organs contain tissue other than muscle fibers and thus deviate slightly from this law. The human muscle fiber can contract to about half its total length. (Oral Physiol.)

regeneration of m. Reproduction or repair of muscle fiber, which is a sequela to many types of muscle damage. Reparation is always associated with the proliferation of sarcolemmic nuclei. Connective tissue elements do not participate in this process except to bridge the gap and to offer support for the regenerative fibers. The regenerative process takes place in two forms: regeneration by budding from the surviving parts of the muscle fibers, which occurs when segments of the muscle fiber and its sheath are destroyed, and regeneration by proliferation of cellular bands, which occurs when the sarcolemmic nuclei are spared and can form a sarcoplasmic band by linkage of the cytoplasmic processes. (Oral Physiol.)

m., sequence of development The pattern of embryologic muscular development. The muscles of the neck and trunk are the first to develop; they are followed by the lingual and facial musculature and then by the distal and proximal appendicular musculature. (Oral Physiol.)

smooth m. The simplest of the three types of muscle (smooth, striated, and cardiac). It is the muscle of the lining of the digestive tract, the ducts of glands, and the viscera associated with the gut. It also supplies the muscles for the genitourinary tract, the structures of the blood vessels, the connective tissues of the mucous membranes, and the skin with its appendages. A typical smooth muscle fiber is a slender spindle-shaped body averaging a few tenths of a millimeter in length. There is a single centrally striated nucleus. The cytoplasm appears homogeneous. The cells are arranged in bands, or bundles, with interspersed connective tissue fibers uniting them into an effective common mass. Smooth muscle fibers are innervated in part by nerve fibers and in part by the contraction of adjacent muscle tissues. The digestive tract, particularly, demonstrates waves of contraction that pass along a band of smooth muscle. (Oral Physiol.)

spasticity of m. Increased muscular tension of antagonists that prevents normal movement; caused by an inability to relax (a loss of reciprocal inhibition) due to a lesion of the upper motor neuron. (Comp. Prosth.; Remov. Part. Prosth.)

striated m. Skeletal muscles forming the bulk of the body; the voluntary muscles derived from the myotomes of the embryo. In general, they are organized as formed muscles that attach to and move the skeletal structures. The cells are large, elongated, and cylindrical, with lengths ranging from 1 mm to several centimeters. The cells have multiple nuclei that are peripherally situated and scattered along the length of the fiber. The fiber contains a large number of elongated fibers which, under the microscope, appear as the alternating light and dark bands that give the characteristic striated appearance of the striated muscle. The dimensional relationships between these light and dark bands are altered during contraction of the muscle fiber. The potential interaction between these bands permits the wide range of selective purposeful, and rapid activity of the skeletal muscles. (Oral Physiol.)

suprahyoid and infrahyoid m. The muscles grouped about the hyoid bone. They aid in depressing and fixing the mandible, the hyoid bone, and the larynx in the performance of their several respective functions. (Oral Physiol.)

tongue m., extrinsic Muscles of the tongue that provide a scaffolding by which the intrinsic muscles can be moved about in the oral cavity while the latter are continuously modifying their dimension and contour. The extrinsic muscles are paired and originate from both sides of the cranial skeleton, the mandible, and the hyoid bone to radiate medially and insert into the body of the tongue, which consists principally of the intrinsic muscles. (Oral Physiol.)

tongue m., intrinsic Muscles of the tongue that have no attachments in bone, terminating either within each other or in the extrinsic muscle group. The fibers of the intrinsic muscles also lie in all three planes of space and are called longitudinal, vertical, and transverse fibers in order to describe their distribution. They are capable of assuming an infinite variety of shapes. They depend, however, on the activity of the extrinsic muscles to be moved bodily through space. (Oral Physiol.)

m. trimming (see **border molding; impression, correctable**)

muscular dystrophy (mŭs′kū-lar dĭs′trō-fē) (see **dystrophy, muscular**)

musculature (mŭs′kū-lah-tūr) Any part of the muscular apparatus of the body; the source of power for the movement of the body or its parts. (Comp. Prosth.)

cheek m. The muscles giving support, form, and function to the cheeks. Should disequilibrium exist between the functional forces exerted on the dentition by the tongue and the cheek musculature, deviations in tooth alignment may occur. (Periodont.)

lip m. The muscles that perform the physiologic or functional activities of the lips. The primary muscles include the orbicularis oris, quadratus labii superiorus, risorius, buccinators, etc. If the tongue and the musculature of the lips do not exert equivalent forces against the teeth, movement of the teeth may occur. (Periodont.)

mimetic m. The facial muscles by which emotion and intelligence are expressed. The facial nerve provides neurologic control over the muscles of the face. Persons who assume a masklike face have greater difficulty in relating to other people and the community at large because the face and its appearance in modern as well as in older cultures have been imputed with many social and cultural values. Thus the mimetic property of the facial musculature expresses the highest form of muscle function. (Oral Physiol.)

musculoskeletal system (mŭs″kū-lō-skĕl′ĕ-tal) (see **system, musculoskeletal**)

mushbite An obsolete type of maxillomandibular record made by introducing a mass of soft wax into the patient's mouth and instructing the patient to bite into it to the desired degree. Not a generally accepted procedure. (Comp. Prosth.; Remov. Part. Prosth.) (see **record, maxillomandibular**)

mutant An individual showing a mutation. (Oral Radiol.)

mutation (mū-tā′shŭn) A departure from the parent type, as when an organism differs from its parents in one or more heritable characteristics; caused by genetic change. (Oral Radiol.)

  gene m. A sudden and permanent change in a gene. The term mutation is sometimes used in a broader sense to include chromosome aberrations. (Oral Radiol.)

  lethal m. A mutation leading to death of the offspring at any stage. (Oral Radiol.)

mutual Interchangeable; reciprocal; joint. (D. Juris.)

mycelium (mī-sē′lē-ŭm) The filamentous network of hyphae of a fungus. (Periodont.)

mydriatic (mĭd″rē-ăt′ĭk) A drug that dilates the pupil. (Anesth.)

myelin (mī′ĕ-lĭn) A fatlike substance forming a sheath around certain nerve fibers. It is associated with volitional nervous system fibers and is thought to be related to the capacity of nerve structures for rapid transmission of nerve impulses. The nerves associated with learned muscular activity, such as sitting, walking, talking, and chewing, are not completely myelinated at birth. For maximum speed and specificity of action associated with these learned functions, the myelination process of the peripheral nerves must be completed. The myelinated fibers lie both inside and outside the brain and spinal cord. (Oral Physiol.)

myeloma (mī″ĕ-lō′mah) A neoplasm characterized by cells normally found in the bone marrow. (Oral Diag.)

  multiple m. An invariably fatal malignant neoplasm of bone marrow cells. It appears as radiolucent lesions in bones, including the jaws. (Oral Diag.)

  — A primary malignant neoplasm of bone marrow characterized by proliferation of cells resembling plasma cells. Circumscribed radiolucencies are seen within the bones, and Bence Jones protein is usually found in the urine. (Oral Path.)

  plasma cell m. A malignant neoplasm characterized by plasma cells. Solitary lesions may appear as radiolucencies in the bone and are sometimes considered benign, although most authorities believe that even these lesions become multiple and terminate fatally. (Oral Diag.)

  solitary p. c. m. An incompletely understood monostotic neoplasm of bone that is histologically identical with multiple myeloma. Laboratory findings, positive in multiple myeloma, are usually negative in solitary plasma cell myeloma. Behavior of the myeloma, though usually benign, may be malignant. (Oral Path.)

myelophthisis (mī″ĕ-lō-thī′sĭs) A displacement of bone marrow by fibrous tissue, carcinoma, leukemia, etc. (Oral Med.)

mylohyoid region (see **region, mylohyoid**)

mylohyoid ridge, cantilevered A condition in which a major undercut occurs inferior to a broad mylohyoid ridge; creating a vertical groove into such an area often causes perforation of the medial cortical plate. (Oral Implant.)

myoblastoma (mī″ō-blăs-to′mah) A benign neoplasm characterized by large polyhedral cells resembling young muscle cells. Occurs most frequently in the tongue. (Oral Diag.)

— A benign tumor composed of granular eosinophilic cells reminiscent of primitive muscle cells. (Oral Path.)

  granular cell m. A benign soft tissue tumor of disputed origin. The tumor cells are large and have a granular eosinophilic cytoplasm and a small nucleus. (Oral Path.)

myodysfunction (mī″ō-dĭs-fŭngk′shŭn) Imbalance or disturbance of muscle function. (Orthodont.)

myofunction Normal muscle function. (Orthodont.)

myolipoma (mī″ō-lĭ-pō′mah) A myxoma containing fatty tissue. (Oral Path.)

myoma (mĭ-ō′mah) A neoplasm characterized by muscle cells. (Oral Diag.)

myopia (mī-ō′pē-ah) A form of defective vision due to excessive refractive power of the eye. In this condition, commonly called nearsightedness or shortsightedness, light rays coming from an object beyond a certain distance are focused in front of the retina. When a patient's vision is distorted, for either optical or neurologic reasons, the dentist is confronted with a difficult treatment experience because it is necessary to evaluate, for his clinical needs, the visual judgment of a patient. (Oral Physiol.)

myotomy (mī-ŏt′ō-mē) Cutting or resection of a muscle. (Oral Surg.)

myxedema (mĭk-sĕ-dē′mah) Generalized edema of the hands and face caused by thyroid deficiency. (Oral Diag.)

— A condition associated with hypothyroidism (primary myxedema) or hypopituitarism (secondary or pituitary myxedema). Characteristics include dry hair and skin; thickened skin of the lips; puffy eyelids; thinning of the eyebrows, especially the lateral half; slow, low-pitched, and hoarse speech; and slowness of thinking. (Oral Med.)

— A condition resulting from hypofunctional activity of the thyroid gland; characterized by anorexia, lethargy, fatigue, dryness of the skin, infraorbital edematous swelling, edematous macroglossia, etc. (Periodont.)

myxofibroma (mĭk″sō-fĭ-brō′mah) A benign neoplasm characterized by mucous and fibroblastic tissues. (Oral Diag.)

— A fibroma containing myxomatous tissue. (Oral Path.)

myxoma (mĭk-sō′mah) A benign neoplasm characterized by mucoid tissue. (Oral Diag.)

— A benign tumor composed of fibroblastic cells that have reverted to embryonic growth and produce a mucoid matrix containing widely dispersed stellate cells that have multipolar processes. (Oral Path.)

myxosarcoma (mĭk′sō-sar-kō′mah) A sarcoma containing myxomatous tissue. (Oral Path.)

N

name A word or combination of words by which a person, object, or idea or a group of persons, objects, or ideas is regularly known or designated.

generic n. A name that is usually descriptive of the substance. Strictly speaking, it is a a name used to designate a class relationship. Often used synonymously with nonproprietary name. (Oral Med.; Pharmacol.)

nonproprietary n. A drug name that is not restricted by a trademark. Nonproprietary names are now selected in the United States by the USAN Council. (Oral Med.; Pharmacol.)

official n. The title under which a drug is listed in *The United States Pharmacopeia* ·(U.S.P.) or *The National Formulary* (N.F.). (Oral Med.; Pharmacol.)

Nance analysis of arch length A method of determining if there is sufficient arch length to accommodate the permanent dentition. (Pedodont.)

nanometer (nm) A billionth of a meter (10^{-9} meter). This term is now preferred over millimicron. (D. Mat.)

narcoma Coma or stupor from narcotics. (Anesth.)

narcosis (nar-kō'sĭs) Drug-induced unconsciousness. (Oral Med.; Pharmacol.)

narcotic (nar-kŏt'ĭk) A drug, usually with strong analgesic action and an addiction potential, which may be synthesized or derived from natural sources. Especially one of the opium alkaloids. (Anesth.; Oral Med.; Pharmacol.)

narcotism (nar'kō-tĭzm) State of stupor induced by a narcotic. (Anesth.)

narcotize (nar'kō-tīz) To render unconscious by use of narcotics. (Anesth.)

nasal cavity (see **cavity, nasal**)

nasal septum (see **septum, nasal**)

nasality The quality of speech sounds when the nasal cavity is used as a resonator, especially when there is too much nasal resonance. (Cleft Palate)

nascent (nās'ĕnt) Literal meaning: recently born. Also, just released from chemical combination. (Oral Med.; Pharmacol.)

nasion (nā'zē-on) The point at which the nasofrontal suture is bisected by the midsagittal plane. (Comp. Prosth.; Remov. Part. Prosth.)

— The point at the root of the nose that is intersected by the median sagittal plane. The root of the nose corresponds to the nasofrontal suture, which is not necessarily the lowest point on its dorsum and which can usually be located with the finger. (Orthodont.)

Nasmyth's membrane (năs'mĭths) (see **cuticle, primary**)

nasoalveolar cyst (nā"zō-ăl-vē'ō-lar) An intraosseous cyst. A form of globulomaxillary cyst in which the epithelial inclusion is in the soft tissue fusion line. (Oral Diag.)

nasomandibular fixation (see **fixation, nasomandibular**)

national health plan Modification of the present method of delivering health care on a national scale, involving the professions, the consumers, and the government. (Pract. Man.)

Nealon's technique (see **technique, Nealon's**)

necessaries Things indispensable or useful for the sustenance of human life; e.g., food, shelter, clothing. (D. Juris.)

n. contracts of infants (minors) Necessaries are those things which are suitable to each individual child according to his circumstances. (D. Juris.)

neck of condyle (see **process, condyloid, neck of**)

necrosis (nē-krō'sĭs) Death of a cell or group of cells in contact with living tissue. (Oral Path.)

— Local death of cells due to loss of blood supply, bacterial toxins, physical and chemical agents, etc. (Periodont.)

caseous n. (kā'sē-ŭs) A change commonly associated with tuberculosis and characterized by death of tissue, resulting in a granular eosinophilic mass with loss of cell detail. (Oral Path.)

n. of epithelial attachment Death of cells comprising the epithelial attachment. It has been proposed that in a specific periodontitis produced by *Actinomyces*-like organisms, there is necrosis of the epithelial attachment, permitting a rapid apical shift of the base of the pocket. (Periodont.)

exanthematous n. An acute necrotizing process involving the gingivae, jawbones, and contiguous soft tissues. It is of unknown cause, affects primarily children, and resembles noma. It differs from noma, however, in that it has a slight odor, a tendency for self-limitation, a low mortality rate, and a normal leukocyte count. (Oral Med.) (see also **noma**)

gingival n. Death and degeneration of the cells and other structural elements of the gingivae; e.g., necrotizing ulcerative gingivitis. (Periodont.)

ischemic n. Death and disintegration of a tissue due to interference with its blood supply, thus depriving the tissues of an avenue of ingress of substances necessary for metabolic sustenance; e.g., a degenerative process occurring in portions of periodontal membrane in occlusal traumatism. (Periodont.)

periodontal membrane n. Necrosis of a portion of the periodontal membrane, usually due to traumatic injury; e.g., in occlusal traumatism. Much of this necrotic change is the result of ischemia. (Periodont.)

radiation n. Death of tissue caused by radiation. (Oral Radiol.)

needle A sharp metal shaft in a variety of forms for penetrating tissue; e.g., in carrying sutures or injecting solutions. (Oral Surg.)

Gillmore n. An instrument used in a penetration type of test for measuring the setting time of materials such as plaster or stone. A ¼-pound needle is used for determining the initial set, and a 1-pound needle is used for defining the final set. (D. Mat.)

n. holder A forceps used to hold and pass the needle through the tissue while suturing with a suture forceps. (Oral Surg.)

n. point tracer (see **tracer, needle point**)

Vicat n. An instrument used for measuring setting time by means of a penetration test. (D. Mat.)

neglect Failure to do something that one is bound to do; lack of due care. (D. Juris.)

negligence Failure to observe, for the protection of another person, that degree of care and vigilance which the circumstances demand, whereby such other person suffers injury. (D. Juris.)

contributory n. Negligence by an injured party that combines as a proximate cause with the negligence of the injurer in producing the injury. May bar recovery or mitigate damages. (D. Juris.)

imputed n. That which is not directly attributable to the person himself but which is the negligence of a person employed by or in association with him and with whose fault he is chargeable; e.g., a dental assistant or other dental employee. (D. Juris.)

neighborhood An adjoining or surrounding district; an immediate vicinity. (D. Juris.)

Nembutal Proprietary name for pentobarbital sodium. (Pharmacol.)

neomycin (nē″ō-mī′sǐn) An antibiotic secured from cultures of *Streptomyces fradiae*. In its sulfate form, it is used for preoperative intestinal sterilization; as a constituent of topically applied ointments, solutions, troches, etc., for its antibacterial action. Prolonged ingestion of neomycin has been associated with the production of a malabsorptive syndrome characterized by azotorrhea, steatorrhea, etc. (Periodont.)

neoplasia (nē″ō-plā′zē-ah) The disease process responsible for neoplasm formation. (Oral Path.)

neoplasm (tumor) An autonomous new growth. (Oral Diag.)
— An abnormal mass of tissue, the growth of which exceeds and is uncoordinated with that of the normal tissues. It persists in the same excessive manner after cessation of the stimuli that evoked the change. Benign and malignant forms are recognized. (Oral Path.) (see also **tumor**)

gingival n. A new and abnormal growth (tumor) on the gingival tissue; e.g., fibroma. Produces localized gingival enlargement subject to irritation by local agents, with subsequent secondary inflammatory change. (Periodont.)

nerve(s) A cordlike structure that conveys impulses between a part of the central nervous system and some part of the body, and that consists of an outer connective tissue sheath and bundles of nerve fibers. (Oral Physiol.)

abducent n. (VI) Sixth cranial nerve; a small, completely motor nerve arising in the pons, supplying the lateral rectus muscle of the eye. (Oral Physiol.)

accessory n. (see **nerve, spinal accessory**)

acoustic n. (VIII) Eighth cranial n.; the vestibulocochlear n.; a sensory nerve consisting of a vestibular position and an auditory (or cochlear) portion. (Oral Physiol.)

branchial n. One of five cranial nerves that supply the derivatives of the branchial arches: trigeminal (V), facial (VII), glossopharyngeal (IX), vagus (X), and spinal accessory (XI). Each branchial nerve may have a variety of functions, including visceral motor and visceral and somatic sensory. (Oral Physiol.)

b. n., functional components The five fiber groups associated with the branchial nerves. Not all of the fiber groups accompany each nerve. The components are the special visceral motor, the general visceral motor, the general visceral sensory, the special visceral sensory, and the general somatic sensory. In some nerves, such as the trigeminal nerve, the general somatic sensory component predominates, whereas in the vagus nerve, the visceral components dominate the fiber groups. (Oral Physiol.)

b. n., f. c., general somatic sensory The nerve fibers that are associated with the branchial nerves and that receive the exteroceptive and proprioceptive impulses from the skin, mucous membrane, and striated musculature of the head, neck and face regions. The trigeminal nerve is the major carrier of these fiber components. The exteroceptive fibers of the trigeminal nerve have their origin in the semilunar ganglion. Pain and temperature are mediated almost exclusively by the spinal tract nucleus of the trigeminal nerve, and tactile sensibility is mediated in part by the main sensory nucleus and in part by the spinal tract nucleus of the trigeminal nerve. The proprioceptive somatic nuclei of the branchial nerves innervate the muscles of mastication. (Oral Physiol.)

b. n., f. c., general visceral motor The nerve fibers that are associated with the branchial nerves and that supply the cardiac and smooth muscles and the glandular tissues of the viscera. The nuclei of this component extend through the medulla and part of the pons. The nerve fibers are small and myelinated and end in autonomic nerve ganglia, where they synapse with other cells that terminate in the effector organs. The nerves that bear this component are the vagus (X), glossopharyngeal (IX), facial (VII), and oculomotor (III). All the nuclei of the visceral motor nerve components of the cranial nerves lie within the medulla, pons, and midbrain. The fibers are distributed among the motor roots of the cranial nerves as they leave the brain. This distribution is similar to that of the motor components of the cerebrospinal nerves, which have their nuclei in the ventral horn of the spinal cord. (Oral Physiol.)

b. n., f. c., general visceral sensory One

of two groups of visceral sensory fibers of the branchial nerves. Both groups—the general and the special visceral sensory fibers—are contained in the facial, glossopharyngeal, and vagus nerves. The general visceral sensory fibers mediate the general sensory impulses from the posterior part of the tongue, pharynx, larynx, and esophagus, and thoracic and abdominal viscera. These afferent fibers provide all the exteroceptive sensory impulses for the structures of the viscera, their smooth muscles, glands, and blood vessels. They also provide information principally for the autonomic nervous system. (Oral Physiol.)

b. n., f. c., special visceral motor The fiber group of the branchial nerves that serves the muscle groups derived from the branchial gill arches. These are the trigeminal nerve (V), which supplies the masticatory muscles from the first branchial arch; the facial nerve (VII), which supplies the muscles from the second branchial arch, chiefly the muscles of facial expression; the glossopharyngeal nerve (IX), which supplies the muscles derived from the third branchial arch, the stylopharyngeus muscle, and the circular and other longitudinal striated muscles of the upper portion of the pharynx; the vagus nerve (X), which supplies the muscles derived from the posterior branchial arches and the muscles of the larynx; the spinal accessory nerve (XI), which is included in the branchial nerve group, but about which there is some doubt as to whether it is of branchial or somatic origin. It supplies the sternocleidomastoid muscle and the upper part of the trapezius muscle. (Oral Physiol.)

b. n., f. c., special visceral sensory The nerve fibers that mediate the sense of taste and serve the taste buds in the tongue. The buds can differentiate between sensations of salt, sweet, bitter, and sour. There are specific papillae that respond only to specific taste experiences. The buds are distributed so that acid response is readily elicited on the lateral margins of the tongue, whereas salt is perceived not only at the margins but also on the dorsum of the tongue. (Oral Physiol.)

chiasma, optic n. The decussation, or crossing, of optic nerve fibers from the medial side of the retina on one side to the opposite side of the brain. (Oral Physiol.)

chorda tympani n. A parasympathetic and special sensory branch of the facial nerve supplying the submandibular and sublingual glands and the anterior two thirds of the tongue (taste). (Oral Physiol.)

cochlear n. One of the two major branches of the eighth cranial nerve; a special sensory nerve for the sense of hearing that transmits impulses from the organ of Corti to the brain. (Oral Physiol.)

c. n. involvement, symptoms Most frequently, tinnitus and deafness associated with the peripheral nerve disorders. The symptoms associated with central brain involvement of the cochlear nerve are sensory aphasias associated with cerebrovascular accidents, the auditory hallucinations associated with psychosis and drug addiction, and the auditory auras associated with epileptic seizures. There are also some unusual reactions to commonly used pharmacologic agents, such as salicylates, quinine, and cinchophen, which affect the cochlear nerve. (Oral Physiol.)

cranial n. Any one of twelve paired nerves, classified in three sets, arising directly in the brain and supplying various tissues of the head and neck. The cranial nerves are the *special somatic sensory nerves:* olfactory (I), optic (II), and acoustic (VIII); the *somatic motor nerves:* oculomotor (III), trochlear (IV), abducent (VI), and hypoglossal (XII); and the *branchial nerves:* trigeminal (V), facial (VII), glossopharyngeal (IX), vagus (X), and spinal accessory (XI). (Oral Physiol.)

origin of the special sensory c. n. The ganglia of the olfactory, optic, and acoustic nerves, which are located in the forebrain, midbrain, and hindbrain, respectively. The olfactory and optic nerves are extensions of the brain structure to the external world. The ganglion of the acoustic nerve are associated with the inner ear. (Oral Physiol.)

facial n. (VII) Seventh cranial nerve; a mixed nerve supplying motor fibers to the facial muscles, the stapedius, and posterior body of the digastricus; sensory fibers from the taste buds in the anterior two thirds of the

tongue (via the chorda tympani); and general visceral autonomic fibers for submaxillary and sublingual salivary glands. (Oral Physiol.)

f. n. disorders Usually, facial paralysis, since the facial nerve is predominantly a motor nerve. Facial paralysis may result from lesions involving (1) tumor of the brainstem or vascular accidents, (2) skull fractures or tumors involving the internal auditory meatus, which usually also involves hearing disorders, (3) injury to the nerve in the facial canal just before it emerges from the cranial skeleton, also involved in fracture and in otitis media when the nerve is inflamed (e.g., in Bell's palsy), and (4) injury to the nerve or its branches after emergence, such as injury resulting from trauma or surgery. The consequence of the paralysis is that muscle imbalances, if prolonged, may cause serious periodontal involvement and occlusal disharmonies. (Oral Physiol.)

f. n. d., symptoms associated with Characteristics evident in lesions outside the stylomastoid foramen: the angle of the mouth droops and may be drawn to one side, there is an inability to whistle effectively, food collects between the teeth and gingivae, there is an inability to wink or to wrinkle the forehead, and there is a loss of sensation deep in the facial muscles. When the lesion is in the facial canal or progressively closer to the nucleus of the facial nerve in the pons, the following symptoms appear, in addition to those just listed: loss of taste at the anterior two thirds of tongue and reduced salivation when the chorda tympani is involved; hyperacusia, a disorder in which there is an increased sense of hearing, with involvement of the nerve to the stapedius; acute pain in the ear; and finally, deafness from involvement of the acoustic nerve. (Oral Physiol.)

f. n. function The activity of the facial nerve, which is of extreme importance in the practice of dentistry. This nerve mediates the activity of taste sense, which is important to salivary function for the control of the oral flora and fauna. It is also an important factor in denture retention and stability and mediates the activity of the lubricating mechanisms so that the tongue and lips may move over each other with extreme facility for speech and for the management of the food bolus in mastication and swallowing. In addition, the facial musculature, particularly the lips and buccinator muscles, must oppose the tongue activity in order to maintain the occlusal arch in a stable relationship. A further consideration is the role of the facial nerve in the maintenance of good muscle tone of the facial musculature to provide the esthetic values of the human face. (Oral Physiol.)

glossopharyngeal n. (IX) Ninth cranial nerve; a mixed motor and sensory nerve arising in the medulla and supplying motor efferents to stylopharyngeal muscles and other pharyngeal muscles; visceral motor efferents via the otic ganglion for the parotid gland; special visceral afferents from the taste buds in the posterior one third of tongue; and general sensory afferents from the pharynx and posterior aspects of the oral cavity. (Oral Physiol.)

hypoglossal n. (XII) Twelfth cranial nerve; a motor nerve that arises in the medulla and supplies extrinsic and intrinsic muscles of the tongue. (Oral Physiol.)

inferior alveolar n. A motor and general sensory branch of the mandibular nerve, with mylohyoid, inferior dental, mental, and inferior gingival branches. (Oral Physiol.)

intermediate n. Parasympathetic and special sensory division of the facial nerve, with chorda tympani and greater petrosal branches. (Oral Physiol.)

lingual n. A general sensory branch of the mandibular nerve having sublingual and lingual branches and connections with the hypoglossal nerve and chorda tympani. (Oral Physiol.)

mandibular n. Mandibular division of the trigeminal nerve, arising in the trigeminal ganglion and supplying general sensory and motor fibers via mesenteric, pterygoid, buccal, auriculotemporal, deep temporal, lingual, inferior alveolar, and meningeal branches. (Oral Physiol.)

maxillary n. Maxillary division of the trigeminal nerve arising in the trigeminal ganglion and supplying general sensory fibers via zygomatic, posterosuperior alveolar, infraorbital, pterygopalatine, and nasopalatine branches. (Oral Physiol.)

oculomotor n. (III) Third cranial nerve; primarily a motor nerve arising from the midbrain and supplying motor efferents to the superior rectus, medial rectus, inferior rectus, and inferior oblique eye muscles, as well as autonomic fibers via the ciliary ganglion to the ciliary body and the iris. (Oral Physiol.)

olfactory n. (I) First cranial nerve; a special sensory nerve for the sense of smell. (Oral Physiol.)

ophthalmic n. Ophthalmic division of the trigeminal nerve, arising in the trigeminal ganglion and supplying general sensory fibers via the frontal, lacrimal, and nasociliary branches. (Oral Physiol.)

optic n. (II) Second cranial nerve; a special sensory nerve for vision passing from the retina of the eye to the optic chiasma. (Oral Physiol.)

somatic motor n. (cranial) The somatic motor nerves—the oculomotor (III), the trochlear (IV), the abducent (VI), and the hypoglossal (XII)—largely comparable to the ventral motor roots of the spinal nerves. They are composed almost entirely of somatic motor fibers that emerge ventrally from the brainstem. Their arrangement is closely correlated to the distribution of the myotomes in the head region. The oculomotor, the trochlear, and the abducent nerves, which supply the eye musculature, have the same myotomic origin and arrangement as the somatic muscles of the trunk and extremities. (Oral Physiol.)

special somatic sensory n. The structural arrangements from typical sensory nerves by which the three main sense organs—nose, eye, and ear—are innervated. The sensory nerves are the olfactory nerve (I), optic nerve (II), and acoustic nerve (VIII). (Oral Physiol.)

spinal n. Any one of 31 pairs of mixed peripheral nerves (8 cervical, 12 thoracic, 5 lumbar, 5 sacral, and 1 coccygeal), being connected segmentally with the spinal cord the dorsal sensory trunk and the ventral motor root. (Oral Physiol.)

spinal accessory n. (XI) Eleventh cranial nerve; a motor nerve that derives its origin in part from the medulla and in part from the cervical spinal cord. Its internal ramus joins with the vagus nerve to supply some of the muscles of the larynx. Its external ramus joins with the spinal nerves to supply the sternocleidomastoid and trapezius muscles. The dentist's principal interest in the spinal accessory nerve is its relation to head posture, which is so important in maintaining stable occlusal relationships of vertical dimension and centric relation. (Oral Physiol.)

s. a. n., disorders and symptoms Atrophy of the sternocleidomastoid muscle, inability to rotate the head from side to side, inability to shrug the affected shoulder, and depression of the shoulder due to atrophy of the trapezius muscle. (Oral Physiol.)

tensor tympani n. A small motor branch of the mandibular nerve. (Oral Physiol.)

trigeminal n. (V) Fifth cranial nerve; a mixed motor and sensory nerve connected with the pons through three roots (motor, proprioceptive, and large sensory), the latter root expanding into the trigeminal ganglion, from which arise the ophthalmic, masseteric and mandibular divisions. (Oral Physiol.)

t. n., disorders and symptoms Pain; loss of sensation; dissociation of senses; paresthesia; paralysis of the muscles of mastication; loss of jaw jerk, sneeze, and eye reflexes; hearing loss from paralysis of the tensor tympani; trismus from rabies, tetanus, epilepsy, and hysteria; occusal imbalances associated with temporomandibular joint syndrome; trophic and secretory disturbances of the nose with anosmia (loss of smell); and ulcerations on the face and mucous membranes. Symptoms vary, depending on whether the lesion affects the nerve ending, the nerve fiber, the trigeminal ganglion, the medulla, the pons, the midbrain, or the cerebrum. The most common disorders are trigeminal neuralgia, which is excruciatingly painful and frequently accompanied by trigger zones and flushing of the face; the effects of tumor or cerebrovascular accident in the brain or along the path of the nerve; and the degenerative changes in the peripheral vascular circulation that cause a heightened irritability of the nerve endings to the mucous membranes of the mouth. Of most significance to the dentist are the exteroceptive and proprioceptive mechanisms of the trigeminal nerve in maintaining occlusal stability in function and in treatment procedures. (Oral Physiol.)

trochlear n. (IV) Fourth cranial nerve; a small motor nerve arising ventrally in the midbrain and supplying the inferior oblique muscle of the eye. (Oral Physiol.)

vagus n. (X) Tenth cranial nerve; a mixed parasympathetic, visceral, afferent, motor, and general sensory nerve with laryngeal, pharyngeal, bronchial, esophageal, gastric, and many other branches. (Oral Physiol.)

v. n., function Principally, the activity of the respiratory, the deglutitive, and the cardiovascular mechanisms. These nerves control the respiratory mechanisms by maintaining the patency of the airway, and they control the deglutitive mechanisms by maintainng a high degree of synchronous and reciprocal muscle activity with the respiratory mechanism, since both the deglutitive and the respiratory functions use a common passage on the oropharynx. The interplay between these two functions requires intricate multivalve action by the soft palate, the tongue, the pharyngeal walls, the oropharynx, and the esophageal-laryngeal muscles. (Oral Physiol.)

v. n., disorders and symptoms Three groups of disorders: (1) motor disorders, in which there are malfunctions of speech (e.g., dysphonia or aphonia), dysphagia, regurgitation of fluids, and pharyngeal, esophageal, and laryngeal spasms, and paralysis of the soft palate; (2) sensory disturbances, in which there are pain or paresthesia of the lower pharynx and larynx, cough and respiratory irregularities, or salivary increments or decrements; and (3) cardiac and gastric disorders. (Oral Physiol.)

vestibular n. (VIII) One of the two major branches of the eighth cranial nerve; a special sensory nerve for the sense of balance and the transmission of space-orientation impulses from the semicircular canals to the brain. (Oral Physiol.)

v. n., disorders and symptoms Most frequently, vertigo (disturbance of equilibrium) and disorientation in space accompanied by giddiness. Vertigo is the result of reflexes of motion; sickness in the air and on the sea; prolonged, bizarre, strained, or abnormal head posture; tumors; degenerative disease; etc. Other symptoms of vestibular nerve disorders are nystagmus (a side-to-side movement of the eyeballs), nausea, vomiting, low blood pressure, and tachycardia. (Oral Physiol.)

vestibulocochlear n. (VII) Seventh cranial nerve; acoustic nerve; a sensory nerve consisting of a vestibular portion and an auditory, or cochlear, portion. (Oral Physiol.)

net Devoid of anything extraneous; free from

all deductions, such as charges, expenses, taxes; remaining after expenses. (D. Juris.)

neuralgia (nū-răl'jē-ah) Pain associated with a nerve or nerves; e.g., trigeminal neuralgia and glossopharyngeal neuralgia. (Oral Diag.)

— Paroxysmal pain occurring in, or radiating along, nerve pathways that do not have apparent structural changes. (Oral Med.; Oral Surg.)

auriculotemporal n. (auriculotemporal causalgia n.) Sharp pain in the distribution of the auriculotemporal nerve. (Oral Surg.)

buccal n. A throbbing, burning, and boring type of pain involving the cheeks, lips, gingivae, nose, and jaws. It may last for a few minutes or as long as several days. No trigger zones are present, although it may be initiated by chewing or thermal changes. (Oral Med.)

causalgia n. Neuralgia characterized by an intense, diffuse burning sensation in a limited area. (Oral Surg.)

auriculotemporal c. n. (see **neuralgia, auriculotemporal**)

facial n. (see **neuralgia, trigeminal**)

atypical f. n. (cluster headache, lower-half headache, sphenopalatine n.) Severe unilateral pain behind the eye that spreads to the temple and behind the ear. It lasts from 30 minutes to 3 hours and occurs once to several times a day and in cycles or clusters lasting several weeks. The clusters may be separated by several months or years. No trigger zones exist. (Oral Med.)

glossopharyngeal n. Pain in the nerves of the tongue, pharynx, ear, and neck precipitated by swallowing, sneezing, coughing, talking, or blowing the nose. (Oral Diag.)

— Paroxysmal pain comparable to that of trigeminal neuralgia. There may be a trigger area in the throat or ear. The distribution of pain in the anterior tonsillar pillar and the upper area of the throat, the base of the tongue, and the soft palate. (Oral Surg.)

Sluder's n. Irritation of the sphenopalatine ganglion. Diffuse pain may affect the eye, the root of the nose, the teeth, and the ear. Also, slight anesthesia and paralysis of the soft palate and palatine arch on the affected side may be present. (Oral Surg.)

sphenopalatine n. (see **neuralgia, facial, atypical**)

trifacial n. (see **neuralgia, trigeminal**)

trigeminal n. (facial n., tic douloureux, trifacial n.) Inflammation of the trigeminal nerve with very severe paroxysms of pain elicited by stimulating a specific trigger point or points. (Oral Diag.)

— Excruciating paroxysmal, stabbing, searing, or lancinating pain usually occurring on the right side of the face and involving the distribution of the three divisions of the trigeminal nerve. It may last for a few seconds, to be followed by additional episodes either spontaneously or from stimulation of trigger zones. Intervals between attacks vary from a few hours to months or years. (Oral Med.)

— Neuralgia due to involvement of the trigeminal ganglion and the root and branches of the trigeminal nerve; marked by pain along the course of the trigeminal nerve. On the face, a trigger zone, which is sensitive to touch, is associated with the initiation of the pain. (Oral Path.)

— Neuralgia characterized by paroxysmal pain along the distribution of any branch of the fifth cranial nerve. Lancinating, sharp, sudden, stabbing pain is associated with trigeminal neuralgia, often causing a characteristic muscle spasm. Characteristically evoked by stimulation of a trigger site. (Oral Surg.)

neurasthenia (nū-răs-thē'nē-ah) A neurotic reaction characterized by chronic physical fatigue, listlessness, mental sluggishness, and often phobias. (Oral Med.)

neurectomy (nū-rĕk'tō-mē) Surgical excision of a nerve or the more traumatic tearing away of nervous tissue from its anatomic position. (Oral Surg.)

neurilemma (nū-rĭ-lĕm'ah) **(nucleated sheath, primitive sheath, sheath of Schwann)** The thin membranous outer covering surrounding the myelin sheath of a medullated nerve fiber or the axis cylinder of a nonmedullated nerve fiber. It is associated with the booster mechanisms for the rapid transmission of impulses. (Oral Physiol.)

neurilemoma (nū'rĭ-lĕ-mō'mah) **(neurinoma, perineural fibroblastoma, schwannoma)** A neoplasm characterized by Schwann cells of the neurilemma. (Oral Diag.)

— A benign tumor of the neurilemma of disputed origin (Schwann cells vs. fibroblasts). May occur in soft tissue and bone. Composed of characteristic Antoni type A and Antoni type B tissue and contains Verocay bodies. A malignant form occurs. (Oral Path.) (see also **body, Verocay; tissue, Antoni type A; tissue, Antoni type B**)

neurinoma (nū-rĭ-nō′mah) (see **neurilemoma**)

neuritis (nū-rī′tĭs) Inflammation of a nerve. The condition is attended by pain and tenderness over the nerves, anesthesia, disturbance of sensation, paralysis, wasting, and disappearance of reflexes. (Oral Diag.; Oral Path.; Oral Surg.)

endemic multiple n. (see **beriberi**)

neuroblastoma (nū″rō-blăs-tō′mah) A malignant neoplasm characterized by proliferating nerve cells. (Oral Diag.)

neurofibroma (nū″rō-fi-brō′mah) (**neurogenic fibroma, perineural fibroblastoma**) A benign neoplasm characterized by the various cells of a peripheral nerve (axon cylinders, Schwann cells, fibroblasts). (Oral Diag.) (see also **neurilemoma**)

— Benign tumor of nerve sheath origin; it is not encapsulated. Also may be seen in multiple neurofibromatosis (von Recklinghausen's disease). (Oral Path.)

— A connective tissue tumor of the nerve fiber fasciculi. Formed by the proliferation of the perineurium and endoneurium. (Periodont.)

neurofibromatosis (nū″rō-fi″brō-mah-tō′sĭs) (**molluscum fibrosum, multiple neuroma, von Recklinghausen's disease of skin**) A disease characterized by multiple neurofibromas that are most frequently seen on the skin but that may involve the oral mucosa. (Oral Diag.)

— An inherited disease characterized by multiple neurofibromas and brownish coffee-colored spots (café-au-lait spots) on the skin. (Oral Med.)

— A hereditary disease characterized by multiple neurofibromas of the peripheral and cranial nerves and associated with skin pigmentation and bone lesions. (Oral Path.)

neuroma (nū-rō′mah) Technically, a benign neoplasm of nerve cells. As used in oral disease, the term usually refers to a traumatic neuroma, which is not a true tumor but an overgrowth of nerves associated with injury. The mental foramina and extraction scars are possible oral sites of this painful lesion. (Oral Diag.; Oral Path.)

amputation n. (see **neuroma, traumatic**)

multiple n. (see **neurofibromatosis**)

traumatic n. (**amputation n.**) Hyperplasia of nerve fibers and their supporting tissues in an exuberant attempt at repair following damage to, or the severing of, a nerve. (Oral Path.)

neuromuscular action (see **action, neuromuscular**)

neuron (nū′ron) Nerve cell; the basic structural unit of the nervous system. There is a wide variation in the shape of nerve cells, but they all have the same basic structures: cell body, protoplasmic processes, axons, and dendrites. The axon, generally only one to a cell, conducts stimuli away from the cell body. Some axons may extend as long as 3 feet from the cell body, and they terminate in a multitude of fine branches in the tissues they serve. Multiple dendrites are attached to the cell body. They are shorter than the axons and terminate closer to the cell body in dense arborization. They have a spiny appearance and form an interlacing arborization with adjacent dendrites and axon termination. They transmit stimuli to the cell body. The neuron is the only body cell whose principal function is the conduction of impulses. The neuron has contact with other neurons only through synaptic contacts, which are highly specialized for the transmission of impulses. Impulses are thus conducted along chains formed from cell units. Neurons cannot regenerate when the cell body is destroyed; however, cell processes such as axons and dendrites often can regenerate. (Oral Physiol.)

neurosis (nū-rō′sĭs) A person's abnormal or altered reaction to his environment; e.g., anxiety, hysteria, and phobias. (Oral Diag.)

— A functional disorder in which there is no gross personality disorganization but in which there is an inability to cope effectively with routine frustrations, anxieties, and other daily problems. (Oral Med.)

habit n. A disorder of the psyche marked by the impulse toward some abnormal or absurd act that may or may not be detrimental to the structures of the body involved in performance of the action; e.g., bruxism may or may not induce traumatic lesions of the attachment apparatus of the teeth. (Periodont.)

occlusal n. An impulsive habit, often due to emotional conflicts, that involves afunctional movements of the mandibular teeth against the maxillary teeth; often results in traumatic lesions of the teeth and their attachment apparatus. (Periodont.)

neurostomatosis (nū″rō-stō″mah-tō′sĭs) An oral condition associated with psychosomatic or other psychologic factors; e.g., lichen planus and benign migratory glossitis may be considered as types of neurostomatoses. (Oral Diag.)

neurosyphilis, paretic (nū″rō-sĭf′ĭ-lĭs) (see **paresis**)

neurotomy (nū-rot′ō-mē) The severance of a nerve process. (Oral Surg.)

neutral A solution that has a pH of 7. Equal numbers of hydrogen and hydroxyl ions are formed on dissociation. (Anesth.)

n. zone (see **zone, neutral**)

neutralization The reaction of an acid with a base. (Oral Med.; Pharmacol.)

neutroclusion Normal anteroposterior relationship of the lower jaw to the upper jaw. (Orthodont.)

complex n. Neutroclusion that involves facial features and complicated treatment. (Orthodont.)

simple n. Neutroclusion that does not involve facial features or complicated treatment. (Orthodont.)

neutron (nū′tron) An elementary particle with approximately the mass of a hydrogen atom but without any electrical charge; one of the constituents of the atomic nucleus. (Oral Radiol.)

n. ray (see **ray, neutron**)

neutropenia (nū″trō-pē′nē-ah) Relative or absolute decrease in the normal number of neutrophils in the circulating blood. Various limits are given; e.g., absolute neutropenia may be said to exist when the total is less than 1700 cells/mm³ regardless of the percentage; whereas relative neutropenia may be said to exist when the total percentage of neutrophils is less than 38% and the total number is not less than 1500/mm³. May be associated with viral infections, pernicious anemia, sprue, aplastic anemia, bone marrow, neoplasms, chronic intoxication with drugs and heavy metals, malnutrition, and non-pyogenic and overwhelming infections. (Oral Diag.; Oral Med.)

cyclic n. A condition in which there is a depression in the number of circulating white cells, especially the neutrophils, at an interval of about 21 days. The neutropenia lasts for approximately 10 days, during which time gingival inflammation and aphthous ulcer occur. (Periodont.)

neutrophilia (nū″trō-fil′ē-ah) Absolute or relative increase in the normal number of neutrophils in the circulating blood. Various limits are given; e.g., an absolute neutrophilia may be said to exist, regardless of percentage, if the total number of neutrophils exceeds 7000/mm³; whereas a relative neutrophilia may be said to exist if the percentage of neutrophils is greater than 70% and the total number of neutrophils less than 7000/mm³.

May be associated with acute infections, chronic granulocytic leukemia, erythemia, therapy with ACTH or cortisone, uremia, ketosis, hemolysis, drug or heavy metal intoxication, or malignancy, or it may follow severe hemorrhage. (Oral Med.)

nevus (nē′vŭs) A circumscribed new growth of congenital origin that may be vascular (due to hypertrophy of blood or lymph vessels) or nonvascular (with epidermal and connective tissue predominating). (Oral Path.)

blue n. A benign neoplasm characterized by heavily pigmented spindle cells deep in the corium; appears clinically as a dark mole. (Oral Diag.)

— A congenital malformation seen on the skin and occasionally on the oral mucosa; consists of melanin-containing nevus cells located in the connective tissue below the basement membrane. (Oral Path.)

cellular pigmented n. A nevus composed of melanin-producing "nevus" cells. (Oral Path.)

compound n. A nevus in which the melanin-producing "nevus" cells are found in the epidermis and dermis. The intradermal nevus plus the junctional nevus. (Oral Path.)

intradermal n. A nevus in which the melanin-producing "nevus" cells are found only in the dermis. (Oral Path.)

junctional n. A nevus in which the melanin-producing "nevus" cells are found within the epidermis at the junction with the dermis. (Oral Path.)

pigmented n. A dark-colored, benign neoplasm characterized by nevus cells. Junctional, intradermal, and compound types are recognized. Melanomas (malignant neoplasms) may develop from the junctional or compound nevi. (Oral Diag.)

n. spongiosus albus mucosa (**white folded gingivostomatitis, white sponge n.**) An inherited disease of the oral mucosa characterized by generalized white mucosal surfaces with a spongelike appearance. (Oral Diag.)

— A hereditary condition characterized by a white, thickened, soft mucosa. Histologically, it shows acanthosis and a washed-out appearance of the epithelium. (Oral Path.)

Newton's law, clinical application (see **law, Newton's, clinical application**)

Ney surveyor (see **surveyor, Ney**)

N.F. *The National Formulary.* (Oral Med.; Pharmacol.)

niacin (nī'ah-sĭn) (see **acid, nicotinic**)

nib The part of a condensing instrument corresponding to the blade of a cutting instrument. The end of the nib is called the face of the condenser. (Oper. Dent.)

nickel-chromium alloy (see **alloy, nickel-chromium**)

nicotinic (nĭk"ō-tĭn'ĭk) Pertaining to an agent that mimics the effects of nicotine, especially at myoneural junctions in skeletal muscle. (Anesth.)

Niemann-Pick disease (nē'măn pĭk) (see **disease, Niemann-Pick**)

night-grinding (see **bruxism**)

night guard (see **guard, night**)

Nikolsky's sign (nĭ-kol'skēz) (see **sign, Nikolsky's**)

nippers Small rongeurs capable of excising small sections of gingiva and bone as well, if necessary. (Periodont.)

nitrogen monoxide (see **nitrous oxide**)

nitrogen monoxidum (see **nitrous oxide**)

nitrogen, nonprotein (see **nonprotein nitrogen**)

nitromersol, tincture (nĭ-trō-mer'sol) A solution used in 1:200 strength as a topically applied antiseptic to temporarily minimize the bacterial count on an area of tissue. (Periodont.)

nitrous oxide (**N₂O, laughing gas, nitrogen monoxide, nitrogen monoxidum**) A gas with a sweet odor and taste; used as an analgesic and anesthetic agent, in combination with oxygen, for the performance of minor operations. It is sometimes called laughing gas because it may excite a hilarious delirium preceding insensibility. (Anesth.; Periodont.)

noble An archaic term referring to inert gases and previous metals. (D. Mat.)

n. metal (see **metal, noble**)

nocardiosis (nō-kar-dē-ō'sĭs) Any of the pathologic entities that may follow infection with the bacterium *Nocardia*. (Oral Diag.)

node(s) (nōd) A swelling or protuberance.

brown n. of hyperparathyroidism A central giant cell lesion of the bone seen in hyperparathyroidism. Its microscopic appearance is similar to giant cell reparative granuloma and giant cell tumor. (Oral Path.)

n. of Ranvier Gaps that are distributed at regularly spaced intervals along a myelinated nerve fiber. The intervals are 1 mm or more in length and function essentially as relay stations to facilitate the passage of an impulse. (Oral Physiol.)

nodule, pulp (nod'ūl) (see **denticle**)

nodules, Bohn's (**Epstein's pearls**) Multiple white ricelike lesions of the mucous membrane; seen in newborn infants. Microscopically each lesion shows a keratin-filled cyst that lies close to the mucosal surface. It disappears spontaneously in 2 to 3 months. (Oral Path.)

noma (nō'mah) A progressive necrotizing process originating in the cheek, with secondary involvement of the gingiva and jawbone. It occurs primarily in debilitated children, in which the mortality rate is high. There is a strong, foul odor present, marked surrounding edema, absence of a specific erythematous halo, marked changes in the white blood cell count, and high temperature. (Oral Med.) (see also **necrosis, exanthematous; stomatitis, gangrenous**)

nomenclature (nō"měn-klā'tūr) The formally adopted terminology of a science, art, or discipline; the system of names or terms used in a particular branch of science. (Oper. Dent.)

non rep. (**non repetatur**) Abbreviation of Latin term; placed on prescriptions that are not to be refilled. (Oral Med.; Pharmacol.)

noncohesive Lacking the property of sticking together, or cohering. (Oper. Dent.)

nonfeasance (non-fē'zěnz) Failure of a person to do some act that he ought to do. (D. Juris.)

nonocclusion A situation in which the tooth or teeth in one arch fail to make contact with tooth or teeth of the other arch. (Orthodont.)

nonprotein nitrogen (**NPN**) The nitrogen of whole blood or serum exclusive of that of the proteins. The concentration of nonprotein nitrogen is a gross measure of renal function. The upper limit of normal is 35 mg/100 ml. (Oral Med.)

nonsuit Failure on the part of a plaintiff to continue the prosecution of his suit; abandonment of a suit. (D. Juris.)

nor- Prefix that indicates lack of a methyl group. (Oral Med.; Pharmacol.)

norepinephrine (nor"ĕp-ĭ-něf'rĭn) The neurohormonal transmitter for neuroeffector junction of adrenergic nerve fibers. Its official drug name in the United States is levarterenol. (Oral Med.; Pharmacol.) (see also **levarterenol**)

norm A structural unit representative of the human species as a whole. (Orthodont.)

normality A reference solution in which the concentration is stated with regard to the number of gram equivalent weights present per liter of solution (D. Mat.)

normoblast A nucleated red blood cell found in

the peripheral bloodstream in severe pernicious anemia and in some leukemias. (Oral Diag.)

nosebleed (see **epistaxis**)

notch An indentation.

buccal n. The notch in the flange of a denture that accommodates the buccal frenum. Buccal notches may be formed on either or both sides of either or both dentures, depending on the size and shape of the buccal frenum in each location. (Comp. Prosth.)

hamular n. (see **notch, pterygomaxillary**)

labial n. The notch in the labial flange of an upper or lower denture that accommodates the labial frenum. (Comp. Prosth.)

mandibular n. A depression of the inferior border of the mandible anterior to the attachments of the masseter muscle where the external facial vessels cross the lower border of the mandible. This landmark may be accentuated by arrested condylar growth and developmental disturbances of the mandible. (Oral Surg.)

pterygomaxillary n. (**hamular n.**) The notch or fissure formed at the junction of the maxilla and the hamular, or pterygoid, process of the sphenoid bone. (Comp. Prosth.; Remov. Part. Prosth.)

sigmoid n. The concavity on the superior surface of the ramus of the mandible, lying between the coronoid and condyloid processes. (Periodont.)

note, promissory A written promise to pay to another, at a specified time, a stated amount of money, or other articles of value. (D. Juris.)

notice Knowledge; information; awareness of facts. (D. Juris.)

Novocain Proprietary brand of procaine hydrochloride. (Pharmacol.)

noxious (nok′shŭs) Hurtful; not wholesome. (Anesth.)

NPN (see **nonprotein nitrogen**)

nucleoprotein (nū″klē-ō-prō′tē-ĭn) Any one of a special group of protein substances in combination with nucleic acid. The essential component is the phosphoric acid radical. The nucleoproteins are generally confined to the nucleus of the cell and are intimately associated with chromosome and gene function. (Oral Physiol.)

nucleus The small central part of an atom in which the positive electric charge and most of the mass are concentrated. (Oral Radiol.)

Nuhn's gland (noonz) The anterior lingual gland embedded in the substance of the tongue near the apex and the midline on the inferior surface of the tongue. (see also **gland, Blandin and Nuhn's**)

nuisance That which produces hurt unlawfully or causes inconvenience or damage. Anything that is injurious to health, is offensive, or prevents the free use of property. (D. Juris.)

number, Brinell hardness (**B.H.N.**) A numerical expression of the hardness of a material, determined by measuring the diameter of a dent made by forcing a hard steel or tungsten carbide ball of standard dimension into the material, under specified load, in a Brinell machine (devised by J. A. Brinell, a Swedish engineer). The larger the indention, the smaller the Brinell hardness number. (Oper. Dent.) (see also **test, Brinell hardness**)

number, Vickers hardness Hardness as measured by the Vickers hardness test. (D. Mat.) (see also **test, Vickers hardness**)

nurse, chairside A dental assistant whose primary duty is to remain with the dentist at the chairside and assist him there. (Pract. Man.)

nutrient canal (see **canal, interdental**)

nutrition The process of assimilation and utilization of essential food elements from the diet—carbohydrates, fats, proteins, vitamins, mineral elements, etc. (Comp. Prosth.; Periodont.; Remov. Part. Prosth.)

nutritional disturbances (see **disturbances, nutritional**)

nutriture (nū′trĭ-tūr) Nutritional status of a patient. (Oral Med.)

nystagmus (nĭs-tăg′mŭs) The state of oscillatory movements of an organ or part, especially the eyeballs; irregular jerking movement of the eyes. Each movement of the cycle consists of a slow component in one direction and a rapid component in the opposite direction. (Oral Diag.; Oral Physiol.)

O

oath A pledge verifying statements made or to be made and with a prayer to deity to witness the words of the party and to punish him if they be false. (D. Juris.)

obdormition (ob″dor-mĭsh′ŭn) Numbness and anesthesia of a part from nerve pressure. (Anesth.)

obesity, adrenocortical (ō-bēs′ĭ-tē) (**buffalo obesity**) One of the symptoms characteristic of Cushing's syndrome; an obesity that is confined chiefly to the trunk, face, and neck. (Oral Med.)

obesity, buffalo (see **obesity, adrenocortical**)

object-film distance (see **distance, object-film**)

obligation The binding power of a promise, oath, or contract or of law. Independent of a promise; a legal or moral duty that renders a person liable to punishment for neglecting it. (D. Juris.)

obtain Exists; is found. (Oper. Dent.)

obtund (ob-tŭnd′) To diminish the ability to perceive pain and/or touch. (Oral Med.; Pharmacol.)

obtundent (ob-tŭn′dĕnt) An agent that obtunds. (Oper. Dent.; Oral Med.; Pharmacol.)

obturation (ob″tū-rā′shŭn) The act of closing or occluding. (Anesth.)

    retrograde o. (see **filling, retrograde**)

    o., root canal filling technique The procedure employed for closing or filling the root canal. (Endodont.)

obturator (ob″tū-rā′tor) A prosthesis used to close a congenital or acquired opening in the palate. (Cleft Palate; Comp. Prosth.; Remov. Part. Prosth.) (see also **aid, prosthetic speech**)

— That portion of a prosthesis that mechanically or functionally closes an acquired, congenital, or developmental opening, as in the palate. (M.F.P.)

— A device used to obliterate defects in the jaws, especially the maxilla, that have congenital, mechanical, or surgical origins. (Oral Surg.)

    o., hollow That portion of an obturator made hollow to minimize its weight. (M.F.P.)

occipital anchorage (ok-sĭp′ĭ-tăl) (see **anchorage, occipital**)

occlude To close together; to close tight. (Anesth.)

— To bring together; to shut. To bring the mandibular teeth into contact with the maxillary teeth. (Comp. Prosth.; Orthodont.; Remov. Part. Prosth.)

occluder A name given to some articulators. (Comp. Prosth.; Remov. Part. Prosth.) (see also **articulator**)

occluding frame (see **articulator; frame, occluding**)

occluding relation (see **relation, occluding**)

occlusal Pertaining to the contacting surfaces of opposing occlusal units (teeth or occlusion rims). Pertaining to the masticating surfaces of the posterior teeth. (Comp. Prosth.; Oper. Dent.; Orthodont.; Remov. Part. Prosth.)

    o. adjustment (see **adjustment, occlusal**)

    o. analysis (see **analysis, occlusal**)

    o. balance (see **balance, occlusal**)

    o. contouring (see **contouring, occlusal**)

    o. correction (see **correction, occlusal**)

    o. curvature (see **curve of occlusion**)

    o. disharmony (see **disharmony, occlusal**)

    o. disturbances (see **disturbances, occlusal**)

    o. embrasure (see **embrasure, occlusal**)

    o. equilibration (see **equilibration, occlusal**)

    o. force (see **force, occlusal**)

    o. form (see **form, occlusal**)

    o. function (see **function, heavy**)

    o. glide (see **glide, occlusal**)

    o. harmony (see **harmony, occlusal**)

    o. load (see **load, occlusal**)

    o. path (see **path, occlusal**)

    o. path registration (see **path, occlusal, registration**)

    o. pattern (see **pattern, occlusal**)

    o. perception (see **perception, occlusal**)

    o. pivot (see **pivot, occlusal**)

    o. plane (see **plane, occlusal**)

    o. position (see **position, occlusal**)

    o. pressure (see **pressure, occlusal**)

    o. recontouring (see **contouring, occlusal**)

    o. rest (see **rest, occlusal**)

    o. splint (see **splint, occlusal**)

    o. stop (see **rest, occlusal**)

    o. surface (see **surface, occlusal**)

    o. system (see **system, occlusal**)

    o. table (see **table, occlusal**)

    o. template (see **template, occlusal**)

    o. trauma (see **trauma, occlusal**)

    o. unit One of two kinds of cusps: (1) a stamp cusp coupled with a fossa and (2) a shear cusp, the occlusal edges of which are coupled with the edges of a stamp cusp, by which it passes closely without sliding contacts. (Gnathol.)

o. wear (see **wear, occlusal**)

occlusion The act of closure or state of being closed. (Anesth.)

— Any contact between the incising or masticating surfaces of the upper and lower teeth. This term should be used to designate any or all contacts between opposing teeth. (Comp. Prosth.)

— The intimate relationship between the cusps of the lower teeth when in normal contact with the upper teeth. (Orthodont.)

— The large genus of good and bad dental closures, ranging from the contacts made by a coupling of canines to the couplings of all the teeth, and to approximations of the following: molars without cusps, rims of intergnathic temporary records, the contiguity of a mucosa and the basal surface in a denture, and the various abnormal relations of malclosures. (Gnathol.)

acentric o. (see **occlusion, eccentric**)

adjusting o. (see **adjusting occlusion**)

anatomic o. The ideal relation of the mandibular and maxillary teeth when closed. (Orthodont.)

anterior determinants of cusp o. The characteristics of the anterior teeth—their occlusion, their alignment, their overlaps, and their capacity to disclude conjointly with the trajectories given the condyles—that determine the cusp elevations and the fossa depressions of the postcanine teeth. (Gnathol.)

attritional o. Occlusion in which each tooth of the dentition wears occlusally and proximally as it erupts. (Orthodont.)

balanced o. The simultaneous contacting of the upper and lower teeth on the right and left sides and in the anterior and posterior occlusal areas of the jaws. This occlusion is developed to prevent a tipping or rotating of the denture base in relation to the supporting structures. This term is used primarily in connection with the mouth, but it may be used in relation to teeth on an articulator. (Comp. Prosth.)

— An occlusion of the teeth that presents a harmonious relation of the occluding surfaces in centric and eccentric positions within the functional range of mandibular positions and tooth size. (Comp. Prosth.; Orthodont.; Remov. Part. Prosth.)

— An occlusion in which stresses generated by the musculature, causing the mandible (and

teeth) to function, fall within the limits of endurance or tolerance of periodontal ligaments. Balancing of occlusion involves adjustment of the direction, magnitude, and distribution of the occlusal forces within physiologic boundaries. (Periodont.)

bilateral b. o. The closure suitable for worn dentitions that either are cuspless or have flat-sided cusps; it permits an increase of the amount of surface contact in centric closure and provides as much closure contact as possible for horizontal chewing. This kind of occlusion is a therapeutic form designed to keep dentures seated when fine-textured foods are chewed horizontally. It is not found in young, unworn natural dentitions. (Gnathol.)

centrically b. o. A centrically related centric occlusion in which the teeth close with even pressures on both sides of the mouth but have no occlusion of the postcanine teeth in attempted eccentric closures. (Gnathol.)

mechanically b. o. An occlusion balanced without reference to physiologic considerations; e.g., on an articulator. (Comp. Prosth.)

physiologically b. o. A balanced occlusion that is in harmony with the temporomandibular joints and the neuromuscular system. (Comp. Prosth.) (see also **occlusion, balanced**)

unilateral b. o. A neospherical form in which unilateral balance is provided by having a right and left spherical arrangement of closure contacts. It has given rise to a technique for using a "chew-in" method of generating, in wax, the grooves for the lateral and the lingual sliding runways for cusps and also for the sliding distal and mesial runways in the fore-and-aft slidings of cusps. The advantages claimed for the unilateral balanced occlusion is that it removes all cross-arch leverage. The disadvantage of the bispherical unilateral balanced occlusion is that it provides no defense against wear that follows bruxism. (Gnathol.)

central o. (see **occlusion, centric**)

centric o. (central o.) The occlusion intended or planned to occur when the jaws are in centric relation. With cusp teeth, (1) each tooth is opposed by two, except the lower central incisors and the upper last molars, (2) the upper teeth overlap the lower teeth, and (3) the long axis of each upper tooth is distal to the long axis of the corresponding lower tooth. All other occlusal contacts are eccentric occlusions. (Comp. Prosth.)

— The relation of opposing occlusal surfaces that provides the maximum planned contact and/or intercuspation. It should exist when the mandible is in centric relation to the maxillae. (Comp. Prosth.; Orthodont.)

— The occlusion of the teeth that is the resultant of mandibular closure, the condyles remaining in their posterior terminal hinge position. (Fixed Part. Prosth.)

— The position in which there are the maximum number of holding contacts of the teeth, both individually and collectively, when the jaws are in centric relation. (Periodont.)

— The occlusion of the teeth when the mandible is in centric relation to the maxillae. (Remov. Part. Prosth.)

faulty c. o. A condition wherein centric occlusion does not correspond to a patient's centric jaw relationship, resulting in premature or interceptive or deflective tooth contacts in the centric path of closure. (Periodont.)

handheld c. o. Dental occlusion obtained by hand coupling the casts of a pair of molars that allow their main stamp cusps to be seated mutually in the central fossae of their opposites. (Gnathol.)

centric relation o. The occlusion of the teeth when the jaws are in centric relation. (Periodont.)

components of o. The various factors that are involved in occlusion;· e.g., the temporomandibular joint, the associated neuromusculature, and the teeth. In denture prosthetics, also the denture-supporting structures. (Comp. Prosth.; Fixed Part. Prosth.; Remov. Part. Prosth.)

convenience o. (convenience jaw relation, convenience relationship of teeth) The assumed position of maximum intercuspation when there is occlusal interference in the centric path of closure. The convenience occlusion may be anterior, lateral, anterolateral, etc. to the true centric occlusion. (Periodont.)

coronary o. Coronary thrombosis resulting in closure of the coronary artery. (Oral Med.)

cross-bite o. An occlusion in which the lower teeth overlap the upper teeth.

determinants of o. The classifiable factors in the gnathic organ that influence occlusion. These factors are divided into two groups: those that are fixed, and those that can be modified by reshaping or repositioning the teeth. The fixed factors most mentioned are the intercondylar distance; anatomy, which influences the paths of the mandibular axes; mandibular centricity; and the mating of the jaws. The changeable factors most mentioned are tooth shapes, tooth positions, vertical dimension, height of cusps, and depth of fossae. (Gnathol.)

eccentric o. Any occlusion other than centric occlusion. A condition in which the habitual voluntary closure pattern of the mandible does not coincide with centric relation, producing primary premature tooth contacts in the centric path of closure. (Comp. Prosth.; Orthodont.; Periodont.; Remov. Part. Prosth.)

acquired e. o. An eccentric occlusion that is the resultant of a proprioceptive mechanism activated by deflective occlusal contacts. (Fixed Part. Prosth.)

edge-to-edge o. An occlusion in which the anterior teeth of both jaws meet along their incisal edges when the teeth are in centric occlusion. (Comp. Prosth.; Fixed Part. Prosth.; Remov. Part. Prosth.)

end-to-end o. (see **occlusion, edge-to-edge**)

functional o. Occlusion in which attention is directed specifically to performance and is differentiated from structure and appearance. The term should be used with modifiers to indicate the degree of function that occlusion achieves. (Comp. Prosth.; Remov. Part. Prosth.)

—Any tooth contacts made within the functional range (according to the size) of the opposing tooth surfaces. An occlusion that occurs during function. (Comp. Prosth.; Orthodont.)

gliding o. Used in the sense of designating contacts of teeth in motion. A substitute for the term articulation. (Comp. Prosth.; Remov. Part. Prosth.)

ideal o. A well-occluded dentition in which the teeth are well arrayed in symmetric arches attached to well-mated jaws so that full automation of the gnathic system is possible and present. (Gnathol.)

key to o. First permanent molar. (Orthodont.)

locked o. An occlusal relationship of such nature that lateral and protrusive mandibular movements are limited. (Orthodont.)

malfunctional o. A disturbance in the normal or proper action of the masticatory apparatus produced by such factors as missing teeth or tilting and drifting of teeth; may be a potent factor in the production of periodontal disease and disturbances in the temporomandibular joints and mandibular musculature. (Periodont.)

normal o. The relation of the opposing dentitions or dentures when brought into habitual apposition. (Orthodont.)

physiologic n. o. The normal relationships of the inclines of the cusps of opposing teeth to each other in occlusion, when the alignment, proximal contacts, and axial positions of all teeth in both arches have resulted from normal growth and development in relation to all associated tissues and parts of the head. An occlusion that operates in harmony and presents no pathologic manifestation in the supporting structures of the teeth. (Periodont.)

pathogenic o. An occlusal relationship capable of producing pathologic changes in the supporting tissues, such as joint pains, noisy joints, spastic masticatory muscles, excessively worn crowns from night grinding, and poorly cared-for periodontium. (Comp. Prosth.; Gnathol.; Remov. Part. Prosth.)

physiologic o. An occlusion in harmony with functions of the masticatory system. (Comp. Prosth.; Remov. Part. Prosth.)

— An occlusion that operates in harmony and presents no pathologic manifestation in the supporting structures of the teeth; the stresses placed on the teeth are dissipated normally, with a balance existing between the stresses and the adaptive capacity of the supporting tissues. (Periodont.)

— An acceptable occlusion found in a healthy gnathic system. (Gnathol.)

plane of o. (see **plane, occlusal**)

posterior determinants of cusp o. The variable factors of occlusion that arise from the nature of the condyle thrusts, such as the sagittal slopes and curvatures of the eminences, the location of the rearmost hinge axis position, the character of the fore-and-aft and the in-and-out condyle paths, and the variable kinds of laterotrusion given in the individual to the bolus condyle. (Gnathol.)

protrusive o. An occlusion of the teeth existing when the mandible is protruded forward from centric position. (Comp. Prosth.; Remov. Part. Prosth.)

rest o. Contradictory term that should not be used in this combination. (Comp. Prosth.; Remov. Part. Prosth.) (see also **position, rest, physiologic**)

o. rim (see **rim, occlusion**)

spherical form of o. Arrangement of teeth that places their occlusal surfaces on the surface of an imaginary sphere (usually 9 inches in diameter), with its center above the level of the teeth, as suggested by Monson. (Comp. Prosth.; Remov. Part. Prosth.)

o. table (see **table, occlusal**)

terminal o. The relation of opposing occlusal surfaces that provides the maximum natural or planned contact and/or intercuspation. (Comp. Prosth.)

traumatic o. An occlusion that results in overstrain and injury to teeth, to periodontal tissues, or to the residual ridge or other oral structures. (Comp. Prosth.; Oper. Dent.; Orthodont.; Remov. Part. Prosth.)

traumatogenic o. A malocclusion capable of producing injury to the residual ridge, the teeth, the temporomandibular joints, the muscles of mastication, and the supporting structures of the teeth. (Comp. Prosth.; Remov. Part. Prosth.)

— An occlusion that produces an injury of the periodontal tissues under biting pressure. (Orthodont.)

working o. The occlusal contacts of teeth on the side toward which the mandible is moved. From the mesial or distal view, the buccal and lingual cusps of the upper teeth appear to be end to end with the buccal and lingual cusps of the lower teeth, respectively. Viewed from the side, each upper cusp is distal to the corresponding lower cusp. The mesial incline of each upper cusp makes contact with the distal incline of the opposing cusp in front of it, and the distal incline of each upper cusp makes contact with the mesial incline of the opposing cusp distal to it. (Comp. Prosth.; Remov. Part. Prosth.)

occupy To hold; to keep for use. (D. Juris.)

odontalgia (ō″don-tăl′jē-ah) Pain in a tooth; toothache. (Oper. Dent.; Oral Diag.; Oral Surg.)

phantom o. (ghost pain) Pain in the area from which a tooth has been removed. (Oral Surg.)

odontectomy (ō″don-těk′tō-mē) Removal of a tooth. (Oral Surg.)

odontexesis (ō″don-těk′sě-sĭs) The thorough scaling of teeth. (Remov. Part. Prosth.)

odontodysplasia (ghost teeth) A developmental anomaly characterized by deficient tooth development. Deficiencies are noted in both enamel and dentin formation. (Oral Diag.) (see also **tooth, shell**)

odontogenesis imperfecta (ō-don″tō-jĕn′ĕ-sĭs) Generic term that includes simultaneous defects in both epithelial and mesenchymal tissue involved in tooth development. (Oral Path.)

odontoma (ō″don-tō′mah) (**gestant anomaly**) An anomaly of the teeth resembling a tumor of hard tissue; e.g., dens in dente, enamel pearl, complex or composite odontoma. It is composed of enamel, dentin, cementum, and pulp tissue that may or may not be arranged in the form of teeth. (Oral Diag.; Oral Path.)

    ameloblastic o. An odontogenic tumor characterized by the occurrence of an ameloblastoma within an odontoma. (Oral Path.) (see also **ameloblastoma; odontoma**)

    composite o. (kom-pos′ĭt) Complex odontoma; an odontogenic tumor characterized by the formation of calcified enamel and dentin in an abnormal arrangement because of lack of morphodifferentiation. Compound odontoma: a tumor of enamel and dentin arranged in the form of anomalous miniature teeth. Several small abnormal teeth surrounded by a fibrous sac. (Oral Diag.)

    cystic o. An odontoma associated with a follicular cyst. (Oral Path.)

    gestant o. (see **dens in dente**)

odontotomy, prophylactic (ō″don-tot′ō-mē) The operation of cutting into a tooth for preventive reasons. (Oper. Dent.)

— Removal of precarious pits and fissures in posterior primary and permanent molars and their restoration with amalgam restorations. (Pedodont.)

office hours (see **business hours**)

office planning The physical arrangement of the rooms available within the limitations of space designed to enable the dentist to practice. (Pract. Man.)

office routine (see **routine, office**)

offset (**set-off**) A deduction; a counterclaim; a demand by which a given claim may be relieved or cancelled. (D. Juris.)

oil An unctuous combustible substance that is liquid, or easily liquefiable on warming, and is soluble in ether but insoluble in water.

    essential o. (**volatile o.**) A volatile, nonfatty liquid of vegetable origin having a distinct aroma and flavor, often pleasant. (Oral Med.; Pharmacol.)

    fixed o. A nonvolatile oil consisting chiefly of glycerides. (D. Mat.)

    mineral o. Any one of the various grades of liquid petrolatum. (D. Mat.)

    volatile o. (see **oil, essential**)

ointment A soft, bland, smooth, semisolid mixture that is used as a lubricant and as a vehicle for external medication. (Oral Med.; Pharmacol.)

    hydrophilic o. An ointment that is miscible with water. (Oral Med.; Pharmacol.)

oligodontia (ol″ĭ-gō-don′shē-ah) The condition of having only a few teeth. (Pedodont.)

oligodynamic (ol″ĭ-gō-dī-năm′ĭk) Effective in extremely small quantities. (Oral Med.; Pharmacol.)

oliguria (ol″ĭ-gū′rē-ah) Decreased output of urine (usually less than 500 ml/day). It may be associated with dehydration from diarrhea or excessive sweating, low fluid intake, lower nephron nephrosis due to burns, heavy metal poisoning, terminal renal disease, or an increase in extracellular fluid volume in untreated renal, cardiac, or hepatic disease. (Oral Med.)

omission A phoneme left out at a place where it should occur. (Cleft Palate)

on account In partial payment; in partial satisfaction of an amount owed. (D. Juris.)

on or about Phrase used in stating the date of an occurrence or conveyance to avoid being bound by the statement of an exact or certain date. (D. Juris.)

oncocytoma (ong″kō-sī-tō′mah) (**acidophilic adenoma, oxyphilic adenoma**) A rare benign tumor usually occurring in the parotid glands in elderly patients. The lesion is encapsulated and is composed of sheets and cords of large eosinophilic cells having small nuclei. (Oral Path.)

onlay An occlusal rest that is extended to cover the entire occlusal surface of a tooth. (Remov. Part. Prosth.)

    o. bone (see **graft, onlay bone**)

ontogeny (on″toj′ĕ-nē) The natural life cycle of an individual as contrasted with the natural life cycle of the race (phylogeny). (Oral Physiol.)

opacity, optical The reciprocal of transmission, which is in turn the ratio of transmitted and incident light intensity. (Not to be confused with radiopacity, the term opacity is used in radiography to characterize those [darker] portions of the image that are relatively impenetrable to light, i.e., that transmit little or no light.) (Oral Radiol.) (see also **density**)

opaque Relatively impenetrable to light. (Oral Radiol.) (see also **opacity, optical**)

open bite (see **bite, open**)

open flap technique The raising of a mucoperiosteal flap for the multiple extraction of teeth; the removal of a root; or the exposure of any area of bone beneath the flap. (Oral Surg.)

open panel The group purchase of dental care wherein both the patient and the dentist enjoy the free selection of dentist and patient. (Pract. Man.)

opening movement (see **movement, mandibular, opening**)

opening, vertical (see **dimension, vertical**)

operating field (see **field, operating**)

operating light (see **light, operating**)

operating procedure (see **procedure, operating**)

operation An act or series of acts performed on the body of a patient for his relief or cure. (D. Juris.)

    Abbé-Estlander o. Transfer of a full-thickness section of one lip of the oral cavity to the other lip, using an arterial pedicle to ensure survival of the graft. (Oral Surg.)

    blind o. A procedure in which the surgeon operates by using his sense of touch and knowledge of surgical anatomy without making a significant mucous membrane or cutaneous incision. (Oral Surg.)

    exploratory o. A surgical procedure used to establish a diagnosis. (Oral Surg.)

    Gillies' o. A technique for reducing fractures of the zygoma and the zygomatic arch through an incision in the temporal hairline. (Oral Surg.)

    Kazanjian's o. (**Kazanjian's procedure**) A technique of surgical extension of the vestibular sulcus for improved prosthetic foundation of edentulous ridges. (Oral Surg.) (see also **extension, ridge**)

    modified flap o. A variation of the flap procedure in oral and periodontal surgery. In this variation the vertical incisions of the flap procedure are not made, but the labial and/or lingual gingival walls are distended as far as possible to assure sufficient access and an unobstructed view for instrumentation. (Periodont.)

    open o. A procedure in which the surgeon operates with full view of the structures before him through mucous membrane or cutaneous incisions. (Oral Surg.)

    Partsch's o. The name applied to a technique of marsupialization. (Oral Surg.)

    pedicle flap o. A procedure in mucogingival surgery designed to relocate or slide gingival tissue from a donor site in close proximity to an isolated defect, usually a tooth surface denuded of attached gingiva. (Periodont.)

    Sorrin's o. A type of flap approach in the treatment of the periodontal abscess; espe-cially suitable when the marginal gingiva appears well adapted and gives no access to the abscess area. A semilunar incision is made below the involved area in the attached gingiva, leaving the gingival margin undisturbed; a flap is raised, allowing for access to the abscessed area for curettage. Suturing follows. (Periodont.)

operatory (op′er-ah-tor″ē) The room or rooms in which the dentist performs his professional services. (Pract. Man.)

operculectomy (ō-per-kū-lĕk′tō-mē) The surgical removal of the mucosal flap partially or completely covering an unerupted tooth. (Oral Surg.)

operculitis (ō-per″kū-lī′tĭs) (see **pericoronitis**)

operculum (ō-per′kū-lŭm) Cover or lid. (Oral Surg.)

opiate A remedy containing or derived from opium; also any drug that induces sleep. (Anesth.)

opinion In the law of evidence, an inference or conclusion drawn by a witness from facts either known to him or assumed. (D. Juris.)

opisthion (ō-pĭs′thē-on) The hindmost point on the posterior margin of the foramen magnum. (Orthodont.)

opisthocheilia (ō-pĭs″thō-kē′ĭl-ĭ-ah) A condition of receding lips. (Orthodont.)

opisthocranion (ō-pĭs″thō-krā′nē-on) The point in the midline of the cranium that projects farthest backward. (Orthodont.)

opium Concrete juice of the poppy, *Papaver somniferum*. It contains morphine, codeine, nicotine, narceine, and many other alkaloids. (Anesth.)

optimal (ŏp′tĭ-mal) The best or most favorable. (Anesth.)

oral Pertaining to the mouth.

    o. digestion Comminution and mixing of foods with saliva and with whatever other enzymes may be released from crushed living cells in the diet. (Oral Physiol.)

    o. environment (see **environment, oral**)

    o. evacuator (**vacuum**) A suction apparatus used to remove any fluids and debris from an operating field. (Oper. Dent.)

    o. hygiene (see **hygiene, oral**)

    o. medicine (see **medicine, oral**)

    o. mucosa (see **mucosa, oral**)

    o. physiology (see **physiology, oral**)

orbital (or′bĭ-tăl) Pertaining to the orbit. (Orthodont.)

    o. exenteration Surgical removal of the entire contents of the orbit. (M.F.P.)

    o. marker A projecting part of a face-bow

that marks the location of the orbitale. It is used in the orientation of casts on an articulator in relation to cranial planes. (Comp. Prosth.)

o. plane (see **plane, orbital**)

orbitale (or″bĭ-tā′lē) The lowest point in the margin of the orbit (directly below the pupil when the eye is open and the patient is looking straight ahead) that may readily be felt under the skin. The eye-ear plane passes through the orbitale and tragion. (Orthodont.)

orbiting condyle The condyle that arcs around the vertical axis of the rotating condyle, formerly called the idling condyle, or the balancing condyle. It is not idling, because it it is tied to the rotating condyle and is satellite to it. Once it was called the advancing condyle, but it may go forward, downward, and inward, all at the same time. It is not idling but moving and helping the rotating condyle. It is also helping the canine on the far side to disclude all other teeth. (Gnathol.)

orders Written or verbal directions of a doctor to a nurse or other assistant detailing the care that is to be given a patient. (Oral Surg.)

organism(s) (or′gah-nĭzm) Any organized body of living economy.

Miller's o. The fusospirochetal organisms present in the flora of oral microorganisms, found by Willoughby D. Miller and Hugo Karl Plaut to be the causative agents in nondiphtheritic membranous angina (necrotizing ulcerative gingivitis, necrotizing ulcerative gingivostomatitis, Vincent's infection, "trench mouth," etc.). (Periodont.)

Vincent's o. The fusospirochetal organisms associated with the initiation of necrotizing ulcerative gingivitis, necrotizing ulcerative stomatitis, and/or Vincent's angina. (Periodont.)

orifice (or′ĭ-fĭs) The entrance or outlet of any body cavity; any foramen, meatus, or opening. (Anesth.)

orodigitofacial dysostosis (**OFD syndrome**) Syndrome characterized by abnormal development of the jaws and tongue, cleft lip and palate, hypoplasia of bones of the skull with ocular hypertelorism, nasal alar deformity, malformation of digits (frequently manifest as brachydactyly and syndactyly), mental retardation, granular skin, and alopecia of the scalp. (Cleft Palate)

oronasal Pertaining to the mouth and nose. (Anesth.)

orthocheilia (or′thō-kē′lē-ah) A condition of straight lips. (Orthodont.)

orthodontia (or-thō-don′shē-ah) (see **orthodontics**)

orthodontic Describing or referring to orthodontics. (Orthodont.)

o. appliance (see **appliance, orthodontic**)

orthodontic space maintainer (see **space maintainer, orthodontic**)

orthodontically Implying an orthodontic manner of action. (Orthodont.)

orthodontics The science that has for its object the prevention and correction of dental and oral anomalies. (Orthodont.)

corrective o. The correction of malocclusion with appliances. (Pedodont.)

interceptive o. The application of early treatment procedures, using appliances, to the primary or mixed dentition for the prevention of serious malocclusion when there are poor cross-bite and oral habits. (Pedodont.)

preventive o. (**prophylactic o.**) The use of space maintainers to preserve satisfactory occlusal relationships. (Pedodont.)

prophylactic o. (see **orthodontics, preventive**)

orthodontist A dentist engaged in the practice of orthodontics. (Orthodont.)

orthognathic (or″thō-năth′ĭk) Having straight jaws and a straight profile. (Orthodont.)

orthognathus (or-thō-năth′ŭs) Straight jaws; no projection of the lower part of the face. The facial angle is from 85° to 90°. (Remov. Part. Prosth.)

orthopantograph (or″thō-păn′tō-grăf) A panoramic radiographic device (Panorex) that permits visualization of the entire dentition, alveolar bone, and other contiguous structures on a single extraoral film. (Oral Surg.)

Orthopantomograph (or″thō-pănt′ō-mō-grăf) A radiographic system (manufactured by Siemens) that utilizes three axes of rotation to obtain a panoramic radiograph of the dental arches and their associated structures. (Oral Radiol.)

orthopnea (or″thop-nē′ah) Inability to breathe except in an upright position. (Anesth.)

Osler's disease (see **erythremia**)

Osler-Weber disease (see **telangiectasia, hereditary hemorrhagic**)

osmosis The passage of pure solvent from the lesser to the greater concentration when two solutions are separated by a membrane that selectively prevents the passage of solute molecules but is permeable to the solvent. The principles of osmosis coupled with the selective permeability of the cell membrane help regulate the transfer of fluids and metabolites to and from the cells. Thus they also maintain the stability of the salt/ion concentration in the extracellular and intracellular fluid. (Anesth.; Oral Physiol.)

osmotic Pertaining to osmosis. (Anesth.)

  o. pressure (see **pressure, osmotic**)

ostectomy (os-tĕk'tō-mē) (**osteoectomy**) Excision of a bone or a portion of a bone. (Oral Surg.)

— Removal of alveolar bone from about the tooth root in order to eliminate an adjacent pocket and to secure physiologic osseous and gingival form. (Periodont.)

osteitis (os"tē-ī'tĭs) Inflammation of the bone; inflammation of the haversian spaces, canals, and their branches but generally not of the medullary cavity. The disease is characterized by tenderness and a dull, aching pain. Enlargement of the bone may occur. (Oral Diag.; Oral Surg.) (see also **osteomyelitis**)

— Inflammation of the bone, such as that of the alveolar process following the extraction of a tooth, commonly referred to as dry socket. (Remov. Part. Prosth.)

  alveolar o., localized (see **socket, dry**)

  condensing o. A bone-thickening chronic inflammation associated with some nonvital teeth or located in the site of extraction of such teeth. (Oral Path.)

  o. deformans (**Paget's disease**) A disease of the bone of unknown cause; characterized by enlargement of the cranial bones and often of the maxillae or the mandible. The x-ray appearance is characterized by a cotton-wool appearance. (Oral Diag.)

— A localized or generalized disease of bone of unknown origin characterized by the replacement of normal bone with soft, poorly mineralized osteoid tissue. In later stages affected bone is replaced by densely sclerotic bone. Bony enlargement, deformities, and sometimes fractures occur. (Oral Med.)

— A generalized disease of bone characterized by the concurrent destruction and formation of bone. The etiology is unknown. (Oral Path.)

— A bone disease characterized by thickening and bowing of the long bones and enlargement of the skull and maxillae. It is represented radiographically by a cotton-wool appearance of the bone; microscopically it presents a mosaic bone pattern. Hypercementosis and loosening of the teeth may be significant manifestations. (Periodont.)

  o. fibrosa cystica, generalized (**von Recklinghausen's disease of bone**) A disease caused by parathyroid adenomas and characterized by cystlike radiolucencies in the bones (in-

cluding the jaws), loosening of teeth, localized swellings, giant cell lesions, increased blood calcium and phosphatase, and lowered blood phosphorus. The term von Recklinghausen's disease (of skin) is also used as a synonym for neurofibromatosis. (Oral Diag.)

— Increased resorption and destruction of bone caused by primary and secondary hyperparathyroidism. (Oral Path.) (see also **hyperparathyroidism**)

osteoarthritis (os"tē-ō-ar-thrī'tĭs) Chronic degeneration and destruction of the articular cartilage leading to bony spurs, pain, stiffness, limitation of motion, and change in size of joints. It is considered to be due to chronic traumatic injury as well as to wear and tear. Heberden's nodes occur in a special form of the disease. (Oral Med.)

— A disorder of joints affecting the cartilage and bone. All joints undergo change during function, but joints subjected to abnormal stresses may develop local disorders of the cartilage and bone, and patients in good health may complain about creaky sounds in the joints. A number of chemical, physical, and structural variables collectively give rise to these symptoms. The symptoms may be associated with hormonal, vascular, and/or nutritional disorders. The structural changes of advanced osteoarthritis may involve erosion of the articular cartilages or the subchondral bone. Osteoarthritis rarely affects the temporomandibular joint beyond the "creaking" state. Osteoarthritis differs principally from rheumatoid arthritis in that the synovitis is a late change in osteoarthritis, whereas it is an early change in rheumatoid arthritis. (Oral Physiol.)

osteoarthropathy, hypertrophic pulmonary (os"tē-ō-ar-throp'ah-thē) Clubbing of the fingers and toes due to deposition of calcium in the subperiosteal tissues about the joint. Related to chronic pulmonary disease and occasionally to circulatory and digestive disease. (Oral Med.)

osteoblast (os'tē-ō-blăst") The cell associated with the growth and development of bone; it is cuboidal in shape and about 15 to 20 μm in width. In active growth osteoblasts form a continuous layer on old bone similar to a sheet of epithelial cells; when the bone growth is arrested, the cells assume an elongated appearance like fibroblasts. (Oral Physiol.)

— The polyhedral-shaped cell that forms osteoid; the mucopolysaccharide protein substance that is later mineralized into bone, with the inclusion of osteoblasts, as osteocytes, in the lacunae of the bone. (Periodont.)

osteocementum (os″tē-ō-sē-měn′tŭm) Secondary cementum; the hard, bonelike cementum deposited after root formation is completed. In man, formed in an exuberant attempt to maintain biologic width of the periodontal membrane of a tooth when opposing occlusal force is absent. (Periodont.) (see also **atrophy of disuse**)

osteoclasia, traumatic (os″tē-ō-klā′zē-ah) (see **cementoma; dysplasia, osseous, focal; fibroma, periapical**)

osteoclast (os′tē-ō-klăst″) A giant cell with a variable number of nuclei (often as many as 15 or 20); the nuclei resemble the nuclei of the osteoblasts and the osteocytes; the cytoplasm is often foamy, and the cell frequently has branching processes. Osteoclasts may arise from the stromal cells of the bone marrow, they may represent fused osteoblasts, or they may include fused osteocytes liberated from resorbing bone. They are usually found in close relationship to the resorption of bone and frequently lie in grooves (Howship's lacunae). (Oral Physiol.)

— A large multinucleated cell associated with the resorption of bone. Seen in irregular concavities within marginal areas of bone undergoing resorption. (Periodont.)

osteoclastoma (see **granuloma, giant cell reparative, peripheral**)

osteocyte (os′tē-ō-sīt″) An osteoblast that has been surrounded by a calcified interstitial substance; the cells are enclosed within lacunae, and the cytoplasmic processes extend through apertures of the lacunae into canaliculi in the bone. Like the osteoblast, the osteocyte may undergo transformations and assume the form of an osteoclast or of a reticular cell. (Oral Physiol.)

osteodystrophy (os″tē-ō-dĭs′trō-fē) A condition marked by defective or deficient bone formation. (Periodont.)

    renal o. A form of dwarfism associated with osteoporosis produced by renal insufficiency during childhood. Periodontal changes include widening of the periodontal membrane space and marked osteoporosis of the mandibular and maxillary bones. Similar to renal rickets. (Periodont.) (see also **rickets, renal**)

osteoectomy (os″tē-ō-ĕk′tō-mē) (see **ostectomy**)

osteofibroma (os″tē-ō-fī-brō′mah) (**calcifying fibroma, fibro-osteoma, ossifying fibroma**) A benign neoplasm characterized by bone developing in a connective tissue mass. A benign neoplasm that develops in the spongiosa of the bone through proliferation of fibroblasts. A benign neoplasm of the bone characterized by unilateral swelling and fibroblastic and osteoclastic activity in marrow spaces. (Oral Diag.) (see also **dysplasia, fibrous; dysplasia, osseous**)

— A fibroma in which areas of calcification are seen; central fibro-osseous lesion of the jaws; fibrous dysplasia occurring within a single bone. Consists of various amounts of fibrous connective tissue and bone. Also called fibroma, monostotic fibrous dysplasia, fibroma with ossification, fibroma with calcification, osteogenic fibroma, fibro-osteoma, localized osteitis fibrosa, localized fibrous osteodystrophy, fibrous osteoma of the jaws, hypertrophic localized osteitis, localized leontiasis ossea, central osteoma, enostosis, and ossifying fibroma. (Oral Path.)

osteogenesis imperfecta (os″tē-ō-jěn′ě-sĭs) (**brittle bone disease, fragilitas ossium, Lobstein's disease, osteopsathyrosis idiopathica**) A disease of the bones characterized by frequent fractures. Dentinogenesis imperfecta may be associated with this bone disturbance. (Oral Diag.)

— A congenital disease of unknown cause characterized by fragile, brittle, and easily fractured bones; presumed to stem from a failure in the formation of bone matrix. Variants of this disease are often hereditary or familial and include such manifestations as blue sclerae, dentinogenesis imperfecta, and otosclerosis. (Oral Med.; Periodont.)

— A disease of unknown etiology but usually hereditary; characterized by abnormal osteogenesis and results in porous bone formation. (Oral Path.)

osteoid (os′tē-oid) The mucopolysaccharide-protein complex laid down by the osteoblasts. It is later calcified, with inclusion of osteoblasts as osteocytes within lacunae, into bone. (Periodont.)

osteolysis (os″tē-ol′ĭ-sĭs) A process of bone resorption, also referred to as halisteresis, whereby the bone salts can be withdrawn by a humoral mechanism and returned to the tissue fluids, leaving behind a decalcified bone matrix. (Periodont.)

osteoma (os″tē-ō′mah) A benign neoplasm of bone or bone tissue. (Oral Diag.; Oral Path.)

osteomalacia (os″tē-ō-mah-lā′shē-ah) (**adult rickets**) A systemic disorder of bone characterized by decreased mineralization of bone matrix. It may be due to vitamin D deficiency, inadequate calcium in the diet, renal disease, and/or steatorrhea. Manifestations include incomplete fractures and gradual resorption of cortical and cancellous bone. (Oral Med.)

— A condition caused by a deficiency of vitamin D in adults and characterized by defective calcification of bone matrix. (Oral Path.)

osteomyelitis (os″tē-ō-mī″ĕ-lī′tĭs) Inflammation of the bone marrow or of the bone, marrow, and endosteum. (Oral Diag.; Oral Surg.)

— Inflammation of bone caused by a pyogenic organism. (Oral Path.) (see also **osteitis**)

osteon (os′tē-on) The three-dimensional reconstruction of concentric lamellae arranged circumferentially about the course of a central blood vessel. (Oral Physiol.; Periodont.)

osteopetrosis (os″tē-ō-pĕ-trō′sĭs) (**Albers-Schönberg disease, marble bone**) Osteosclerosis of unknown origin that obliterates the bone marrow regions, with resultant anemia. Delayed tooth eruption and severe osteomyelitis or necrosis following dental infection may be associated with the disease. (Oral Diag.)

— An uncommon hereditary disorder believed to be transmitted as a mendelian recessive trait and characterized by overgrowth and sclerosis of bone. Manifestations include brittle bones that tend to fracture, anemia due to fibrosis and obliteration of marrow cavities, reduced bone resorption, optic atrophy, deafness, osteomyelitis of the jaws, and delayed eruption of the teeth. (Oral Med.; Oral Path.)

osteoplasty (ŏs′tē-ō-plăs″tē) Surgical procedure to modify or change the configuration of a bone. (Oral Surg.)

— The recontouring or plastic reshaping of bone to secure a functional form of the bone and overlying soft tissues. The procedure does not involve removal of alveolar bone. (Periodont.)

osteoporosis (os″tē-ō-po-rō′sĭs) (**Schüller's disease**) Enlargement of the soft marrow and haversian spaces due to a decreased rate of formation of the hard bone matrix. With the exception of immobilized parts, it is a systemic disorder that occurs in advanced age (senile osteoporosis), during ACTH and cortisone therapy, during and after menopause, in limited physical activity, in Cushing's syndrome, during malnutrition, and in other disorders of matrix formation such as hyperadrenalism, hyperthyroidism, vitamin C deficiencies, and deficiency of androgenic steroids. (Oral Med.; Oral Physiol.) (see also **atrophy, bone; bone rarefaction**)

— Abnormal porosity of bone caused by a failure of osteoid formation. Among the causes are excessive stress applied to bone; insufficient functional stimulation; disturbances of metabolism of calcium, phosphorus, and vitamin D; lack of estrogenic stimulation; dietary deficiencies of protein and the vitamin B complex; hyperthyroidism; etc. (Periodont.)

osteopsathyrosis idiopathica (os″tē-op-săth″ĭ-rō′sĭs) (see **osteogenesis imperfecta**)

osteoradionecrosis (os″tē-ō-rā″dē-ō-nĕ-krō′sĭs) Bone necrosis secondary to irradiation and superimposed infection. (Oral Diag.)

osteosarcoma A malignant neoplasm of the bone-forming tissues. (Oral Diag.)

— Term applied to a group of malignant neoplasms of the bone. (Oral Path.)

osteosclerosis (os″tē-ō-sklĕ-rō′sĭs) Increased bone formation resulting in reduced marrow spaces and increased radiopacity. (Oral Diag.)

osteotomy (os″tē-ot′ō-mē) Surgical cutting or transection of a bone. (Oral Surg.)

blind o. Osteotomy performed indirectly by touch. (Oral Surg.)

open o. Osteotomy performed under direct vision. (Oral Surg.)

perforation o. Osteotomy performed through intact overlying mucosa by means of a bur. (Oral Implant.)

segmental alveolar o. A surgical procedure in which the bone is cut horizontally apical to the apices of teeth to facilitate repositioning of segments of the alveolus and dentition. (Oral Surg.)

otalgia dentalis (ō-tăl′jē-ah) Reflex pain in the ear due to dental disease; usually propagated along the auriculotemporal nerve. (Oral Surg.)

otic ganglion (see **ganglion, otic**)

otitis media (ō-tī′tĭs mē′dē-ah) Inflammation of the middle ear that may be marked by pain, fever, abnormalities of hearing, deafness, tinnitus, and vertigo. It may originate in the pharynx and be transmitted by the eustachian tubes. (Oral Physiol.)

otosclerosis (ō″tō-sklĕ-rō′sĭs) A disorder of the middle ear that generally results in hardening and fusion of the ossicles of the ear, with resultant immobilization, so that sound waves cannot be conducted along their paths. (Oral Physiol.)

outline form (see **form, outline**)

ovalocytosis (ō-văl″ō-sī-tō′sĭs) (see **elliptocytosis**)

overbite (see **overlap, vertical**)

deep o. (see **overlap, vertical, deep**)

overclosure Raising of the mandible too far before the teeth make contact; loss of occlusal vertical dimension is the cause. (Orthodont.) (see also **distance, interarch, reduced**)

overextended Pertaining to any extrusion beyond the apical opening into the periapical area. May be with instrumentation, medication, or root canal filling. (Endodont.)

overfilled Pertaining to extrusion or overextension of the root canal filling material beyond the apical opening. (Endodont.)

overhang Excess filling material projecting beyond cavity margins. (Oper. Dent.)

overhead Production costs required to be expended by the dentist in order to practice his profession; e.g., rent, utilities, salaries, laundry, etc. Costs involved in management, supplies, equipment, salaries (taxes), and maintenance. Amounts deducted from the gross receipts of a dental practice before the dentist's net income (take-home pay) is received. (Pract. Man.)

overjet (see **overlap, horizontal**)

overjut (see **overlap, horizontal**)

overlap, horizontal (**overjet, overjut**) Projection of the anterior and/or posterior teeth of one arch beyond their antagonists in a horizontal direction. (Comp. Prosth.; Remov. Part. Prosth.)

overlap, vertical (**overbite**) Extension of the upper teeth over the lower teeth in a vertical direction when the opposing posterior teeth are in contact in centric occlusion. This term is used especially to designate the distance the upper incisal edges drop below the level of the lower ones, but it may also be used to describe the vertical relations of opposing cusps of posterior teeth. (Comp. Prosth.; Remov. Part. Prosth.)

  deep v. o. (**closed bite, deep bite, deep overbite**) Excessive vertical overlap of the anterior teeth. (Orthodont.)

overlay A cast intracoronal restoration that includes the restoration of one or more cusps. May also designate extension of another material to include one or more cusps. (Oper. Dent.)

  o. denture A removable prosthesis constructed over existing natural teeth or implanted studs. (Cleft Palate)

overshooting accident The result of seating an endosteal implant beyond its normal host site (through the inferior mandibular border, into the mandibular canal or nasal or antral floor). (Oral Implant.)

ovoid arch (see **arch, ovoid**)

owner The person holding ownership, dominion, or title of property. (D. Juris.)

Owren's disease (see **parahemophilia**)

oxidation The combination of oxygen with other elements to form oxides. The process in which an element gains electrons. (Anesth.)

  o. of metal The formation of a surface oxide during the casting or soldering of a metal or during subsequent use by the patient. (Remov. Part. Prosth.)

oxide divinyl (see **ether, divinyl**)

oxycephaly (ŏk″sē-sĕ-fă′lē) (**steeple head**) A high conical crown resulting from early closure of sutures and disturbed cranial development. (Oral Diag.)

oxygenate (ŏk′sē-jĕ-nāt) To saturate with oxygen. (Oral Surg.)

oxyhemoglobin (ŏk″sē-hē″mō-glō′bĭn) A compound of hemoglobin with two atoms of oxygen. (Anesth.)

oxytocin (ŏk″sē-tō′sĭn) A hormone of the posterior pituitary gland that is the principal uterus-contracting hormone. It is used in obstetrics to induce uterine contractions. (Oral Med.)

P

PAB, PABA Abbreviation for para-aminobenzoic acid.

PAC (see **aspirin, phenacetin, caffeine**)

pachyderma oralis (păk″ĭ-der′mah ō-rā′lĭs) An appearance of the buccal mucosa suggestive of elephant hide. (Oral Diag.)

pachyderma oris (păk″ĭ-der′mah or′ĭs) (**focal keratosis, hyperkeratosis**) A benign white lesion of the mucous membrane characterized by a thick layer of keratin overlying stratified squamous epithelium, the cells of which are normal. (Oral Path.)

pachymucosa alba (păk″ĭ-mū-kō′sah ăl′bah) An appearance of the buccal mucosa resembling elephant hide with a white surface. (Oral Diag.)

Pacini's corpuscle (pah-chē′nēz) (see **corpuscle, Pacini's**)

pack A material used to protect tissue, to fill space, or to prevent hemorrhage. (Oral Med.; Pharmacol.)

> **periodontal p.** A surgical dressing applied to the necks of teeth and the adjacent tissue to cover and protect the surgical wound, thus serving as a matrix for the regenerating tissues and offering some protection against postoperative discomfort. (Periodont.)

packing The act of filling a mold. (Comp. Prosth.; Remov. Part. Prosth.)

> **denture p.** The laboratory procedure of filling and compressing a denture base material into a mold in a flask. (Comp. Prosth.; Remov. Part. Prosth.)

pad, Passavant's (**Passavant's bar, Passavant's ridge**) The bulging "cross roll" of the posterior pharyngeal wall produced by the upper portion of the superior pharyngeal constrictor muscle during the act of swallowing or during vocal effort. A ridge of erectile tissue on the posterior wall of the pharynx. (Comp. Prosth.; Remov. Part. Prosth.)

— (An objectionable term.) (Cleft Palate) (see **pharynx, activities of posterior and lateral pharyngeal wall**)

pad, retromolar (**pear-shaped area**) A mass of soft tissue, frequently pear shaped, that is located at the distal termination of the mandibular residual ridge. It is made up of fibers of the buccinator muscle, the pterygoman-dibular raphe, the superior constrictor muscle, the temporal tendon, and mucous glands. (Comp. Prosth.; Remov. Part. Prosth.)

pad, rubber dam (**rubber dam mask**) An absorbent piece of flannelette, bird's-eye cloth, or gauze of suitable shape to interpose between a rubber dam and the face to protect the face from contact with the rubber and with the clips of the dam holder. (Oper. Dent.)

Paget's disease (păj′ĕtz) (see **osteitis deformans**)

pain An unpleasant sensation created by a noxious stimulus mediated along specific nerve pathways to the central nervous system, where it is interpreted as such. (Anesth.)

— A sharp, prickling, burning, or aching sensation perceived as the result of a noxious stimulus. Pain stimuli, which may be initiated by chemical, electrical, and/or mechanical injury, have one property in common: they cause a threatened injury, with resultant withdrawal of a part. The sensation of pain is a protective mechanism that warns of· danger without giving too much information about the specific nature of the danger. It gives rise to nociceptive reflexes. (Oral Med.; Oral Physiol.)

> **chest p.** Pain that occurs in the chest region due to disorders of the heart (e.g., angina pectoris, myocardial infarction, and pericarditis), pulmonary artery (pulmonary embolism or hypertension), lungs (pleuritis), esophagus ("heartburn"), abdominal organs (aerophagia, biliary tract disease, splenic infarction, and gaseous distention in splenic flexure), or the chest wall (neoplasia, costochondral strains, and trauma, hyperventilation, and muscular tension). (Oral Med.)

> **deep p.** Dull, aching, or boring pain originating in muscles, tendons, and joints. It is poorly localized and tends to radiate. (Oral Med.)

> **ghost p.** (see **odontalgia, phantom**)

> **habit reference p.** Pain referred from one area to another area that has previously been the site of pain; e.g., aerodontalgia. (Oral Med.)

> **p. nerve ending** A receptor nerve ending that is relatively primitive and ends in an undifferentiated arborization. The nerve end-

ing for the sensation of pain is essentially a protective mechanism that warns of danger without giving too much information about the specific nature of the danger. The danger stimuli give rise to nociceptive reflexes, which are characterized by defensive, protective, or withdrawal movements. The nociceptive reflexes supercede other, less urgent reflexes that are thus inhibited. (Oral Physiol.)

p. perception The physiologicoanatomic process whereby the nerve impulse reaches the central nervous system. There is a sharp distinction between the reactions and sensations produced by pain from skin lesions and those produced by pain from deep visceral disorders. Sensations in the viscera are much less specific in character and localization than those in the mouth. Pain is poorly localized in intestinal colic, abdominal stress, labor pains, and a blow to the solar plexus or the testes. It is generally associated with generalized reactions of faintness, blanching, apnea, and vomiting. Somatic pain, however, is localized even when intense and is usually referable to a specific stimulus; e.g., pain from periodontosis or an aphthous ulcer in the buccal mucosa can usually be localized without difficulty. (Anesth.; Oral Physiol.)

projected pathologic p. Pain erroneously perceived to arise in a peripheral region because of a stimulus from end-organs supplying the region; e.g., sciatic pain. Actually, the stimulus has occurred somewhere along the pain pathway from the nerve to the cortex. (Oral Med.)

p. reaction The individual's manifestation of the unpleasant sensation. (Anesth.)

referred p. Pain caused by an agent in one area but manifested in another; e.g., pain caused by caries in the maxillary third molar may be referred to the mandible, so that the source of pain appears to be in the mandible. (Oral Diag.)

— Pain that is erroneously projected to a site distal and superficial to the point of stimulus of the peripheral end-organs of a pain pathway. (Oral Med.)

— Neuralgic pain sensed in other areas innervated by a sensory nerve rather than in the area stimulated. (Oral Surg.)

pair, ion (see **ion**)

palatal Relating to the palate.

p. bar (see **bar, palatal**)

p. perforation (see **perforation, palatal**)

p. plate (see **connector, major**)

p. seal (see **seal, posterior palatal**)

palate The roof of the mouth. It consists of a hard anterior part (the hard palate) and a soft movable part (the soft palate). (Comp. Prosth.)

cleft p. (**palatoschisis**) Congenital fissure of the soft palate and roof of the mouth, sometimes extending through the premaxilla and upper lip. (Cleft Palate)

— A cleft in the palate between the two palatal processes. If both hard and soft palates are involved, it is a uranostaphyloschisis; if only the soft palate is divided, it is a uranoschisis. The term cleft palate is often erroneously applied to clefts between the median nasal and maxillary processes through the alveolus. This type of cleft is properly termed cleft jaw, or gnathoschisis. (Oral Diag.)

— A deformity of the palate resulting from improper union or lack of union, during the second month of intrauterine development, of the maxillary process with the nasomedial process. (Orthodont.)

acquired c. p. Noncongenital defect of soft and/or hard tissues of the hard and soft palate. (Cleft Palate)

congenital c. p. Congenital nonunion or inadequacy of soft and hard tissues related to the lip, nose, alveolar process, hard palate, and velum. The extent of these deformities varies among individuals. Varieties of classifications are available to identify the extent of the cleft. (Cleft Palate)

soft p., redivision Surgical incision or removal of a V-shaped area of tissue from the soft palate to facilitate the proper placement of the pharyngeal section of the prosthetic speech aid. (Cleft Palate)

palatine arch (păl'ah-tīn) (see **arch, palatine**)

palatine mucosa (see **mucosa, palatine**)

palatine suture, median (see **suture, intermaxillary**)

palato- (păl'ah-tō) Prefix meaning pertaining to the palate. (Oral Surg.)

palatoplasty (păl'ah-tō-plăs"tē) Surgical repair of palatal defects. (Oral Surg.)

palatorrhaphy (păl"ah-tor'ah-fē) Surgical closure of a cleft palate with suturing. (Oral Surg.)

palatoschisis (păl"ah-tos'kĭ-sĭs) (see **palate, cleft**)

palinesthesia (păl"ĭn-ĕs-thē'zē-ah) Rapid termination of the anesthetic state and restoration to consciousness of a person under general anesthesia. (Anesth.)

pallesthesia (păl″ĕs-thē′zē-ah) (**bone sensibility**) Sensibility to vibrations; the vibrating sensation felt when a tuning fork is placed against a subcutaneous bony prominence. (Anesth.)

palliate (păl′ē-āt) To reduce the severity of. (Anesth.)

palliative (păl′ē-ā″tĭv) An alleviating measure. (Orthodont.)

pallor (păl′or) Paleness; absence of skin coloration. (Anesth.)

　perioral p. Paleness of soft tissues surrounding the mouth; an indication of impending syncope. (Oral Surg.)

palpate (păl′pāt) To examine the soft tissues digitally. (Oral Diag.)

palpation (păl-pā′shŭn) The act of feeling with the hand. (Anesth.)

— The use of the sense of touch for examination. (Oral Diag.)

—. A phase of the examination procedure in which the sense of touch is used to gather data essential for diagnosis. (Periodont.)

palpitation (păl″pĭ-tā′shŭn) Unduly rapid action of the heart that is perceptible to the patient. (Anesth.)

palsy (pawl′zē) Synonym for paralysis but preferred by some to refer to certain types of paralysis. (Oral Med.)

　Bell's p. A peripheral, unilateral type of facial paralysis that is usually transitory. (Oral Diag.)

　— Facial paralysis thought to be due to inflammation in or around the facial nerve. One side of the face sags, the corner of the mouth droops, the eyelid will not close, and saliva dribbles from the corner of the mouth on the affected side. (Oral Med.) (see also **paralysis, facial**)

　— A characteristic facial paralysis due to a lesion or an injury of the facial nerve. (Oral Surg.)

　cerebral p. Collective term for neurologic defects with associated disturbances of motor function. The disturbances vary in cause and anatomic type; e.g., acquired, hereditary, natal, postnatal, or congenital palsy. (Oral Med.)

　— Nonspecific term standing for a group of pathologies having the following common related characteristics: agenesis or a lesion of nervous tissue within the cranium; interference with voluntary muscular movements; disabling disorders of a chronic nature, neither acute nor progressive; and occurrence of the original lesion at the date of birth of the patient or before the development of learned human muscular function. (Oral Path.)

　— A condition caused by damage to the motor centers of the brain, resulting in varying disturbances of motor function and often accompanied by mental subnormality. (Pedodont.)

　creeping p. (see **gait, spastic**)

　facial p. Paralysis of the muscles supplied by the seventh cranial nerve. It may be associated with peripheral lesions, neoplasms invading the temporal bone, herpes zoster involving the geniculate ganglion, acoustic neuromas, and pontine disease. Bilateral paralysis may occur in uveoparotid fever and polyneuritis. (Oral Med.)

　lead p. Weakness and paralysis of the hand, wrist, and fingers associated with lead poisoning. (Oral Med.)

pamplegia (păm-plē′jē-ah) Total paralysis. (Anesth.)

panesthesia (păn″ĕs-thē′zē-ah) The sum of the sensations experienced. (Anesth.)

panhypopituitarism (păn-hī″pō-pĭ-tū′ĭ-tăr-ĭzm″) A deficiency involving all the hormonal functions of the pituitary gland. (Oral Med.) (see also **disease, Simmonds'**)

panneuritis endemica (păn″nū-rī′tĭs ĕn-dĕm′ē-kah) (see **beriberi**)

Panoramix A radiographic system in which the source of radiation is placed inside the mouth to expose a large film placed extraorally around the face. (Oral Radiol.)

Panorex A radiographic system (manufactured by the S. S. White Co.) that utilizes two axes of rotation to obtain a panoramic radiograph of the dental arches and their associated structures. (Oral Radiol.) (see also **pantomography**)

pansinusitis (păn″sī-nŭ-sī′tĭs) Inflammation of all the sinuses, as of the facial bones. (Oral Surg.)

pantograph (păn′tō-grăf) Figurative term given to a pair of face-bows fixed to both jaws and designed to inscribe centrically related points and arcs leading to them on segments of planes relatable to the three craniofacial planes of space. The maxillary planes are attached to the maxillary bow, and the inscribing styluses are attached to the mandibular bow. (Gnathol.)

pantomography (păn-tō-mŏg′rah-fē) Panoramic radiography by which radiographs of the maxillary and mandibular dental arches and their associated structures may be obtained. Three x-radiation generating devices are now in use for pantomography: the Panorex, the Ortho-pantomograph, and the General Electric 3000. (Oral Radiol.)

paper, articulating (see **articulating paper**)

paper point A cone of absorbent paper so formed that it can be inserted into the length of the root canal and used to absorb fluid, to carry medication into the canal, or to inoculate cultures. (Endodont.)

papilla(e) (pah-pĭl′ah) Any small, nipple-shaped elevation. (Comp. Prosth.; Remov. Part. Prosth.)

incisive p. The elevation of soft tissue covering the foramen of the incisive or naso-palatine canal. (Comp. Prosth.; Orthodont.; Remov. Part. Prosth.)

interdental p. The part of the gingivae filling the interproximal spaces between adjacent teeth, consisting partly of free and partly of attached gingivae. (Periodont.)

interproximal p. The cone-shaped projection of the gingiva filling the interdental spaces up to the contact areas when viewed from the labial, buccal, and lingual aspects. When viewed buccolingually or labiolingually, the crest of the interproximal papilla presents a rounded concavity at an area below the contact point of the teeth. If recession has occurred, this concavity may become an area of pathology, and the entire papilla may require reshaping in order to restore health. (Periodont.) (see also **papilla, interdental**)

palatine p. A convexly rounded and elliptically shaped pad of soft tissue lying palatal to the upper central incisors. (Periodont.)

pseudo-p. False papillae formed by the presence of deeply depressed lines or grooves on the interdental papillae or the marginal gingivae but *without* the separation of the tissue seen with cleft formation. (Periodont.)

papillary-marginal-attached (păp′ĭ-lăr″ē) (see **PMA**)

papilloma (păp″ĭ-lō′mah) A benign neoplasm of epithelium often having a warty appearance. (Oral Diag.)

— A benign, exophytic, pedunculated, cauliflower-like neoplasm of epithelium. (Oral Path.)
   basal cell p. (see **keratosis, seborrheic**)

papillomatosis, inflammatory (păp″ĭ-lō′mah-tō′sĭs) (see **hyperplasia, papillary, inflammatory**)

papillomatosis, multiple (see **hyperplasia, papillary, inflammatory**)

Papillon-Lefevre syndrome (see **syndrome, Papillon-Lefevre**)

papule (păp′ūl) A small, circumscribed, solid elevation of the skin. (Oral Surg.)

split p. A secondary lesion of syphilis seen at the angle of the lips, with part on each lip. (Oral Diag.)

— A secondary syphilid at the angle of the mouth, resulting from the formation of a papule that becomes fissured because of its position. (Oral Med.)

— Fissured papillary lesions that resemble those of perlèche; found at the corners of the mouth in secondary syphilis. (Periodont.)

paradontosis (par″ah-don-tō′sĭs) (see **periodontosis**)

parafunction Synonym for bruxism. In medicine the term "parakinesia" is used for identifying motor functional disorders that result in strange and harmful movements. (Gnathol.)

— Movements (such as bruxism, clenching, and rocking of teeth) that are considered outside or beyond function and that result in worn facets. (Periodont.)

parahemophilia (par″ah-hē″mō-fĭl′ē-ah) (**ac-globulin deficiency, hemophilioid state A, Owren's disease**) A hemorrhagic disorder due to a deficiency of proaccelerin. Manifestations include mild to severe bleeding after extraction of teeth or other surgical procedures, epistaxis, easy bruisability, menorrhagia, and hematomas. The one-stage prothrombin time is prolonged, but the bleeding time is ordinarily normal. (Oral Med.)

parakeratosis (par″ah-kĕr″ah-tō′sĭs) Persistence of nuclei in the stratum corneum of stratified squamous epithelium. (Oral Path.)

— Presence of an epithelial surface of a layer of cells with flattened nuclei. (Periodont.)

parakinesia Literally a state of wild motions. This term characterizes well the seizures of mandibular muscles in both procursive and laterocursive night grinding of the teeth during disturbed sleep. (Gnathol.)

paralgesia (păr″al-jē′zē-ah) (**paralgia**) Any condition marked by abnormal and painful sensations; a painful paresthesia. (Anesth.)

paralgia (păr-ăl′jē-ah) (see **paralgesia**)

parallel attachment (see **attachment, parallel**)

parallelism The condition of two or more surfaces which, if extended to infinity, could never meet. In removable partial prosthodontics such a condition is created on vertical tooth surfaces to act as guiding planes. (Remov. Part. Prosth.)

parallelometer (par″ah-lĕl-om′ĕ-ter) An apparatus used to determine parallelism or a lack of parallelism or to make a part or an object parallel with some other part or object. (Comp. Prosth.; Remov. Part. Prosth.) (see also **surveyor**)

paralysis Cessation of cell function. (Anesth.)
— Loss or impairment of the motor control or function of a part or region. (Oral Diag.; Oral Med.)

   facial p. Paralysis of the muscles of facial expression due to supranuclear, nuclear, or peripheral nerve disease. (Oral Med.) (see also **palsy, Bell's**)
   — Paralysis of the facial musculature that may be due to disease of the peripheral nerve branches of the facial nerve. When the paralysis is mild and the face is at rest, the disorder is not readily observed. However, during muscular contraction (e.g., wrinkling the forehead, blinking the eyes, pursing the lips, or speaking), the disorder is very marked. Only one lid may close, and the asymmetry of the mouth is pronounced because the normal buccinator muscle contracts and is unopposed by the weakness on the paralyzed side. This imbalance produces a marked asymmetry. The affected side remains smooth, and the normal side shows marked contraction. (Oral Physiol.)

   infantile p. (see **poliomyelitis**)

   motor p. A loss of the power of skeletal muscle contraction due to interruption of some part of the pathway from the cerebrum to the muscle. (Oral Med.)

paramolar A supernumerary molar tooth located buccal or lingual to a normal molar, as distinguished from a distomolar, which is behind the third molar. (Oral Diag.; Oral Path.)

paranalgesia (par″ăn-ăl-jē′zē-ah) Analgesia of the lower part of the body, including the lower limbs. (Anesth.)

paranesthesia (par″ăn-ĕs-thē′zē-ah) Anesthesia of the lower part of the body and limbs. (Anesth.)

paranoia (par″ah-noi′ah) Mental derangement characterized by delusions and hallucinations that are well systematized. (Oral Med.)
— The irrational belief that one is the object of special persecution by others or by fate. (Oral Physiol.)

paraproteinemia (par″ah-prō″tē-ĭ-nē′mē-ah) An increase in protein in the blood due to aberrant protein synthesis. (Oral Med.)

paraspasmus faciale (par-ah-spăz′mŭs fā″cē-ăl′ē) A painless motor disturbance affecting both sides of the face. (Oral Diag.)

parasympatholytic (par″ah-sĭm″pah-thō-lĭt′ĭk) (see **anticholinergic**)

parasympathomimetic (par″ah-sĭm″pah-thō-mĭ-mĕt-ĭk) (see **cholinergic**)

Para-thor-mone (păr″ah-thor′mōn) Proprietary brand of parathyroid hormone. (Pharmacol.)

Parathyrin (păr″ah-thī′rĭn) Proprietary brand of parathyroid hormone. (Pharmacol.)

parenteral (pah-rĕn′ter-ăl) Not through the alimentary canal (literally, aside from the gastrointestinal tract); i.e., by subcutaneous, intramuscular, intravenous, or other nongastrointestinal route of administration. (Anesth.; Oral Med.; Pharmacol.)

paresis (pah-rē′sĭs) (**dementia paralytica, paretic neurosyphilis**) A progressive psychosis associated with neurosyphilis. (Oral Med.)

paresthesia (păr″ĕs-thē′zē-ah) Morbid or perverted sensation; sensation such as burning or prickling. (Anesth.)
— A perverted sensation causing itching, numbness, or tingling. Often associated with injury, resection, or regeneration of nerves. (Oral Diag.; Oral Med.)
— An altered sensation reported by the patient in an area where the sensory nerve has been afflicted by a disease or an injury; the patient may report burning, prickling, formication, or other sensations. (Oral Surg.)

parol (pah-rōl′) Oral or verbal; expressed by speech only; not expressed in writing. (D. Juris.)

parotitis (par″ō-tī′tĭs) Inflammation of the parotid gland. (Oral Diag.; Oral Med.; Oral Path.) (see also **mumps**)

   endemic p. (**epidemic p., infectious p., mumps**) An acute viral infection characterized by unilateral or bilateral swelling of the salivary glands, especially the parotid. (Oral Path.)

   epidemic p. (see **parotitis, endemic**)

   infectious p. (see **parotitis, endemic**)

paroxysmal (păr″ok-sĭz′mal) Recurring in paroxysms. (Anesth.)

Parry's disease (see **goiter, exophthalmic; hyperthyroidism**)

partial anodontia (see **oligodontia**) Congenital absence of some of the primary and permanent teeth. May be accompanied by other evidence of ectodermal dysplasia. (Pedodont.)

partial denture retention (see **retention, denture, partial**)

particle A small amount of material.
   alpha p. (**alpha ray, alpha radiation**) Positively charged particulate ionizing radiation consisting of helium nuclei (two protons and two neutrons) traveling at high speeds. Such

rays are emitted from the nucleus of an unstable element. (Oral Radiol.)

beta p. (**beta ray, beta radiation**) Particulate ionizing radiation consisting of either negative electrons (negatrons) or positive electrons (positrons) emitted from the nucleus of an unstable element. Such a phenomenon is called beta decay. (Oral Radiol.)

parties The persons who take part in the performance of any act, or who have a direct interest in any contract or conveyance, or who are actively involved in the prosecution and defense of any legal proceeding. (D. Juris.)

partnership The association of two or more persons for the purpose of carrying on business (or practice) together and dividing its profits. (D. Juris.)

— A legal, binding agreement for sharing all aspects of a professional dental practice. (Pract. Man.)

    notice of dissolution of p. Intelligence, by whatever means communicated, to creditors and the public that a partnership has been dissolved. (D. Juris.)

Partsch's operation (see **operation, Partsch's**)

parulis (pah-roo'lĭs) (**gumboil**) An elevated nodule at the site of a fistula draining a chronic periapical abscess. These nodules occur most frequently in relation to pulpally involved deciduous teeth. (Oral Diag.)

Pascal's law (see **law, Pascal's**)

P.A. skull (see **examination, radiographic, extraoral, posteroanterior**)

Passavant's bar (see **pad, Passavant's**)

Passavant's pad (see **pad, Passavant's**)

Passavant's ridge (see **pad, Passavant's**)

passer, foil (see **foil passer**)

passive Referring to an orthodontic appliance that has been adjusted to apply no effective tooth moving force to the teeth. (Orthodont.)

passivity The quality or condition of inactivity or rest assumed by the teeth, tissues, and denture when a removable denture is in place but is not under masticatory pressure. (Comp. Prosth.; Remov. Part. Prosth.)

passive reciprocation (see **reciprocation, passive**)

paste A soft, smooth, semifluid mixture, often medicated. (Oral Med.; Pharmacol.)

    p. filler A semisoft mixture of materials used to fill the root canal system, as opposed to solid filling material such as silver or guttapercha cones. (Endodont.)

    pressure-indicating p. A soft mixture used to disclose areas of contact or pressure in restorations. (Fixed Part. Prosth.)

patch, mucous An ulcerated lesion of the mucous membrane having a mucoid appearance. It is a secondary lesion of syphilis. (Oral Diag.)

— A lesion of secondary syphilis occurring on the oral mucosa and consisting of a pearl-gray translucent elevation of mucous membrane. (Oral Med.)

— Multiple gray-white patch overlying an area of ulceration and occurring on the oral mucosa as an expression of secondary syphilis. Highly infectious. (Oral Path.; Periodont.) (see also **syphilis**)

path A certain course that is ordinarily followed.

    p. of appliance insertion and removal (see **insertion, path of**)

    p. of closure (see **closure, centric path of**)

    condyle p. (see **condyle path**)

    lateral c. p. (see **condyle path, lateral**)

    idling p. The path that a stamp cusp travels when the bolus is being treated on the other side of the mouth. (Gnathol.)

    p. of insertion (see **insertion, path of**)

    milled-in p. Any one of the contours carved by various mandibular movements into the occluding surface of an occlusion rim by teeth or studs placed in the opposing occlusion rim. The curves or contours may be carved into wax, acrylic resin, modeling compound, or plaster of paris. (Comp. Prosth.; Remov. Part. Prosth.)

    occlusal p. A gliding occlusal contact. The path of movement of an occlusal surface. (Comp. Prosth.)

    generated o. p. A registration of the paths of movement of the occlusal surfaces of teeth on a wax, plastic, or abrasive surface attached to the opposing dental arch. (Comp. Prosth.; Fixed Part. Prosth.; Remov. Part. Prosth.)

    o. p. registration The cutting of a wax record by the teeth of the opposing dental arch when the record is worn by the patient. (Remov. Part. Prosth.)

    p. of placement The direction in which a removable dental restoration is positioned in relation to the planned location on its supporting structures. The restoration is removed in the opposite direction. (Remov. Part. Prosth.) (see also **placement, choice of path of**)

    working p. The path that the stamp cusps make when working on the bolus. At first the bolus deflects the direction of these cusps, but after the fibers of the food have been reduced enough to be almost ready for swallowing, the travel coincides directionally with the working groove. (Gnathol.)

pathfinder (see **broach, smooth**)

pathogenic occlusion (păth-ō-jĕn'ĭk) (see **occlusion, pathogenic**)

pathognomonic (păth″ŏg-nō-mŏn'ĭk) A sign or symptom significantly unique to a disease; distinguishes it from other diseases. (Oral Med.)

pathology (pah-thol'ō-jē) The branch of medical science that deals with disease in all its relations, especially with its nature and the functional and material changes it causes. (Comp. Prosth.; Remov. Part. Prosth.)

— In medical jurisprudence, the science of diseases; the part of medicine that deals with the nature of disease, their causes, and their symptoms. (D. Juris.)

   experimental p. The study of disease processes induced usually in animals; undertaken to ascertain the effect of local environmental changes and/or systemic disorders on particular tissues, parts, and organs of the body. This branch of medical science also attempts to correlate the interplay of local and systemic factors in the production, modification, and continuance of a disease. (Periodont.)

   p. of joint (see **joint pathology**)

   speech p. The study and treatment of all aspects of functional and organic speech defects and disorders. (Cleft Palate)

pathosis (pah-thō'sĭs) A disease entity. Not to be called pathology. (Comp. Prosth.; Remov. Part. Prosth.)

— A pathologic condition. A patient is said to have a pathosis rather than pathology, which is the study of disease. (Oral Diag.)

pathway of inflammation The route of extension of chronic gingival inflammation into the subjacent structures, extending into the interdental septum from the gingivae, along the interdental vessels, and/or following the course of these blood vesesls onto the periosteal side of the bone as well as into the bone marrow spaces. (Periodont.)

patient A person under medical or dental care. (D. Juris.)

pattern A form used to make a mold, as for a denture, an inlay, or a partial denture framework. (Comp. Prosth.; Remov. Part. Prosth.)

   occlusal p. The form or design of the occluding surfaces of a tooth or teeth. These forms may be based on natural or modified anatomic or nonanatomic concepts of teeth. (Comp. Prosth.; Fixed Part. Prosth.; Remov. Part. Prosth.)

   trabecular p. The trabecular arrangement of alveolar bone in relation to marrow spaces; may be radiographically interpreted. (Periodont.)

   p. vision (see **vision, pattern**)

   wax p. A wax form of a denture (trial denture) that, when it is invested in a flask and the wax is eliminated, will form the mold in which the resin denture is formed. (Comp. Prosth.)

   — A wax form of a shape that, when invested and eliminated, will produce a mold in which the casting is made. (Comp. Prosth.; Fixed Part. Prosth.; Remov. Part. Prosth.)

   — A wax model for making the mold in which the metal will be formed in casting. (D. Mat.; Oper. Dent.)

   wear p. The topographic attributes and distribution of areas of tooth wear (facets) that are due to attritional effects of food, tooth contacts during swallowing, the terminal aspects of the masticatory cycle, and the habits of occlusal neuroses. Wear patterns may be used to determine many of the functional and afunctional movements the mandible has been passing through in preceding years. Occlusal wear occurs with aging. The type of wear is termed the wear pattern. (Periodont.)

Paul-Bunnell test (see **test, Paul-Bunnell**)

pauperissimus (paw-per-ĭs'sē-mŭs) (**Pp**) Latin term meaning poorest. Sometimes written on prescriptions to indicate to the pharmacist that the patient is being charged less than the usual fee by the dentist or physician. (Oral Med.; Pharmacol.)

payable Pertaining to an obligation to pay at a future time; when used without restriction or modification, the term means that the debt is payable at once. (D. Juris.)

payment The performance of a duty or promise, or the discharge of a debt or liability by the delivery of money or something else of value. (D. Juris.)

payroll record A printed form on which detailed records are kept of the amounts of money paid to auxiliaries. The record has columns for all the necessary tax deductions so that a detailed record is available for tax reporting and cost accounting. (Pract. Man.)

PBI (see **iodine, protein-bound**)

p.c. (**post cibum**) Latin term meaning after meals. The abbreviation may be used in writing prescriptions. (Oral Med.; Pharmacol.)

PDL (see **ligament, periodontal**)

peak, buccal Outer high point of the normal interproximal tissue that rises to a peak; connected interdentally to lingual peak by a triangular ridge, with a depression termed a col. (Periodont.)

pearl, enamel (enameloma) A small focal mass of enamel formed apical to the cementoenamel junction and resembling pearls. The bifurcation of molar roots is a favorite site for this aberration in tooth development. (Oral Diag.; Oral Path.)

pearls, Epstein's (see **nodules, Bohn's**)

pedicle flap (see **flap, pedicle**)

pedodontics (pĕ″dō-don′tĭks) (**dentistry for children**) The branch of dentistry that includes training the child to accept dentistry; restoring and maintaining the primary, mixed, and permanent dentitions; applying preventive measures for dental caries and periodontal disease; and preventing, intercepting, and correcting various problems of occlusion. (Pedodont.)

pegs, epithelial (rete pegs) Papillary projections of epithelium into the underlying stroma of connecting tissue that normally occur in mucous membrane and dermal tissues subject to functional stimulation. They occur to excess where epithelium-lined tissues are irritated and inflamed. (Periodont.)

pegs, rete (see **pegs, epithelial**)

pellagra A nutritional deficiency due to faulty intake or metabolism of nicotinic acid, a vitamin B complex factor. (Oral Diag.)

— A nutritional disease due to a deficiency of nicotinic acid. It is characterized by glossitis, dermatitis of sun-exposed surfaces, stomatitis, diarrhea, and dementia. Thiamine, riboflavin, and tryptophan deficiencies may be associated. (Oral Med.)

— A condition due to deficiency of niacin and characterized by keratotic skin lesions, mental changes, diarrhea, and oral changes, which include scarlet glossitis, atrophy of the papillae of the tongue, and glossopyrosis. (Oral Path.)

— A deficiency syndrome due to a lack of niacin and other vitamin B complex fractions in the diet; characterized by weakness, debility, digestive disturbances, convulsions, melancholia, erythema of the skin, burning sensations of the tongue and mucous membranes of the mouth, hypertrophied papillae on the tongue, diffuse burning erythema of the oral mucous membranes, desquamation of the papillae of the tongue, massive periodontal breakdown, and a gingival condition resembling acute necrotizing ulcerative gingivitis. (Periodont.)

pellet A small, rounded mass of material. (Oper. Dent.)

cotton p. A rolled ball of cotton varying in diameter from approximately ⅜ to ⅛ inch (larger size is cotton ball; smaller size is pledget). (Oper. Dent.)

foil p. A loosely rolled piece of gold foil of various thicknesses; prepared from a portion—1/128, 1/96, 1/64, 1/48, 1/32, 1/16—cut from a 4-inch square of foil. (Oper. Dent.)

pellicle A film or membrane. (Oral Diag.)

brown p. A specific name for a brownish gray to black film formed over a period of time on the surfaces of the teeth of 20% to 25% of the population as a result of not using an abrasive-containing dentifrice. (Oral Diag.)

pemphigoid, benign mucous membrane (pĕm′fĭ-goid) A bullous disease that resembles pemphigus but is more chronic in nature. The oral mucosa, especially the gingiva where it resembles desquamative gingivitis, and the conjunctiva are the sites of predilection. Skin is involved in about 20% of the cases. (Oral Diag.)

pemphigus (pĕm′fĭ-gŭs) A fatal disease characterized by bullae on the skin and oral mucosa. (Oral Diag.)

— A rare, grave skin disease of unknown etiology characterized by the development of bullae on the skin and mucous membrane. (Oral Path.) (see also **bulla; sign, Nikolsky's**)

acute disseminated p. A dread disease of unknown etiology, temporarily controlled by the administration of corticosteroids. Manifested by bullous formation on the skin and mucous membranes. Desquamation of the epithelium exposes a raw, burning, oozing submucosa. Adequate nutritional status is difficult to maintain; secondary infection is common; with progressive debility, pneumonia is common and is usually the cause of death. (Periodont.)

pen grasp (see **grasp, pen**)

penetrability (pĕn″ĕ-trah-bĭl′ĭ-tē) The ability of a beam of x radiation to pass through matter. The degree of penetrability is determined by kilovoltage and filtration. (Oral Radiol.)

penetrating (pĕn′ĕ-trā-tĭng) Piercing; entering deeply. (Oral Surg.)

penetration (pĕn″ĕ-trā′shŭn) The ability of radiation to extend down into and go through substances. The degree of penetration is determined by the kilovoltage. (Oral Radiol.)

penetrometer (pĕn″ĕ-trom′ĕ-ter) An aluminum step wedge or ladder exposed over a film to determine the quality or penetrating ability of a specific beam of x radiation. (Oral Radiol.)

penicillin An antibiotic secured from cultures of *Penicillium notatum*, being bacteriocidal for gram-positive cocci, some gram-negative cocci (gonococcus and meningococcus), the clostridia, and the spirochetal organisms. Its topical application to the oral mucous membranes is discouraged because of the high risk of sensitization from local application of antibiotic substances. (Periodont.)

pentobarbital sodium (pĕn″tō-bar′bĭ-tal) Monosodium ethyl (1-methylbutyl) barbiturate, used for its sedative and hypnotic effects; usual dosage, ¾ to 1½ gr. Useful as a preoperative sedative in dentistry. (Periodont.)

penumbra, geometric (pĕ-nŭm′brah) Partial or imperfect shadow about the umbra, or true shadow, of an object. In radiography, it is influenced by the size of the focal spot, the focal-film distance, and the object-film distance. (Oral Radiol.) (see also **geometric unsharpness**)

   g. transmission p. The region of free space irradiated by photons that have traversed only part of the thickness of the collimator (i.e., the part of the collimator at its lower edge). (Oral Radiol.)

   g. p., width The width of the penumbra in a plane perpendicular to the central ray at any distance of interest from the source. (Oral Radiol.)

perception, occlusal The patient's cognizance of occlusal patterns and disharmonies, mediated by the proprioceptive sense of the nerve fibers of the periodontal membrane. (Periodont.)

percolation Extraction of the soluble parts of a drug by causing a liquid solvent to flow slowly through it. (Oper. Dent.)

percussion (per-kŭsh′ŭn) The act of striking an area, a structure, or an organ as an aid in diagnosing a diseased condition by the sensations reported by the patient and by the sounds heard by the examiner. (Oral Surg.; Periodont.)

perfectionism (per-fĕk′shŭn-ĭzm) A behavior pattern that reveals an exaggerated independence and frequently demands perfectionist goals. The trait of perfectionism is exhibited when the patient attempts too much too rapidly in learning to masticate with a new fixed or removable prosthesis. He may disregard the instructions to ingest small morsels of food and to avoid chewing bread crusts and biting bones before the proprioceptor mechanism can adjust to the new occlusal pattern. (Oral Physiol.)

perforation osteotomy (see **osteotomy, perforation**)

perforation, palatal A perforation that exists in the palatal area after the surgical repair of a cleft. (Cleft Palate)

perforation, radicular An artificial opening or hole made by boring or cutting through the lateral aspect of the root. Also occurs as the result of internal or external resorption. (Endodont.)

perforation, sublabial A perforation existing in the upper labial sulcus after surgical repair of the area. The perforation communicates between the oral and nasal cavities. (Cleft Palate)

performance Fulfillment of a promise, contract, or other obligation. (D. Juris.)

periadenitis mucosa necrotica recurrens (per″ē-ăd-ĕ-nī′tĭs) (**Mikulicz' aphthae, Mikulicz' ulcer, recurrent scarring aphthae, Sutton's disease**) A recurrent aphthous ulcer on the oral mucosa that clinically simulates herpes simplex but heals slowly by scar formation. (Oral Diag.; Oral Path.)

— Involvement of the oral mucosa with deep-seated aphthouslike ulcers that tend to heal with scars. It may be impossible to differentiate the disease from Behçet's syndrome in the absence of a diagnosis of cyclic neutropenia. (Oral Med.)

perialveolar wiring (see **wiring, perialveolar**)

periapex (per″ē-ā′pĕks) That area of tissue which immediately surrounds the root apex. (Endodont.)

periapical (per″ē-ā′pĭ-kal) Enclosing or surrounding the apical area of a tooth root. (Oper. Dent.; Oral Surg.)

   p. radiograph A radiograph demonstrating tooth apices and surrounding structures in a particular intraoral area. (Oral Radiol.)

   p. radiographic survey A series of intraoral radiographs depicting periapical areas of interest. A complete mouth radiographic survey may consist of seventeen or more intraoral radiographs that demonstrate all areas of the oral cavity. (Oral Radiol.)

periauricular (per″ē-aw-rĭk′ū-lar) Surrounding the external ear. (Oral Surg.)

pericementitis (per″ē-sē″mĕn-tī′tĭs) (see **periodontitis**)

pericervical saucerization (see **saucerization, pericervical**)

pericoronitis (per″ē-kor″ō-nī′tĭs) (**operculitis**) Inflammation of the operculum or tissue flap over a partially erupted tooth, particularly a third molar. Inflammation around a crown, particularly the inflammation of a partially erupted tooth. (Oral Diag.)

— Inflammation of the soft tissues surrounding

the crown of an erupting tooth. Frequently seen in association with erupting mandibular third molars and usually accompanied by infection. (Oral Surg.)

— An acute inflammation of the gingivae surrounding teeth that are incompletely erupted or that, because of their location in the arch, cannot be completely freed of enveloping gingivae. Characterized by edema, severe inflammation of the enveloping tissues, trismus, lymphadenopathy, etc. (Periodont.)

peridens (per-ē-dĕnz') An accessory tooth located buccal or labial to the dental arch. (Oral Path.)

peri-implant space The space between an implant and its investing tissues. (Oral Implant.)

peri-implantoclasia (per″ē-ĭm-plăn″tō-klā′zē-ah) A general term defining disease surrounding and/or involving implanted foreign materials. Peri-implantoclasia is a catabolic condition surrounding an implant with or without sepsis or suppuration. (Oral Implant.)

— A general term defining disease surrounding and/or involving implanted foreign material. It is a catabolic condition surrounding an implant with or without sepsis or suppuration. (Oral Implant.)

exfoliative p. A condition wherein the implant is exfoliating, exposing the struts, and causing localized tissue inflammation. (Oral Implant.)

resorption p. A condition in which the supporting bone structure has resorbed under either vertical or lateral stresses. This may be due to pressure atrophy from excessive masticatory pressures, excessive increase of the vertical dimension, or insufficient metal coverage of the supporting bone structures. (Oral Implant.)

traumatic p. A condition in which constant abuse or an injury has dislodged, distorted, fractured, or disturbed an implant. (Oral Implant.)

ulcerative p. An inflammatory condition that presents various degrees of ulceration; characterized by hyperplasia, hyperemia, edema, and pain. Suppuration may exist from the abscesses. Etiology may be oral sepsis, a loose screw, latent surgical infection, galvanic action of improper metal, etc. (Oral Implant.)

necrotic u. p. An inflammatory and infectious condition that presents various degrees of necrosis, ulceration, hyperplasia, hyperemia, edema, sloughing, and tendency to bleed easily. The etiology is usu-

ally oral sepsis, combined with food impaction and large deposits of salivary calculus. (Oral Implant.)

perineural fibroblastoma (per″ĭ-nū′ral) (see **neurilemoma; neurofibroma**)

period, latent The area of delay between the time of exposure of an organism to radiation and the manifestation of the changes produced by that radiation. This delay is dependent on many factors, but particularly on the magnitude of the dose. The larger the dose, the earlier the appearance of the injury. In some instances the latent period for some effects may be as long as twenty-five years or more. (Oral Radiol.)

periodontal (per″ē-ō-don′tal) Relating to the periodontium.

p. atrophy (see **atrophy, periodontal**)

p. chisel (see **chisel, periodontal**)

p. pack (see **pack, periodontal**)

p. pocket (see **pocket, periodontal**)

p. probe (see **probe, periodontal**)

p. prosthesis (see **prosthesis, periodontal**)

p. therapy (see **therapy, periodontal**)

p. treatment planning The sequential arrangement of therapeutic procedures required to obtain a healthy gingival attachment and an intact, functioning attachment apparatus. Periodontal therapy cannot be performed on an empiric basis but rests on an integrated knowledge of the theory and practice of periodontology. (Periodont.)

periodontia (per″ē-ō-don′shē-ah) (see **periodontics**)

periodontics (per″ē-ō-don′tĭks) The art and science of examination, diagnosis, and treatment of diseases affecting the periodontium; a study of the supporting structures of the teeth, including not only the normal anatomy and physiology of these structures but also the deviations from normal. (Periodont.)

concept of cure in p. The idea that a successful result in periodontal therapy consists of restoring any tooth or collection of teeth to functional capability, regardless of whether they are able to function alone or require stabilization to survive. The concept of cure does not include the salvaging of hopelessly involved teeth. (Periodont.)

periodontitis (per″ē-ō-don-tī′tĭs) (**periodontal inflammation**) Inflammation of the periodontium. (Oral Diag.; Oral Path.)

— The alterations occurring in the periodontium with inflammation. Gingival changes are those of gingivitis, with the clinical signs described under gingivitis. Periodontitis presents histologic characteristics such as ulceration of the sulcular epithelium, epithelial hyperplasia, proliferation of epithelial rete pegs into the gingival corium, apical migration of the epithelial attachment after lysis of the gingival fiber apparatus, cellular and exudative infiltrate into tissues, and increased capillarity. With the extension of gingival inflammation into bone, bone resorption ensues. With resorption of bone in an apical direction, attachment of the periodontal fibers to the bone is progressively lost. A transseptal band of reconstituted periodontal fibers walls off the gingival inflammation from the underlying bone. A chronic, progressive disease of the periodontium. (Periodont.)

acute p. A sharply localized acute inflammatory process involving the interproximal and marginal areas of two or more adjacent teeth, characterized by severe pain, purulent exudate from edematous inflamed gingivae, general malaise, fever, and sequestration of the crestal aspects of the alveolar process. (Periodont.)

bacteria in p. Role of microorganisms in the initiation of chronic inflammatory lesions of the periodontium. There is little evidence for a direct role; however, the general authoritative consensus holds that microorganisms and their toxic products play a major part in the modification and perpetuation of periodontitis. (Periodont.)

p. in children (see **periodontitis, juvenile**)

chronic periapical p. Periapical inflammation characterized by dental granuloma formation. (Oral Diag.)

juvenile p. Marginal periodontitis present in children or adolescents, with radiographic and clinical findings similar to those observed in the adult, including gingivitis, periodontal pocket formation, bone resorption, etc. (Periodont.)

marginal p. The sequela to gingivitis in which the inflammatory process has spread apically to involve the alveolar process. An inflammation of the marginal periodontium with resorption of the crest of alveolar bone; there is apical migration of the epithelial attachment with suprabony and/or infrabony pocket formation and cuplike resorptions and marginal translucence of the alveolar crest. In children the process may be more rapid and destructive than in adults. (Periodont.)

   diagnosis of m. p. Determination of marginal periodontitis by consideration of the salient

diagnostic features: loss of uniform coloration of gingival tissues, loss of gingival stippling, thickening and retraction of the gingival margin, presence of calculus and/or other etiologic factors, formation of a periodontal pocket, and resorption of the interdental alveolar crest and/or buccal, labial, palatal, or lingual alveolar crest. The tissues affected in periodontitis are the gingivae, alveolar bone, supporting bone, and the part of the periodontal membrane above and adjacent to the alveolar crest. (Periodont.)

   epithelium in m. p. Epithelial changes noted in marginal periodontitis, including ulceration of the sulcular (cervical) epithelium and pseudoepitheliomatous hyperplasia (downward proliferation of epithelium caused by hyperplasia of the stratum spinosum epidermidis). (Periodont.)

   exudate in m. p. The substance of serous, fibrinous, or purulent nature that passes through the ulcerated epithelium of the pocket from the underlying soft tissue corium when those tissues are inflamed. The purulent fibrinous or serous substance present in the area of the pocket formed in marginal periodontitis. The exudate forms as a result of inflammation involving the ulcerated sulcular epithelium and underlying connective tissue. (Periodont.)

   inflammatory cells in m. p. The lymphocytes and plasma cells, with occasional histiocytes, comprising the primary substance of the infiltrate in marginal periodontitis. If the acute phase should occur, polymorphonuclear leukocytes are present. (Periodont.)

   pocket in m. p. (see **pocket in marginal periodontitis**)

periodontium (per″ē-ō-don′shē-ŭm) The tissues that invest (or help to invest) and support the teeth; i.e., the gingivae, the cementum of the tooth, the periodontal ligament, and the alveolar and supporting bone. (Periodont.)

dietary influences on p. The role of the patient's nutritional status in periodontal disease. Nutritional inadequacies may initiate degenerative changes in the periodontium or may modify previously existing periodontal disease; e.g., protein depletion may produce osteoporotic changes in supporting bone, resorption of alveolar bone, and disintegration of the alveolar group of periodontal fibers. The superimposition of protein depletion will produce more rapid periodontal destruction in an individual with periodontitis that was initiated by local factors such as calculus. (Periodont.)

endocrine influences on p. The alterations induced in the periodontium as a result of hormonal imbalances; e.g., the excessive production of thyroxin in hyperthyroidism can produce catabolic tissue changes resulting in osteoporosis of the supporting bone of the alveolar process; decreased estrogenic stimulation as a result of menopause may affect epithelial integrity, with resultant desquamative gingival lesions. (Periodont.)

local influence on p. Factors within the oral cavity or the stomatologic system that may initiate, perpetuate, or modify periodontal disease; e.g., dental calculus, by acting as a physical irritant, may produce ulceration of sulcular epithelium and other changes. (Anesth.)

physiology of p. Study of the individual and integrated functional attributes of the structures comprising the periodontium. The periodontium serves to invest and support the teeth; portions thereof serve as an attachment apparatus for function (cementum, periodontal membrane, and bone), whereas the gingivae serve as a covering and protective tissue. (Periodont.)

systemic influences on p. Diseases affecting bodily structures (other than those of the stomatologic system), which may initiate, perpetuate, or modify lesions of the periodontium; e.g., emotional stress, through the mediation of the adrenal cortex with increased production of glucocorticoids, may decrease antibody formation and thus permit overgrowth of the fusospirochetal organisms producing necrotizing ulcerative gingivitis. (Periodont.)

periodontosis (per″ē-ō-don-tō′sĭs) **(diffuse alveolar atrophy)** Degeneration of the periodontium. (Oral Diag.)

— A noninflammatory condition affecting the periodontium in which principal fibers of the periodontal membranes degenerate, alveolar bone is resorbed, and the epithelial attachment is proliferated along the root surface. The result is the loosening and migration of teeth. (Oral Path.)

— A rare disease of young people (occurring primarily in women) that represents an idiopathic destruction of the periodontium. Originates in one or more of the periodontal structures and is characterized clinically by migration and loosening of one or more teeth, with irregular bone resorption in a vertical pattern. Apical proliferation of the epithelial attachment occurs only with the secondary inflammatory complications. Characteristically, the first permanent molars and incisors are the most severely involved. (Periodont.)

bone involvement in p. Resorptive or regressive changes in the alveolar and supporting bone, with osteoclastic action exceeding osteoblastic activity. Results in the loss of a portion of the attachment apparatus and the loosening and migration of teeth. (Periodont.)

gingiva in p. Inflammatory changes in the gingiva in the various stages of periodontosis. In the initial phase of periodontosis, gingival changes are either absent or of such a nature that one cannot attribute the loosening and migration of teeth to periodontosis. In the later stages, gingival inflammatory changes occur due to action of local etiologic agents. (Periodont.)

pocket formation in p. A sequela that is not inherent in the degenerative state produced by periodontosis. May be the result of gingival inflammation induced by local etiologic agents superimposed on previously existing degenerative lesions of the attachment apparatus. (Periodont.)

periodontal membrane in p. Dystrophic or degenerative changes of the periodontal membrane, along with the alveolar and supporting bone. The periodontal fibers principally affected are the alveolar fiber groups that are replaced by heterogeneously and indifferently located loose connective tissue without functional orientation. Capillarity is increased. The cemental group of periodontal fibers is affected much later by degenerative change. (Periodont.)

periorbital Surrounding the eyes. The periorbital soft tissues are easily contused and will produce marked inflammatory responses to trauma. (Oral Surg.)

periosteal elevator (per″ē-os′tē-al) (see **elevator, periosteal**)

periosteum (per″ē-os′tē-ŭm) The layer of connective tissue that varies considerably in thickness in the different areas of bone. It is thick over the surfaces that do not serve as areas of muscle attachment, especially on surfaces that are covered only by skin and subcutaneous tissue. In these areas it is loosely connected with the bone itself and is easily lifted from it. Muscles either are attached to bones directly, or they end on the periosteum. When muscles or tendons are attached to the bone itself, connective tissue extends into the bone as Sharpey's fibers. In such areas a periosteum may be lacking. When muscles are attached to the periosteum and thus are indirectly attached to the bone, the periosteum is relatively thin but is strongly fixed to the bone. The periosteum consists of two layers: an outer layer, which is rich in blood vessels and nerves and shows a dense arrangement of collagenous fibers, and an inner layer, the cambium, in which the fibers are loosely arranged, the cells numerous, and the blood vessels relatively sparse. During active growth, this layer of osteoblasts covers the periosteal surface of the bone. In the quiescent state in the adult the periosteum serves primarily in a supporting function. However, the inner layer retains its osteogenetic potencies and in fractures is activated to form osteoblasts and new bone. (Oral Physiol.)

periostitis (per″ē-os-tī′tĭs) An inflammation of the periosteum in which the membrane may become detached from the underlying bone due to exudates produced by inflammation or infection. (Oral Diag.; Oral Surg.)

peripheral circulation (pě-rĭf′er-al) (see **circulation, peripheral**)

periphery (pě-rĭf′er-ē) (see **border, denture**)

peritonsillar Surrounding the tonsils. Generally used in reference to the pharyngeal tonsils. (Oral Surg.)

perlèche (per-lĕsh′) An ulcerative inflammation of the angles of the lips associated with the habit of licking the lips. (Oral Diag.)

— A general term applied to superficial fissures occurring at the angles of the mouth. Lesions may be due to a variety of causes but most often can be related to deep labial commissures, with associated drooling, licking of the lips, unhygienic conditions, and the overgrowth of bacteria, yeast, or fungi. The term has also been applied to angular cheilosis due to riboflavin deficiency but not to the split papule of syphilis or to herpetic lesions. (Oral Med.)

— A condition characterized by fissures or cracks at the angles of the mouth. Monilial infection, avitaminosis, and loss of vertical dimension are complicating etiologic factors. (Oral Path.) (see also **cheilitis**)

— Eroded fissures at the angles of the mouth due to a deficiency disease (e.g., a deficiency of the B complex vitamins), monilial infection, decreased vertical dimension, drooling of saliva from the corners of the mouth, or a combination of two or more of these causative factors. (Periodont.)

permanent Of a lasting or durable nature (opposite of temporary). (Oper. Dent.)
  p. dentition (see **dentition, permanent**)

permissible dose (see **dose, maximum permissible**)

perneiras (pār-nā′răs) (see **beriberi**)

peroral Through or about the mouth. (Comp. Prosth.)

personal Belonging to an individual; limited to the person; having the nature of the qualities of human beings or of movable property. (D. Juris.)

personality The sum total of a patient's ideas, emotions, and behavior, including the rational and irrational, the conscious and unconscious, and the defensive and learned behavior patterns. Personality develops from both genetic factors and environmental factors. Thus the patient brings to a dental office his individual personality syndrome. It may be a well-adjusted, stable personality, a depressed, anxious, neurotic personality, or a manic, schizophrenic, psychotic personality. Patients present a broad spectrum of healthy and disordered personalities. (Oral Physiol.)

— The characteristics of a person by which other people evaluate him. (Pract. Man.)

  p. and reflex mechanisms The relationship between personality and the actions governing motor responses to sensory perception. In all human behavior there is a universality about these reflex mechanisms. Every stimulus impressed on a human organism results in a direct motor response, the nature of which depends on the nature of the stimulus, the nature of the organism's past experience, and the current activity of the organism. A stimulus is an impression received from the external environment through one of the sensory end-organs and conveyed to the brain by the sensory nerves and a remembered or imagined internal stimulus that arises within the brain as a result of memory or experience and is capable of inducing a motor response. (Oral Physiol.)

personnel monitoring (see **monitoring, personnel**)

perversion Impacted tooth. (Orthodont.)

petechiae (pē-tē′kē-ē) Capillary hemorrhages producing small red or purplish pinhead-sized discolorations of the mucous membrane and skin. Petechiae are typical of blood dyscrasias, vitamin C deficiency, positive Rumpel-Leede test, liver disease, and subacute bacterial endocarditis. (Oral Diag.)

petrolatum (pĕt″rō-lā′tŭm) (**petroleum jelly**) A mixture of hydrocarbons obtained from petroleum. In its semisolid form it is utilized as a protective covering to prevent gingival dehydration and inflammation during mouth breathing. A lubricant; protective covering for burns, etc. (Periodont.)

Peutz-Jeghers syndrome (pūtz-jĕg′erz) (see **syndrome, Peutz-Jeghers**)

pH The concentration of hydrogen ions expressed as the negative logarithm of base 10. (Anesth.)

phagocyte (făg′ō-sīt) Any cell that ingests microorganisms, cells, or other substances. (Oral Path.)

phagocytosis (făg″ō-cī-tō′sĭs) The engulfing of microorganisms, cells, and other substances by phagocytes. (Oral Path.) (see also **phagocyte**)

phantom (făn′tom) A device that absorbs and scatters x radiation in approximately the same way as the tissues of the body. It may be made of a gallon of water, a set of pressed wood sheets, a sack of rice, a cocoanut, or other similar substances. Readings taken without a patient or phantom in the examining position are meaningless for personnel protection because they do not take into account the effect of the patient's body in scattering radiation throughout the room. (Oral Radiol.)

pharmacodynamics (far″mah-kō-dī-năm′ĭks) The science of drug action. (Oral Med.; Pharmacol.)

pharmacology (far″mah-kol′ō-jē) The total science of drugs, including their use in therapeutics. (Oral Med.; Pharmacol.)

pharmacy The art and science of preparing and dispensing drugs. (Oral Med.; Pharmacol.)

pharyngeal arch (fah-rin′jē-al) (see **arch, pharyngeal**)

pharyngeal flap A pedicle flap usually raised on the posterior pharyngeal wall and attached to the soft palate in order to reduce the size of the velopharyngeal gap. (Cleft Palate)

pharyngitis (far″in-jī′tĭs) Inflammation of the pharynx. (Oral Surg.)

pharyngoplasty (fah-rĭng′gō-plăs″tē) Reconstructive operation to alter the size and shape of the nasopharyngeal orifice. (Cleft Palate)

pharyngospasm (fah-rĭng′gō-spăzm) Spasm of the phayngeal muscles. (Oral Surg.)

pharynx (făr′ingks) The least specialized and most primitive structure of the head and neck region. It is a simple, funnel-shaped tube of muscle tissue that is wide at the head end and narrow at the esophageal end. The constrictor muscles are so arranged by interlocking fibers that a wave of constricting impulses propels the food toward the stomach. The pharynx is the common pathway for the air and food; consequently, food cannot long be retained there but must be either passed down to the esophagus or regurgitated back into the mouth. Hence the gag and cough reflexes are very sensitive in response to this requirement for maintaining the patency of the airway. The soft palate action provides the valve for separating the pharynx from the oral cavity. (Oral Physiol.)

p., activities of posterior and lateral pharyngeal wall The bulging of the posterior and lateral pharyngeal wall produced by the superior pharyngeal constrictors and palatopharyngeus during the acts of swallowing and phonation; seen in individuals with a congenitally short soft palate, operated soft palate, or unoperated cleft of the soft palate. These activities are rarely present in the individual with the normal soft palate. (Cleft Palate)

phase Any one of the varying aspects or stages through which an anesthetic or process may pass. (Anesth.)

implant surgical p. *First stage:* A major oral operation in which the mucoperiosteum is elevated, exposing the oral surface of the jawbone; the surgical jaw relations are established and an impression is made of the exposed bone surfaces. *Second stage:* A major oral surgical operation in which the mucoperiosteum is reelevated, the prepared implant is placed on the bone surface, and the mucoperiosteum is coapted and sutured about the posts of the protruding implant abutments. (Oral Implant.)

phenacetin, caffeine, aspirin (fĕ-năs′ĕ-tĭn) (see **aspirin, phenacetin, caffeine**)

phenol (fē′nol) (**carbolic acid**) An organic compound in which one or more hydroxyl groups are attached to a carbon atom in an aromatic ring that contains conjugated double bonds. (Oral Med.; Pharmacol.)

phenomenon, Hamburger's (**chloride shift**) The conversion of carbon dioxide (CO_2) to carbonic acid (H_2CO_3) by the enzyme carbonic anhydrase, which occurs when CO_2 enters the blood from the tissues and passes into the red blood cells. The HCO_3-ion passes into the plasma. The NaCl of the plasma provides Cl ions that enter the cell, where they form KCl.

The Na ion in the plasma joins with the HCO_3-ion to form bicarbonate. Reverse changes occur in the lungs when CO_2 is eliminated from the blood. (Anesth.)

— The diffusion of chloride ions into red blood cells to compensate for the diffusion of bicarbonate ions into the blood plasma. (Oral Med.)

phenotype (fē'nō-tīp) Term referring to the expression of genotypes that can be directly distinguished; e.g., by clinical observation of external appearance or serologic tests. (Oral Med.)

phlebectasia (flĕb″ĕk-tā′zē-ah) Dilation of a vein. (Oral Diag.; Oral Path.)

phlebolith (flĕb'ō-lĭth) A calcified thrombus in a vein. (Oral Diag.; Oral Path.)

phlegmon (flĕg′mon) An intense inflammation spreading through tissue spaces over a large area. (Oral Diag.)

— A diffuse, purulent inflammatory lesion without definite limits. Clinically, a hard, boardlike swelling without gross pus. (Oral Surg.) (see also **cellulitis**)

phobia (fō′bē-ah) A specific fear of a hysterical nature. (Oral Diag.)

phonation (fō-nā′shŭn) The production of voiced sound by means of vocal cord vibrations. (Cleft Palate)

   speech p. Modification, by the vocal folds, of the airstream as it leaves the lungs and passes through the larynx, for the purpose of producing the various sounds that are the basis of speech. By opposing each other with different degrees of tension and space, the vocal folds create a slitlike aperture of varying size and contour, and by creating resistance to the stream of air, they set up a sequence of laryngeal sound waves with characteristic pitch and intensity. (Oral Physiol.)

phoneme (fō′nēm) A group or family of closely related speech sounds all of which have the same distinctive acoustic characteristics in spite of their differences; often used in place of the term speech sound. (Cleft Palate)

phonetic values (see **values, phonetic**)

phonetics The study of the production and perception of speech sounds, including individual and group variations, and their use in speech. (Cleft Palate)

— The science of sounds used in speech. (Comp. Prosth.; Remov. Part. Prosth.)

phosphatases (fos′fah-tā-sĕz) The enzymes particularly associated with bone growth and destruction. Normally the blood alkaline phosphatase is 0.1 to 0.2 unit (Jenner-Kay) or 1.5 to 4.5 units (Bodansky). The phosphatase level is raised in rickets and osteitis fibrosa cystica and is lowered in osteitis deformans. (Oral Diag.)

   alkaline p. An enzyme that liberates inorganic phosphates, causing an increase in the blood level in certain diseases affecting bone, such as hyperparathyroidism, osteitis deformans, and rickets. (Oral Diag.)

phosphates (fos′fāts) The organic compounds of phosphorus. The blood phosphate level is normally 2.5 to 5.0 mg/100 ml. It is low in rickets and early hyperparathyroidism and high in tetany and nephritis. (Oral Diag.)

phosphorus (fos′for-ŭs) A nonmetallic element; atomic weight, 30.98. It is essential, as the phosphate, for the mineralization of the organic matrix of teeth and bone. It is also essential in the intermediary metabolism of carbohydrates as a vital constituent of the various intermediary compounds (e.g., glucose 6-phosphate) and of the enzyme systems (e.g., adenosine triphosphate [ATP]). (Periodont.)

phossy jaw (fos′sē) (see **poisoning, phosphorus**)

photon A bullet or quantum of electromagnetic radiant energy emitted and propagated from various types of radiation sources. The term should not be used alone but should be qualified by terms that will clarify the type of energy; e.g., light photon and x-ray photon. (Oral Radiol.)

physical Relating to the body, as distinguished from the mind. (D. Juris.)

   p. plant The entire architectural and decorated suite of offices in which the dentist operates. (Pract. Man.)

physician A person duly trained and authorized, or licensed, to treat diseases. (D. Juris.)

physiologic occlusion (see **occlusion, physiologic**)

physiologic rest position (see **position, rest, physiologic**)

physiology (fĭz″ē-ol′ō-jē) Study of tissue and organism behavior. The physiologic process is a dynamic state of tissue as compared to the static state of descriptive morphology (anatomy). Physiology is differentiated from descriptive morphology by the following qualifying properties: rate, direction, and magnitude. Physiologic processes are thus morphologic alterations in the three dimensions of space associated with a temporary (time) sequence. Physiologic processes relate to a wide spectrum of life activities on three levels: biochemical and biophysical activity of a subcellular nature, the activity of cells and tissues aggregated into organ systems, and multiorgan system activity as expressed in human behavior. (Oral Physiol.)

oral p. Physiology related to clinical manifestations in the normal and abnormal behavior of oral structures. The principal clinical functions in which the oral structures participate are deglutition, mastication, respiration, speech, and head posture. These functions may be altered by pathologic modifications in the gross or microscopic anatomy of the tissues, in the neurologic and hormonal mechanisms that activate and regulate tissues, or in the biochemical processes associated with cellular activity. (Oral Physiol.)

— The functionally integrated and dynamic activities of the structures comprising the stomatologic system necessary for the self-preservation of an individual and for the performance of such vital actions as swallowing, mastication, sucking, and speech. Also includes the individual functions of the various members of the system. (Oral Med.)

— The science that deals with the independent and interrelated functions of the structures comprising the stomatologic system: the teeth and their attachment and supporting apparatus, the tongue, the mandible, the temporomandibular articulation, etc. (Periodont.)

pathologic p. Altered, disturbed, and abnormal physiologic processes of tissue. The pathologic relationships between the functional activity and the structural changes of a tissue are often not easily defined or described. Virchow's description of pathology best describes the clinical state of disturbed pathologic physiology: "Disease is life under altered conditions." (Oral Physiol.)

p. p., signs and symptoms The clinical manifestations of alterations in normal physiology. In practice, these changes have been regarded traditionally as the result of either organic or functional disorders. Such a separation, however, is an oversimplification of a complex phenomenon; in life there is generally no function without organic integrity. Similarly, there is no vital organic substance or tissue without some level of functional activity. Thus, when a disorder is categorized as functional, the implication is that it is so categorized only because available diagnostic agents or the acceptable concepts of the structure are inadequate. (Oral Physiol.)

physioprints (fiz-ē-ō-prĭnts) Photographs obtained by projecting a grid on the subject's face and superimposing two exposures. The resultant picture gives a three-dimensional approach for the diagnosis of facial contours and swelling. (Oral Diag.)

physiotherapy, oral (fiz"ē-ō-ther'ah-pē) The collective procedures properly performed for the maintenance of personal hygiene of the mouth; those procedures necessary for cleanliness, tissue stimulation, and tone and for the preservation of the dentition. (Periodont.) (see also **aid in physiotherapy**)

pickling The process of cleansing from metallic surfaces the products of oxidation and other impurities by immersion in acid. (Comp. Prosth.; Oper. Dent.; Remov. Part. Prosth.)

Pick's disease (see **disease, Niemann-Pick**)

pickup impression (see **impression, pickup**)

picture, x-ray (objectionable) (see **radiograph**)

pier (pēr) An intermediate retaining or supporting abutment for a prosthesis. (Fixed Part. Prosth.; Remov. Part. Prosth.) (see also **abutment**)

Pierre Robin syndrome (pē-air' rō'bǎn) (see **retrognathism; syndrome, Pierre Robin**)

pigmentation, gingival (see **gingiva, pigmentation**)

pigmentation, melanin The discoloration of tissues produced by the deposition of melanin. Seen normally in the oral mucous membranes (especially gingivae) of dark-complexioned individuals and abnormally in such conditions as adrenal hypofunction (Addison's disease). (Periodont.)

pilocarpine (pī"lō-kar'pĭn) An alkaloid that causes parasympathetic effects; e.g., secretion of the salivary, bronchial, and gastrointestinal glands. It stimulates the sweat glands and also causes vasodilation and cardiac inhibition. (Oral Physiol.)

pin A small cylindrical piece of metal. (Fixed Part. Prosth.)

cemented p. A metal rod cemented into a hole drilled into dentin to enhance retention. (Oper. Dent.)

friction-retained p. A metal rod driven or forced into a hole drilled into dentin to enhance retention. It is retained solely by elasticity of dentin. (Oper. Dent.)

incisal guide p. A metal rod that is attached to the upper member of an articulator and that touches the incisal guide table. It maintains the established vertical separation of the upper and lower arms of the articulator. (Comp. Prosth.; Remov. Part. Prosth.)

retention p. The frictional grip of small metal projections extending from a metal casting into the dentin of the tooth. (Fixed Part. Prosth.)

self-threading p. A pin screwed into a hole prepared in dentin to enhance retention. (Oper. Dent.)

sprue p. A solid or hollow length of metal used to attach a pattern to the crucible former. A metal pin used to form the hole that provides the pathway through the refractory investment to permit the entry of metal into a mold. (Oper. Dent.)

Steinmann p. A firm metal pin that is sharpened on one end; used for the fixation of fractures. It is sometimes passed through the maxillae or mandible to provide external points for attachment of upward-supporting devices. (Oral Surg.)

pit A small depression in enamel, usually located in a developmental groove where two or more enamel lobes are joined. A depression in a restoration due to nonuniform density. (Oper. Dent.)

pit and fissure cavity (see **cavity, pit and fissure**)

pit and fissure sealant (see **sealant, pit and fissure**)

Pituitrin (pĭ-tū′ĭ-trĭn) Proprietary name for an extract of the posterior lobe of the pituitary gland. (Oral Med.)

pityriasis rosea (pĭt″ĭ-rī′ah-sĭs rō′zē-ah) A noncontagious skin disease with reddish, scaly patches, and moderate fever. (Oral Diag.; Oral Med.)

pivot, occlusal An elevation artificially developed on the occlusal surface, usually in the molar region, and designed to induce sagittal mandibular rotation. (Comp. Prosth.; Remov. Part. Prosth.)

adjustable o. p. An occlusal pivot that may be adjusted vertically by means of a screw or by other means. (Comp. Prosth.; Remov. Part. Prosth.)

placement The act of placing an object, e.g., a removable denture, in its planned location on the dental arch. (Remov. Part. Prosth.)

choice of path of p. Determination of the direction of placement and removal of a removable partial denture on its supporting oral structures, which can be varied by altering the plane to which the guiding abutment surfaces are made parallel. The choice is a compromise to best fulfill five demands: to subject abutment teeth to a minimum or no torquing force, to encounter the least interference, to provide needed retention, to establish adequate guiding-plane

surfaces, and to provide acceptable esthetics. (Remov. Part. Prosth.)

placebo (plah-sē′bō) A substance that resembles medicine superficially and is believed by the patient to be medicine but that has no intrinsic drug activity. (Oral Med.; Pharmacol.)

— An inert substance, usually a drug, administered to satisfy a person who desires medication although no need for medication has been established. Refers also to a control in place of a drug being tested. (Oral Med.)

p. effect The real or imagined effect of a placebo, which may actually be the same effect ordinarily associated with the administration of a therapeutically active agent. (Oral Med.)

plaintiff A person who brings an action; the party who sues in a personal action and is so designated on the record. (D. Juris.)

plan, bank (see **bank plan**)

plan, treatment The sequence of procedures planned for the treatment of a patient. (Comp. Prosth.; Fixed Part. Prosth.; Remov. Part. Prosth.)

— The sequential arrangement of the therapeutic measures to be utilized in the restoration of the oral cavity to health. (Periodont.)

— The prescription for the treatment indicated for a patient. (Pract. Man.)

provisional t. p. Tentative treatment plan that is capable of modification or continuance after reevaluation of periodontal status after initial therapeutic procedures. (Periodont.)

plane Term used to describe an ideal flat surface that is supposed to intersect solid bodies, extend in various directions, or be determined by the position in space of three points. (Oper. Dent.)

axial p. A hypothetical plane parallel to the long axis of an object. (Oper. Dent.)

axial wall p. An instrument used to plane and true the axial wall of a Class 3 preparation. (Oper. Dent.)

bite p. (bite plate) An appliance that covers the palate. It has an inclined or flat plane at its anterior border that offers resistance to the mandibular incisors when they come into contact with it. (Orthodont.) (see also **guide, bite**)

Bolton-nasion p. (nā′zē-ahn) A plane passing through the upper face and lower cranium. Its anterior termination is at the junction of the frontal and nasal bones in the midplane. In the profile, the posterior termination is the highest point of the notches at the posterior end of the condyles on the occiptal bone. (Orthodont.)

Broca's p. (brŏ'kahz) (**French plane**) A plane extending from the tip of the interalveolar septum between the upper central incisors to the lowermost point of the occipital condyle. (Orthodont.)

Camper's p. A plane extending from the inferior border of the ala of the nose to the superior border of the tragus of the ear. (Orthodont.)

eye-ear p. (see **plane, Frankfort horizontal**)

Frankfort horizontal p. The eye-ear plane. A plane passing through the lowest point in the margin of the orbit (the orbitale) and the highest point in the margin of the auditory meatus (the tragion). (Comp. Prosth.; Remov. Part. Prosth.)

— The eye-ear plane seen in profile by drawing a line from the orbitale to the ear point. (Oral Diag.)

— A craniometric plane determined by the inferior borders of the bony orbits and the upper margin of the auditory meatus. It passes through the two orbitales and the two tragions. (Orthodont.)

guide p. (**guiding p.**) A mechanical device, part of an orthodontic appliance, having an established inclined plane that, when in use, causes a change in the occlusal relation of the maxillary and the mandibular teeth and permits their movement to a normal position. (Orthodont.)

— A plane developed in the occlusal surfaces of occlusion rims to position the mandible in centric relation. (Comp. Prosth.)

— Two or more vertically parallel surfaces of abutment teeth, so shaped as to direct the path of placement and removal of a remarkable partial denture. (Remov. Part. Prosth.)

guiding p. (see **plane, guide**)

Hamy's p. A plane extending from glabella to lambda. (Orthodont.)

His's p. A plane extending from anterior nasal spine to opisthion. (Orthodont.)

horizontal p. A plane that is parallel to the horizon and perpendicular to the vertical plane. (Oper. Dent.)

Huxley's p. A plane extending from nasion to basion (basicranial axis). (Orthodont.)

mandibular p. (see **border, mandibular**)

Martin's p. A plane extending from nasion to inion. (Orthodont.)

mean foundation p. The mean of the inclination of the denture-supporting (basal seat) tissues. Since the tissues constituting the denture foundation are irregular in form and consistency, and since there is only one direction from which force may be applied if it is to comply with the law of statics, which requires the exertion of force at a right angle to maintain support, the mean foundation plane forms a right angle with the most favorable direction of force. The ideal condition for denture stability exists when the mean foundation plane is most nearly at right angles to the direction of force. (Comp. Prosth.; Remov. Part. Prosth.)

median-raphe p. The median plane of the head. (Orthodont.)

Montague's p. The plane extending from nasion to porion. (Orthodont.)

occlusal p. An imaginary surface that is related anatomically to the cranium and that theoretically touches the incisal edges of the incisors and the tips of the occluding surfaces of the posterior teeth. It is not a plane in the true sense of the word but represents the mean of the curvature of the surface. (Comp. Prosth.; Oper. Dent.; Remov. Part. Prosth.) (see also **curve of occlusion**)

— A line drawn between points representing one half of the incisal overbite (vertical overlap) in front and one half of the cusp height of the last molars in back. (Orthodont.)

— Metaphoric term made popular when dentistry first became interested in relating chewing surfaces to a horizontal plane of space. It has been variously defined as (1) an imaginary plane determined by a point in the lower incisor and the points of the distobuccal cusps of both mandibular second molars; (2) an imaginary plane determined by points in the edges of the upper incisors and the cuspal points of the postcanine teeth; or (3) unilaterally, a cord of the "curve of Spee." (Gnathol.)

orbital p. A plane perpendicular to the eye-ear plane and passing through the orbitale. (Orthodont.)

— The plane that passes through the visual axis of each eye. (Remov. Part. Prosth.)

p. of reference A plane that acts as a guide to the location of other planes. (Comp. Prosth.; Remov. Part. Prosth.)

sagittal p. The anteroposterior median plane of the body. (Oper. Dent.)

—A plane that divides the body in the midline into right and left sides. (Oral Radiol.)

median s. p. A plane passing through the median raphe of the palate at right angles to the Frankfort horizontal plane. (Orthodont.)

Schwalbe's p. (shvahl'behz) A plane that extends from glabella to inion. (Orthodont.)

p. of teeth For descriptive purposes, three planes are considered in the teeth proper: buccolingual, horizontal, and mesiodistal.

axial p. of t. Term that applies to either the mesiodistal or the buccolingual plane. (Oper. Dent.)

axiobuccolingual p. of t. (see **plane of teeth, buccolingual**)

axiomesiodistal p. of t. (see **plane of teeth, mesiodistal**)

buccolingual p. of t. (**axiobuccolingual p.**) A plane that passes through the tooth buccolingually parallel with its long axis. In incisors and cuspids this is the labiolingual plane. (Oper. Dent.)

horizontal p. of t. A plane that is perpendicular to the long axis of the tooth and may be supposed to cut through the crown at any point in its length. (Oper. Dent.)

mesiodistal p. of t. (**axiomesiodistal p.**) A plane that passes through the tooth mesiodistally parallel with its long axis. (Oper. Dent.)

vertical p. of t. An upright plane that is perpendicular to the horizon. (Oper. Dent.)

Von Ihring's p. A plane extending from orbitale to the center of the bony external auditory meatus. (Orthodont.)

plaque (plăk) A flat plate or tablet. Leukoplakia is a white plaque, and dentobacterial plaques are flat plates or masses of bacteria and debris on tooth surfaces. (Oral Diag.)

mucin p. A sticky substance that accumulates on the teeth; composed of mucin derived from the saliva and of bacteria and their products; often responsible for the inception of caries and for gingival inflammation. (Oper. Dent.; Periodont.)

plasma (plăz'mah) The fluid portion of the blood, in which the cellular elements are suspended. (Anesth.)

— The fluid portion of the blood that, after centrifugation contains all the stable components except the cells. It is obtained from centrifuged whole blood that has been prevented from clotting by the addition of anticoagulants such as citrate, oxalate, or heparin. (Oral Med.)

p. accelerator globulin (see **proaccelerin; accelerator, prothrombin conversion, I**)

p. ac-globulin (see **factor V; proaccelerin**)

normal human p. Pooled sterile plasma from a number of persons to which a preservative has been added. It is stored under refrigeration or desiccated for later use as a substitute for whole blood. (Oral Med.)

p. proteolytic enzyme (see **plasmin**)

p. thromboplastin antecedent (**antihemophilic factor C, factor XI, PTA, p. thromboplastin factor C**) A factor required for the development of thromboplastic activity in plasma. (Oral Med.)

p. thromboplastin component (**antihemophilic factor B, autoprothrombin II, Christmas factor, factor IX, platelet cofactor II, PTC**) A clotting factor in normal blood necessary for the development of thromboplastic activity in plasma. A deficiency results in Christmas disease. (Oral Med.) (see also **factor IX**)

plasmacytoma (plăz"mah-sī-tō'mah) Term usually reserved to indicate the primary soft tissue plasma cell tumors of the oral, pharyngeal, and nasal mucous membranes. The lesion consists of typical and atypical plasma cells, and its behavior is unpredictable. (Oral Path.)

soft tissue p. A primary plasma cell tumor of the nasal, pharyngeal, and oral mucosa that has no apparent primary bone involvement. The lesions are sessile or polypoid sessile masses in the mucous membrane. The majority remain localized, but metastases have been reported. (Oral Path.)

plasmin (plăz'mĭn) (**fibrinolysin, lysin, plasma proteolytic enzyme, tryptase**) Collective term for one or more proteolytic enzymes found in the blood. The proteolytic enzymes are capable of digesting fibrin, fibrinogen, and proaccelerin. Plasminogen, the inactive form, may become active spontaneously in shed blood. An activator, fibrinokinase (fibrinolysokinase), is found in many animal tissues. (Oral Med.)

plasminogen (plăz-mĭn'ō-jĕn) (**profibrinolysin**) The precursor of plasmin found in plasma. It is probably activated by a tissue factor or by a blood activator which first must be activated by a blood or tissue fibrinolysokinase. (Oral Med.)

plasmokinin (plăz-mō-kĭn'ĭn) (see **factor VIII**)

plaster (plăs'ter) Colloquial term applied to dental plaster of paris. (Comp. Prosth.; Remov. Part. Prosth.)

p. headcap (see **headcap, plaster**)

impression p. Plaster used for making impressions. Sets rapidly and is characterized by low setting expansion and strength. (D. Mat.)

model p. Plaster used for diagnostic casts and as an investing material. (D. Mat.)

p. of paris The hemihydrate of calcium sulfate that, when mixed with water, forms a paste that subsequently sets into a hard mass. (Comp. Prosth.; Remov. Part. Prosth.) (see also **beta-hemihydrate**)

— Calcined calcium sulfate in the form of a fine powder, in which about half of the water crystallization has been driven off. When water is mixed with the powder, the mixture solidifies to a porous mass that is used extensively in dentistry and in surgery. (Oper. Dent.)

plastic Capable of being molded. A restorative material (e.g., amalgam, cement, gutta-percha, resin) that is soft at the time of insertion and may then be shaped or molded, after which it will harden or set. (Oper. Dent.)

p. base (see **base, plastic**)

p. closure Suturing of tissues that involves their displacement by sliding or rotation to create a surgical closure. (Oral Implant.)

modeling p. (**modeling composition, modeling compound**) A thermoplastic material usually composed of gum dammar, prepared chalk, and other materials; used especially for making dental impressions. An impression material sold under the name of modeling compound. (Comp. Prosth.; Oper. Dent.; Remov. Part. Prosth.)

p. strip A clear plastic strip of Celluloid or acrylic resin used as a matrix when silicate cement or acrylic is inserted into proximal prepared cavities in anterior teeth. (Oper. Dent.)

plasticity (plăs-tĭs'ĭ-tē) The quality of being moldable or workable. The degree of permanent deformation resulting from stress application; usually associated with substances that are classed as solids or semirigid liquids. (Oper. Dent.)

plate, bone An approximation plate of bone. Also referred to as finger, small bone plates, or have plate; used with interosseous screws or wires for bone immobilization. (Oral Surg.)

Sherman b. p. A chrome-cobalt alloy or stainless steel bone plate that can be affixed to a fracture site with screws; frequently used in open reduction of mandibular fractures. (Oral Surg.)

plate, lingual (see **connector, major, linguoplate**)

plate, occlusal plane A metal plate used in checking or establishing the occlusal plane of the teeth. (Remov. Part. Prosth.)

plate, palatal (see **connector, major**)

platelet (plăt'lĕt) A disk found in the blood of mammals that is concerned in the coagulation and clotting of blood. (Oral Physiol.)

p. ac-globulin (see **factor, platelet, I**)

p. cofactor I (see **factor VIII**)

p. cofactor II (see **factor IX; plasma thromboplastin component**)

p. disorders (see **disorder, platelet**)

platinocyanide crystals (plăt"ĭ-nō-sī'ah-nīd) (see **crystals, platinocyanide**)

platinum matrix (see **matrix, platinum**)

pleadings Written allegations of what is affirmed on the one side or denied on the other, disclosing the real matter to the court or jury having to try the cause. (D. Juris.)

Pleasure curve (see **curve, Pleasure**)

pledget (plĕj'ĕt) A minute pellet of absorbent cotton used for accurately controlled placement of medication or base. (Oper. Dent.) (see also **cotton, absorbent**)

pleomorphic adenoma (plē"ō-mor'fĭk ăd"ĕ-nō'mah) (**mixed salivary gland tumor**) A benign tumor of the salivary gland containing varying proportions of epithelial and mesenchymal elements. The intermediate type of epithelial cells are in sheets, cords, and acini. The mesenchymal tissue varies from myxomatous to cartilaginous to densely hyalinized connective tissue. The marked variations in histologic pattern are responsible for the designation of pleomorphic. (Oral Diag.)

plethora (plĕth'or-ah) A nonspecific increase in blood bulk. Clinically, the patient is flushed and has a feeling of tenseness in the head; the blood vessels are full, and the pulse is firm. (Oral Physiol.)

pleurisy (ploo'rĭ-sē) Inflammation of the pleura, with exudation into its cavity and on its surface. (Anesth.)

plexus (plĕk'sŭs) A network or tangle, especially of nerves, lymphatics, or veins. (Anesth.)

Haller's p. A nerve plexus of sympathetic filaments and branches of the external laryngeal nerve on the surface of the inferior constrictor muscle of the larynx. (Anesth.)

intermediate p. The area of the periodontal membrane approximating in the midsection of the periodontal membrane, where the fiber bundles of the alveolar and cemental groups of periodontal fibers are woven together by small, thick strands of collagen fibers. The interweaving of fiber bundles of the intermediate plexus allows for tooth eruption and tooth movement between the cemental and alveolar periodontal fibers. (Periodont.)

pliers (plural noun, but singular or plural in construction, as a pair of pliers) A tool of pincer design with jaws of varying shapes; used for holding, bending, stretching, contouring, cutting, etc. (Oper. Dent.)

contouring p. Pliers with jaws curved to permit developing tooth contours in banding metal. (Oper. Dent.)

cotton p. A slender, tweezerlike instrument used to hold cotton pellets or pledgets, to apply medicaments, and to carry small objects to and from the mouth. (Oper. Dent.)

stretching p. Pliers whose jaws are designed as a hammer and anvil, with the handles sufficiently long to develop a high leverage ratio; used to enlarge metal bands (gold, aluminum, copper) or to thin the contact area of matrix bands. (Oper. Dent.)

plosive (plō′sĭv) Any speech sound made by creating air pressure in the air tract and suddenly releasing it. (Cleft Palate)

— Any speech sound made by impounding the airstream for a moment until considerable pressure has been developed and then suddenly releasing it; e.g., in the pronunciation of "d," "p," and "g." (Oral Physiol.)

plug A lumpy mass. (Anesth.)

plugger An instrument used to compress the filling material in an apical and lateral direction when a root canal is being filled. (Endodont.) (see also **condenser**)

plugging (objectionable as a synonym for inserting or condensing) (Oper. Dent.)

pluglet (**billet**) A compressed tablet designed for use in pressure anesthesia of the dental pulp. (Oral Med.; Pharmacol.)

plumbism (plŭm′bĭzm) (**lead poisoning, saturnism**) Acute or chronic intoxication due to the ingestion, inhalation, or skin absorption of lead. Manifestations of acute poisoning include abdominal pain, paralysis, metallic taste, and collapse. Chronic manifestations include gastrointestinal disturbances, headache, peripheral neuropathy (foot drop and wrist drop), lead in the urine and blood, basophilic granular degeneration, coproporphyrinuria, and stomatitis. (Oral Med.) (see also **stomatitis, lead**)

— An occupational disease characterized by digestive disturbances, loss of weight and muscular strength, constipation, backache, arthralgia, anemia, colic, anorexia, motor paralysis, metallic taste in the mouth, hypertension, chest pain, and the presence of a lead line on the gingival tissues, with occasional patches, representing deposits of lead sulfide, on the mucous membrane of the lips and cheek. (Periodont.)

Plummer-Vinson syndrome (see **syndrome, Plummer-Vinson**)

plunger cusp A stamp cusp, the tip of which is made to occlude in an embrasure; its shoulder has not been restored to occlude in a fossa. The much-used picture by Turner of the lingual aspects of occlusion unintentionally displays plunger cusps (Angle: Text 1902, p. 11). (Gnathol.)

PMA (**papillary-marginal-attached**) A system of epidemiologic scoring of periodontal disease devised by Schour and Massler in which the symbols denote the areas involved in gingival inflammation. (Periodont.)

pneumatic condenser (nū-măt′ĭk) (see **condenser, pneumatic**)

pneumatodyspnea (nū″mah-tō-dĭsp′nē-ah) Difficulty in breathing due to emphysema. (Anesth.)

pneumocyst (nū′mō-sĭst) An operation to reduce the size of dental periapical cysts prior to their removal. (Endodont.)

pneumonitis (nū″mō-nī′tĭs) Inflammation of the lungs of an acute, localized nature. (Oral Med.)

pneumothorax (nū″mō-thō′răks) An accumulation of air or gas in the pleural cavity. The air enters by way of an external wound, a lung perforation, a burrowing abscess, or rupture of a superficial lung cavity. Pneumothorax is accompanied by sudden, severe pain and rapidly increasing dyspnea. (Anesth.)

pocket Diseased gingival attachment, characterized by gingival discoloration, retraction of gingivae from the tooth, bleeding, presence of an exudate, loss of the presence of stippling, etc. A space bordered on one side by the tooth and on the opposite side by ulcerated crevicular epithelium, and limited at its apex by the epithelial attachment. Pseudopockets and periodontal pockets have been described. (Periodont.)

p., abscess formation Formation of a periodontal abscess within a periodontal pocket. The cause may be blockage of the pocket orifice, which prevents egress of suppurative material. It is attended by pain, swelling, and the formation of a fluctuant area on the gingival tissues. The abscesses are localized and consist of a combined acute and chronic inflammatory infiltrate, exudative substances, and necrotic tissue elements. (Periodont.)

p., bleeding An occurrence that denotes ulcerations of the pocket epithelium, with hemorrhaging through the broken surface from exposed connective tissue capillaries. (Periodont.)

p. bottom The base of the pocket, marked or limited by the epithelial attachment to the cementum of the root (periodontal pocket) or the enamel of the crown (gingival pocket). (Periodont.)

p., calculus Calcified deposits that usually occupy the entire pocket. It is attached to the tooth structure, with the gingival tissues tightly adapted to the surface of the calculus. (Periodont.)

p., deepening Increase of the depth of the pocket, which is dependent on apical proliferation of the epithelial attachment alongside the cementum, with subsequent separation from the tooth, or on hyperplasia of the gingivae resulting from inflammation. (Periodont.)

depth of p. The measurement, usually expressed in millimeters, of the distance between the gingival crest and the base of the pocket. (Periodont.)

p. elimination The application of therapeutic measures to obtain a healthy gingival attachment and an intact, functioning attachment apparatus. The procedures employed include curettage (root and gingival), reattachment or new attachment operations, gingivectomy and gingivoplasty, and osseous and mucogingival surgical procedures. (Periodont.)

gingival p. A gingival sulcus of abnormal depth; a pathologic condition as opposed to the normal sulcus about the tooth. (Oral Diag.)

—A pseudopocket; gingival inflammation with edema, hyperplasia, and ulceration of the sulcular epithelium but without apical proliferation of the epithelial attachment. (Periodont.)

infrabony p. (infracrestal p., intra-alveolar p., intrabony p.) A periodontal pocket extending apically from the alveolar bone crest. (Oral Diag.)

— A periodontal pocket, the base of which is apical to the crest of the alveolar bone. Consists basically of a vertical resorptive defect in alveolar and supporting bone, overlying which are a band of transseptal fibers connecting adjacent teeth, disintegrated fibers of gingival corium, inflammatory cellular infiltrate, and hyperplastic pocket epithelium, accompanied by apical migration of the epithelial attachment. Clinical signs are those of periodontitis, associated with

radiographic evidence of vertical bone resorption. The infrabony pocket has been classified according to the number of remaining osseous walls supporting it for the purpose of therapeutic rationale. (Periodont.)

epithelial attachment in i. p. In therapy of the infrabony pocket the epithelial attachment to the tooth must be completely eliminated so as to prevent an epithelial barrier to new attachment. (Periodont.)

etiologic factors in i. p. Factors responsible for the genesis and perpetuation of the infrabony pocket; e.g., inconsistent marginal impaction and occlusal traumatism, remembering that the superimposition of a local environmental factor (with subsequent inflammation of the gingival tissue) is necessary to convert the infrabony defect, produced by occlusal trauma, into an infrabony pocket. (Periodont.)

— The agents responsible for the genesis of the infrabony pocket, including inflammatory changes superimposed on vertical bone loss, tilted teeth, food impaction, broad interdental septal lesions, etc. (Periodont.)

reattachment of i. p. The process that may occur after enucleation of the contents of the infrabony pocket, root planing or curettage, and associated periodontal procedures, in which a portion of the attachment apparatus and the supporting bone are newly constituted so as to provide increased attachment and investment for the tooth. Reattachment is a predictable occurrence after appropriate treatment of the infrabony pocket presenting three osseous walls, with variable results in other varieties of infrabony pockets. New attachment. (Periodont.)

treatment of i. p. The therapeutic procedures employed in the elimination of the infrabony pocket. Treatment includes enucleation of the contents of the infrabony defect, root curettage, tooth stabilization, etc., and the procedures necessary to gain access to the pocket for appropriate treatment. (Periodont.)

infracrestal p. (see **pocket, infrabony**)

intra-alveolar p. (see **pocket, infrabony**)

intrabony p. (see **pocket, infrabony**)

p. ionization chamber (see **chamber, ionization, pocket**)

p. in marginal periodontitis A condition in which the inflammatory process has progressed from the gingival tissues to the underlying alveolar process. The changes are those associated with gingivitis plus resorptive bone lesions. The base of the pocket is at the marginal point of the union of the epithelial attachment to the cementum of the root. (Periodont.)

p. marker, Crane-Kaplan An instrument used to delineate the depths of gingival and periodontal pockets prior to gingivectomy incision. The straight beak of the instrument is inserted to the limit of the pocket while the sharp angulated beak is pressed into the tissue until a small bleeding point is seen. The resultant series of bleeding points is used as a guide for the gingivectomy incision. (Periodont.)

marking p. The accurate determination and delineation of pocket depth and topography as an aid to diagnosis and prognosis or to provide a guide for the gingivectomy incision. (Periodont.)

p. in occlusal trauma Pocket formation, not as a sequela of occlusal traumatism but as a secondary phenomenon associated with induction of gingival inflammation by local etiologic factors on an attachment apparatus previously damaged by traumatic injury. (Periodont.)

periodontal p. A pathologically deepened gingival sulcus associated with periodontal disease. (Oral Diag.)

— A pathologic deepening of the gingival sulcus produced by destruction of the supporting tissues and apical proliferation of the epithelial attachment. Ulceration of the pocket epithelium lining is characteristic. (Periodont.)

p., purulent discharge The discharge of exudate from the subepithelial tissues through ulcerations in the epithelial lining of the pocket. The degree of exudation depends on the amount of destruction of the sulcular epithelium and the amount of cellular infiltration of the subepithelial tissues as well as the resistance of those tissues to infection. (Periodont.)

reattachment of p. A desirable result of periodontal therapy in which, after complete débridement of the diseased gingival attachment, there is formation of a new attachment of the investing and supporting tissues to the tooth. This new attachment involves the formation of a new gingival attachment placed more coronally to the tooth and, in the case of the repair of infrabony defects,

the additional reconstitution of a new, more coronally situated attachment apparatus. (Periodont.)

suprabony p. A pocket whose base is coronal to the alveolar crest. Includes the gingival pocket (pseudopocket) where there is gingival inflammation and ulceration of the sulcular epithelium, but apical proliferation of the epithelial attachment and the periodontal pocket is associated with the pocket. This apical proliferation may be described as a pathologic deepening of the gingival sulcus produced by destruction of the gingival fibers and apical proliferation of the epithelial atttachment. (Periodont.)

p., trifurcation involvement The extension of pocket formation into the intraradicular areas of the trirooted teeth; i.e., the maxillary molar teeth. (Periodont.)

pogonion (pō-gō′nē-on) The most anterior, prominent point on the chin. (Orthodont.)

poikilocytosis (poi″kĭ-lō-sī-tō′sĭs) Irregular shape of the red blood cells. (Oral Diag.)

point A small spot; a minute area; a rotating instrument having a small cutting end or surface.

p. A The most retrusive point of the maxillary alveolar process. (Orthodont.)

abrasive p., rotary Mounted carborundum, diamond, etc. Small abrasive instruments used either in straight or contra-angle handpieces. (Oper. Dent.; Periodont.)

p. angle (see **angle, point**)

p. B The most retrusive point of the mandibular alveolar process. (Orthodont.)

bleeding p. (see **bleeding points**)

boiling p. The temperature at which the vapor pressure within a liquid equals atmospheric pressure. (Anesth.)

Bolton p. The highest point of the curvature between the occipital condyle and the basilar part of the occipital bone; located behind the occipital condyle. The highest point of the curvature behind the occipital condyle. A substitute for the basion point when it cannot be ascertained on cephalometric headplates. (Orthodont.)

central-bearing p. The contact point of a central-bearing device. (Comp. Prosth.; Remov. Part. Prosth.)

p. of centricity If the point of the buccal cusp of the lower right molar, put in lateral position, is arced about the upright axis of the right condyle, it will reach a station where further muscular efforts leftward will change the cusp's direction so that it will arc about the left condyle. The station where the right arc ends and the left arc begins is a point of mandibular centricity. While the right cusp point was orbiting (arcing) about the near vertical axis, all other points in the jaw joined in orbiting (arcing). The left condyle arced rearward until it reached a cranial backstop; then the muscles started rotating it and carrying it leftward, and the right condyle began arcing forward, downward, and medially. In the right and left swings of the jaw, a condyle reciprocally alternates between being a rotator and an orbiter. The point of centricity of the mandible is demonstrated usually on a horizontal plane, but it can be demonstrated on all three planes of projection. The point of centricity may be confused with median planes of the face or the midsagittal plane. Points of centricity can be found outside the face and are as truly of mandibular joint and muscular directions as those determined within the face. The point of centricity is rearmost, midmost (between the arcs of motion), and uppermost. (Gnathol.) (see also **face-bow; relation, centric**)

condenser p. The nib of a condensing instrument. A short instrument, for condensing foil or amalgam, that is inserted into a mechanical condenser or into a cone socket handle. (Oper. Dent.)

contact p. (**contact area**) The area of contact of approximating surfaces of two adjacent teeth. The areas of contact are located at the line of junction between the occlusal and middle thirds of the posterior teeth and the incisal and middle thirds of the anterior teeth. (Periodont.)

  faulty c. p. Defective contact between the proximal surfaces of adjacent teeth, produced by wearing of the contact areas, dental caries, improper restoration, altered tooth position, etc. (Periodont.)

  loss of c. p. Failure of contact of convex proximal surfaces of adjacent teeth; produced by tooth migration, dental caries, improper restoration, etc. (Periodont.)

  c. p. of teeth The contact of the convex proximal surfaces of adjacent teeth in such a manner that food is deflected away from the tissues of the interdental papillae. (Periodont.)

convenience p. (see **point, starting**)

p. D The center of the body of the symphysis. (Orthodont.)

gutta-percha p. (see **gutta-percha points**)

hinge axis p. A point placed on the skin corresponding with the opening axis of the mandible. (Comp. Prosth.)

Hirschfeld's silver p. A calibrated silver rod used to record the clinical depth of periodontal pockets radiographically for the purpose of diagnosis. (Periodont.)

incisor p. The intersection of the lower occlusal plane and the midsagittal plane. The point at the mesioincisal angles of the two mandibular central incisors. (Comp. Prosth.)

median mandibular p. A point on the anteroposterior center of the mandibular ridge in the median sagittal plane. (Comp. Prosth.)

p., paper (see **paper point**)

registration p. Any point considered as fixed for a particular pattern of analysis. Also, the midpoint of a perpendicular line from the sella turcica to the Bolton-nasion plane. (Orthodont.)

starting p. (**convenience p.**) A small undercut in the cavity wall convenient for placing and retaining the first portion of a filling material. (Oper. Dent.)

  s. p. for foil Any one of the small undercuts or penetrations in the cavity wall placed at strategic positions convenient for starting and building a triangular bar of cohesive gold foil. (Oper. Dent.)

transition p. (see **Tg value**)

treatment p. A piece of paper point, selected for the root canal being treated, that carries or holds the medication in place. (Endodont.)

trial p. A cone of filling material placed in a canal and radiographed to check on the length and fit of the filling. (Endodont.)

yield p. The place on the stress-strain curve where marked permanent deformation occurs; it is just beyond the proportional limit. (D. Mat.)

— The point where permanent deformation starts in a metal. (Remov. Part. Prosth.)

pointing Term associated with fluctuation pertaining to the area where the purulent exudate is eroding through tissues to an external surface. It is at this point that an incision and drainage operation usually is performed. (Oral Surg.)

poison In medical jurisprudence, a substance that, on being applied to the human body, internally or externally, has the capability of destroying life. (D. Juris.)

— A substance that, when ingested, inhaled, absorbed, injected into, or developed within the body, will cause damage to structures of the body and impair or destroy their function. (Periodont.)

poisoning The morbid condition caused by poison. (Oral Med.; Oral Path.)

arsenic p. Acute or chronic intoxication from the ingestion of insecticides or administration of organic arsenicals. Manifestations of acute poisoning include abdominal pain, nausea, vomiting, and collapse. Chronic manifestations include weakness, peripheral neuropathy, hyperkeratosis, skin rashes, and oral manifestations secondary to liver dysfunction and bone marrow depression. (Oral Med.) (see also **stomatitis, arsenical**)

bismuth p. (see **bismuthosis**)

chemical p. A form of poisoning caused by ingestion of a toxic chemical agent. As exemplified by bismuth or other systemic poisoning, a purplish blue line appears along the gingiva at about the height of the alveolar crest and extends to the cervical margin. (Periodont.)

iodine p. (see **iodism**)

lead p. (see **plumbism**)

mercury p. (see **mercurialism**)

metallic p. A toxic condition produced by excessive exposure to or intake of metals. In the oral cavity there may be definite signs of arsenic, bismuth, lead, phosphorus, radium, and other metals. Fluorides produce changes in developing teeth at levels far below those which are toxic for the rest of the human economy. (Oral Diag.)

phosphorus p. The result of the ingestion of phosphorus, especially yellow phosphorus. Manifestations include burning of the mouth and throat, abdominal pain, vomiting, jaundice, liver damage, and death. In chronic poisoning, necrosis of the jaws (phossy jaw) occurs. (Oral Med.)

police power The authority of the state to enact laws to protect the public, such as a dental practice act. It is the police power reserved to the states under the United States Constitution. (D. Juris.)

poliomyelitis (pō″le-o-mī″e-lī′tĭs) A disease produced by a small viral organism that enters the body via the alimentary tract and produces upper pharyngeal, pharyngeal, and intestinal inflammation in its mentor form. In the more severe variety, a subsequent viremia is produced, with extension of the infection to the anterior pulp horn cells and ganglia of the spinal cord, producing a flaccid paralysis. In bulbar poliomyelitis the viral infection involves the medulla, resulting in impairment of swallowing, respiration, and/or circulation. It is now recognized that three types of viruses are responsible for the nonparalytic, paralytic, and bulbar varieties of poliomyelitis. Excellent immunization procedures have been provided by use of killed viruses (Salk) and attenuated mutant vaccines (Sabin). (Periodont.)

polishing, *n.* The art or process of making a denture or casting smooth and glossy. (Comp. Prosth.; Remov. Part. Prosth.)

—, *v.* Making smooth and glossy, usually by friction; giving luster to. (Comp. Prosth.; Remov. Part. Prosth.)

p. brush (see **brush, polishing**)

coronal p. Removal of mucinous film, superficial stain, deposits, etc. to provide a smooth enamel surface that will be more resistant to future accumulations of foreign substances (materia alba, calculus, mucinous plaque, etc.). (Periodont.)

p. disk (see **disk, polishing**)

pollakiuria (pol″ah-ke-u′re-ah) Unduly frequent urination. It may be due to partial obstruction (e.g., in prostatic enlargement), or it may be of nervous origin. (Oral Diag.; Oral Med.)

pollen A fertilizing element of plants that travels in the air and produces seasonal allergic responses (e.g., hay fever and asthma) in sensitive individuals. (Oral Med.)

polyantibiotic (pol″e-ăn″tĭ-bī-ot′ĭk) A combination of two or more antibiotics used to eliminate bacteria from a root canal. (Endodont.)

polychromatophilia (pol″e-krō-măt″o-fil′e-ah) Irregular staining of cells, particularly red blood cells. (Oral Diag.)

polycythemia (pol″e-sī-the′me-ah) Increase in blood volume as a result of an increase in the number of red blood cells, the erythrocytes. It may be due to a blood-forming disease that increases cell production, or it may be a physiologic response to an increased need for oxygenation in high altitudes, in cardiac disease, or in respiratory disorders. (Oral Physiol.)

primary p. (see **erythremia**)

p. rubra (see **erythremia**)

secondary p. (see **erythrocytosis**)

p. vera (see **erythremia**)

polydipsia (pol″e-dĭp′se-ah) Abnormally increased thirst. (Oral Diag.)

polymer (pol′ĭ-mer) A long-chain hydrocarbon. In dentistry, the polymer is supplied as a powder to be mixed with the monomer for fabrication of appliances and restorations. (D. Mat.)

polymerization (pō-lĭm″er-ĭ-zā′shŭn) The forming of a compound from several single molecules of the same substance, the molecular weight of the new compound being a multiple equal to the number of single molecules that have been combined. (Comp. Prosth.; Remov. Part. Prosth.)

— The chaining together of similar molecules to form a compound of high molecular weight. (D. Mat.)

addition p. A compound formed by a combination of simple molecules without the formation of any new products; e.g., methyl methacrylate $A + A = A - A - (A_n)$. (D. Mat.)

condensation p. Combination of simple, dissimilar molecules, with the formation of byproducts such as water or ammonia; e.g., vulcanite. (D. Mat.)

cross p. (cross linkage, cross-linked p.) The formation of chemical bonds between linear molecules, resulting in a three-dimensional network. Used for artificial teeth and denture bases because of superior craze resistance. (D. Mat.)

cross-linked p. (see **polymerization, cross**)

polymyxin (pol″ē-mĭk′sĭn) An antibiotic substance derived from cultures of *Bacillus polymyxa*. Used topically, in troche form, in combination with bacitracin and neomycin in the treatment of various oral infections. Not used systemically; therefore, sensitization is minimized. Systemic use may be attended by renal dysfunction and toxicity. (Periodont.)

polyneuritis, endemic (pol″ē-nū-rī′tĭs) (see **beriberi**)

polyostotic (pol″ē-os-tot′ĭk) Affecting more than one bone. (Oral Path.)

polyp (pol′ĭp) A smooth, pedunculated growth from a mucous surface such as from the nose, bladder, or rectum. (Anesth.)

pulp p. (see **pulpitis, hypertrophic**)

polypharmacy The prescription or dispensation of unnecessarily numerous or complex medicines. (Oral Med.; Pharmacol.)

polypnea (pol″ĭp-nē′ah) A rapid or panting respiration. (Anesth.)

polyposis, multiple (pol″ĭ-pō′sĭs) (see **syndrome, Peutz-Jeghers**)

polystyrene (pol″ē-stī′rēn) A polymer of styrene, which is a derivative of ethylene; $[-CH(C_6H_5)CH_2-]n$. Often one of the resins present in materials designed for denture construction by the injection molding technique. (D. Mat.)

polysulfide polymer (pol″ē-sul′fĭd pol′ĭ-mer) A rubber base impression material utilizing a mercaptan bondage. Prepared by mixing a base material (mercaptan) with either an in-

organic catalyst (lead peroxide) or an organic catalyst (benzoyl peroxide). (D. Mat.)

polyuria (pol″ē-ū′rē-ah) The passage of an abnormally increased volume of urine. It may be due to increased intake of fluids, inadequate renal function, uncontrolled diabetes mellitus or diabetes insipidus, diuresis of edema fluid, or ascites. (Oral Diag.; Oral Med.)

pons A structure dorsal to the medulla and intimately related to the pathways to the cerebrum. The cranial nerves whose nuclei lie in the pons are the trigeminal, the abducens, the facial, and part of the acoustic. The pons is intimately related to the medulla, has the same blood vessel supply, and is involved in many lesions that affect the medulla. It is especially involved with the cerebellar manifestations of disease and may cause serious muscular incoordination in motor function of the head, neck, and facial structures. (Oral Physiol.)

pontic (pon′tĭk) The suspended member of a fixed partial denture; an artificial tooth on a fixed partial denture or an isolated tooth on a removable partial denture. It replaces a lost natural tooth, restores its function, and usually occupies the space previously occupied by the natural crown. (Comp. Prosth.; Fixed Part. Prosth.; Remov. Part. Prosth.)

porcelain A material formed by the fusion of feldspar, silica, and other minor ingredients. Most dental porcelains are glasses and are used in the manufacture of artificial teeth, facings, jackets, and occasionally denture bases and inlays. (D. Mat.)

— A vitreous, tooth-colored material used in restorative dentistry. It is composed principally of selected clays and silica and maintains its form by virtue of a pyrochemical reaction under critical heat control. Its widest use in dentistry is in the form of commercially manufactured teeth. (Fixed Part. Prosth.)

baked p. (see **porcelain, dental**)

dental p. (baked p., fired p.) A fused mixture that is glasslike and more or less transparent. Classification of the type of porcelain employed in inlays and crowns is based on the fusion temperature of the porcelain: high fusing, 2350° to 2500° F; medium fusing, 2000° to 2300° F; low fusing, 1600° to 2000° F. (Oper. Dent.)

fired p. (see **porcelain, dental**)

synthetic p. (see **cement, silicate**)

porion (pō′rē-on) The upper edge of the external auditory meatus. (Orthodont.)

porosity (pō-ros′ĭ-tē) Presence of pores or voids within a structure. (D. Mat.)
— The state or quality of having minute pores, openings, or interstices. (Oper. Dent.)
   back-pressure p. Porosity produced in castings due to the inability of gases in the mold to escape through the investment. (D. Mat.)
   occluded gas p. Porosity produced by improper use of the blowpipe; i.e., heating the metal in the oxidizing portion of the flame. (D. Mat.)
   shrink-spot p. An area of porosity in cast metal that is caused by shrinkage of a portion of the metal as it solidifies from the molten state without flow of additional molten metal from surrounding areas. (Oper. Dent.)
   solidification p. A porosity that may be produced by improper spruing or improper heating of either the metal or the investment. (D. Mat.)
porphyria, congenital (see **porphyria, erythropoietic**)
porphyria, erythropoietic (por-fi′rē-ah) (**congenital p., photosensitive p.**) An inborn error of metabolism (porphyrin synthesis) characterized clinically by skin photosensitivity, hypertrichosis, and reddish brown staining of the primary teeth. (Oral Med.)
porphyria, photosensitive (see **porphyria, erythropoietic**)
port The opening through which x-ray photons or the useful beam of radiation exits from the head of a dental x-ray machine. (Oral Radiol.)
position The placement of body members.
   border p., posterior The most posterior position of the mandible at any specific vertical relation of the maxillae. (Comp. Prosth.)
   centric p. The position of the mandible in its most retruded relation to the maxillae at the established vertical relation. (Comp. Prosth.)
   — The constant position into which the patient will close his jaws; this relationship may be either his convenience relationship or his true centric relationship. (Periodont.)
   — Abbreviation used in captioning an item or listing. If the cusp of the lower first molar, when occluded by the hands, occupies the most centric part of the centric fossa of the upper molar, it has centric position in its coupling with the upper molar. (Gnathol.)
   eccentric p. (**eccentric jaw p.**) Any position of

the mandible other than that in centric relation. (Comp. Prosth.) (see also **relation, jaw, eccentric**)
   e. jaw p. (see **position, eccentric; relation, jaw, eccentric**)
finger p. (see **finger positions**)
gingival p. (see **gingival position**)
hinge p. The orientation of parts in a manner permitting hinge movements between them. (Comp. Prosth.; Fixed Part. Prosth.; Remov. Part. Prosth.)
   condylar h. p. Mandibular joints at which a hinge movement of the mandible is possible. (Comp. Prosth.)
   —The maxillomandibular relation from which a consciously stimulated true hinge movement can be executed. (Comp. Prosth.; Remov. Part. Prosth.)
   mandibular h. p. Any position of the mandible that exists when the condyles are so situated in the temporomandibular joints that opening or closing movements can be made on the hinge axis. (Comp. Prosth.; Remov. Part. Prosth.)
   terminal h. p. The mandibular hinge position from which further opening of the mandible would produce translatory rather than hinge movement. (Comp. Prosth.; Remov. Part. Prosth.)
   — The posterior terminal position of the mandibular condyles effecting hinge movement, as in opening and closing of the jaws without translation of the condyles. (Fixed Part. Prosth.) (see also **position, hinge**)
intercuspal p. Term applied to the cuspal contacts of teeth when the mandible is in centric relation. Also referred to as centric occlusion. (Periodont.)
occlusal p. The relation of the mandible to the maxillae when the jaw is closed and the teeth are in contact. This mandibular position may or may not coincide with centric occlusion. (Comp. Prosth.; Remov. Part. Prosth.)
protrusive p. Occlusion of the teeth as the mandible and lower central incisors are moved straight forward toward the incisal edges of the upper central incisors; the normal anteroclusal relationship; the forward end position, with the upper and lower incisors in edge-to-edge contact. (Periodont.)
rest p. The position of the mandible when the jaws are in rest relation. (Comp. Prosth.; Fixed Part. Prosth.; Remov. Part. Prosth.)

(see also **position, rest, physiologic; relation, jaw, rest**)

— A position of the mandible in which the teeth are uncoupled during times when the gnathic organ, between swallowings, is being used for the following: breathing; draining of the oral secretions; speaking or humming; or toileting of the teeth with the tongue. However much the gap between the uncoupled teeth varies with changes in posture from proneness to sitting poses, or during sleep, it seems that the function of chewing or biting can recommence quickly from any such variations in the amounts of interocclusal distance. It is agreed that "rest" position, sometimes specified as the upright posture of chewing idleness, is the base from which mandibular chewing activities start and to which the mandible returns after eating ends. (Gnathol.)

—The position that the mandible passively assumes when the mandibular musculature is relaxed. (Orthodont.)

— A postural position of the mandible under the influence of the resting length of the muscles that elevate or depress the mandible. (Periodont.)

mandibular r. p. The normal postural position of the mandible at rest with the teeth apart. In this position, the mandible is under the influence of the resting length of the muscles that elevate or depress the jaws. (Periodont.)

physiologic r. p. The habitual postural position of the mandible when the patient is resting comfortably in the upright position and the condyles are in a neutral, unstrained position in the glenoid fossae. The mandibular musculature is in a state of minimum tonic contraction to maintain posture and to overcome its force of gravity. (Comp. Prosth.; Remov. Part. Prosth.) (see also **relation, jaw, rest**)

tooth p. The placement or location of the tooth in the dental arch in relation to the bone of the alveolar process, its adjacent teeth, and the opposing dentition. (Periodont.)

Trendelenburg p. A position in which the patient is on his back with his head and chest lowered and his legs elevated. (Oral Surg.)

positioner (tooth positioner) A resilient removable appliance covering the maxillary and mandibular teeth; used to effect limited repositioning of the teeth. (Orthodont.)

positioning, surgical The surgical repositioning of a tooth or the tilting of a tooth without injuring its blood supply. (Oral Surg.)

positions at the chair Posture and relative location of dentist or chairside assistant in respect to the dental chair and patient. Classified as standing or sitting and as right side behind, right side in front, left side behind, left side in front, and directly behind. The position used should permit the most efficient performance of the current procedure and also keep paramount the health and comfort of the dentist and the patient. (Oper. Dent.)

possession The control or custody of anything that may be the subject of property, either as owner or as one who has a qualified right in it. (D. Juris.)

post cibum (pōst sī'bŭm) (see **p. c.**)

postdam area (see **area, posterior palatal seal**)

post, implant (see **substructure, implant, neck**)

postcondensation (aftercondensation) The procedure of completing the condensation or compaction of the surface of a gold-foil restoration after all the gold has been placed. Usually a condenser with a large face and fine serrations is used. (Oper. Dent.)

posterior Situated behind. (Orthodont.)

p. nasal spine (see **spine, posterior nasal**)

p. palatal bar (see **connector, major, posterior palatal**)

p. palatal seal (see **seal, posterior palatal**)

p. palatal seal area (see **area, posterior palatal seal**)

posteroanterior extraoral radiographic examination (see **examination, radiographic, extraoral, posteroanterior**)

postpalatal seal (see **seal, posterior palatal**)

p. s. area (see **area, posterior palatal seal**)

postperception (afterperception) The perception of a sensation after the stimulus producing it has ceased. (Anesth.)

postresection The performance of an apicoectomy after the filling of a root canal. (Endodont.)

postsensation (aftersensation) A sensation lasting after the stimulus that produced it has been removed. (Anesth.)

posture, normal The configuration of the body in the upright position, which varies considerably among individuals. However, normal posture can be described as follows: the shoulder, pelvis, and eyes are level; the sagittal plane is between the feet, and the line of gravity passes through the center of gravity at the lumbosacral joint. When observed from the following positions, the line of gravity intersects the following structures: *lateral posi-*

tion—anterior border of the ear, and the shoulder, hip, knee, and ankle joints; *anterior position*—nose, symphysis pubis, and between knees and feet; *posterior position*—occiput, spinous processes, gluteal crease, and between knees and feet. (Oral Physiol.)

potassium sulfate An accelerator used to speed the setting of gypsum products. Hydrocolloid impressions are fixed in a 2% solution of potassium sulfate. (D. Mat.)

potency (pŏ'ten-sē) Power. (Anesth.)

potential, action (see **action potential**)

potentiation (pō-těn″shē-ā'shŭn) (**synergism**) Increase in the action of a drug by the addition of another drug that does not necessarily possess similar properties. (Anesth.)

— Enhancement of action, e.g., of a drug. (Oral Med.; Pharmacol.)

Potter-Bucky diaphragm (see **grid, Potter-Bucky**)

Potter-Bucky grid (see **grid, Potter-Bucky**)

Pott's disease (see **disease, Pott's**)

pour hole An aperture in a refractory investment or other mold material leading to the pattern space into which prosthetic material is deposited. (M.F.P.)

powdered gold (see **gold, powdered**)

power stroke (see **stroke, power**)

Pp (see **pauperissimus**)

PPCF (see **factor V**)

practice To follow or work at, as a profession, trade, or art. (D. Juris.)

p. administration The organization, operation, and supervision of the business and professional aspects of a dental practice. (Pract. Man.)

p. building Increasing the number of patients and the number of services without sacrificing quality, by means of observing the principles of constantly improving professional care and maintaining effective human relations with patients. (Pract. Man.)

p. goal The planning of the objectives of a dental practice and the method of reaching those objectives. To be ascertained by the dental practitioner before or immediately on entering dental practice. (Pract. Man.)

group p. A large partnership formed for the purpose of practicing dentistry; may or may not include the services of the recognized specialties in dentistry. (Pract. Man.)

p. growth Increase in the size, scope, and quality of service within a dental practice. (Pract. Man.)

private p. The business and profession in which dental services are administered for a fee. (Pract. Man.)

Prausnitz-Küstner test (prows'nĭts kĭst'ner) (see **test, skin, indirect**)

preanesthetic (prē″ăn-ĕs-thĕt'ĭk) A medicine for producing preliminary anesthesia; e.g., Avertin. (Anesth.)

precipitate (prē-sĭp'ĭ-tāt) An insoluble solid substance that forms from chemical reactions between solutions. (Anesth.)

precision attachment (see **attachment, intracoronal**)

precision rest (see **rest, precision**)

precordial Pertaining to the region over the heart or stomach; the epigastrium and lower thorax. (Anesth.)

precursor, fifth plasma thromboplastin (see **factor XII**)

precursor of serum prothrombin conversion accelerator (**cothromboplastin, factor VII, pro-SPCA**) A clotting factor found in serum plasma and thought to be needed for the optimal action of tissue thromboplastin. Formerly, with the Stuart factor, it was known as proconvertin or stable factor. (Oral Med.) (see also **proconvertin**)

prednisone (prĕd'nĭ-sōn) A steroid used systemically and topically as an anti-inflammatory agent. Useful also in the treatment of adrenal hypocorticism and the various collagen diseases. (Periodont.)

preextraction cast (see **cast, diagnostic; cast, preextraction**)

preextraction record (see **record, preoperative**)

prematurities (see **contact, deflective occlusal; contact, interceptive occlusal**)

grinding of p. Selective reduction of interfering tooth surfaces in the centric path of closure, lateral mandibular excursive movement, protrusive mandibular movement, etc., when there is evidence that these contacts are contributing to traumatic lesions of the attachment apparatus. (Periodont.)

premaxilla, floating (see **premaxilla, loose**)

premaxilla, loose (**floating premaxilla**) Nonunion of the premaxillary process with the lateral maxillary segments, so that the premaxilla is loose, or floating. The position of the loose premaxilla in relation to the lateral maxillary segments varies among patients. (Cleft Palate)

premedication The use of a single drug or a combination of drugs to allay fear and reduce muscular tension in children who are difficult to handle during dental procedures. (Pedodont.)

— The administration of a tranquilizing drug, a drug that influences blood-clotting time, or any other drug that produces a preplanned set of conditions and is administered preceding any dental procedures. (Pract. Man.)

premolar (bicuspid) One of the eight teeth in man, four in each jaw, between the cuspids and the first molars; usually has two cusps; replaces the molars of the deciduous dentition. (Oper. Dent.)

preoperative cast (see **cast, diagnostic**)

preoperative record (see **record, preoperative**)

preparation The selected form given to a natural tooth when it is reduced by instrumentation to receive a prosthesis; e.g., an artificial crown or a retainer for a fixed or removable prosthesis. The selection of the form is guided by the clinical circumstances and the physical properties of the materials that make up the prosthesis. (Fixed Part. Prosth.) (see also **preparation, mouth**)

cavity p. One of the various operations in which carious material is removed from teeth and biomechanically correct forms are established in the teeth to receive and retain restorations. A constant requirement is provision for prevention of failure of the restoration through recurrence of decay or inadequate resistance to applied stresses. (Oper. Dent.)

initial p. One of a number of procedures aimed at preparing the patient for final treatment. The objectives consist of eliminating or reducing all the local etiologic factors and environmental influences prior to the operative procedures and establishing a sequence of therapy for the patient. (Periodont.)

mouth p. One of the various necessary procedures applied to the oral structures preparatory to the making of a final impression for a prosthesis. (Remov. Part. Prosth.)

slice p. A type of cavity preparation for Class 2 cast restorations. The proximal portion is formed by removing a sufficient slice of the proximal convexity of the tooth to achieve cleansable margins and a line of draw; there is a tapered keyway or two keyed grooves or channels in the proximal surface to provide retention form. (Oper. Dent.)

surgical p. Any modification that utilizes surgical procedures that may be required for preparing the oral structures for prosthodontic treatment. (Remov. Part. Prosth.)

preponderance In evidence, outweighing. (D. Juris.)

presbyopia (prĕs″bē-ō′pē-ah) A form of optical distortion affecting the vision of patients, particularly those of advancing age. It is dependent on diminution of the power of the accommodation of the lens as a result of loss of elasticity of the crystalline lens, causing the near point of distinct vision to be removed farther from the eye. When a patient's vision is distorted by presbyopia, the dentist may encounter difficulty when the patient is called upon to exercise judgment in determining the preferred shade and form of teeth during a clinical procedure. This type of of optical distortion is commonly called farsightedness, longsightedness, or hyperopia. (Oral Physiol.)

prescription A written direction for the preparation and use of medicine or appliance; a medical recipe; a prescribed remedy. (D. Juris.)

— An order issued to a pharmacist, a dental laboratory, or the patient, ensuring that the dentist's judgment requiring certain medications or procedures be carried out accurately. Also used in dentistry to describe the treatment plan. (Pract. Man.)

extemporaneous p. (magistral p.) A prescription for a nonofficial drug. (Oral Med.; Pharmacol.)

— A prescription that directs the pharmacist to compound the specified medication according to his art, as contrasted with a prescription that specifies medication available in precompounded form. (Oral Med.; Pharmacol.)

magistral p. (see **prescription, extemporaneous**)

official p. A prescription for an official drug. (Oral Med.; Pharmacol.)

preservation A neurologic phenomenon such as the involuntary repetition of motor response or the continuation of a sensation after the adequate external stimulus has ceased. (Oral Physiol.)

preservative A substance added to prevent deterioration. (Oral Med.; Pharmacol.)

— An ingredient, sodium sulfite, of the fixing solution that dissolves residual salts on the film and also aids in preventing decomposition of the fixing solution. It is also an ingredient of the developing solution; its function prevents oxidation in the presence of air. (Oral Radiol.)

pressure A stress or strain that may occur by compression, pull, thrust, etc.; an applied force.

p. area (see **area, pressure**)

p. atrophy (see **atrophy, pressure**)

biting p. The actual or potential power used in bringing the teeth into contact. (Comp. Prosth.; Remov. Part. Prosth.) (see also **pressure, occlusal**)

blood p. The pressure of the blood on the walls of the arteries as determined by the amount of heart action, the elasticity of the walls of the arteries, the resistance in the capillaries, and the volume and viscosity of the blood. (Anesth.)

— The pressure exerted on arterial walls by the blood when the heart is in systole (systolic pressure) and the pressure maintained by the elasticity of the arteries when the heart is in diastole (diastolic pressure). A consistent arterial pressure greater than 140/90 is considered abnormally high and suggestive of hypertensive vascular disease. (Oral Med.)

deeper p. Any pressure to the body—in excess of that which stimulates Meissner's corpuscles, Merkel's disks, or the hair receptors of light touch—that stimulates the deeper receptors such as the pacinian corpuscles. These latter deep-pressure perception organs lie in the inner layers of the dermis and in the muscle and tendon groups. (Oral Physiol.)

equalization of p. The act of distributing pressure evenly. (Comp. Prosth.)

hand p. Force applied by an instrument held in the hand. (Oper. Dent.)

hydraulic p. The pressure exerted by a column of liquid in a root canal when solid materials are introduced. (Endodont.)

hydrostatic p. The pressure in the circulatory system exerted by the volume of blood when it is confined in a blood vessel. The hydrostatic pressure, coupled with the osmotic pressure, within a capillary is opposed by the hydrosatic and osmotic pressure of the surrounding tissues. Fluids flow from the higher pressure areas to the lower pressure areas. (Oral Physiol.)

intrapleural p. Pressure within the pleura. (Anesth.)

occlusal p. Any force exerted on the occlusal surfaces of teeth. (Comp. Prosth.) (see also **force, occlusal; load, occlusal**)

osmotic p. The stress that develops when solutions containing different concentrations of solute in a common solvent are separated by a membrane that is permeable to the solvent but not the solute. (Oral Med.; Pharmacol.)

partial p. The pressure exerted by each of the constituents of a mixture of gases. (Anesth.)

pulse p. The difference between systolic and diastolic pressure. (Anesth.; Oral Med.)

p. sensibility The ability to detect light touch and deep pressure. (Oral Physiol.) (see also **corpuscle, Meissner's; corpuscle, Merkel's; corpuscle, Pacini's**)

presumption A deduction that the law expressly directs to be made from certain facts; a consequence that the law or the judge draws from a known fact to one unknown. (D. Juris.)

presurgical impression An overextended impression of the intact mandible prior to the first surgical stage. The cast made for this impression is altered so that the surgical tray may be fabricated on it. (Oral Implant.) (see also **tray, surgical**)

prevention The steps necessary in preventing the prepathogenesis and pathogenesis of the disease process in periodontal disease. (Periodont.)

preventive Avoiding occurrence. (Oper. Dent.)

prima facie (prī′mah fā′shē-ē″) On the face of it; so far as can be judged from the first appearance; presumably. (D. Juris.)

primary First in time; first in order in any series. (Oper. Dent.)

p. beam (see **radiation, primary**)

p. fixation Immediate postoperative fastening of an implant to bone by means of wires, screws, or a superstructure until, through natural healing and adhesion, final fixation occurs. (Oral Implant.)

p. intention healing The healing of a wound directly at the incision site. (Oral Implant.)

p. radiation (see **radiation, primary**)

principal Chief; highest in rank; the source of authority. (D. Juris.)

p. in law of agency The employer; the person who gives authority to an agent to act for him. (D. Juris.)

p.r.n. (see **pro re nata**)

pro re nata (**p.r.n.**) (prō rē nā′tah) A Latin phrase meaning occasionally as needed, or according to circumstances. (Oral Med.; Pharmacol.)

proaccelerin (factor V, labile factor, plasma accelerator globulin, plasma ac-globulin, prothrombinase, prothrombin conversion accelerator I) An unstable protein found in the blood; the precursor of accelerin. (Oral Med.)

proandrogens (prō-ăn′drō-jĕnz) Compounds that are not androgenic when applied locally but that have androgenic activity when metabolized in the organism. Included are cortisone and cortisol, which may be converted within the organism to androgens such as adrenosterone, 11-ketoandrosterone, and 11-hydroxyandrosterone. (Oral Med.)

probative (prō′bah-tĭv) In the law of evidence, tending to prove or actually proving. (D. Juris.)

probe A slender, flexible instrument designed for introduction into a wound or cavity for purposes of exploration. (Oral Surg.)

calibrated p. A periodontal instrument calibrated in millimeters; used to measure the depth of gingival sulci and gingival and periodontal pockets. (Periodont.)

cross p. A fine-caliber instrument used to ascertain the presence of calculus or other foreign materials on the root surface of the gingival sulcus, gingival pocket, or periodontal pocket. (Periodont.)

lacrimal p. An instrument useful in probing the lumen of duct structures, such as the nasolacrimal or salivary gland ducts. (Oral Surg.)

periodontal p. A fine calibrated instrument designed and used for measuring the depth and topography of gingival and periodontal pockets. Also used to determine the degree of attachment and adaptation of the gingival tissues to the tooth. (Periodont.)

Williams' p. A periodontal probe used to measure retractable gingival tissue and locate the base of the pocket. (Periodont.)

procaine hydrochloride A local anesthetic agent; 2-diethylaminoethyl 4-aminobenzoate hydrochloride. (Periodont.)

procedure A series of steps, followed in a regular, orderly, definite way, by which a desired result is accomplished. (Comp. Prosth.)

dental prosthetic laboratory p. The steps in the fabrication of a dental prosthesis that do not require the presence of the patient for their accomplishment. (Comp. Prosth.; Fixed Part. Prosth.; Remov. Part. Prosth.)

Kazanjian's p. (see **operation, Kazanjian's**)

open p. Procedure in which the overlying tissues are surgically reflected and the host site is exposed in order to insert an implant. (Oral Implant.)

operating p. The technique or method of conducting or performing an operation or form of treatment. (Oper. Dent.)

order of p. The sequence of steps made in performing an operation or following through a technique. In cavity preparation the sequence is as follows: (1) obtain the required outline form, (2) obtain the required resistance form, (3) obtain the required retention form, (4) retain the required convenience form, (5) remove any remaining carious dentin, (6) finish the enamel walls, and (7) make the débridement. (Oper. Dent.)

orthodontic p. Therapeutic measures employed to correct malalignment and malposition of the teeth and to immobilize and stabilize periodontally involved or previously moved teeth. (Periodont.)

restorative p. A method or mode of action that reestablishes or reforms a tooth or teeth or portions thereof to anatomic or functional form and health. (Oper. Dent.)

process In anatomy, a marked prominence or projection of a bone. In dentistry, a series of operations that convert a wax pattern, such as that of a denture base, into a solid denture base of another material. (Comp. Prosth.; Remov. Part. Prosth.) (see also **denture curing**)

alveolar p. The part of the bone that surrounds and supports the teeth in the maxillae and the mandible. (Oper. Dent.)

— The cancellous bony structure that supports the teeth. (Orthodont.)

— The portion of the maxillae or mandible that forms the dental arch and serves as a bony investment for the teeth. Its cortical covering is continuous with the compact bone of the body of the maxillae or mandible, whereas its trabecular portion is continuous with the spongiosa of the body of the jaws. (Periodont.) (see also **ridge, alveolar**)

dehiscence of a. p. A dipping of the crestal bone margin, exposing an abnormal amount of root surface. (Periodont.)

fenestration of a. p. A circumscribed hole, located in the cortical plate over the root, that does not communicate with the crestal margin. (Periodont.)

condyloid p. (kahn′dĭ-loid) (**capitulum mandibulae**) A projection of the mandible arising on the posterosuperior aspect of the mandibular ramus. It consists of a neck and an elliptically shaped head or condyle that enters into the formation of the temporomandibular joint in conjunction with the articular disk and the glenoid fossa of the temporal bone. (Periodont.)

neck of c. p. The part of the condyloid process that connects the condyle to the main part of the ramus. The term "neck of the condyloid process" is preferred by anatomists. It is not the neck of the mandible, but rather the portion of the mandible to which the condyle is attached. (Comp. Prosth.)

coronoid p. The thin triangular rounded eminence originating from the anterosuperior surface of the ramus of the mandible. Provides insertion for the various fiber bundles of the temporal muscle. (Periodont.)

hamular p. (pterygoid p.) The pterygoid process of the sphenoid bone; appears as a vertical projection distal to the maxillary tuberosity. (Periodont.)

horizontal resorptive p. The pattern of bone resorption, occurring with periodontal disease, in which the resultant level of bone is more or less flat or level in nature. (Periodont.)

pterygoid p. (see **process, hamular**)

processing (prăh'sĕs-ĭng) Term that usually refers to the procedure of bringing about polymerization of appliances; processing of dentures. (D. Mat.) (see also **film processing**)

denture p. The conversion of a wax pattern of a denture or trial denture into a denture with a base made of another material, e.g., acrylic resin. (Comp. Prosth.) (see also **process**)

p. tank (see **tank, processing**)

procheilia (prō-kēl'ē-ah) A condition of protruding lips. (Orthodont.)

proconvertin (autoprothrombin I, cofactor V, cothromboplastin, factor VII, precursor of serum prothrombin conversion accelerator [pro-SPCA], stable factor) Variously described as the inactive precursor of convertin. Recently proconvertin has been considered as a collective term for pro-SPCA and Stuart factor. (Oral Med.)

proconvertin-convertin (see **thromboplastin, extrinsic**)

procumbency (prō-cŭm'bĕn-sē) Excessive labioaxial inclination of the incisor teeth. (Orthodont.)

product, contact activation (see **factor C**)

production The amount of work that can be accomplished in a specific length of time. (Pract. Man.)

products, fission (see **fission products**)

profession A calling; vocation; a means of livelihood or gain. (D. Juris.)

profibrin (prō-fī'brĭn) (see **fibrinogen**)

profibrinolysin (prō-fī''brĭ-nol'ĭ-sĭn) (see **plasminogen**)

profile An outline or contour, especially one representing a side view of a human head. (Comp. Prosth.; Remov. Part. Prosth.)

p. extraoral radiographic examination (see

examination, radiographic, extraoral, profile)

facial p. The sagittal outline form of the face. (Comp. Prosth.)

p. record (see **record, profile**)

progeria (prō-jē'rē-ah) (see **syndrome, Hutchinson-Gilford**)

progesterone (prō-jĕs'tĕ-rōn) The ovarian hormone produced by the corpus luteum and responsible for preparing the endometrium for nidation and nourishment of the ovum. It also suppresses the production of the pituitary luteinizing hormone, estrus, and ovulation and stimulates the mammary glands. (Oral Med.)

prognathic (prŏg'năth'ĭk) Pertaining to a forward relationship of the jaws to the head (anterior to the skull); denoting a protrusive lower face. (Orthodont.)

prognathism (prŏg'nah-thĭzm) Prominence of the mandible. (Oral Diag.)

— Facial disharmony in which one or both jaws project forward. Prognathism may be real or imaginary. Mandibular prognathism may exist when both the maxillae and the mandible increase in length or when the maxillae are of normal length but the mandible increases in length. Prognathism may be imaginary when the maxillae are underdeveloped and short and the mandible is of normal length or when the maxillary and mandibular dental relationships are normal but there is an increase in the mental prominence of the mandible. (Oral Surg.; Orthodont.)

prognathus (prŏg-năth'ŭs) The condition of having a marked projection of the mandible, usually resulting in a horizontal overlap of the lower anterior teeth in relation to the maxillary anterior teeth. (Remov. Part. Prosth.)

prognosis (prog-nō'sĭs) A forecast of the probable result of treatment. (Orthodont.; Pract. Man.)

— An evaluation of the condition present, based on the etiologic factors responsible for the disease process and the benefit from therapeutic measures to be instituted, as well as the possibility of maintaining the status of a functionally dynamic reparation. A calculated prediction of the future condition of the tissues and/or the organism as a whole, based on an evaluation of the present state and knowledge of the therapeutic techniques to be employed and the probable results of such therapy. (Periodont.)

— A forecast as to the probable result of an attack of disease; the prospect as to recovery is afforded by the nature and symptoms of the disease entity. In prosthodontics, an opinion of the prospects for the success of a restoration. (Comp. Prosth.; Remov. Part. Prosth.)

denture p. An opinion or judgment, given in advance of treatment, of the prospects for success in the construction and usefulness of dentures. (Comp. Prosth.; Remov. Part. Prosth.)

factors in p. The combination of factors on which prognosis depends: (1) extent and type of the disease process; (2) causative factors, including (a) local environmental factors—correctable or noncorrectable, (b) physical health—correctable or noncorrectable—of the patient as it influences periodontal therapy, and (c) habits—correctable or noncorrectable; (3) occlusal factors; (4) number and distribution of remaining teeth; (5) age of patient; (6) cooperation of patient; and (7) ability of the dentist. (Periodont.)

projection, orthographic A projection made on the assumption that the projection lines from the object to the plane of projection are at right angles to the plane. (Gnathol.)

gnathic planes of o. p. The three planes of projection to which gnathologically mounted casts are oriented: the horizontal, vertical, (frontal), and profile. The horizontal plane is the axis-orbital plane. The hinge axis is the line of intersection for both the horizontal and the frontal planes. The profile plane is the mechanical midsagittal plane of the articulator. (Gnathol.)

prolactin (see **hormone, lactogenic**)

proliferation (prō-lĭf″ĕ-rā′shŭn) Growth by reproduction of similar cells. (Periodont.)

epithelial p. A characteristic finding in inflammatory lesions affecting the gingival tissues; consists of hyperplasia of the pocket epithelium, with extension and elongation of epithelial rete pegs into the submucosa. Accompanying the hyperplastic changes in the crevicular epithelium, it is noticed that the epithelial attachment proliferates onto and alongside the cementum. Also, the multiplication of epithelial cells resulting either in increased thickness or new epithelial covering of a wound or an ulcer. (Periodont.)

promissory (prom′ĭ-sōr″ē) A promise; stipulation for a future act or course of conduct. (D. Juris.)

pronasion (prō-nā′zē-on) The most prominent point on the tip of the nose when the head is placed in the eye-ear (horizontal) plane. (Orthodont.)

proof The establishment of a fact by evidence. To find the truth. (D. Juris.)

convincing p. That which is sufficient to establish the matter in question beyond ambiguity or reasonable doubt. (D. Juris.) (see also **evidence**)

prop A device inserted between the jaws to maintain an open position of the mandible. (Oral Surg.)

propagation The reproduction or continuance of an impulse along a nerve fiber in an afferent or efferent direction. (Anesth.)

property Rightful ownership; the exclusive right to a thing. (D. Juris.)

prophylactic (prō-fĭ-lăk′tĭk) A remedy that tends to ward off disease. (Oral Surg.)

prophylaxis (prō-fĭ-lăk′sĭs) Prevention of disease of the mouth and teeth. A procedure of removing extraneous materials from tooth surfaces by scaling and polishing techniques. (Oper. Dent.)

— Prevention of disease. Preventive therapy. (Oral Med.; Pharmacol.)

proportional limit (see **limit, elastic**)

proprietary Controlled by a private interest. (Oral Med.; Pharmacol.)

proprioceptive influence (prō″prē-ō-sĕp′tĭv) Influence of the muscle sense (kinesthetic sense) in guiding the jaw to close in such a way as not to be injurious to the teeth. (Gnathol.)

proprioceptive neuromuscular mechanism A biomechanical hookup of sensory and motor nerve trunk lines that control or help automate the muscular activities of posture. The muscular sensation and memory of jaw motions, relations, and positions in space should be studied to understand better the disorderly actions (ataxia) of the mandible. Appreciation of the automaticity of gnathic procedure grows as the student studies the well-ordered relations of the organically fit mouth (eutaxia). The outer informants of jaw movements and positions are receptors in the periodontium, the jaw joint capsules, and the important chewing muscles. What these reporters discover is "wired" to centers in either the brain or the spinal cord. These centers of recorded neural learning command the effectors to care for the needs of the jaw, if possible, by stimulating the correct controls of jaw action. Even after the effectors begin, other signals from receptors such as those of touch, pain, and pressure join with the proprioceptors in monitoring both further corrections of the amount of force and the directions in which the vector is running. Such monitoring is called feedback. (Gnathol.)

proprioceptors (prō″prē-ō-sĕp′torz) Sensory nerve receptors situated in the muscles, tendons, and joints that furnish information to the central nervous system concerning the movements and positions of the limbs, the trunk, the head and neck, and, more specifically for the dentist, the mandible and its associated oral structures. As a result of these stimuli received by the nerve centers, the contractions of individual muscles and groups of muscles are coordinated to produce smooth, finely adjusted, effective movements that would be impossible in the absence of such information. (Oral Physiol.)

proprothrombinase (prō″prō-throm′bĭn-ās) (see **factor V**)

proptosis (prop-tō′sĭs) Forward displacement or protrusion of the eyeball. (Oral Diag.) (see also **exophthalmus**)

pro-SPCA (see **precursor of serum prothrombin conversion accelerator**)

prosthesis (pros′thĕ-sĭs; pros-thē′sĭs) The replacement of an absent part of the human body by an artificial part. (Comp. Prosth.; Remov. Part. Prosth.)

cleft palate p. A restoration to correct congenital or acquired defects in the palate and related structures if they are involved. (Comp. Prosth.; Remov. Part. Prosth.)

complete denture p. (see **denture, complete**)

cranial p. An artificial material (alloplast) used to replace a portion of the skull. (M.F.P.)

dental p. An artificial replacement for one or more natural teeth and/or associated structures. (Comp. Prosth.; Remov. Part. Prosth.)

definitive p. A permanent type of substitute for missing tissue. (M.F.P.)

exercise p. A temporary, removable dental prosthesis, usually without teeth and always without occluding contact, used for the purpose of reconditioning the supporting structures (especially the alveolar process) by means of light intermittent biting pressure applied against bilaterally interposed fingers. (Remov. Part. Prosth.)

expansion p. A prosthesis used to expand the lateral segment of the maxilla in unilateral or bilateral cleft of the soft and hard palates and alveolar processes. (Cleft Palate)

fixed e. p. A prosthesis that cannot be readily removed and stays in position for the required length of treatment. (Cleft Palate)

removable e. p. A prosthesis that can be removed from the mouth and replaced when indicated. (Cleft Palate)

feeding p. A prosthesis worn by a young infant with a cleft palate to increase sucking power and to eliminate the escape of food through the nose. (Cleft Palate)

improper p. An inadequate or faulty fixed or removable partial prosthesis which, by virtue of its faulty characteristics, is capable of contributing to and/or producing injury and abuse of the gingivae, attachment apparatus, teeth, oral mucosa, or bone. (Periodont.)

partial denture p. (see **denture, partial**)

periodontal p. Any restorative and replacement device which, by its intent and nature, is used as a therapeutic aid in the treatment of periodontal disease; it is an adjunct to other forms of periodontal therapy and does not cure periodontal disease by itself. (Periodont.)

postsurgical p. An artificial replacement for a missing part or parts after surgical intervention. (Comp. Prosth.; Remov. Part. Prosth.)

surgical p. An appliance prepared to assist in surgical procedures and placed at the time of surgery. (Comp. Prosth.; M.F.P.; Remov. Part. Prosth.)

temporary p. A fixed or removable restoration for which a more permanent appliance is planned within a short period of time. (Comp. Prosth.; Remov. Part. Prosth.)

prosthetic appliance (pros-thĕt′ĭk) (see **appliance, prosthetic**)

prosthetic restoration (see **prosthesis**)

prosthetic speech aid (see **aid, speech, prosthetic**)

prosthetics (pros-thĕt′ĭks) The art and science of supplying, fitting, and servicing artificial replacements for missing parts of the human body. (Comp. Prosth.; Remov. Part. Prosth.)

complete denture p. The restoration of the natural teeth and their associated parts in the dental arch by artificial replacements. (Comp. Prosth.)

— The phase of dental prosthetics dealing with the restoration of function when one or both dental arches have been rendered edentulous. (Remov. Part. Prosth.)

dental p. (see **prosthodontics**)

full denture p. (see **prosthetics, complete denture**)

maxillofacial p. The branch of prosthodontics concerned with the restoration of stomatognathic and associated facial structures that have been affected by disease, injury, surgery, or congenital defect. (Fixed Part. Prosth.; M.F.P.)

partial denture p. The dental service that, by replacing one or more but less than all the teeth of a dental arch, avoids the degenerative changes resulting from tooth movement and may thus achieve preventive measures of maximum benefit toward the maintenance of optimal oral health as well as reasonable restoration of dental functions. (Remov. Part. Prosth.)

prosthetist (pros'thĕ-tĭst) The principal responsible individual involved in the construction of an artificial replacement for any part of the human body. (Comp. Prosth.; Remov. Part. Prosth.)

prosthion (pros'thē-on) The point of the upper alveolar process that projects most anteriorly in the midline. (Orthodont.)

prosthodontia (pros"thō-don'shē-ah) (see **prosthodontics**)

prosthodontics (pros"tho-don'tĭks) (**prosthetic dentistry**) The branch of dentistry which is concerned with the diagnosis, planning, making, and insertion of artificial devices intended for the replacement of one or more teeth and associated tissues. (Comp. Prosth.)
— The branch of dental science pertaining to the restoration and maintenance of oral function by the replacement of missing teeth and associated structures, as well as orofacial structures, with artificial substitutes. (Remov. Part. Prosth.)
— The part of dentistry pertaining to the restoration and maintenance of oral function, comfort, appearance, and health of the patient by the replacement of missing teeth and contiguous tissues with artificial substitutes. Prosthodontics has three main branches: removable prosthodontics, fixed prosthodontics, and maxillofacial prosthetics. (Fixed Part. Prosth.)
　fixed p. The branch of prosthodontics concerned with the replacement and/or restoration of teeth by artificial substitutes that are not readily removable. (Fixed Part. Prosth.)

prosthodontist (pros"thō-don'tĭst) A dentist engaged in the practice of prosthodontics. A specialist in the practice of prosthodontics. (Comp. Prosth.; Remov. Part. Prosth.)

protective A medication, varnish, pack, or covering designed to shield a tissue from its environment. (Oral Med.; Pharmacol.)
　p. apron (see **apron, lead**)
　p. tube housing (see **tube, protective, housing**)

protein(s) (prō'tē-ĭn) Any one of a group of complex organic nitrogenous compounds; the principal constituent of cell protoplasm. (Oral Physiol.)
　anabolic p. (see **steroid, C-19 cortico-**)
　Bence Jones p. A special protein found in the

blood and urine of patients with multiple myeloma and occasionally other diseases involving bone marrow, such as sarcoma and leukemia. (Oral Diag.; Oral Med.)
— A protein found in urine in certain disease states, particularly multiple myeloma. Protein coagulates when urine is heated to 40° to 60° C and disappears on boiling, reappearing as the urine is allowed to cool. (Oral Path.)

cell p. The compounds that form the principal constituents of the cell protoplasm. Proteins are characterized by the inclusion of a nitrogen radical in the complex carbon and hydrogen molecules and are composed chiefly of the amino acids and their derivatives. Ingestion of foods with high protein composition is facilitated by healthy dentition, whereas faulty dentition is usually associated with a high carbohydrate diet. (Oral Physiol.)

C-reactive p. A mucoprotein whose presence in serum is always abnormal. It may be present in a variety of inflammatory or necrotic disease processes. It is almost always present in the serum in acute rheumatic fever. (Oral Med.)

p. deficiency (see **deficiency, protein**)

plasma p. Blood serum contains 6.5 to 8 gm% of a complex mixture of proteins, including albumin, globulin, and fibrinogen. (Oral Med.)

p. specificity The arrangement of protein molecules in numerous spatial configurations to suit the special needs of the physical and chemical activity of the cell. The wide degree of variability of protein structures permits a high degree of specificity of tissue within one body. This characteristic of protein specificity is of great significance in blood transfusions, tissue grafts, and many allergic manifestations. (Oral Physiol.)

thromboplastic p. (see **factor III**)

proteinuria (prō"tē-ĭ-nū'rē-ah) (see **albuminuria**)
　orthostatic p. (**postural proteinuria**) Proteinuria that occurs during daily activities but does not occur when the individual is recumbent. (Oral Med.)

physiologic p. (see **proteinuria, transient**)

postural p. (see **proteinuria, orthostatic**)

transient p. (**physiologic proteinuria**) Proteinuria that occurs in normal subjects after a high-protein meal, violent exercise, severe emotional stress, or syncope. It may occur after an epileptic seizure or during pregnancy. It disappears after the cause subsides. (Oral Med.)

proteuria (prō″tē-ū′rē-ah) (see **albuminuria**)

Prothero "cone" theory (see **retention**)

prothrombase (prō-throm′bās) (see **factor II; prothrombin**)

prothrombin (prō-throm′bĭn) (**factor II, prothrombase, thrombogen**) A glycoprotein precursor of thrombin that is produced in the liver and is necessary for the coagulation of blood. A prothrombin deficiency is uncommon but may occur in liver disease. Vitamin K is essential for the synthesis of prothrombin. (Oral Med.)

p. B (see **factor II**)

component A of p. (see **factor V**)

component B of p. (see **factor VII**)

prothrombinase (prō-throm′bĭn-ās) (**complete thromboplastin, direct activator of prothrombin, extrinsic prothrombin activator**) An inferred direct activator of prothrombin common to tissue and plasma coagulation systems. (Oral Med.) (see also **factor V**)

prothrombinogen (prō″throm-bĭn′ō-jĕn) (see **factor VII**)

prothrombokinase (prō-throm″bō-kī′nās) (see **factor VIII**)

prothromboplastin, beta (prō-throm″bō-plăs′tĭn) (see **factor IX**)

proton (prō′ton) An elementary particle having a positive charge equivalent to the negative charge of the electron but possessing a mass approximately 1845 times as great; the proton is a nuclear particle, whereas the electron is extranuclear. (Oral Radiol.)

protoplasm (prō′tō-plăzm″) A colloid; a fluid, watery sol with particles of living organic materials in solution. The solution varies greatly in viscosity and sometimes reaches a gel state. It has three levels of organization: its gross and histologic appearance, its physical constitution, and its underlying chemical activity. Protoplasm must be viewed as two phenomena in interaction: (1) the structural aspects of solutions in the cells wherein aggregates of mineral salt ions as well as huge, complex protein ions create and respond to ion and molecular atmospheres; these charged areas respond to any change in position and form in accordance with cellular function; (2) particulate systems, which are aggregates of molecules not in solution and which can be separated out by centrifugal action. They are the large-granule fractions such as mitochondria (0.05 to 10 μm) and the small-granule

fractions associated with enzyme function. (Oral Physiol.)

protraction (prō-trak′shŭn) A condition in which teeth or other maxillary or mandibular structures are situated anterior to their normal position. (Orthodont.)

mandibular p. A type of facial anomaly in which the gnathion lies anterior to the orbital plane. (Comp. Prosth.; Fixed Part. Prosth.)

maxillary p. A type of facial anomaly in which the subnasion lies anterior to the orbital plane. (Comp. Prosth.; Remov. Part. Prosth.)

protrusion A position of the mandible forward or laterally forward from the centric position. (Comp. Prosth.; Remov. Part. Prosth.)

bimaxillary p. A relatively forward position, or prognathism, of the maxillary and mandibular teeth, alveolar processes, or jaws. (Orthodont.)

double p. A definite labioversion of the maxillary and mandibular anterior teeth. (Orthodont.)

forward p. A protrusion forward from the centric position. (Comp. Prosth.; Remov. Part. Prosth.)

lateral p. A protrusion to the side from the centric position. (Comp. Prosth.; Remov. Part. Prosth.)

mandibular p. Abnormal protrusion of the mandible, as in a Class III malocclusion. (Oral Diag.)

maxillary p. Abnormal protrusion of the maxillae. (Oral Diag.)

protrusive checkbite (see **record, interocclusal, protrusive**)

protrusive occlusion (see **occlusion, protrusive**)

protrusive position (see **position, protrusive**)

protrusive record (see **record, protrusive**)

protrusive relation (see **relation, jaw, protrusive**)

provisional prosthesis An interim prosthesis worn for varying periods of time. (M.F.P.)

provisional splint (see **splint, provisional**)

proximal surface (see **surface, proximal**)

proximate cause One that directly produces an effect; that which in ordinary, natural sequence produces a specific result with no agencies intervening. (D. Juris.)

pruritus (proo-rī′tŭs) Itching. (Oral Med.; Pharmacol.)

pseudarthrosis (sū″dar-thrō′sĭs) A false joint; sometimes seen after a fracture. (Oral Surg.)

pseudocooperation A behavior pattern that is deceptive because the patient appears to be the ideal patient. He is prompt and cooperative and is pleasant and friendly to everyone. He listens to instruction and yet fails to carry out any of the obligations and self-care that he agrees to execute. He may be the patient who listens to instructions for home care in periodontal treatment, nods in agreement to every suggestion, and yet shows no improvement even though there is no apparent physical or physiologic reason for the lack of improvement in the gingival condition. (Oral Physiol.)

pseudohemophilia (sū″dō-hē″mō-fil′ē-ah) Term used to describe several hemorrhagic states: (1) von Willebrand's disease, pseudohemophilia type B, vascular hemophilia; (2) a hereditary disease in which prolonged bleeding is the only consistent abnormality detected by currently available tests. (Oral Med.) (see also **purpura, thrombocytopenic**)

pseudomembrane A loosely adherent, grayish false membrane typical of intracellular coagulation necrosis. It is formed by necrotic epithelium embedded in fibrin, leukocytes, and erythrocytes. It is seen in Vincent's infection and diphtheria. Removal leaves a raw, bleeding surface. (Oral Med.)
— A clinical and histologic sign of necrotic ulcerative gingivitis. The color of the membrane may be whitish, yellowish, or gray due to the destructive process present. (Periodont.)

pseudopocket A pocket formed by gingival hyperplasia and edema without apical migration of the epithelial attachment. (Periodont.) (see also **pocket, gingival**)

psoriasis (sō-rī′ah-sĭs) A papulosquamous inflammatory skin disease of unknown etiology. Rare oral lesions consist of red patches with white, scaly surfaces. (Oral Path.)

PSP test (see **test, phenolsulfonphthalein**)

psychasthenia (sī″kǎs-thē′nē-ah) A functional neurosis in which there are abnormal and pathologic fear and anxiety, with fixed ideas, failure to face reality, self-accusation, and obsessions. (Oral Med.)

psychoneurosis (sī″kō-nū-rō′sĭs) Abnormal reaction to the environment, including anxieties, phobias, hysteria, and hypochondria. (Oral Diag.)
— Term that includes neurasthenia, hysteria, psychasthenia, and mental disorders short of insanity. (Oral Med.)

psychosedative (sī″kō-sĕd′ah-tĭv) A calming agent that reduces anxiety and tension without depressing mental or motor functions. (Anesth.)

psychosis (sī-kō′sĭs) A functional or organic kind of mental derangement marked by a severe disturbance of personality involving autistic thinking, loss of contact with reality, delusions, and/or hallucinations. (Oral Med.)
manic-depressive p. (**cyclothymia**) A psychosis characterized by varying periods of depression and excitement. One state may predominate; e.g., manic-depressive reaction, manic type. (Oral Med.)

psychosomatic Pertaining to the mind-body relationship; having bodily symptoms of a psychic, emotional, or mental origin. (Anesth.; Comp. Prosth.; Remov. Part. Prosth.) (see also **disease, psychosomatic**)
— Referring to anatomic or physiologic abnormalities produced by mental disturbances or reactions. (Oral Diag.)
p. factors (see **factor, psychosomatic**)

PTA (see **plasma thromboplastin antecedent**)

PTC (see **plasma thromboplastic component**)

pterygoid process (ter′ĭ-goid) (see **process, hamular**)

pterygomaxillary fissure (see **fissure, pterygomaxillary**)

pterygomaxillary notch (see **notch, pterygomaxillary**)

PTF (see **factor, plasma thromboplastic**)

PTF-A (**plasma thromboplastin factor A**) (see **factor VIII**)

PTF-B (**plasma thromboplastin factor B**) (see **factor IX**)

PTF-C (**plasma thromboplastin factor C**) (see **factor XI**)

PTF-D (see **factor, plasma thromboplastin, D**)

ptosis (tō′sĭs) (**blepharoptosis**) A drooping of the upper eyelid. (Oral Diag.)

ptyalectasis (tī″ah-lĕk′tah-sĭs) (see **sialoangiectasis**)

ptyalism (tī′ah-lĭzm) (see **sialorrhea**)

puberty (pū′ber-tē) The age at which the reproductive system becomes functional, with concurrent development of secondary sex characteristics. Marked by increased estrogenic activity in the female and rise of androgenic activity in the male. (Periodont.)

pulp (**dental p., tooth p.**) The vascular connective tissue, with all its cellular elements, that fills the pulp chambers and root canals of a tooth. (Endodont.)
— The highly vascular connective tissue contained within the pulp cavity of a tooth; made up of gelatinous ground substance, collagenous and argyrophilic fibers, cellular elements, terminal blood vessels, and nerves. (Oper. Dent.)
— The connective tissue contained within the pulp chamber and root canal(s) of a tooth, which is richly vascularized and innervated.

The dentinal periphery of the pulp is formed by a layer of columnar cells (odontoblasts) that possess protoplasmic processes extending into the dentinal tubules. (Periodont.)

p. amputation (see **pulpotomy**)

p. canal (see **canal, pulp**)

p. capping (see **capping, pulp**)

p. cavity (see **cavity, pulp**)

p. chamber (see **chamber, pulp**)

dental p. (see **pulp**)

p. extirpation (see **pulpectomy**)

p. horn (see **horn, pulp**)

p. involvement (see **involvement, pulp**)

mummification of p. Dry gangrene of the dental pulp in which the pulp dries and shrivels. (Oper. Dent.)

p. removal (see **pulpectomy**)

p. stone (see **denticle**)

p. tester (**vitalometer**) An electric instrument of either high or low frequency designed to determine the response of a pulp to an electrical stimulus. (Endodont.)

tooth p. (see **pulp**)

p. vitality The health status of the pulp. When the pulp tissue of a tooth has undergone complete degeneration or has been removed, the tooth is termed pulpless or nonvital. (Periodont.)

pulpal Relating to the pulp or the pulp cavity. (Oper. Dent.)

pulpalgia (pul-păl′jē-ah) The sensitivity of the pulp to pain. (Endodont.)

pulpectomy (pul-pĕk′tō-mē) (**pulp extirpation, pulp removal**) The complete removal of a pulp from the pulp chamber and root canal. The removal of vital or inflamed pulp tissue. This term is not used in reference to the removal of necrotic pulp tissue. (Endodont.)

— Complete surgical removal of a vital pulp from the pulp cavity of a tooth. (Oper. Dent.; Pedodont.)

complete p. Surgical removal of the pulp to the dentinocemental junction at the apex of the root. (Pedodont.)

partial p. Surgical removal of only a part of the contents of the canal(s). (Pedodont.)

pulpitis (pul-pī′tĭs) Inflammation of the pulpal tissue of a tooth. (Oral Diag.; Oral Path.)

anachoretic p. Inflammation of the pulp resulting from the entrance of infection into the pulp from the bloodstream. (Oral Diag.)

hypertrophic p. (**pulp polyp**) Formation and proliferation of granulation tissue from the surface of an exposed pulp. (Oral Diag.)

pulpless (pulp′lĕs) Having a nonfunctioning pulp (untreated) or a pulp that has been replaced

with an inert material (treated). (Endodont.)

p. tooth (see **tooth, pulpless**)

pulpotomy (pul-pot′ō-mē) (**pulp amputation**) Surgical amputation of the dental pulp coronal to the dentinocemental junction. (Endodont.; Pedodont.)

— A technique involving the removal of the coronal portion of an exposed vital pulp in an effort to retain the radicular part of the pulp in a healthy, vital state. (Oper. Dent.)

partial p. Surgical removal of only a part of the tissue in the pulpal chamber. (Pedodont.)

total or complete p. Surgical removal of the entire contents of the pulpal chamber at the entrance of the root canal(s). (Pedodont.)

pulse Rhythmical expansion and contraction of arteries due to the surges of blood through the arteries. The pulse can be felt by the fingers in arteries that are close to the skin. (Oral Med.; Oral Physiol.)

arterial p. Pulsation of an artery produced by the rise and fall in blood pressure as the heart goes into systole and diastole. (Oral Med.)

— Pulsation of an artery. The transmission of the pulsatile phenomenon resulting from intermittent contraction of the heart is observed clinically by palpation of the radial artery. The frequency of its beat and the regularity of its rate reflect the condition of the heart and circulatory system in health and disease. The pulse rate at birth is approximately 130 beats/min, diminishing to approximately 70 beats/min in the healthy adult. The range of normalcy is from 50 or 60 to 80 or 90 beats/min. (Oral Physiol.)

p. pressure (see **pressure, pulse**)

venous p. Pulsation of a vein; most easily felt in the right jugular vein. (Oral Med.)

pumice (pŭm′ĭs) A type of volcanic glass used as an abrasive. Prepared in various grits and used for finishing and polishing in dentistry. Also used in the prophylaxis of natural teeth. (D. Mat.)

— A polishing agent in powdered form, used for the teeth, fixed and removable restorations, etc. Derived from volcanic lava. (Periodont.)

punch, rubber dam A hand instrument that has a circular plate with holes of different sizes and a punch to fit these holes; used to make holes in rubber dams. (Endodont.)

— An instrument used to punch holes of varying sizes in a rubber dam so that it may be applied to the teeth. (Oper. Dent.)

pupil, Argyll Robertson Pupillary abnormalities

associated with tabes dorsalis (neurosyphilis), manifested by miosis, the absence of a ciliospinal reflex, and a reaction to accommodation but not to light. (Oral Med.)

purchasing cooperative A group of dentists pooling their financial resources for the purchase of large quantities of supplies and equipment for the purpose of obtaining a discount. (Pract. Man.)

purpura (per'pū-rah) Extravasation of blood into the tissues, resulting in blue to black lesions of the skin or mucosa. (Oral Diag.)

— Bleeding into the skin and mucous membrane, forming petechiae and ecchymoses. (Oral Med.)

— A condition characterized by formation of purple-blue patches on the skin and mucous membrane due to subcutaneous extravasation of blood. (Oral Path.)

allergic p. (anaphylactoid p.) Any thrombocytopenic or nonthrombocytopenic purpura related to an allergic reaction. Manifestations other than ecchymoses and petechiae associated with erythema and inflammation include the common symptoms of allergy. (Oral Med.)

anaphylactoid p. (see **purpura, allergic**)

essential p. (see **purpura, thrombocytopenic, idiopathic**)

p. hemorrhagica (see **purpura, thrombocytopenic; purpura, thrombocytopenic, idiopathic**)

nonthrombocytopenic p. Purpura usually related to increased capillary permeability. Included are allergic purpuras and those due to vitamin C deficiency, bacterial toxins (scarlet fever, typhoid), drug intoxications, and metabolic toxins (nephritis, liver disease). (Oral Med.)

primary p. (see **purpura, thrombocytopenic, idiopathic**)

secondary p. (see **purpura, thrombocytopenic, symptomatic**)

thrombocytopathic p. Bleeding associated with qualitative abnormalities of the platelets. (Oral Med.)

thrombocytopenic p. (essential thrombopenia, pseudohemophilia, hemorrhagica, Werlhof's disease) Severe ecchymoses and petechiae associated with marked reduction in the numbers of blood platelets. (Oral Diag.)

— An idiopathic or symptomatic purpura in which there is a significant reduction in platelets. There is a prolonged bleeding time and poor clot retraction, but the coagulation and prothrombin times are normal. (Oral Med.)

— A severe form of purpura with copious hemorrhage from the mucous membranes; due to a marked decrease in the number of blood platelets. Constitutional symptoms are also present. (Oral Path.)

— A disease of the blood in which extravasations of blood are in or under the skin and mucous membranes. The condition may be brought about by aplastic anemia such as that occurring with chemical poisonings (e.g., benzoyl poisoning), but for the most part its etiology is unknown. There is marked diminution of the number of blood platelets. Hemorrhage may occur spontaneously from any area of the oral mucosa. This disease may be acute and fatal, whereas in other instances it may run a chronic course with intermittent attacks. (Periodont.)

idiopathic t. p. (essential purpura, land scurvy, primary purpura, purpura hemorrhagica) A thrombocytopenic purpura of unknown cause. (Oral Med.)

symptomatic t. p. (secondary purpura) Purpura due to the effect of chemical, physical, vegetable, or animal agents, infections, or related blood disorders. (Oral Med.)

thrombotic t. p. A febrile disease of unknown cause characterized by hemolytic anemia, neurologic symptoms, hemorrhage into the skin and mucous membranes, icterus, hepatosplenomegaly, low platelet count, and platelet thrombi occluding capillaries and arterioles. (Oral Med.)

purulent discharge (pū'roo-lĕnt) (see **pus**)

pus (purulent discharge) An inflammatory exudate formed within the tissues; consists of polymorphonuclear leukocytes, degenerated and liquefied tissue elements, microorganisms, tissue fluids, etc. It may form within the tissues in periodontitis and escape via the ulcerated pocket epithelium into the oral environment. The suppurative material may be retained within the tissues when the orifice of the periodontal pocket is blocked, thus creating a favorable circumstance for the formation of a periodontal abscess. (Periodont.)

pyknik (pĭk'nĭk) A constitution characterized by a short, squat appearance. (Oral Diag.)

pyknosis (pĭk-nō'sĭs) Increased basophilia and shrinkage of the nucleus of a dying cell. (Oral Path.)

pyogenic (pī″ō-jĕn′ĭk) Pus producing.

pyorrhea (pī″ō-rē′ah) Term used to designate periodontal disease. Generally it means flow of pus, which previously was a feature of periodontal disease. Prior to the use of the term pyorrhea, periodontitis was designated as Rigg's disease and Fauchard's disease. (Oral Diag.)

pyrexia (pī-rĕk′sē-ah) (see **fever**)

pyridoxine (pĭr″ĭ-dok′sēn) (see **vitamin B₆**)

pyrometer (pī-rom′ĕ-ter) An instrument for measuring temperature by the change of electrical resistance within a thermocouple. It is a millivoltmeter calibrated in degrees of temperature. (D. Mat.)

pyuria (pī-ū′rē-ah) Abnormal numbers of white blood cells in the urine. Without proteinuria, it suggests infection of the urinary tract; with proteinuria, it suggests infection of the kidney (pyelonephritis). (Oral Med.)

Q

q. 4 h. (quaque 4 hora) Latin phrase meaning every 4 hours. (Oral Med.; Pharmacol.)

q.i.d. (quater in die) Latin phrase meaning four times a day. (Oral Med.; Pharmacol.)

q.s. (quantum satis, quantum sufficiat) Latin phrase meaning a sufficient quantity. (Pharmacol.)

quack One who professes to have medical or dental skill that he does not possess; one who practices medicine or dentistry without adequate preparation or proper qualification. (D. Juris.)

qualified Having the required ability; fitted; entitled. (D. Juris.)

quality When applied to the voice, the acoustic characteristics of vowels resulting from their overtone structure or the relative intensities of their frequency component. (Cleft Palate)

q. of radiation (see **radiation quality**)

quantity of radiation (see **radiation quantity**)

quantum A discrete unit of electromagnetic energy or of an x ray. A quantity becomes quantized when its magnitude is restricted to a discrete set of values as opposed to a continuous set of values. (Oral Radiol.)

q. theory (see **theory, quantum**)

quartz (see **silica**)

fused q. A form of silica that is amorphous and exhibits no inversion at any temperature below its fusion point. Of little use in dentistry. (D. Mat.)

quasi contract (kwah′ze̅ kon′tră̆kt) An obligation that the law imposes on a person; in general, corresponding to those obligations not arising from tort or from true contracts. (D. Juris.)

quaternary (kwah′ter-năr″e̅) Having four elements. Molecules containing one or more nitrogen atoms, each having four alkyl or aryl groups attached. (Oral Med.; Pharmacol.)

quench To cool a hot object rapidly by plunging it into water or oil. (D. Mat.)

question, hypothetical A combination of assumed or proved facts and circumstances stated in such form as to constitute a coherent and specific situation or state of facts, on which the opinion of an expert is asked by way of evidence at a trial. (D. Juris.)

questionnaire A form usually filled out by patients that provides data concerning their dental and general health. (Pract. Man.)

health q. A list of key questions, answered by the patient, that permits an interpretation by the diagnostician of the general and oral health of the patient. (Periodont.)

quick-cure resin (see **resin, autopolymer**)

Quincke's disease (kwĭnk′ĕz) (see **edema, angioneurotic**)

R

racemic (rā-sē'mĭk) Referring to a mixture of equal quantities of the dextro- and levo-isomers of a compound. (Oral Med.; Pharmacol.)

rachianesthesia (rā"kē-ăn"ĕs-thē'zē-ah) Spinal anesthesia; anesthesia produced by the injection of the anesthetic into the spinal canal. (Anesth.)

rachiodynia (rā"kē-ō-dĭn'ē-ah) Pain in the spinal column. (Anesth.)

rachiresistance (rā"kē-rē-zĭs'tăns) A condition in which the injection of a spinal anesthetic produces little or no effect. (Anesth.)

rachiresistant (rā"kē-rē-zĭs'tănt) Abnormally insensitive to spinal anesthetics. (Anesth.)

rachisensibility (rā"kē-sĕn"sĭ-bĭl'ĭ-tē) The condition of being abnormally sensitive to spinal anesthetics. (Anesth.)

rachisensible (rā"kē-sĕn'sĭ-b'l) Abnormally sensitive to spinal anesthetics. (Anesth.)

rad (răd) (see **dose, radiation-absorbed**)

radiate (rā'dē-āt) To diverge or spread from a common point; arranged in a radiating manner. (Anesth.)

— To expose to radiation, as x radiation. (Oral Radiol.)

radiation(s) The emission and propagation of energy through space or through a material medium in the form of waves, quanta, or a phantom; e.g., the emission and propagation of electromagnetic waves, of sound and elastic waves, or of nuclear particles. (Oral Radiol.)

actinic r. Radiation capable of producing chemical change; e.g., the effect of light and x rays on photographic emulsions. (Oral Radiol.)

background r. Radiation arising from radioactive material other than the one directly under consideration. Background radiation due to cosmic rays and natural radioactivity is always present. There may also be background radiation due to the presence of radioactive substances in other parts of the building, in the building material itself, etc. (Oral Radiol.)

backscatter r. (see **radiation, scattered**)

biologic effectiveness of r. The ability of a particular type of ionizing radiation to produce biologic effects on an organism with small absorbed doses. (Oral Radiol.)

relative b. e. of r. (RBE) A comparison between one type of ionizing radiation and another with respect to the ability to produce biologic effects with small doses. All ionizing radiations have the ability to produce the same kinds of biologic effects, but certain types of radiation are more effective than others in that smaller absorbed doses of these radiations are required to produce a particular effect. The RBE is expressed in numerals, usually from 1 to 10. (Oral Radiol.)

Bremsstrahlung r. ("breaking x radiation") Radiation produced by the sudden deceleration of electrons (cathode rays) when the tungsten target of an x-ray tube is bombarded. (Oral Radiol.)

characteristic r. Radiation that originates from an atom after removal of an electron or excitation of the nucleus. The wavelength of the emitted radiation is specific, depending only on the element concerned and the particular energy levels involved. Also, the specific type of secondary radiation resulting when rays from a radio ray tube strike another substance, such as copper. (Oral Radiol.)

corpuscular r. Subatomic particles such as electrons, protons, neutrons, or alpha particles that travel in streams at various velocities. All the particles have definite masses, and they travel at various speeds. The properties are in opposition to electromagnetic radiations, which have no mass and travel in wave forms at the speed of light. (Oral Radiol.) (see also **radiation, electromagnetic**)

cosmic r. (see **ray, cosmic**)

decelerated r. (see **radiation, Bremsstrahlung**)

r. dermatitis (see **dermatitis, radiation**)

r. detector Any device for converting radiant energy to a form more suitable for observation and/or recording. Examples include x-ray films and radiometers. (Oral Radiol.)

direct r. (primary r.) Radiation emanating from a tube aperture and comprising the useful beam, as compared with any stray radiation such as may come from the tube container. (Oral Radiol.)

electromagnetic r. Forms of energy propagated by wave motion, such as photons or discrete quanta. The radiations have no matter associated with them, as opposed to corpuscular radiations, which have definite masses. They differ widely in wavelength, frequency, and photon energy and have strikingly different properties. Covering an enormous range of wavelengths (from 10^{17} to 10^{-6} Å), they include radio waves, infrared waves, visible light, ultraviolet radiation, gamma rays, and cosmic radiation. (Oral Radiol.) (see also **radiation, corpuscular**)

r. field (see **x-ray beam, field size**)

gamma r. (see **ray, gamma**)

genetic effects of r. (see **genetic effects of radiation**)

grenz r. (see **ray, grenz**)

hard r. Radiation consisting of the short wavelengths (higher kilovolt peak equals greater penetration). (Oral Radiol.)

r. hazard (see **hazard, radiation**)

heterogeneous r. A beam or "bundle" of radiation containing photons of many wavelengths. (Oral Radiol.)

homogeneous r. A beam of radiation consisting of photons all of which have the same wavelength. (Oral Radiol.)

r. hygiene (see **hygiene, radiation**)

r. intensity (see **intensity, radiation**)

ionizing r. Electromagnetic radiation such as x rays and gamma rays; particulate radiation such as alpha particles, beta particles, protons, and neutrons; and all other types of radiations that produce ionization directly or indirectly. (Oral Radiol.)

r. leakage (**stray r.**) The escape of radiation through the protective shielding of the x-ray unit tube head. This radiation is detected at the sides, top, bottom, or back of the tube head; it does not include the useful beam. (Oral Radiol.)

monochromatic r. (see **radiation, homogeneous**)

r. necrosis (see **necrosis, radiation**)

neutron r. (see **ray, neutron**)

primary r. All radiation produced directly from the target in an x-ray tube. (Oral Radiol.) (see also **radiation, direct**)

r. protection Provision designed to reduce exposure of persons to radiation. For external radiation this provision consists in the use of protective barriers of radiation-absorbing material, in ensuring adequate distances from the radiation sources, in reducing exposure time, or in combinations of these measures. For internal radiation it involves measures to restrict inhalation, ingestion, or other modes of entry of radio-

active material into the body. (Oral Radiol.)

r. quality The ability of a beam of x rays to allow the production of diagnostically useful radiographs. Usually measured in half-value layers of aluminum and controlled by the kilovolt peak. (Oral Radiol.)

r. quantity Amount of radiation. The amount of exposure is expressed in roentgens (R), whereas quantity of dose is expressed in rads. (Oral Radiol.)

remnant r. The radiation that passes through an object or part being examined and that is available either for recording on a radiographic film or for measurement. (Oral Radiol.)

scattered r. (**backscatter r.**) Radiation whose direction has been altered. It may include secondary and/or stray radiation. (Oral Radiol.)

secondary r. The new radiation created by primary radiation acting on or passing through matter. (Oral Radiol.)

r. shield (see **shield, radiation**)

r. sickness A self-limited syndrome characterized by varying degrees of nausea, vomiting, diarrhea, and psychic depression after exposure to very large doses of ionizing radiation, particularly doses to the abdominal region. Its mechanism is not completely understood. It usually occurs a few hours after treatment and may subside within a day. It may be sufficiently severe to necessitate interrupting the treatment series, or it may incapacitate the patient. (Oral Radiol.)

soft r. Radiation consisting of the long wavelengths (lower kilovolt peak = lesser penetrability). (Oral Radiol.)

speed of r. The speed of light, or approximately 186,000 miles per second. (Oral Radiol.)

stray r. (see **r. leakage**)

r. survey (see **survey, radiation**)

r. therapy (see **therapy, radiation**)

total body r. The exposure of the entire body to penetrating radiation. In theory, all cells in the body receive the same overall dose. (Oral Radiol.)

useful r. (**useful beam**) That part of the primary radiation which is permitted to pass from the tube housing through the tube head port, aperture, or collimating device. (Oral Radiol.)

radiculalgia (rah-dĭk″ū-lăl′jē-ah) Neuralgia of the nerve roots. (Anesth.)

radicular (rah-dĭk′ū-lar) Pertaining to the root; in restorative dentistry, where the form of both the preparation and the restoration for the coronal portion of the natural tooth extends into the treated root canal of the pulpless tooth; e.g., radicular preparation or radicular restoration (dowel crown). (Fixed Part. Prosth.)

— Referring to the root aspect of a tooth. (Endodont.)

radio- Prefix used to denote radiation from any source. (Oral Radiol.)

radioactive decay (see **decay, radioactive**)

radioactive isotope (see **radioisotope**)

radioactivity (ră″dē-ō-ăk-tĭv′ĭ-tē) Spontaneous nuclear disintegration with emission of corpuscular or electromagnetic radiations. The principal types of radioactivity are alpha disintegration, beta decay (negatron emission, positron emission, and electron capture) and isometric transition. Double beta decay is another type of radioactivity that has been postulated, and spontaneous fission and the spontaneous transformations of mesons are sometimes considered to be types of radioactivity. To be considered radioactive, a process must have a measurable lifetime between approximately 1 to 10 seconds and 1017 years, according to present experimental techniques. Radiations emitted within a time too short for measurement are called prompt; however, prompt radiations, including gamma rays, characteristic x rays, conversion and auger electrons, delayed neutrons, and annihilation radiation, are often associated with radioactive disintegrations because their emission may follow the primary radioactive process. (Oral Radiol.)

— A particular radiation component from a radioactive source, such as gamma radioactivity; a radionuclide, such as radioactivity produced in a bombardment. (Oral Radiol.)

— The process whereby certain unstable nuclides undergo spontaneous disintegration with energy liberation, generally resulting in the formation of new nuclides. The process is accompanied by emission of one or more types of radiation; e.g., alpha particles, beta particles, and gamma photons. (Oral Radiol.)

radiogram (see **radiograph**)

radiograph(s), *n.* An image or picture produced on a radiation-sensitive film emulsion, by exposure to ionizing radiation directed through an area, region, or substance of interest, followed by chemical processing of the film. It is basically dependent on the differential absorption of radiation directed through heterogeneous media. (Oper. Dent.; Oral Radiol.; Periodont.)

bite-wing r. A form of dental radiograph that reveals approximately the coronal halves of the maxillary and mandibular teeth and portions of the interdental alveolar septa on the same film. (Oper. Dent.; Oral Radiol.; Periodont.)

body-section r. Radiograph produced by rotation of the film and x-ray source around the region of interest in opposite directions during exposure, so as to blur interposed anatomic structures outside the region of interest. (Oral Radiol.)

cephalometric r. Extraoral radiographs produced under conditions assuring maximum dimensional accuracy and reproducible film-object-beam relationship for purposes of cephalometric study. (Oral Radiol.)

composite r. Radiograph made by superimposing a radiograph of osseous tissue, whose exposed border has been cut away, on a radiograph of soft tissue for the purpose of detecting radiographic information concerning both the soft tissues and the osseous tissues of the head and face from a single radiographic view. (Oral Radiol.)

contrast media r. Radiograph that records the shadow images of the secretory apparatus of any of the salivary glands, body cavities, or fistulous tracts after the injection of a liquid radiopaque solution. (Oral Radiol.)

extraoral r. Radiograph produced on a film placed extraorally. (Oral Radiol.)

follow-up r. Radiographs made during and after therapy in order to follow the progress or regress of a disease, to determine the course of healing, or to ascertain the results of treatment. (Oral Radiol.)

intraoral r. Radiograph produced by placing a radiographic film within the oral cavity. (Oral Radiol.)

r., microscopic examination (see **microradiography**)

occlusal r. A special type of intraoral radiograph made with the film held between the occluded teeth. (Oral Radiol.)

oral r. Radiographic representation of shadow images of all the tissues, structures, and regions of the oral cavity and its adjacent areas and associated parts. (Oral Radiol.)

panoramic r. A large radiograph depicting the curvatures of the maxillae and mandible and associated structures. (Oral Radiol.)

salivary gland r. (see **sialograph**)

stereoscopic r. A pair of radiographs of a structure made by shifting the position of the x-ray tube a few centimeters between each of two exposures. Such pairs provide a three-dimensional, or stereoscopic, presentation of the recorded images. (Oral Radiol.)

Towne projection r. Radiographic view of the mandibular condyles and the midfacial skeleton.

—, *v.* To produce a shadow image on a photographic emulsion. (Oral Radiol.)

radiographer A specialist or technician in radiography. (Oral Radiol.)

oral r. A specialist or technician in oral radiography. (Oral Radiol.)

radiographic Relating to process of radiography, the finished product, or its use.

r. anatomy (see **anatomy, radiographic**)

r. contrast (see **contrast, radiographic**)

r. density (see **density, radiographic**)

r. detail (see **detail, radiographic**)

r. diagnosis (see **diagnosis, radiographic**)

r. examination (see **examination, radiographic**)

r. grid A clear plastic device with the horizontal and vertical wires crossing one another at intervals of 1 mm; used in x-ray techniques for the purpose of measurement. (Oral Implant.)

r. interpretation (see **interpretation, radiographic**)

r. localization (see **localization, radiographic**)

r. survey (see **survey, radiographic**)

radiography (rā″dē-og′rah-fē) The making of shadow images on photographic emulsion by the action of ionizing radiation. The image is the result of the differential attenuation of the radiation in its passage through the object being radiographed. Roentgenography refers to production of film by the use of x rays only; radiography refers to films produced by any source of radiation. (Oral Radiol.)

bone in r. Radiography of bone and marrow tissue. Translucencies and opacities in bone in radiographs are dependent on the different densities that bone and marrow spaces present to the x rays. The configuration of bone tissue represents the topography and arrangement of bone trabeculae, which register as opaque in contrast to the translucency of the marrow spaces. (Periodont.)

oral r. The specialized operative and technical procedures and practices for making successful radiographic surveys, with the understanding that it involves the selection of the dental x-ray unit and its adjustments as well as the generation and application of x rays to all phases of interest to the dental profession. It also takes into consideration all the

processes necessary for the production of finished radiographs of the teeth, their supporting tissues, adjacent regions, and associated parts. (Oral Radiol.)

radioisotope (rā″dē-ō-ī′sō-tōp) A chemical element that has been made radioactive through bombardment of neutrons in a cyclotron or atomic pile or found in a natural state. (Oral Radiol.)

radiologist A person who has special experience in the science of radiant energy and radiant substances (including roentgen rays); especially, a person engaged in the branch of medical science that deals with the use of radiant energy in the diagnosis and treatment of disease. (Oral Radiol.)

oral r. A specialist in the art and science of oral radiology. (Oral Radiol.)

radiology (1) That branch of medicine dealing with the diagnostic and therapeutic applications of ionizing radiation. (2) The science of radiant energy, its use toward the extension of present knowledge, and its diverse applications for the benefit of mankind. (Oral Radiol.)

oral r. All phases of the science and art of radiology that are of interest to the dental profession. It involves the generation and application of x rays for the purpose of recording shadow images of teeth, their supporting tissues, adjacent regions, and associated parts. It also includes the interpretation of the radiographic findings. (Oral Radiol.)

radiolucence Relative term indicating the comparatively low attenuation of an x-ray beam produced by materials of relatively low atomic number. (The image on a radiograph of such materials will be relatively dark due to the greater amount of radiation that penetrates to reach the film.) (Oral Radiol.)

radiolucency A radiographic representation of decreased density of hard and/or soft tissue structures. (Endodont.)

radiolucent (rā″dē-ō-lū′sĕnt) Partly penetrable by roentgen rays; the image of such a material on the radiogram ranges from dark gray to black. (Oper. Dent.)

— Permitting the passage of radiant energy, with relatively little attenuation by absorption. (Oral Radiol.)

radionuclide An unstable or radioactive type of atom characterized by the constitution of its nucleus and capable of existing for a measurable time. The nuclear constitution is specified by the number of protons (Z), number of neutrons (N), and energy content; or alternatively by the atomic number (Z), the mass number (A – N + Z), and the atomic mass. (Oral Radiol.)

radiopacity (ră″dē-o-păs′ĭ-tē) Relative term referring to the considerable attenuation of an x-ray beam produced by materials of relatively high atomic number. It should be noted that the image on a radiograph of such materials will be relatively translucent, or transparent, less radiation passing through them to produce blackening of the film. (Oral Radiol.)

radiopaque (ră″dē-ō-pāk′) Highly resistant to penetration by roentgen rays. The image of such a material appears on the radiogram within the range of gray to white. (Oper. Dent.) (see also **medium, radiopaque**)

— Permitting the passage of radiant energy but only with considerable or extreme attenuation of the radiation by absorption. (Oral Radiol.)

radioparent Made visible by means of roentgen rays or other means of radiation. Permitting the passage of x rays or other radiation. (Oral Radiol.)

radioresistance (ră″dē-ō-rē-zĭs′tăns) The relative resistance of cells, tissues, organs, or organisms to the injurious effects of ionizing radiation. (Oral Radiol.) (see also **radiosensitivity**)

radiosensitivity Relative susceptibility of cells, tissues, organs, organisms, or any substances to the injurious action of radiation. Radioresistance and radiosensitivity are employed at present in a qualitative, comparative sense rather than in a quantitative, absolute sense. (Oral Radiol.)

radiotherapy (see **therapy, radiation**)

radon seed (rā′don) A small sealed container or tube for carrying radon. It is made of gold or glass, is inserted into the tissues for the treatment of certain disease entities, and is visible radiographically. (Oral Radiol.)

rale (rāl) Abnormal sound that originates from the trachea, bronchi, or lungs. (Oral Diag.)

ramify (răm′ĭ-fī) To branch; to diverge in various directions; to traverse in branches. (Anesth.)

ramitis (rah-mī′tĭs) Inflammation of a nerve root. (Anesth.)

ramulus (răm′ū-lŭs) A small branch or terminal division. (Anesth.)

ramus (rā′mus) A branch, as of an artery, nerve, or vein. Any constant branch of a fissure, or sulcus, of the brain. In the *Basle Nomina Anatomica* terminology, the term ramus is given to a primary division of a nerve or blood vessel. (Anesth.)

range, melting The temperature range from the time an alloy begins to melt until it is completely molten. It varies from 100° to 200° F in gold-platinum-palladium alloys. (Remov. Part. Prosth.)

ranula (răn′ū-lah) A large mucocele in the floor of the mouth. It is usually due to obstruction of the ducts of the sublingual salivary glands. Less frequently it is due to obstruction of the ducts of the submandibular salivary glands. (Oral Diag.)

— A large, mucus-containing pathologic space (mucocele) located in the floor of the mouth. It may be associated with submaxillary (submandibular) or sublingual gland secretions. (Oral Path.)

Ranvier, nodes of (rahn-vē-ā′) (see **node of Ranvier**)

raphae, midpalatine (rā′fē) The ridge of mucous membrane that marks the median line of the hard palate. (Orthodont.)

rarefaction, bone (see **bone rarefaction**)

rash, wandering (see **tongue, geographic**)

ratchet wrench An instrument that when seated over a spiral implant abutment, twists it into its bony seat or, by the snapping of a reversal lever, untwists it. The wrench is supplied with a variety of adapters and extension tips. (Oral Implant.)

rate Measurement of a thing by its ratio or given in relation to some standard.

basal metabolic r. (see **basal metabolic rate**)

DEF r. An expression of dental caries experience in deciduous teeth. The DEF rate is calculated by adding the number of decayed primary teeth requiring filling (D), decayed primary teeth requiring extraction (E), and primary teeth successfully filled (F). Missing primary teeth are not included in the count since it is frequently impossible to determine whether they were extracted because of caries or were exfoliated normally. (Pedodont.)

DMF index r. A method of classifying the condition of the teeth based on the number of teeth in a given mouth that are decayed, missing or indicated for removal and of those filled or bearing restorations. The DMF index rate is calculated by adding together the number of carious permanent teeth requiring filling (D), the carious permanent teeth requiring extraction (Mr), the permanent teeth previously extracted because of caries (Mp), and the filled permanent teeth (F). Thus the number of DMF teeth per child of a specific age or age group can be calculated by using the following formula (Oper. Dent.; Pedodont.):

$$\frac{\text{D teeth + Mr teeth + Mp teeth + F teeth (in age or ages studied)}}{\text{Number of children examined (in specified age or ages)}} = \text{DMF rate per child in age groups}$$

erythrocyte sedimentation r. The rate of settling of erythrocytes by gravity under conditions in which all factors affecting the rate are corrected, standardized, or eliminated except for alterations in the physicochemical properties of the plasma proteins. These alterations are the basis for interpretation of the rate. There is an increase in the rate in most infections. Sedimentation velocity is useful in prognosis to determine recovery from infection. Normal values vary with the method used in the determination. (Oral Med.)

heart r. The rate of the heartbeat, expressed as the number of beats per minute. The heart rate is reflected in the pulse rate. The cardiac rate of contraction is described as normal (70 beats/min), rapid (above 100 beats/min), or slow (below 55 beats/min). Disturbances in heart rate and rhythm may be paroxysmal or persistent. Descriptive terms are tachycardia (increased, shallow heart rate to compensate for inadequate cardiac output) and bradycardia (slow, firm heart rate caused by cardiac sinus mechanisms and by the vagal effect over the sympathetic innervation of the heart). (Oral Physiol.)

ratification Confirmation of a previous act. (D. Juris.)

ratio Proportion; comparison.

A:G r. The ratio of the protein albumin to globulin in the blood serum. On the basis of differential solubility with neutral salt solution, the normal values are 3.5 to 5 g% for albumin and 2.5 to 4 g% for globulin. (Oral Med.)

clinical crown:clinical root r. The proportion of the length of the portion of the tooth lying coronal to the epithelial attachment to the length of the portion of the root lying apical to the epithelial attachment. The proportion of the length of the anatomic crown to the length of the anatomic root. Radiographically, the clinical crown is that portion of a tooth coronal to the alveolar crest; the clinical root is that part of the root apical to the alveolar crest. The radiographic crown:root ratio is highly significant in evaluation and prognosis of periodontal disease. (Periodont.)

grid r. The relation of the height of the lead strips to the width of the nonopaque material between them. Common grid ratios are 1:8, 1:12, and 1:16. (Oral Radiol.)

water:powder r. Relative amounts of water and powder (usually gypsum products) in a mixture.

ray(s) A line of light, heat, or other form of radiant energy. A ray is a more or less distinct or isolated portion of radiant energy, whereas the word rays is a very general term for any form of radiant energy, whether vibratory or particulate. (Oral Radiol.)

alpha r. (see **particle, alpha**)

beta r. (see **particle, beta**)

cathode r. (see **electron stream**)

central r. The envisioned photon or photons in the geometric center of an x-ray beam. (Oral Radiol.)

cosmic r. Radiation that has its origin outside the earth's atmosphere. Cosmic rays have extremely short wave-lengths. They are able to produce ionization as they pass through the air and other matter and are capable of penetrating many feet of material such as lead and rock. The primary cosmic rays probably consist of atomic nuclei (mainly protons), some of which may have energies of the order of 1010 to 1015 electron volts. Secondary cosmic rays are produced when the primary cosmic rays interact with nuclei and electrons, e.g., in the earth's atmosphere. Secondary cosmic rays consist mainly of mesons, protons, neutrons, electrons, and photons that have less energy than the primary rays. Practically all the primary cosmic rays are absorbed in the upper atmosphere. Almost all cosmic radiation observed at the earth's surface is of the secondary type. (Oral Radiol.)

gamma r. Photons that have a shorter wave-length than those ordinarily used in diagnostic medical and dental radiography, and that originate in the nuclei of atoms. A quantum of electromagnetic radiation emitted by a nucleus as a result of a quantum transition between two energy levels of the nucleus; e.g., as a radioisotope decays, it gives off energy, some of which may be in the form of gamma radiation. (Oral Radiol.)

grenz r. (grĕntz) Roentgen rays that are greater in length than 1 Angström unit; used in radiography of soft tissues, insects, flowers, and microscopic sections of teeth and surrounding tissues. They are the result of using approximately 10 to 20 kilovolts in a specially constructed radiation generating device. They have a wavelength of about 2 Å. (Oral Radiol.)

neutron r. Particulate ionizing radiation consisting of neutrons which, on impact with nuclei or atoms, possess enough kinetic energy to set the nuclei or atoms in motion with sufficient velocity to ionize matter or which enter into nuclear reactions that result in the emission of ionizing radiation. The former variety is usually called the fast neutron and the latter the thermoneutron, with gradations of epithermal and slow neutrons between them. (Oral Radiol.)

roentgen r. (x ray) Electromagnetic vibrations of photons of short wavelengths that are produced when electrons moving at a high velocity strike at target of heavy metal. (Oral Radiol.) (see also **x ray**)

Raynaud's phenomenon Spasm of the digital arteries with blanching and numbness of the extremities, induced by chilling, emotional states, or other diseases. (Oral Diag.)

RBE (see **radiation, biologic effectiveness of, relative**)

RDA The Recommended Dietary Allowances of the Food and Nutrition Board of the National Research Council. (Oral Med.; Pharmacol.)

reaction Opposite action or counteraction; the response of a part to stimulation; a chemical process in which one substance is transformed into another substance(s). (Anesth.)

alarm r. The first stage of the general adaptation syndrome of Hans Selye; occurs in response to severe physical and psychologic distress. Complete mobilization of body resources occurs in association with activity of the pituitary and adrenal glands and the sympathetic nervous system. (Oral Med.) (see also **syndrome, general adaptation**)

anaphylactoid r. A reaction that resembles anaphylactic shock. Probably caused by the liberation of histamine, serotonin, or other substances as a consequence of the injection of colloids or finely suspended material. (Oral Med.)

Arthus' r. (see **anaphylactic hypersensitivity**)

heterophil r. A heterophil agglutination test that measures the agglutination of the red blood cells of sheep by the serum of patients with infectious mononucleosis. (Oral Med.)

-id r. Secondary skin eruptions occurring at a distance from the primary lesion; e.g., the tuberculid. (Oral Med.)

immune r. Altered reactivity of the tissues to a foreign substance that has previously been introduced into the body or was previously in contact with it. (Oral Med.)

leukemoid r. An increase in normal and/or abnormal white blood cells in nonleukemic conditions. Simulates myelogenous, lymphatic, and, rarely, monocytic leukemia. (Oral Med.)

Schwartzman r. An antigen AB local tissue response that occurs when an intravenous injection or challenge of a bacterial endotoxin that had previously been inoculated intradermally results in a hemorrhagic, often necrotic inflammatory lesion. (Periodont.)

tissue r. The response of tissues to altered conditions. (Comp. Prosth.; Fixed Part. Prosth.; Remov. Part. Prosth.)

reactor An apparatus in which nuclear fission may be sustained in a self-supporting reaction at a controlled rate. (Oral Radiol.)

reagin(s) (rē'ah-jĭn) Noncommittal term used for antibodies or antibody-like substances that differ in several respects from ordinary antibodies. It refers to the antibodies of allergic conditions (atopy) and to the antibody (reagin) concerned with the flocculation and complement fixation tests for syphilis. (Oral Med.)

reamer An instrument with a tapered metal shaft, more loosely spiraled than a file; used to enlarge and clean root canals. (Endodont.)

rebase A process of refitting a denture by replacing the denture base material without changing the occlusal relations of the teeth. (Comp. Prosth.)

— A process of adding to the denture base to compensate for the resorptive change that has occurred in the subjacent structures. (Remov. Part. Prosth.)

rebound An outbreak of fresh reflex activity after withdrawal of a stimulus. (Anesth.)

recall The procedure of advising or reminding a patient to have his oral health reviewed or reexamined; an important phase of preventive dentistry. (Oper. Dent.)

— A systematic method of notifying patients that it is time for them to return to the office for professional service. (Pract. Man.)

receipt A written acknowledgment by one person of his having received money or something of value from another. (D. Juris.)

r. book. The book in which the dentist or one of his auxiliaries fills out forms verifying to the patient that he has paid a specific amount of money on his account. (Pract. Man.)

reception room The area within the physical plant of the dental establishment through which patients enter the office. This is also the room in which patients await the attentions of the dentist and/or the receptionist. (Pract. Man.)

receptor(s) A hypothetical group in a cell that has the power of combining with and thus anchoring a haptophore group of a toxin or other substance. Receptors may remain attached to cells or may be cast off into the blood serum. In either case, they retain their combining power and so function as antibodies; a sensory nerve terminal that responds to stimuli of various kinds. (Anesth.)

— A cell, cellular process, or tissue that is sensitive to factors in the environment and that transmits impulses to some part of the central nervous system. Distinguished from the effector. (Oral Physiol.)

adrenergic r. Alpha and beta "units" associated with sympathetic neuroeffectors that react with sympathomimetic drugs to elicit the response of the effector cells. (Oral Med.; Pharmacol.)

sensory r. Receptor system built on the theoretic basis that receptor organs are specialized and respond to the law of specific nerve energies; i.e., each type of end-organ, no matter what stimulus is applied, will respond (if it responds) with only a single appropriate type of sensation. Common experience shows this to be true; e.g., when a person receives a blow in the eye, light is experienced as a consequence of the blow. Another factor is that the impulse will travel in only one direction, from the receptor organ back to the central nervous system. The receptor system is thus the summation in the brain of all the sensory stimuli that come from the special senses, the general senses, the mucous membrane, the skin, and the deeper tissues and is the basis for instruction sent to the musculoskeletal system for action, as in the masticatory phenomenon. (Oral Physiol.)

r. site An area that, after trephining, permits insertion of the head of the intramucosal insert. After healing, the receptor site becomes epithelialized and acts as the female attachment for the intramucosal insert. (Oral Implant.)

recess, rest (see **area, rest**)

recession A moving back or withdrawal.

bone r. Apical progression of the level of the alveolar crest associated with inflammatory and/or dystrophic periodontal disease. A bone resorption process that results in de-creased osseous support for the tooth. (Periodont.)

gingival r. Apical withdrawal of the level of the gingivae; may be physiologic or pathologic. (Oper. Dent.)

—Atrophy of the gingival margin associated with inflammation, apical migration (proliferation) of the epithelial attachment, and resorption of the alveolar crest. (Periodont.)

recipient site The site into which a graft or transplant material is placed. (Periodont.) (see also **donor site**)

reciprocal arm (see **arm, reciprocal**)

reciprocation The means by which one part of a removable partial denture framework is made to counter the effect created by another part of the framework. (Remov. Part. Prosth.)

active r. Reciprocation in a clasp unit achieved by the use of two opposing and balanced retentive clasp arms. Reciprocation cannot be achieved unless there is a similar and balanced arrangement on the opposite side of the dental arch. (Remov. Part. Prosth.)

passive r. Reciprocation in a clasp unit achieved by the use of a rigid part of the clasp, located on or above the height of contour line or on a guiding plane and opposite to the retentive arm. However, reciprocation cannot be achieved by a single clasp alone—there must be a similar action by another component of the removable partial denture located across the arch. (Remov. Part. Prosth.)

Recklinghausen's disease (rĕk'lĭng-how"zĕnz) (see **neurofibromatosis; osteitis fibrosa cystica**)

recontouring, occlusal The reshaping of an occlusal surface of a natural or artificial tooth after extensive grinding that may have been necessary to reestablish the proper level of the occlusal plane. (Comp. Prosth.; Remov. Part. Prosth.)

record Information committed to, and preserved in, writing. (D. Juris.)

r. base (see **baseplate**)

face-bow r. Registration, by means of a face-bow, of the position of the mandibular axis and/or the condyles. The face-bow record is used to orient the maxillary cast to the opening and closing axis of the articulator. (Remov. Part. Prosth.)

functional chew-in r. (1) A record of the natural chewing movement of the mandible made on an occlusion rim by teeth or scribing studs. (2) A record of the movements of the mandible made on the occluding surface of the opposing occlusion rim by teeth or scribing studs and produced by simulated chewing movements. (3) A record of certain lateral and protrusive movements of the mandible made on the occlusal surface of an occlusion rim by teeth or scribing studs on an opposing rim; produced during simulated movements of bruxism. (Comp. Prosth.) (see also **path, occlusal, registration; path, milled-in**)

interocclusal r. A record of the positonal relation of the teeth or jaws to each other; made on occlusal surfaces of occlusion rims or teeth in a plastic material that hardens, such as plaster of paris, wax, zinc oxide–eugenol paste, or acrylic resin. (Comp. Prosth.; Remov. Part. Prosth.)

centric i. r. A record of the centric jaw position (relation). (Comp. Prosth.; Remov. Part. Prosth.)

eccentric i. r. A record of a jaw relation other than the centric relation. (Comp. Prosth.; Remov. Part. Prosth.)

lateral i. r. A record of a lateral eccentric jaw position. (Comp. Prosth.; Remov. Part. Prosth.)

protrusive i. r. A record of a protruded eccentric jaw position. (Comp. Prosth.)

jaw relation r. A registration of any positional relationship of the mandible in reference to the maxillae. The record may be of any of the many vertical, horizontal, or orientation relations. (Comp. Prosth.)

mandibular movement r. (see **path, occlusal, registration**)

maxillomandibular r. (**maxillomandibular registration**) A record of any one of the many positional relations of the mandible to the maxillae. (Comp. Prosth.; Remov. Part. Prosth.)

centric m. r. A record of the relation of the mandible to the maxillae when the mandible is in centric position. (Comp. Prosth.; Remov. Part. Prosth.)

eccentric m. r. A record of the relation of the mandible to the maxillae when the mandible is in any position other than centric position. (Comp. Prosth.; Remov. Part. Prosth.)

occluding centric relation r. A registration of centric relation made at the vertical dimension at which the teeth make contact or are to make contact. (Comp. Prosth.; Remov. Part. Prosth.)

preoperative r. Any record or records made for the purpose of study, diagnosis, or use in treatment planning, or for comparison of treatment results with the pretreatment status of the patient. (Comp. Prosth.; Remov. Part. Prosth.)

profile r. A registration or record of the profile of a patient's face. (Comp. Prosth.; Remov. Part. Prosth.)

protrusive r. A registration of the relation of the mandible to the maxillae when the mandible is anterior to its centric relation with the maxillae. (Comp. Prosth.; Remov. Part. Prosth.)

r. rim (see **rim, occlusion**)

terminal jaw relation r. A record of the relationship of the mandible to the maxillae made at the vertical relation of the occlusion and at the centric position. (Comp. Prosth.; Fixed Part. Prosth.; Remov. Part. Prosth.)

three-dimensional r. (3-D r.) A maxillomandibular interocclusal record. (Comp. Prosth.)

recording The act of making a written record of the data collected during examination. (Pract. Man.)

recovery In a suit at law, the obtaining or restoration of a right to something by a verdict, decree, or judgment of court. (D. Juris.)

recrystallization The return of a wrought metal to crystalline form due to excessive cold working or excessive application of heat. (Remov. Part. Prosth.)

rectification Conversion of electric current from alternating to direct (unidirectional). (Oral Radiol.)

rectifier A device used for converting an alternating current to a direct current; it also prevents or limits the flow of current in the opposite direction. (Oral Radiol.)

full-wave r. An apparatus for rectifying the entire wave of an alternating current in an x-ray machine by means of a mechanical rectifier or valve tube. (Oral Radiol.)

half-wave r. An apparatus used in the rectifying of half of the sine wave in x-ray units. (Oral Radiol.)

redressment (rē-drĕs′mĕnt) Replacement of a part or correction of a deformity. (Oral Surg.)

reduced interarch distance (see **distance, interarch, reduced**)

reducer A solution used to remove some silver from the image on a radiograph so as to produce a less intense image; an oxidizing agent used to remove excess density. (Oral Radiol.)

reduction in area A test to assess ductibility, whereby the cross-sectional area of the fractured end of a wire or rod is compared to the original area. A tensile test is used to break the wire. (D. Mat.)

referred pain (see **pain, referred**)

referred sensation (see **sensation, referred**)

reflected Caused by nervous transmission to a center and thence by a motor nerve to the periphery. (Anesth.)

reflection The act of elevating and folding back the mucoperiosteum, thereby exposing the underlying bone. (Oral Implant.)

   mucobuccal r. (see **fold, mucobuccal**)

reflex(es) A reflected action or movement; the sum total of any specific involuntary activity. (Anesth.)

   allied r. Reflexes that can join to effect a common purpose such as mastication. They may arise from diverse stimuli, such as smell, taste of food, and texture, shape, and resistance of the food bolus. Collectively, they encourage salivation and a sequence of masticatory closures of the mandible, followed by deglutition. (Oral Physiol.)

   antagonistic r. Reflexes that cannot occupy the final pathway simultaneously. The weaker of these reflexes will give way to the stronger, especially if the latter is a protected reflex; e.g., a hot or nauseating food will cause involuntary retching or even vomiting rather than the pleasurable gustatory experience associated with chewing and swallowing tasty food. (Oral Physiol.)

   r. arc (see **arc, reflex**)

   Breuer r. (see **reflex, Hering-Breuer**)

   Cheyne-Stokes r. (see **respiration, Cheyne-Stokes**)

   flexion-extension r. The reflexes based on the principle of reciprocal innervation. When a voluntary or reflex contraction of a muscle occurs, it is accompanied by the simultaneous relaxation of its antagonist. For example, when the jaw reflex is initiated by tapping the mandible downward, the masseter and other elevators of the mandible are stretched. Then reflex flexion-contraction of the elevators takes place, the mandible is elevated, and the depressor muscles of the mandible are stretched. There are many combinations, not only between the agonists and the antagonists about a given joint but also between reflexes that cross over to muscle groups of contralateral extremities, joints, and muscles. (Oral Physiol.)

   Hering-Breuer r. The nervous mechanism that tends to limit the respiratory excursions. Stimuli from the sensory endings in the lungs (and perhaps in other parts) pass up the vagi and tend to limit both inspiration and expiration during ordinary breathing. (Anesth.)

   jaw r. An extension-flexion reflex that is initiated by tapping the mandible downward. The masseter and other elevators of the mandible are the first stretched; then the reflex flexion-contraction elevates the mandible by flexion of elevator muscles while there is a simultaneous stretching (extension) of the depressor muscles of the mandible. (Oral Physiol.)

   pathologic r. Those reflexes observed in the abnormal or inappropriate motor responses of controlled stimuli initiated in the sensory organ that is appropriate to the reflex arc. They may be initiated in the superficial reflexes of the skin and the mucous membrane, in the deep myotatic reflexes of the joints, tendons, and muscles, and in the visceral reflexes of the viscera and other organs of the body. The pathologic reflexes are thus syndromes of abnormal responses to otherwise normal stimuli. (Oral Physiol.)

   pharyngeal r. Contraction of the constrictor muscles of the pharynx, elicited by touching the back of the pharynx. (Oral Surg.)

   stretch r. One of the most important features of tonic contraction of muscle. It is the reflex contraction of a healthy muscle that results from a pull. It has been found that stretching a muscle by as little as 0.8% of its original length is sufficient to evoke a reflex response. It is significant that a stretch of constant degree causes a maintained steady contraction, that the muscle spindles and the stretch receptors in the tendons show very slow adaptation, and that the reflex ceases immediately on withdrawal of the stretching force. The stretch reflex ceases immediately on withdrawal of the stretching force. The stretch reflex is obtained predominantly from those muscles that maintain body posture, among which are the masticating muscles that maintain the position of the mandible and the neck muscles that hold the head erect. Together, the masticating muscles and the neck muscles are responsible for the maintenance of the air and food passages. (Oral Physiol.)

   vagovagal r. A reflex in which the afferent and efferent impulses travel via the vagus nerve. The afferent impulses travel centrally via the sensory nucleus of the vagus. The efferent impulses travel via the motor fibers of the vagus nerve. (Anesth.)

refractory Pertaining to the ability to withstand high temperatures used in certain dental laboratory procedures. (Remov. Part. Prosth.) (see also **cast, refractory**)

regeneration The renewal or repair of lost tissue or parts. (Oral Physiol.)

cell r. (see **cell regeneration**)

muscle r. Repair of muscle tissue. When surgical intervention or inflammatory disease of dental structures injures the facial and masticatory muscles, two types of repair take place: repair by budding and repair by proliferation. (Oral Physiol.)

m. r. by budding Regeneration that takes place in destructive lesions of muscle, traumatic necrosis, hemorrhage, infarction, and suppurative myositis. The buds consist of undifferentiated plasmodial masses and certain sarcolemma nuclei. The rebuilt architecture is not classic and presents bizarre and sometimes fibrous extensions that look like scarred defects. (Oral Physiol.)

m. r. by proliferation Regeneration in degenerating muscles by proliferation of bands of sarcoplasm in which the sarcolemma and its nuclei are preserved. (Oral Physiol.)

region, mylohyoid (mī″lō-hī′oid) The region on the lingual surface of the mandible marked by the mylohyoid ridge and the attachment of the mylohyoid muscle. A part of the alveololingual sulcus. (Comp. Prosth.; Fixed Part. Prosth.; Remov. Part. Prosth.)

regional Pertaining to a region or regions. (Anesth.)

registration The record of desired jaw relations that is made in order to transfer casts, having these same relations, to an articulator. (Comp. Prosth.; Fixed Part. Prosth.; Remov. Part. Prosth.)

r. of functional form (see **impression, functional**)

maxillomandibular r. (see **record, maxillomandibular**)

occlusal r. Clinical examination of the patterns and disharmonies of occlusion by the interposition of wax, articulation paper, etc. between the mandibular and maxillary teeth during the various mandibular excursive movements. (Periodont.)

tissue r. The accurate record of the shape of tissues under any condition by means of

suitable material. (Comp. Prosth.; Fixed Part. Prosth.; Remov. Part. Prosth.)

regurgitation (rē-ger″jĭ-tā′shŭn) A backward flowing; e.g., the casting up of undigested food, or the backward flowing of blood into the heart or between the chambers of the heart. (Anesth.)

rehabilitation (rē″hă-bĭl″ĭ-tā′shŭn) Restoration of form and function. (Fixed Part. Prosth.; M.F.P.)

mouth r. Restoration of the form and function of the masticatory apparatus to a condition as nearly normal as possible. (Comp. Prosth.; Fixed Part. Prosth.; Remov. Part. Prosth.)

oral r. Reconstruction of the teeth; restoration of all decayed surfaces and replacement of all missing teeth; interpreted by some to mean the complete coverage of all the teeth remaining in the mouth. (Pract. Man.)

rehalation Rebreathing. (Anesth.)

reimplant Replacement of a lost or extracted tooth back into its alveolus. (Oral Implant.)

reimplantation (see **replantation**)

reinforcement The increasing of force or strength. (Anesth.)

reintubation (rē″ĭn-tū-bā′shŭn) Intubation performed a second time. (Anesth.)

Reiter's syndrome (rī′terz) (see **syndrome, Reiter's**)

relapse Return of features of the original malocclusion after correction. (Orthodont.)

relation(s) The designation of the position of one object as oriented to another; e.g., centric relation of the mandible to the maxillae. (Comp. Prosth.)

acentric r. (see **relation, jaw, eccentric**)

centric r. (centric jaw r.) (1) The most posterior relation of the mandible to the maxillae at the established vertical relation. (2) The relation of the mandible to the maxillae when the condyles are in their most posterior unstrained positions in the glenoid fossae, from which lateral movements can be made at the occluding vertical relation normal for the individual. Centric relation is a relation that can exist at any degree of jaw separation. It is a designation of a horizontal relation of the mandible to the maxillae. (Comp. Prosth.; Orthodont.; Remov. Part. Prosth.)

— The maxillomandibular relation when the mandibular condyles are in their most posterior and superior positions in their fossae. (Fixed Part. Prosth.)

acquired c. r. (see **relation, jaw, eccentric**)

cusp-fossa r. (see **cusp-fossa relations**)

dynamic r. Relations of two objects involving the element of relative movement of one object to another; e.g., the relationship of the mandible to the maxillae. (Comp. Prosth.)

eccentric r. (see **relation, jaw, eccentric**)

intermaxillary r. The relation between the right and left maxilla. (Comp. Prosth.; Remov. Part. Prosth.) (see **relation, maxillomandibular**)

jaw r. Any relation of the mandible to the maxillae. (Comp. Prosth.; Remov. Part. Prosth.)

  centric j. r. (see **relation, centric**)

  convenience j. r. (**convenience relationship**) The arch-to-arch or tooth-to-tooth relationship assumed on closure of the mandible, which is eccentrically placed in relation to the true centric relation or to the true centric occlusion. (Periodont.) (see also **occlusion, convenience**)

  eccentric j. r. (**convenience relationship, eccentric r., eccentric jaw position**) Any jaw relation other than centric relation. (Comp. Prosth.; Remov. Part. Prosth.)

    acquired e. j. r. An eccentric relation that is assumed by habit in order to bring the teeth into a convenient occlusion. (Comp. Prosth.; Remov. Part. Prosth.)

  median j. r. Any jaw relation existing when the mandible is in the median sagittal plane. (Comp. Prosth.; Remov. Part. Prosth.)

  posterior border j. r. The most posterior relation of the mandible to the maxillae at any specific vertical relation. (Comp. Prosth.)

  protrusive j. r. (**protrusive r.**) A jaw relation resulting from a protrusion of the mandible. (Comp. Prosth.; Remov. Part. Prosth.)

  rest j. r. (**rest r.**) The postural relation of the mandible to the maxillae when the patient is resting comfortably in the upright position, the condyles are in a neutral unstrained position in the glenoid fossae, and the mandibular musculature is in a state of minimum tonic contraction to maintain posture. (Comp. Prosth.; Fixed Part. Prosth.; Remov. Part. Prosth.)

  surgical j. r. The establishing and recording of the correct vertical relation and centric relation between the surgically exposed bone surface and the opposite jaw at the time of the surgical bone impression. (Oral Implant.)

unstrained j. r. Any jaw relation that is attained without undue or unnatural force and that causes no undue distortion of the tissues of the temporomandibular joints. (Comp. Prosth.)
— The relation of the mandible to the skull when a state of balanced tonus exists between all the muscles involved. (Comp. Prosth.; Remov. Part. Prosth.)

lateral r. The relation of the mandible to the maxillae when the lower jaw is in a position on either side of centric relation. (Comp. Prosth.)

maxillomandibular r. (măk-sĭl″ō-măn-dĭb′ū-lar) Any one of the many relations of the mandible to the maxillae, such as centric maxillomandibular relation or eccentric maxillomandibular relation. (Comp. Prosth.; Remov. Part. Prosth.)

median r. (see **relation, centric**)

median retruded r. (see **relation, centric**)

occluding r. The jaw relation at which the opposing teeth contact or occlude. (Comp. Prosth.; Remov. Part. Prosth.)

protrusive r. (see **relation, jaw, protrusive; position, rest, physiologic**)

public r. The opinion held by laymen concerning the individuals, personalities, and services rendered by the profession of dentistry. (Pract. Man.)

rest r. (see **relation, jaw, rest**)

ridge r. The positional relation of the mandibular ridge to the maxillary ridges. (Comp. Prosth.; Remov. Part. Prosth.)

static r. The relationship between two parts that are not in motion. (Comp. Prosth.; Remov. Part. Prosth.)

vertical r. The relative position of the mandible in a vertical direction. One of the basic jaw relations. (Comp. Prosth.)

relationship The condition of being associated or interconnected.

  buccolingual r. (bŭk″kō-lĭng′gwahl) The position of a space or tooth in relation to the tongue and cheek. (Comp. Prosth.; Remov. Part. Prosth.)

  convenience r. of teeth (see **occlusion, convenience**)

  normal r. A relationship in which structures conjoin as they should. (Orthodont.)

  occlusal r. The individual and collective relationships of the mandibular teeth to the maxillary teeth, and the relationship of the adjacent teeth in the same dental arch. (Periodont.)

    abnormal o. r. Occlusal relationships that

deviate from the regular and established type in such a manner as to produce esthetic disharmonies, interference with mastication, occlusal traumatism, and/or speech difficulties. (Periodont.)

patient-dentist r. A relationship based on the freedom of the patient to select his own dentist and the freedom of the dentist to accept or reject a patient for dental services. (Pract. Man.)

structure-activity r. (**SAR**) The relationship between the chemical structure of a drug and its activity. (Oral Med.; Pharmacol.)

tissue-base r. The relationship of the base of a removable prosthesis to the structures subjacent to it. There are three different possibilities: the base may be entirely tissue-borne, it may be completely tooth-borne, or support may be shared by both the tissue subjacent to its base and the abutment that bounds the edentulous space at one terminus. (Remov. Part. Prosth.)

relaxant An antispasmodic; a drug that relaxes spasms of smooth or skeletal muscle. (Anesth.)
— A drug that minimizes or prevents contraction of muscles. (Oral Med.; Pharmacol.)
— A drug used to eliminate muscle spasms, thus facilitating the establishment of centric relation, centric occlusion, rest position, etc. Also used in the treatment of painful muscle spasms associated with occlusal traumatism. Examples are mephenesin, the meprobamates, and methocarbamol (Robaxin). (Periodont.)

muscle r. A drug that specifically aids in lessening muscle tension. (Comp. Prosth.; Remov. Part. Prosth.)

release To give up, as a legal claim; to discharge or relinquish a right to. (D. Juris.)

sustained r. (see **medication, sustained release**)

relief The mitigation or removal of pain or distress. (Anesth.)
— The reduction or elimination of pressure from a specific area under a denture base. (Comp. Prosth.; Remov. Part. Prosth.)
— The reduction or elimination of pressure from a specific area under a denture base or component of a removable partial denture. (Comp. Prosth.; Remov. Part. Prosth.)

r. chamber (see **chamber, relief**)

gingival r. Relief given to removable partial denture units at all gingival crossings to avoid impingement. (Remov. Part. Prosth.)

r. space (see **space, relief**)

relieve To mitigate or remove pain or distress. (Anesth.)
— The procedure of placing hard wax in stra-

tegic areas on a master cast to be duplicated so that a refractory cast can be made. The purpose of relieving the master cast with wax is to provide space between certain components of the framework and the adjacent oral structures; e.g., the minor connector to which the denture base will be attached. (Remov. Part. Prosth.)
— The procedure of adding wax or other substances to casts to block out or eliminate undesirable undercuts. (Comp. Prosth.)

reline To resurface the tissue side (basal surface) of a denture with new base material so that it will fit more accurately. (Comp. Prosth.) (see also **rebase**)

rem (see **roentgen-equivalent-man**)

remedial (rē-mē'dē-al) Curative; acting as a remedy. (Anesth.)

remit To send; to relinquish. (D. Juris.)

remodeling The rearrangement of rooms and equipment within a given space, usually done to permit more efficient operation of a dental practice. (Pract. Man.)

removable lingual arch (see **arch, removable lingual**)

removable partial denture (see **denture, partial, removable**)

removal, pulp (see **pulpectomy**)

remuneration Pay; recompense; salary. (D. Juris)

Rendu-Osler-Weber disease (see **telangiectasia, hereditary hemorrhagic**)

rent A payment made by a tenant to an owner for the use of land or a building. (D. Juris.)

rental The fee paid by the dentist for the utilization of space in a building owned by someone else. (Pract. Man.)

reoxidation The act of taking up oxygen again, as the hemoglobin of the blood. (Anesth.)

rep (see **roentgen-equivalent-physical**)

repair The process of reuniting or replacing broken parts of a denture. A means for extending the usefulness of a denture. (Comp. Prosth.; Remov. Part. Prosth.)
— To make sound; to mend; restoration to former condition. (D. Juris.)
— Formation of new tissues, by such processes as fibroplasia, osteogenesis, and endothelioplasia, to replace tissues damaged by disease or injury. (Periodont.)

cemental r. Repair of areas of cemental resorption and/or cemental tears by apposition of cementum. Repair may be by formation of either cellular or acellular cementum. (Periodont.)

replacement, prosthetic (see **prosthesis**)

replantation (reimplantation) Replacement of teeth that have been removed from the alveolus either accidentally or unintentionally. (Endodont.)

— Reinsertion into the alveolar socket of a tooth accidentally extracted or dislodged. (Oral Surg.)

replasticize To manipulate dental amalgam by rubbing each portion in a squeeze cloth to restore its workability before expressing the excess mercury. (Oper. Dent.)

replenisher A concentrated developing solution designed to maintain the active strength of developer through periodic addition to maintain original volume. (Oral Radiol.)

reposition, muscle Surgical replacement of a muscle attachment into a more acceptable functional position. (Oral Surg.)

repositioning, jaw The changing of any relative position of the mandible to the maxillae, usually by altering the occlusion of the natural or artificial teeth. (Comp. Prosth.; Remov. Part. Prosth.)

repository Referring to long-acting drugs, usually when administered intramuscularly. (Pharmacol.) (see also **medication, repository**)

rapid r. Mixtures of rapid-acting and slow-acting drugs, usually administered intramuscularly. (Oral Med.; Pharmacol.)

reputation A person's credit, honor, character, good name. Injuries to one's reputation, which is a personal right, are defamatory and malicious words, libel, and malicious indictments or prosecutions. (D. Juris.)

res ipsa loquitur (rēz ĭp'sah lok'wĭ-ter) Latin phrase meaning the thing speaks for itself. Used in actions for injury by negligence where the happening itself is accepted as proof. (D. Juris.)

res judicata (rēz joo'dĭ-kā"tah) Decided or determined by judicial power; a thing judicially decided. (D. Juris.)

resection Excision of a considerable portion of an organ. (Oral Surg.)

root r. (see **apicoectomy**)

reserve Something kept in store for future use. (Anesth.)

alkali r. (see **reserve, alkaline**)

alkaline r. (alkali r.) The amount of buffer compounds (e.g., sodium bicarbonate, dipotassium phosphate, and proteins) in the blood capable of neutralizing acids. One of the buffer systems of the blood that can neutralize the acid valences formed in the body. It is made up of the base of weak acid salts and usually is measured by determining the bicarbonate concentration of the plasma. (Anesth.)

— The concentration of bicarbonate ions (HCO_3) in the blood. These ions serve as a reserve in that they may be displaced by anions, e.g., CL^-, $SO_4^=$, and $PO_4^{\equiv}$. Displacement of bicarbonate ions occurs predominantly by means of the chloride shift (Hamburger's phenomenon). The role of the buffer system is such that a large influx of acid or base ions from either metabolic function or ingestion can be neutralized by the alkaline reserves from the mineral and protein salts in the blood and tissue fluids. A strong acid is transformed into a weak base. Consequently, the pH of the blood fluctuates very little, and the tissue cells are constantly bathed in a continuously buffered solution. (Oral Med.; Oral Physiol.)

cardiac r. The reserve strength or pumping ability of the heart, which may be called on in an emergency. (Anesth.)

resident A graduate and licensed dentist or physician who has completed an internship and is serving and residing in the hospital while pursuing advanced didactic and clinical studies in special disciplines of knowledge. (Oral Surg.)

residual ridge (see **ridge, residual**)

residue Remainder; that which remains after the removal of other substances. (Anesth.)

resilience (rē-zĭl'ē-ĕns) The amount of energy absorbed by a structure when it is stressed, not to exceed its proportional limits. Energy absorbed due to elastic deformation. (D. Mat.; Oper. Dent.)

modulus of r. The amount of energy stored up by a body when one unit volume is stressed to its proportional limit. (D. Mat.)

resin (rĕz'ĭn) Broad term used to indicate organic substances that are usually translucent or transparent, and that are soluble in ether, acetone, etc. but not in water. They are named according to their chemical composition, physical structure, and means for activation or curing. Examples are acrylic resin, autopolymer resin (cold-curing resin), synthetic resin, styrene resin, and vinyl resin. (Comp. Prosth.; Oper. Dent.; Remov. Part. Prosth.)

— Amorphous solid or semisolid substance. May be of natural (resins) or synthetic origin. (D. Mat.) (see also **methyl methacrylate; varnish, cavity**)

— A thermoplastic, amorphous, solid, organic, dielectric material. Natural resins are derived from plants. (Oral Med.; Pharmacol.)

acrylic r. General term applied to a resinous material of the various esters of acrylic acid. It is used as a denture base material and also for trays and other dental restorations. (Comp. Prosth.)

— An ethylene derivative that contains a vinyl group; e.g., polymethacrylate (methyl methacrylate), the principal ingredient of many plastics used in dentistry. (D. Mat.; Oper. Dent.)

    a. r. appliance (see **appliance, acrylic resin and copper band**)

    direct restorative a. r. (see **resin, autopolymer**)

activated r. (see **resin, autopolymer**)

autopolymer r. (**activated r., autopolymerizing r., cold-curing r., direct restorative acrylic r., self-curing r.**) Any resin that can be polymerized by an activator and a catalyst without the use of external heat. (Comp. Prosth.)

— A resin whose molecules are in a reactive state. Usually considered to be a molecule whose double bonds are open. (D. Mat.)

— A resin that sets, or cures, at room or body temperature. Tinted to match tooth color, it serves as a temporary restoration or crown. (Oper. Dent.)

cold-curing r. (see **resin, autopolymerizing**)

composite r. A resin used for restorative purposes and usually formed by a reaction of an ether of bisphenol-A (an expoxy molecule) with acrylic resin monomers, initiated by a benzoyl peroxide–amine system, to which is added as much as 75% inorganic filler (glass beads and rods, lithium aluminum silicate, quartz, and/or tricalcium phosphate). (Oper. Dent.)

— A restorative material composed of a high percentage of inorganic filler bonded to a resin matrix. The resin matrix is a polymer formed by reacting an ether of bisphenol-A with an acrylic monomer. The fillers generally are some form of silica such as quartz. The fillers are coated with an agent such as silane, which bonds to both the filler and the matrix. (D. Mat.)

copolymer r. A synthetic resin that is the product of the concurrent and joint polymerization of two or more different monomers of polymers. (Comp. Prosth.)

epoxy r. A resin molecule characterized by reactive epoxy, or ethoxyline, groups that serve as terminal polymerization points. Used in dentistry for denture bases. (D. Mat.)

heat-curing r. Any resin that requires heat to activate its polymerization. (Comp. Prosth.)

quick cure r. (see **resin, autopolymer**)

self-curing r. (see **resin, autopolymer**)

thermoplastic r. A synthetic resin that may be softened by heat and hardened by cooling. (Comp. Prosth.)

vinyl r. An ethylene-derivative copolymer of vinyl chloride and vinyl acetate. Used at one time for denture bases. (D. Mat.; Oper. Dent.)

resin-filled Pertaining to a resin, usually poly (methylmethacrylate), to which has been added some inert material such as glass beads or glass rods. (D. Mat.)

resistance A state in which an organism is insensitive to a drug or a noxious influence. (Oral Med.; Pharmacol.)

— Ability of an individual to ward off the damaging effects of physical, chemical, or microbiologic injury. An immeasurable factor controlled and qualified by numerous local, systemic, and metabolic processes such as blood supply to tissues, nutritional status, age, and antibody formative ability. (Periodont.)

    cross-r. A state in which an organism is insensitive to several drugs of similar chemical nature. (Oral Med.; Pharmacol.)

    r. form (see **form, resistance**)

resolution The discernible separation of closely adjacent radiographic image details. (Oral Radiol.)

resonance (rĕz′ō-năns) The vibratory response of a body or air-filled cavity to a frequency imposed on it. (Cleft Palate)

    speech r. The resonance of the body cavities and surfaces involved in the production of speech. The sound waves produced at the vocal folds are still far from the finished product heard in speech. The resonators give the characteristic quality to the voice. The resonating structures are the air sinuses, the organ surfaces, the cavities such as the pharynx, oral cavity, and nasal cavity, and the chest wall. The resonating structures contribute no energy to the stream of air; they act to conserve and concentrate the energy already present in the laryngeal tone rather than to let it dissipate into the tissues. However, the resonated laryngeal tone still is not speech. (Oral Physiol.)

resorption (rē-sorp′shŭn) Loss of substance (bone) by physiologic or pathologic means. The reduction of the volume and size of the residual alveolar portion of the mandible or maxillae. (Comp. Prosth.; Remov. Part. Prosth.)

— The cementoclastic and dentinoclastic action that often takes place on the root of a re-planted tooth. (Endodont.)

— Removal by absorption. (Oper. Dent.)

r. of bone Destruction or solution of the elements of bone. (Orthodont.)

— Loss of bone due to the activity of multi-nucleated giant cells, the osteoclasts, which are noted in irregular concavities on the periphery of the bone (Howship's lacunae). During the resorptive phase, multinucleated osteoclasts can be seen in irregular con-cavities in the bone margin. Excessive bone resorption, or disequilibrium with bone re-sorption exceeding bone formation, is seen in such conditions as hyperparathyroidism, hyperthyroidism, marginal periodontitis, oc-clusal traumatism, disuse atrophy, and peri-odontosis. Resorption may be physiologic or pathologic. (Periodont.)

pressure r. of b. Osteoclastic destruction of bone as a result of the application of sustained, excessive force upon it. Re-modeling of bone may occur in order to better adapt to these forces, or destruc-tion may continue if the stresses are re-peated and excessive. (Periodont.)

cemental r. Destruction of cementum by cementoclastic action. Noted as the presence of irregular concavities in the cemental sur-faces in such conditions as occlusal trauma-tism and periodontitis. (Periodont.)

frontal r. Osteoclastic resorption of alveolar bone (lamina dura) by multinucleated cells on the osseous margin adjacent to the peri-odontal ligament. (Periodont.)

horizontal r. A pattern of bone resorption in marginal periodontitis in which the marginal crest of the alveolar bone between adjacent teeth remains level; in these instances the bases of the periodontal pockets are supra-crestal. A pattern of bone loss in which the crestal margins of the alveolar bone are resorbed. A horizontal pattern, rather than vertical loss along the root, is the typical type of bone loss in periodontitis. (Peri-odont.)

idiopathic r. Resorption that is not attributable to any known disease or is without an apparent cause. (Oper. Dent.)

internal r. (idiopathic internal resorption, pink tooth) A special form of idiopathic root resorption from within the pulp cavity; granulation tissue is present within the tooth,

apparently with the resorption of the dentin occurring from the inside outward. The cause is unknown. (Oper. Dent.; Oral Path.)

lacunar r. Presence of irregular concavities on the surface of bone that represent areas of osteoclastic bone resorption; they usually contain multinucleated osteoclasts. (Peri-odont.)

osteoclastic r. Loss of bone by cellular activity; osteoclasts are large, multinucleated cells seen in irregular concavities in the margin of the bone (Howship's lacunae) and cur-rently believed to be directly responsible for the active destruction of bone. (Periodont.)

rear r. Osteoclastic resorption of the support-ing bone of the alveolar process from within the marrow spaces, producing thinning and ultimate fragmentation of trabeculae and cortex of bone. (Periodont.)

root r. Destruction of cementum (and possibly the underlying dentin) by cementoclastic or osteoclastic activity, as noted in such entities as occlusal traumatic lesions and neoplasms. Radiographically, root resorption is repre-sented by blunting of root tips. (Periodont.)

— Destruction of the cementum and/or dentin by cementoclastic or osteoclastic activity. (Endodont.)

apical r. r. Dissolution of the apex of a tooth, resulting in a shortened, blunted root. (Orthodont.)

surface r. r. Localized resorptive areas on the cemental surface of the tooth root. (Orthodont.)

undermining r. Indirect, as opposed to frontal, removal of alveolar bone where pressure applied to a tooth has resulted in loss of vitality of localized areas of the periodontal membrane. (Orthodont.)

vertical r. A pattern of bone loss. Seen in oc-clusal traumatism, marginal periodontitis, periodontosis, etc. A pattern of bone loss in which the alveolar bone adjacent to a tooth is destroyed without simultaneous crestal loss, so that a vertical rather than a hori-zontal pattern of loss is observed. (Peri-odont.)

respirable Suitable for respiration. (Anesth.)

respiration The gaseous exchange between the cells of the body and its environment. (Anesth.)

artificial r. Maintenance of respiratory move-ments by artificial means. When respiration has been arrested and no mechanical device is available, resuscitation by means of arti-ficial respiration is the only practical means of ventilating the lungs. The technique of applying back pressure and lifting the arms or hips is an accepted procedure. The subject is placed in a prone position, and the operator kneels at his head. Expiration is produced by pressing the palms against the posterior thorax. Expansion of the thorax and inspiration are produced by elevating the arms. The result is a tidal air volume of over 500 cc, which is quite adequate for normal ventilation. The procedure can be performed after minimal training and must be initiated immediately and continued until spontaneous respiration has been restored or further hope for revival abandoned. (Anesth.; Oral Physiol.)

Cheyne-Stokes r. (chān stōks) (**Cheyne-Stokes reflex**) A type of breathing characterized by rhythmic variations in intensity that occur in cycles; rhythmic acceleration, deepening, and stopping of breathing movements. (Anesth.)

controlled r. Maintenance of adequate pulmonary ventilation in apneic patients. (Anesth.)

external r. Ventilation of the lungs and oxygenation of the blood. (Anesth.)

internal r. The mechanism of gaseous exchange between blood and tissues. (Anesth.)

r. in speech In normal speech, the action of the respiratory apparatus during exhalation, which provides a continuous stream of air with sufficient volume and pressure (under adequate voluntary control) to initiate phonation. The stream of air is modified in its course from the lungs by the facial and oral structures, giving rise to the sound symbols that are recognized as speech. (Oral Physiol.)

stertorous r. Snoring. (Anesth.)

stridulous r. A high-pitched sound occurring during respiration, due to adduction of the vocal cords. (Anesth.)

respirator (rĕs′pĭ-rā″tor) An apparatus that qualifies the air that is breathed through it; a device for giving artificial respiration. (Anesth.)

respirometer An instrument for determining the character of the respiratory movements. (Anesth.)

respondeat superior Latin phrase meaning let the superior answer. Refers to the responsibility of a principal for his agent's acts; the liability of a master for the acts of his servant. (D. Juris.)

response Action or movement due to the application of a stimulus. (Anesth.)

rest An extension from a prosthesis that affords vertical support for a restoration. (Remov. Part. Prosth.)

r. area (see **area, rest**)

auxiliary r. The rest other than the one used as a component part of a primary direct retainer. (Remov. Part. Prosth.)

finger r. (see **finger rest**)

incisal r. A metallic extension onto the incisal angle of an anterior tooth to supply support and/or indirect retention for a removable partial denture. (Remov. Part. Prosth.)

lingual r. A metallic extension onto the lingual surface of an anterior tooth to provide support or indirect retention for a removable partial denture. (Remov. Part. Prosth.)

occlusal r. (**occlusal lug**) A rest placed on the occlusal surface of a posterior tooth. (Remov. Part. Prosth.)

r. occlusion (see **position, rest, physiologic**)

r. position (see **position, rest**)

precision r. A unit consisting of two closely fitted parts, the insert of which rests firmly against the gingival portion of the tubelike receptacle. (Remov. Part. Prosth.)

r. relation (see **relation, jaw, rest**)

r. seat (see **area, rest**)

restoration (**prosthetic restoration**) Broad term applied to any filling, inlay, crown, bridge, partial denture, or complete denture that restores or replaces lost tooth structure, teeth, or oral tissues. A prosthesis. (Comp. Prosth.; Oper. Dent.)

— Term applied to the end result of repairing and restoring or reforming the shape, form, and function of part or all of a tooth, with consideration given to the prevention of recurrence or continuation of the breakdown. (Oper. Dent.)

— The careful reforming of the contours and restoring of the function of parts of teeth destroyed by decay or accident. (Pract. Man.)

r. of cusps (preferred to tipping, capping, or shoeing cusps) Reduction and inclusion of cusps within a cavity preparation and their restoration to functional occlusion with restorative material. (Oper. Dent.)

dental prosthetic r. (see **prosthesis, dental**)

faulty r. Restoration in which there are imperfections or incorrect attributes; e.g., overhanging or deficient fillings, incorrect anatomy of occlusal and marginal ridge areas, and faulty clasps. Such faults may be present in individual tooth restorations, fixed bridges, removable partial dentures, etc. and are conducive to the initiation and perpetuation of inflammatory and dystrophic diseases of the teeth and/or periodontium. (Periodont.)

implant r. The single-tooth implant crown or the multiple-tooth implant, crown, or bridge that replaces a missing tooth or teeth. (Oral Implant.)

inconspicuous Class 3 r. A gold-foil or gold-inlay restoration in the proximal surface of an anterior tooth, wherein the labial extension is restricted so that the metal will not be detected on casual observation. (Oper. Dent.) (see also **foil, lingual approach**)

prosthetic r. (see **prosthesis**)

restorative Promoting a return to health or to consciousness; a remedy that aids in restoring health, vigor, or consciousness. (Anesth.)

— Pertaining to rebuilding, repairing, or reforming. (Oper. Dent.)

rest position (see **position, rest**)

restrainer A chemical ingredient (potassium bromide) of the photographic developing solution. Its function is to inhibit the fogging tendency of the solution. Like the activator, the restrainer also controls the rate of development. (Oral Radiol.)

restrictive covenant Common clause found in a contract for the sale of a dental practice. The seller contracts that he will not practice dentistry within a certain time and area. A junior partner may be asked to sign such a covenant to guarantee that he will not compete with the partnership for a period of time after he leaves the partnership. Also used in an employment situation. (Pract. Man.)

resuscitation (rē-sŭs″ĭ-tā′shŭn) Restoration of life or consciousness to one who appears to be dead. (Oral Physiol.)

resuscitator (rē-sŭs′ĭ-tā″tor) An apparatus for initiating respiration in asphyxia. (Anesth.)

retainer (**retaining appliance**) The part of a dental prosthesis that unites the abutment tooth with the suspended portion of the bridge. It may be an inlay, partial crown, or complete crown. (Fixed Part. Prosth.)

— An appliance for maintaining the positions of the teeth and jaws gained by orthodontic procedures. (Orthodont.)

— The portion of a fixed prosthesis attaching a pontic(s) to the abutment teeth; e.g., an inlay or a three-quarter crown. (Periodont.)

— Any form of clasp, attachment, or device used for the fixation or stabilization of a prosthetic appliance. (Remov. Part. Prosth.)

continuous bar r. A metal bar that is attached to a major connector and that contacts

lingual surfaces of anterior teeth, on or incisal to cingula; it aids in the stabilization of a distal extension removable partial denture. (Remov. Part. Prosth.)

direct r. A clasp, attachment, or assembly applied to an abutment tooth for the purpose of maintaining a removable restoration in its planned position in relation to oral structures. (Remov. Part. Prosth.)

extracoronal r. The type of retainer in which the preparation and its cast restoration lie largely external to the body of the coronal portion of the tooth and complement the contour of the crown. The retention or resistance to displacement is developed between the inner surfaces of the casting and the external walls of the prepared tooth. The extracoronal retainer may be a partial crown, a complete crown, etc. (Fixed Part. Prosth.)

— A direct retainer of the clasp type that engages an abutment tooth on its external surface in such a way as to afford retention and stabilization to a removable partial denture. A direct retainer of the manufactured type, the male portion of which is attached to the external surface of a cast crown on an abutment tooth; for example, the Dalbo and Crismani attachments. (Remov. Part. Prosth.)

Hawley r. A wire and acrylic resin removable appliance designed to stabilize teeth after tooth movement; to serve as a basis for tooth movement by providing an anchorage for wires, rubber dam elastics, etc. used in orthodontic tooth movement; etc. (Periodont.)

intracoronal r. The type of retainer in which the prepared cavity and its cast restoration lie largely within the body of the coronal portion of the tooth and within the contour of the crown; e.g., an inlay. The retention or resistance to displacement is developed between the casting and the internal walls of the prepared cavity. (Fixed Part. Prosth.)

— The type of direct retainer used in the construction of removable partial dentures; it consists of a female portion within the coronal portion of the crown of an abutment and a fitted male portion attached to the denture proper. These retainers may be fabricated or machined in the dental office or obtained through commercial sources. (Remov. Part. Prosth.)

matrix r. (**matrix holder**) A mechanical device designed to engage the ends of a matrix band or strip and to tighten the matrix around the tooth. (Oper. Dent.)

radicular r. The type of retainer that lies within the body of the tooth and is usually confined to the root portion of the tooth; e.g., a dowel crown. The retention or resistance to displacement and shear is developed by extending an attached dowel into the root canal of the tooth. (Fixed Part. Prosth.)

retaining ring A ring that holds the arch wire against the bicuspid bracket to allow free sliding and tipping. (Orthodont.)

retardation, mental (see **subnormality, mental**)

retarder A chemical added to a certain substance to slow a chemical reaction, to prolong the set of the material, and to provide more working time. (D. Mat.)

rete pegs (see **pegs, epithelial**)

retention (rē-těn′shŭn) Resistance of a denture to removal in a direction opposite that of its insertion. The quality inherent in the denture that resists the force of gravity, the adhesiveness of foods, and the forces associated with the opening of the jaws. (Comp. Prosth.)

— Power to retain; capacity for retaining. The inherent property of a restoration to maintain its position without displacement under stress; results from close adaptation of the restoration to the prepared form of the tooth, usually aided by cement. (Fixed Part. Prosth.)

— Term relating to the provision, in cavity preparation, for preventing displacement of a restoration. Retention supplements resistance form and is specifically created to resist any lateral or tipping force that may be brought against the restoration during and after its insertion. (Oper. Dent.)

— The characteristic of a denture that resists forces that tend to alter the relationship between the denture base and the soft tissues to which it is attached. (Remov. Part. Prosth.)

— The period of treatment during which the individual is wearing an appliance to maintain the teeth in the position into which they have been moved. (Orthodont.)

r. arm (see **arm, retention**)

circumferential r. Frictional resistance to displacement derived from completely veneering the exposed tooth surface. (Fixed Part. Prosth.)

denture r. The means by which dentures are held in position in the mouth. The maintenance of a denture in its position in the mouth. The resistance to the movement of a denture from its basal seat in a direction

opposite that in which it was inserted. (Comp. Prosth.)

— The characteristic of a denture to resist forces that tend to alter the relationship between the denture and the soft tissues to which it is attached. (Remov. Part. Prosth.)

— The resistance of a denture to vertical movement in the occlusal direction from its basal seat. (Remov. Part. Prosth.)

partial d. r. The fixation of a fixed partial denture by means of crowns, inlays, and/ or other retainers. (Remov. Part. Prosth.)

removable p. d. r. The resistance to movement of a removable partial denture from its supporting structures, gained by the use of direct and indirect retainers and/or other attachments. (Remov. Part. Prosth.)

direct r. Retention obtained in a removable partial denture by the use of attachments or clasps that resist removal from abutment teeth. (Oper. Dent.; Remov. Part. Prosth.)

r. form (see **form, retention**)

indirect r. Retention obtained in a removable partial denture through the use of indirect retainers. (Oper. Dent.; Remov. Part. Prosth.)

r. lug (see **lug, retention**)

r. pin (see **pin, retention**)

pinhole r. One or more small holes, 2 to 3 mm in depth, placed in suitable areas of a cavity preparation parallel with the general line of draft to provide or supplement resistance and retention form. (Oper. Dent.)

Prothero "cone" theory of r. An explanation of clasp retention advanced by Prothero in 1916. He noted that crowns of posterior teeth roughly conformed to two cones, one projecting from the occlusal and the other from the cervical direction, meeting in a common base at the line of greatest tooth contour (later called "height of contour" by Kennedy). He further pointed out that a clasp terminal placed on the surface of a cervically sloping cone would resist displacement—would be retentive. (Remov. Part. Prosth.)

radicular r. Retention derived from projections of metal into the root canals of pulpless teeth. (Fixed Part. Prosth.)

r. terminal (see **clasp, circumferential, arm; clasp, circumferential, arm, retentive**)

retention, water and salt The keeping in the body of excessive amounts of water and salt. Water intoxication may be caused by pituitary disturbances and by the ingestion of large quantities of water in the presence of low salt concentration. Ingestion of seawater causes respiratory disorders and central nervous system impairment. It accelerates the loss of intracellular water, with resultant disorganization of the cells. (Oral Physiol.)

reticulation of film emulsion A network of wrinkles or corrugations in the emulsion of an x-ray or photographic film, resulting from sharp temperature differences between processing solutions. (Oral Radiol.)

reticulocytosis (rē-tĭk′ū-lō-sī-tō″sĭs) An increase in the normal number of reticulocytes in the circulating blood. Normal values range from 0.5% to 1.5% of the red blood cells. (Oral Med.)

reticuloendotheliosis, nonlipid (rē-tĭk″ū-lō-ĕn″dō-thē″lē-ō′sĭs) (see **disease, Letterer-Siwe**)

retraction A drawing or shrinking back; the laying back of tissues to expose a given part. (Oper. Dent.)
— Distal movement of teeth. A distal or retrusive position of the teeth, the dental arch, or the jaw. (Orthodont.)

 delayed r. (interrupted r.) Progressive interrupted laying back of tissues; applied especially to the setting of the labial jaw of the gingival clamp to secure a field for a restoration in a gingival third, or Class 5, type of restoration without lacerating the soft tissues. (Oper. Dent.)

 gingival r. Laying back of the free gingival tissue to expose the gingival margin area of a preparation by mechanical, chemical, or electrical means. (Oper. Dent.)
 — Reflections of gingival tissue from the tooth surface; seen in gingival inflammation as a result of destruction of the gingival fiber apparatus. (Periodont.)
 — The displacement of the marginal gingiva away from a tooth. (Remov. Part. Prosth.)

 interrupted r. (see **retraction, delayed**)

 mandibular r. A type of facial anomaly in which the gnathion lies posterior to the orbital plane. (Comp. Prosth.; Remov. Part. Prosth.)

retractor An instrument for retracting tissues to assist in gaining access to an area of operation or observation. (Oral Surg.)

 beaver-tail r. A broad-bladed periosteal elevator. (Oral Implant.)

 rake r. A metallic instrument with prongs set transversely for engaging and retracting soft tissues. (Oral Surg.)

 vein hook r. A metallic instrument ending in a rounded flange set transversely for engaging and retracting soft tissues. (Oral Surg.)

retrofill Obturation of the apex of a tooth root by the direct surgical approach. (Endodont.)

retrognathic (rĕt″rō-năth′ĭk) Having a recessive lower face. (Orthodont.)

retrognathism (rĕt″rō-năth′ĭzm) (**bird-face**) Facial disharmony in which one or both jaws (usually the mandible) are posterior to normal facial relationships. This condition may be real or imaginary. (Oral Surg.)

 bird-face r. Typical facial profile associated with an underdeveloped mandible. A retrognathia and small mandible usually associated with interference of condylar growth because of trauma or infection affecting the condyles. Surgical intervention is necessary for improvement. (Oral Surg.)

 micrognathic r. (see **micrognathism**)

 Pierre Robin r. (see **syndrome, Pierre Robin**)

retromolar pad (see **pad, retromolar**)

retromylohyoid eminence (see **eminence, retromylohyoid**)

retromylohyoid space (see **space, retromylohyoid**)

retroversion (rĕt″rō-ver′zhŭn) A condition in which teeth or other maxillary and mandibular structures are located posterior to the normal or generally accepted standard. (Orthodont.)

retrusion Retraction of the mandible from any given position. (Comp. Prosth.; Remov. Part. Prosth.)

 mandibular r. Abnormal retrusion of the mandible, as in a Class II malocclusion. (Oral Diag.)

 maxillary r. Abnormal retrusion of the maxillae. (Oral Diag.)

reverse curve (see **curve, reverse**)

reversible Capable of going through a series of changes in either direction, forward or backward; e.g., a reversible chemical reaction. (Anesth.)

 r. hydrocolloid (see **hydrocolloid, reversible**)

reversion (falling back) A return to a deeper color after bleaching. (Endodont.)

rhabdomyosarcoma (răb″dō-mī″ō-sar-kō′mah) A malignant tumor of striated, or voluntary, muscle. (Oral Path.)

rhagades (răg′ah-dēz) Cracks, fissures, or scars radiating from the angles of the lips. They occur in infancy as manifestations of congenital syphilis. (Oral Diag.; Oral Med.)
— Fissures or cracks in the skin seen around body orifices and in regions subjected to frequent movement. (Oral Path.)

rheology (rē-ol′ō-jē) The study of blood flow, pressure, and velocity through the vascular system. The variables are under the continuous control of the neurologic and hormonal systems that regulate the pumping system, the condition of the blood vessels when blood passes through, the amount of blood in the system, and the resistance to its flow. (Oral Physiol.)

rheonome (rē′ō-nōm) An apparatus for determining the effect of irritation on a nerve. (Anesth.)

rheostat (rē′ō-stăt) A resistor for regulating the current of an x-ray tube by means of variable degrees of resistance. The rheostat is controlled on a dental x-ray machine by the milliampere adjusting knob. (Oral Radiol.)

rheumatic fever (see **fever, rheumatic**)

rheumatism (roo′mah-tĭzm) (**rheumatic disease**) Nonspecific term indicating any painful disorder related to joints, muscles, bone, or nerves; acute rheumatic fever; or, as used by lay persons, rheumatoid arthritis, bursitis, myositis, or degenerative joint disease. (Oral Med.)

rhinoanemometer (rī″nō-ăn-ē-mom′ĕ-ter) An apparatus for measuring the air passing through the nose during respiration. (Anesth.)

rhinolalia (rī″nō-lā′lē-ah) Nasalized speech, of which there are two types: rhinolalia clausa (closed port) and rhinolalia aperta (open port). (Oral Physiol.)

rhizanesthesia (rī′zăn″ĕs-thē′zē-ah) Nerve root anesthesia; spinal anesthesia produced by injecting a local anesthetic into the cavity of the spinal arachnoid. (Anesth.)

rhizotomy, retrogasserian (rī-zot′ō-mē, rĕt″rō-găs-sē′rē-ăn) Intracranial sectioning of the sensory root of the trigeminal nerve posterior to the semilunar ganglion. Used in the treatment of a severe trigeminal neuralgia. (Oral Surg.)

rhythm A measured movement; the recurrence of an action or function at regular intervals. (Anesth.)

heart r. The rhythm pattern in the sequence of heart beats, which which may be altered in the presence of cardiac disease. The various irregularities of rhythm and rate are encountered in patients who generally have serious forms of heart disease or who have had excessive doses of digitalis, quinidine, or other stimulants or depressants. (Oral Physiol.)

riboflavin (rī″bō-flā′vin) (see **vitamin B₂**)

rickets A condition caused by deficiency of vitamin D in infants and children. Characterized by defective calcification of bone matrix. (Oral Path.) (see also **osteomalacia**) — A condition produced by a deficiency of calcium and/or vitamin D in the diet, especially in infants and children, with disturbance in the mineralization of osseous and dental tissues. Marked by bending and bowing of bones, nodular enlargements at the ends of bones, myalgia, delay in closure of fontanels, etc. Osteomalacia of childhood. (Periodont.)

adult r. (see **osteomalacia**)

deficiency r. (**ordinary r.**) A nutritional disease of infancy and childhood characterized by skeletal weakness and deformities such as craniotabes, rachitic rosary, enlargement of joints, bowing of the legs, knock-knee, and pigeon-chest deformity. It is due to a deficiency of vitamin D, resulting in the failure of calcium salts to be deposited in growing bones. Old bone is destroyed, but new osteoid fails to calcify. (Oral Med.)

late r. (see **rickets, resistant**)

ordinary r. (see **rickets, deficiency**)

refractory r. (see **rickets, resistant**)

renal r. A disturbance marked by excessive excretion of phosphorus and calcium due to a lowered renal threshold of excretion of these mineral elements. (Periodont.) (see also **osteodystrophy, renal**)

resistant r. (**late r., refractory r.**) Rickets that responds only to extremely large amounts of vitamin D. (Oral Med.)

ridge The remainder of the alveolar process after the teeth are removed. (Comp. Prosth.; Orthodont.; Remov. Part. Prosth.)

alveolar r. The bony ridge of the maxillae or mandible that contains the alveoli (sockets of the teeth). (Comp. Prosth.; Remov. Part. Prosth.) (see also **process, alveolar**)

center of r. The buccolingual midline of the residual ridge. (Comp. Prosth.; Remov. Part. Prosth.)

crest of r. The highest continuous surface of the ridge but not necessarily the center of the ridge. The top of a residual or alveolar ridge. (Comp. Prosth.; Remov. Part. Prosth.)

r. extension (see **extension, ridge**)

key r. (**zygomaxillare**) The lowest point of the zygomaticomaxillary ridge. (Orthodont.)

r. lap The part of an artificial tooth that is adjacent to the residual ridge. The part of the artificial tooth that laps the ridge. (Comp. Prosth.)

marginal r. A ridge or elevation of enamel

that forms the boundary of a surface of a tooth. (Oper. Dent.)

mental r. A dense ridge extending from the symphysis to the bicuspid area on the anterolateral aspect of the body of the mandible. (Periodont.)

mylohyoid r. A dense line or ridge of bone on the medial surface of the body of the mandible that extends obliquely upward and posteriorly from the symphysis, covers the cervical portion of the third molar, and then goes upward and backward onto the vertical ramus. The mylohyoid muscle is inserted into this ridge of bone. (Periodont.)

Passavant's r. (see **pad, Passavant's**)

r. relation (see **relation, ridge**)

residual r. The portion of the alveolar ridge that remains after the alveoli have disappeared from the alveolar process after extraction of the teeth. (Comp. Prosth.; Remov. Part. Prosth.)

r. support (see **area, supporting**)

Riga-Fede disease (rē'gah fā'dah) (see **disease, Riga-Fede**)

right-angle technique (see **technique, parallel**)

right of action The right to sue; a legal right to maintain an action, based on a happening or state of fact. (D. Juris.)

rigidity The characteristic of being nonflexible, which is essential in a connector, a reciprocal arm, or an indirect retaining unit of a removable partial denture. (Remov. Part. Prosth.)

Riley-Day syndrome (see **syndrome, Riley-Day**)

rim The outer edge; often curved or circular.

occlusion r. (**record r.**) An occluding surface built on temporary or permanent denture bases for the purpose of making maxillomandibular relation records and for arranging teeth. (Comp. Prosth.; Fixed Part. Prosth.)

surgical o. r. A conventional occlusion rim, the base of which has been reduced until it is smaller than the surgical impression tray with which the surgical jaw relations are recorded. (Oral Implant.)

record r. (see **rim, occlusion**)

rinse bath A tank or container of water used in film processing to wash residual developer from the film prior to its being placed in the fixer. (Oral Radiol.)

rinsing (**balneotherapy**) (băl″nē-ō-thĕr'ah-pē) Water irrigation employed in the treatment of periodontal disease. (Periodont.)

Risdon wire (see **wire, Risdon**)

Risdon's incision (see **incision, Risdon's**)

Roach clasp (see **clasp, bar**)

Rockwell test (see **test, Rockwell**)

rod A straight, slim, cylindric form of material, usually metal. (D. Mat.)

analyzing r. The vertical part of a dental cast surveyor that is brought into contact with the surface contour of a tooth as a tangent related to a curve. It is used to determine the relative parallelism of one surface of a cast to other surfaces of the same cast. It is also used to estimate the cervical convergence of an infrabulge area of a tooth as it slopes from the contacting point of the surveying rod toward the cervical line, permitting evaluation of the retentiveness of the surface. (Remov. Part. Prosth.)

condyle r. The adjustable pointers of a facebow, which are placed over the condyles or at points on the face, marking the opening axis of the mandible. (Comp. Prosth.)

enamel r. A calcified column or prism, with an average diameter of 4 μ; extends in a wavy pattern through the entire thickness of the enamel and generally is perpendicular to the surface of the tooth. (Oper. Dent.)

roentgen (**r**) (rĕnt'gĕn) An international unit based on the ability of radiation to ionize air. The exposure to x or gamma radiation such that the associated corpuscular emission per 0.001293 g of air produces, in air, ions carrying 1 esu of quantity of electricity of either sign (2.083 billion ion pairs). (Oral Radiol.)

r.-equivalent-man (**rem**) The dose of any ionizing radiation that will produce the same biologic effect as that produced by 1 roentgen of high-voltage x radiation. (Oral Radiol.)

r.-equivalent-physical (**rep**) An unofficial unit of dose used with ionizing radiation other than x rays or gamma rays. It is defined as that dose which produces an energy absorption of 93 ergs/g of tissue. For most purposes it can be considered equal to the rad; the latter is gradually replacing the use of rep. (Oral Radiol.)

r. ray (see **ray, roentgen**)

roentgeno- (rĕnt'gĕn-ō) Prefix used to denote radiation originating only from an x-ray tube. (Oral Radiol.)

roentgenogram (rĕnt'gen-ō-grăm″) (see **radiograph** and subentries)

roentgenograph (rĕnt'gĕn-ō-grăf) (see **radiograph**)

roentgenographer (rĕnt″gĕ-nog′rah-fer) (see **radiographer**)

oral r. (see **radiographer, oral**)

roentgenographic detail (see **detail, radiographic**)

roentgenography (rĕnt″gĕn-og′rah-fē) (see **radiography** and subentries)

roentgenologist (rĕnt″gĕn-ol′ō-jĭst) (see **radiologist**)

oral r. (see **radiologist, oral**)

roentgenology (rĕnt″gĕn-ol′ō-jē) (see **radiology**)

roentgenolucent (rĕnt″gĕn-ō-lū′sĕnt) (see **radiolucent**)

roentgenopaque (rĕnt″gĕn-ō-pāk′) (see **radiopaque**)

roentgenoparent (rĕnt″gĕn-ō-păr′ĕnt) (see **radioparent**)

roentgenotherapy (rĕnt″gĕn-ō-thĕr′ah-pē) (see **therapy, radiation**)

Roger-Anderson pin fixation (see **appliance, fracture**)

Roger's syndrome (see **syndrome, Roger's**)

root A nerve root; the part of a nerve adjacent to the center with which it is connected; in spinal and cranial nerves, the part of the nerve betwen the cells of origin or termination and the ganglion. (Anesth.)

— The part of a human tooth covered by cementum. (Endodont.)

r. amputation (see **apicoectomy**)

r. canal instrument stop A device placed on a root canal instrument to mark the measured depth of instrument penetration. (Endodont.)

r. curettage (see **curettage, root**)

intra-alveolar r. The portion of a tooth root enclosed in and supported by alveolar bone. (Remov. Part. Prosth.)

r. resection (see **apicoectomy**)

retained r. A root, or part of a root, remaining in the soft tissue or in bone after a traumatic incident, extensive tooth decay, or incomplete extraction. (Oral Surg.)

r. rubber dam clamp (see **clamp, rubber dam, root**)

rosary, rachitic A beading of the ribs at the costochondral junction such as occurs in rickets. (Oral Med.)

Rosenthal's syndrome (see **hemophilia C**)

rotameter (rō-tăm′ĕ-ter) A flow-rate meter of variable area with a rotating float in a tapered tube; used for measuring the gas administered in anesthesia. (Anesth.)

rotary cutting instrument (see **instrument, cutting, rotary**)

rotating anode (see **anode, rotating**)

rotating condyle Either condyle as it rotates about a vertical and a sagittal axis when it is moved to aid and direct the chewing motions in biting off foods with the canines or in making a bolus. As soon as the chewing side is chosen, its condyle moves upward, backward, and usually outward to be braced. The other condyle is pulled forward, downward, and inward. The motions on the food side turn the bolus over and cock the jaw to bite the bolus in an upward and sagittal direction that becomes more vertical as the stamp cusps near their fossae in successive strokes. (Gnathol.)

rotating spring An auxiliary wire used in conjunction with arch wire to rotate a tooth into proper position. (Orthodont.)

rotation Movement of a tooth around its longitudinal axis. (Orthodont.)

— The turning of a rigid body about an axis in such a way that all points describe circles whose centers lie in the axis. (Gnathol.)

— The act of turning about an axis or a center. The mandible has a condylar axis for opening and closing the jaw. As each condyle "works," or turns, the rotation is about two axes—the vertical and the sagittal. In certain movements the mandible rotates about three axes simultaneously, which is possible when all three axes intersect at a common point. (Gnathol.)

r. center (see **center, rotation**)

Rothera's test (see **test, ketone bodies**)

round-wire appliance (see **appliance, light round-wire**)

routine A fixed pattern of procedures used in any phase of treatment. (Pract. Man.)

office r. A series of steps, to be followed in a carefully planned sequence, that provide a means of dealing with situations commonly developing in dental practice. (Pract. Man.)

rubber dam (see **dam, rubber**)

rubber dam clamp (see **clamp, rubber dam**)

rubber dam clamp holder An instrument used to place a clamp on a tooth or to adjust a clamp or remove it from a tooth. It engages the holes or notches of the flanges of the clamp. (Oper. Dent.)

rubber dam holder In endodontics, a rubber dam *frame* holder; in operative dentistry, a rubber dam *frame*. (Endodont.; Oper. Dent.)

rubella (**German measles, three-day measles**) A viral disease with eruptions resembling those seen in measles (rubeola). The lesions are less intense and usually disappear in one week. Oral lesions are red macules. (Oral Diag.)

— A highly contagious disease spread chiefly by direct contact and having an incubation period of about 18 days. Manifestations include pharyngitis, regional lymphadenopathy, mild constitutional symptoms, and a maculopapular rash that becomes scarlatiniform. (Oral Med.)

rubeola (see **measles**)

Ruffini's corpuscles (see **corpuscle, Ruffini's**)

rugae (ru′gī; rū′jē) The irregular ridges in the mucous membrane covering the anterior part of the hard palate. (Comp. Prosth.; Fixed Part. Prosth.; Remov. Part. Prosth.)

  r. area (see **area, rugae**)

rule, Cieszynski's, of isometry (sē-zin′skē) The geometric theorem that two triangles are congruent when they have two equal angles and a common side, as applied to the technique of bisecting an angle. (Oral Radiol.) (see also **technique, bisection of the angle**)

rule, Clark's A formula used estimating the dosage of a drug for individuals whose weight varies from the arbitrarily selected official standard of 150 pounds (Oral Med.; Pharmacol.):

$$\frac{\text{Weight of patient}}{150} \times \text{Usual adult dose} = \text{Dose}$$

— A rule for the orientation of structures portrayed in dual or multiple radiographs, first published by Clark, C. A.: Proc. Roy. Soc. Med., Odont. Sect. **3**:87-90, 1909-1910. (Oral Radiol.)

rule, Young's A mathematic expression used to determine dosage for children (Pedodont.; Pharmacol.):

$$\frac{\text{Age of child}}{\text{Age} + 12} \times \text{Adult dose} = \text{Child's dose}$$

Rumple-Leede test (see **test, capillary resistance**)

❦ S ❧

Sabouraud's medium (săb'oo-rōz) (see medium, Sabouraud's)

saddle (see base, denture)

  s. connector (see connector, major)

  metal s. (see base, metal)

safe-light A source of illumination in a darkroom of a color and intensity that will not fog a radiographic film. (Oral Radiol.)

sagittal (săj'ĭ-tăl) Shaped like or resembling an arrow; straight; situated in the direction of the sagittal suture. Said of an anteroposterior plane or section parallel to the long axis of the body. (Anesth.)

  s. plane (see plane, sagittal)

  s. splitting of mandible Intraoral osteotomy of the ascending ramus and posterior body of the mandible in the sagittal plane for the correction of prognathism, retrognathism, or apertognathia. An alternative procedure confines the split to the body of the mandible. (Oral Surg.)

St. Vitus' dance (sănt vī'tŭs) (see chorea)

Sainton's disease (săn'tōnz) (see dysostosis, cleidocranial)

salary A fixed regular compensation paid for service rendered involving professional knowledge or skill or emploment above the degree of mechanical labor. (D. Juris.)

— The amount of take-home pay received by the dentist from the practice. (Pract. Man.)

  s. arrangements The clear understanding between the dentist and his auxiliaries concerning the amount of money they will be paid, the increase in pay they may expect, and the time interval between pay increases. (Pract. Man.)

salicylism (săl'ĭ-sĭl''ĭzm) A toxic state resulting from excess ingestion of salicylates. (Oral Med.; Pharmacol.)

saline (sā'lĭn) Salty; of the nature of a salt; containing a salt or salts. (Anesth.)

saliva (sah-lī'vah) The clear, slightly acid mucoserous secretion formed in the parotid, submaxillary, sublingual, and smaller oral mucous glands. It has lubricative, cleansing, bactericidal, excretory, and digestive functions and is also an aid to deglutition. Its pH is slightly acid—6.3 to 6.9. Emotional disturbances affect the rate of salivary secretion either by stimulation of secretion or by inhibition of activity, leading to xerostomia. Lowered rate of flow has been noted in depressed patients, whereas a higher degree of salivary activity has been exhibited in manic patients. (Periodont.)

  lingual s. Saliva secreted by Ebner's glands and other serous glands of the tongue. (Oral Surg.)

  loss of CO_2 in s. A theory of calculus formation in which the loss of CO_2 from saliva reduces the salivary carbonic acid content and causes the calcium phosphate in solution in the saliva to become supersaturated; calcium phosphate then precipitates in areas of stasis of the saliva. (Periodont.)

  parotid s. Saliva produced by the parotid gland. It is thinner and less viscous than the other varieties, containing no mucin. (Oral Surg.)

  pH of s. Term referring to the slightly acid reaction of human saliva; pH is normally between 6.3 and 6.9. Saliva is probably buffered principally by carbonic acid and sodium bicarbonate systems, but it is thought that proteins and phosphate present in the saliva also play a role. (Periodont.)

  supersaturated s. Saliva overladen with mineral elements associated with calculus formation. With a loss of CO_2 and a rise in the pH of saliva, precipitation of calcium, phosphates, magnesium carbonate, etc. will occur, thus providing the mineral components of salivary calculus. (Periodont.)

salivant (săl'ĭ-vănt) Provoking a flow of saliva. (Anesth.)

salivary lactobacillus count Determination of the number of lactobacilli per milliliter of saliva; used as an indicator of caries susceptibility. High lactobacillus counts are indicative of high caries activity. (Oral Diag.)

salivation (săl''ĭ-vā'shŭn) Excessive discharge of saliva; ptyalism. (Anesth.)

salt A compound of a base and an acid; a compound of an acid, some of whose replaceable hydrogen atoms have been substituted. (Anesth.)

  basic s. A salt containing replaceable, or hydroxyl, groups. (Anesth.)

  s. depletion (see depletion, salt)

  mineral s. A mineral substance such as calcium phosphate or calcium carbonate that forms the inorganic portion of calcified tissues such as bone and teeth. (Periodont.)

Sandwith's bald tongue (see **tongue, bald, Sandwith's**)

SAR (see **relationship, structure-activity**)

sarcoidosis (sar″koi-dō′sĭs) (**Besnier-Boeck-Schaumann disease, Boeck's sarcoid**) A chronic granulomatous disease of unknown etiology. Causes noncaseating granulomas in the skin, lymph nodes, salivary glands, eyes, lungs, and bones. (Oral Path.)

sarcoma (sar-kō′mah) A malignant neoplasm of connective tissue elements. (Oral Diag.)
— A malignant neoplasm arising from mesenchyme or its derivatives. (Oral Path.)

   ameloblastic s. A rare mixed tumor of odontogenic origin in which the mesenchymal component has undergone malignant transformation. (Oral Path.)

   Ewing's s. (see **tumor, Ewing's**)

   Kaposi's s. A condition affecting blood vessels believed to be of a neoplastic nature and of multicentric origin. Skin lesions appear as multiple red-brown nodules ranging from a few millimeters to 1 cm in size. Histologically, endothelial proliferation in sheets or small vessels, hemosiderin deposits, fibroblastic proliferation, and an inflammatory infiltrate of lymphocytes are seen. (Oral Path.)

   neurogenic s. (**malignant schwannoma**) The malignant form of neurilemoma. (Oral Path.)

   osteoblastic s., osteogenic s. An osteosarcoma in which atypical bone formation is the most evident histopathologic feature. (Oral Path.) (see also **osteosarcoma**)

   osteogenic s. A malignant connective tissue tumor that produces bone. (Oral Diag.)

   reticulum cell s. A malignant neoplasm characterized by reticulum cells of the bone marrow, lymph nodes, or other hematopoietic regions. This is a lymphoma and may develop into monocytic leukemia. (Oral Diag.)
— A malignant tumor of reticulum cells. It may occur as a primary neoplasm in soft tissue or bone. (Oral Path.)

sarcophagization (sar-kahf′ah-jī-zā′shŭn) (Entombment of the pulp by a calcified bridge. (Endodont.)

satin finish (see **finish, satin**)

satisfaction Discharge of an obligation by actual payment of what is due or by legal presumption. (D. Juris.)

saturated Having all the chemical affinities satisfied; unable to hold in solution any more of a given substance. (Anesth.)

saturation, color The quality of color that distinguishes the degree of vividness of hue; e.g., differing in degree from gray. (Oper. Dent.)

saturnism (see **plumbism**)

saucerization Excavation of the tissue of a wound, forming a shallow, saucerlike depression. (Oral Surg.)

   pericervical s. The circular bone resorption that occurs about the necks of endosteal implants shortly after their insertion and that continues slowly during the time of the implant's biologic presence. (Oral Implant.)

saw A cutting blade with a toothed edge used to cut material too hard to slice with a knife; e.g., a plaster saw. (Oper. Dent.)

   Gigli's wire s. A flexible wire with teeth used for osteotomy procedures, frequently as a blind operation. (Oral Surg.)

   gold s. An instrument with a thin sawlike blade used for removing surplus metal from the contact area of gold-foil restorations. (Oper. Dent.)

   Joseph's s. A nasal saw often used in a ramusotomy of the mandible. (Oral Surg.)

   Koeber's s. A saw consisting of a thin, replaceable blade held in a frame; used to trim gross excess from the proximal portion of a Class 2 foil restoration in the preliminary stages of finishing and contouring. (Oper. Dent.)

   oscillating (Stryker-type) s. An oscillating blade in an electrical or compressed gas–driven unit, used to cut bone.

   rotary s. A rotary blade on a shaft in an electrical or compressed gas–driven unit, used to cut bone. (Oral Surg.)

SBE (see **endocarditis, subacute bacterial**)

scaffold A support, either natural or artificial, that maintains tissue contour. (M.F.P.)

scaler (skā′ler) An instrument used in the operation of removing calculus from teeth. (Periodont.)

   sickle s. A hook-shaped instrument available in various sizes and shapes, designed to be used for the removal of tenacious supragingival deposits of calculus. (Periodont.)

   wing s. A variation of the sickle scaler. Consists of a short, cudved blade with a flare at the very edge, thus presenting a wide blade similar to a hoe. Used for the removal of supragingival calculus. (Periodont.)

scaling The removal of calcareous deposits from

the teeth by utilizing suitable instruments. (Periodont.)

coronal s. The removal of deposits of calculus, heavy stains, materia alba, etc. from the crowns of the teeth by suitable instrumentation. (Periodont.)

electrosurgical s. (see **electrosurgery; scalpel, electrosurgical**)

epithelial attachment removal in s. Removal of the epithelial attachment during scaling; invariably occurs in the elimination of subgingival calculus when conventional hand instruments, such as scalers, curets, and hoes, are used. The proximity of subgingival calculus to the epithelial attachment, as evidenced by histologic preparations, precludes the elimination of the calculus without at least partial removal of the attachment. (Periodont.)

root s. A technique of root surface cleansing designed to remove accretions of calculus and debris in the supragingival uninvested areas of a tooth. (Periodont.)

sulcular and pocket epithelium in r. s. Removal of portions of sulcular epithelium during root scaling; may be necessary because of the size and shape of the instrument used. The use of ultrasonic techniques in the removal of calculus may cause some cauterization or coagulation of the sulcular epithelium. (Periodont.)

subgingival s. The removal of accretions and debris from the surfaces of the tooth apical to the gingival margin. This process accomplishes the removal of primary irritants to the gingival tissues and permits the reduction of inflammation in these tissues. (Periodont.)

supragingival s. The technique of meticulous cleansing of the surfaces of the teeth coronal to the gingival margin. (Periodont.)

scalpel A delicate, sharp, straight knife that may be sterilized. (Oral Surg.)

electrosurgical s. A scalpel that severs tissue by means of an electrically heated wire. (Oral Surg.)

s. for gingivectomy A scalpel with a blade that may be either broad or narrow. Broad-bladed, round knives are bent at an angle to permit cutting efficiency from the facial and lingual aspects of the area to be operated on. Narrow-bladed scalpels are bent to allow for interproximal incisions. The instruments are used to remove the detached gingival tissues and thus to eliminate soft tissue pockets. (Periodont.)

scar (see **cicatrix**)

apical s. (ā′pĭ-kal) The end product of wound repair. A radiolucent area characterized histologically by dense fibrous connective tissue. (Endodont.)

scarlatina (see **fever, scarlet**)

scarlet fever (see **fever, scarlet**)

scattered radiation (see **radiation, scattered**)

Schaumann's body (see **body, Schaumann's**)

Schaumann's disease (see **sarcoidosis**)

schedule The division of the working day into segments of time to enable the dentist to render treatment. (Pract. Man.)

schema, Hamberger's (skē′mah) The bodily arrangement by which the external intercostal and intercartilaginous muscles are inspiratory muscles, and the internal intercostal muscles are expiratory muscles. (Anesth.)

scheme, occlusal (see **system, occlusal**)

Schick test (shĭk) (see **test, Schick**)

schistometer (skĭs-tom′ĕ-ter) An instrument for measuring the aperture between the vocal cords. (Anesth.)

schistosomiasis (skĭs″tō-sō-mī′ah-sĭs) (**bilharziasis**) Infestation with blood flukes of the genus *Schistosoma*, causing cystitis, chronic dysentery, hepatosplenomegaly, and esophageal varices. (Oral Med.)

schizophrenia (skĭz″ō-frē′nē-ah) (**dementia precox**) A functional psychosis (split personality) characterized by emotional distortion, withdrawal from reality, and disturbances of thought processes. It includes such disorders as hebephrenia, catatonia, and paranoia. (Oral Med.)

— A psychic disorder or dementia characterized by disinterest in reality, hallucinations and delusions, autism, and a feebleness of emotional reactions. (Oral Physiol.)

Schüller-Christian disease (see **disease, Hand-Schüller-Christian**)

Schüller's disease (shĭl′erz) (see **osteoporosis**)

schwannoma (shwah-nō′mah) (see **neurilemoma**)
malignant s. (see **sarcoma, neurogenic**)

scillaren B (sĭl′ah-rĕn) A mixture of squill glycosides used experimentally in animals to induce a typical picture of necrotizing ulcerative gingivitis. (Periodont.)

scissors, Fox Delicate, fine-pointed scissors designed to gain access to interproximal areas for the removal of small tissue tabs or slight soft issue deformities during gingivoplasty and/or gingivectomy. Can also be used to smooth the cut gingival surfaces. (Periodont.)

scleroderma (sklĕ-rō-der′mah) (**dermatosclerosis, hidebound disease**) A diffuse collagen disease of unknown cause. Stiffening of the skin with fixed features and uniform thickening of the periodontal membrane are among the classic symptoms. (Oral Diag.)

— A dermatologic disease of unknown etiology characterized by fixation of the epidermis to the deeper subcutaneous structures due to thickening and hyalinization of the collagen fibers of the skin. (Oral Path.)

— A collagen disease of unknown etiology; skin lesions are characterized by thickening, rigidity, and pigmentation in patches or diffuse areas. Dermal atrophy may also be seen. Periodontal lesions may simulate those of periodontosis, with widening of periodontal membrane space (verified by radiographic evidence) due to bone resorption, loss of architectural arrangement, and degeneration of periodontal fibers, with absence of inflammatory change in the gingivae and remaining periodontium. (Periodont.)

sclerosis (sklĕ-rō'sĭs) Hardening. As applied to the jaws, sclerosis usually indicates an increased calcification centrally, with radiopacity. Tracts of increased density in the dentin are referred to as areas of dentinal sclerosis. Sclerosis occurs beneath caries, and with abrasion, attrition, or erosion. (Oral Diag.)

— Hardening, thickening, and/or increased density of a tissue due to hyperplasia of connective tissue; occurs in soft tissue as a result of increased deposition of calcium salts (in bone), etc. (Periodont.)

multiple s. A chronic paralytic disease characterized by spotty areas of degeneration in the central nervous system, with weakness, limb-jerking, etc. (Oral Diag.)

— A remitting and relapsing disease of the central nervous system affecting principally the white matter. Manifestations include sensory and motor incoordination and paresthesias; ultimately there is often dementia, blindness, paraplegia, and death. (Oral Med.)

—A chronic crippling condition in which the myelin surrounding the nerve pathways is destroyed and is replaced by scar tissue, preventing nerve impulses from passing from the brain to the muscles. (Pedodont.)

scoliosis (skō''lē-ō'sĭs) A lateral curvature of the spine. (Oral Diag.)

scorbutus (skor-bū'tŭs) (see **scurvy**)

scrap amalgam That portion of a mix of amalgam that is left after the prepared cavity is filled. (Oper. Dent.)

screen, intensifying A layer of fluorescent crystals

(usually calcium tungstate) supported on a flat base. Used in intimate contact with a light-sensitive radiographic film in a cassette. The crystals fluoresce when exposed to x radiation and subsequently expose the film with light. (Oral Radiol.)

screen, oral A Plexiglas or acrylic resin appliance that fits into the vestibule of the mouth for the correction of mouth breathing. (Pedodont.)

screwdriver (see **instrument, screwdriver**)

screw, expansion An orthodontic mechanism for achieving movement of teeth or arch segments, consisting of a threaded shaft and sleeve arrangement that permits controlled separation of elements of the appliance. (Orthodont.)

screw, implant A small screw 3 to 5 mm long that is used as a means for primary retention of the implant. (Oral Implant.)

scribe To write, trace, or mark by making a line or lines with a pointed instrument or carbon marker. (Comp. Prosth.; Remov. Part. Prosth.)

scrofula (skrof'ū-lah) A primary tuberculosis complex occurring in the orocervical region and consisting of tuberculous cervical lymphadenopathy and tuberculosis of adjacent skin (lupus vulgaris), with chronic draining sinuses below the angle of the jaw and cervical region. (Oral Med.)

scurvy (**scorbutus**) A condition resulting from an ascorbic acid deficiency that is severe enough to desaturate the tissues. The development and manifestations depend on tissue storage of ascorbic acid and factors that influence the rate at which it is utilized in or released from the tissues. Manifestations of frank scurvy include weakness, poor wound healing, anemia, and hemorrhage under the skin and mucous membranes. Presence or severity of gingival changes is directly related to the presence of local irritants such as calculus. In a severe form and in infantile scurvy, painful subperiosteal hemorrhages occur. (Oral Med.)

— A condition caused by deficiency of vitamin C and characterized by defects in bone formation, wound healing, and the integrity of blood vessels, with a resultant hemorrhagic diathesis. (Oral Path.)

— A deficiency disease caused by lack of an adequate amount of ascorbic acid in the diet; marked by weakness, anemia, gingivitis with marked hemorrhagic tendencies, petechial hemorrhages of the skin and mucous membranes, subperiosteal bleeding, etc. (Periodont.)

infantile s. (**Barlow's disease, Cheadle's disease, Moeller's disease**) A nutritional disease of infants caused by a deficiency of vitamin C in the diet. It has the same symptoms as scurvy in adults. (Oral Path.)

land s. (see **purpura, thrombocytopenic, idiopathic**)

seal A material, usually plastic, that hardens in the mouth; used to close the coronal opening in a tooth during endodontic treatment. (Endodont.)

border s. (see **border seal**)

double s. A seal consisting of gutta-percha underneath another material (e.g., temporary cement); used to close the coronal opening in a tooth during endodontic treatment. (Endodont.)

hermetic s. Perfect and absolute obliteration of all space within a tooth. (Endodont.)

peripheral s. (see **border seal**)

posterior palatal s. The seal at the posterior border of a denture produced by displacing some of the soft tissue covering the palate by extra pressure developed in the impression or by scraping a groove along the posterior seal area in the cast on which the denture is to be processed. (Comp. Prosth.; Remov. Part. Prosth.)

postpalatal s. (see **seal, posterior palatal**)

sealant, pit and fissure A resinous material designed for application to the occlusal surfaces of posterior teeth in order to seal the surface irregularities to prevent ingress of oral fluids, food, and debris. (D. Mat.)

sealer A substance used to fill the space around silver or gutta-percha points in a pulp canal. (Oral Med.; Pharmacol.)

seat, basal (see **basal seat**)

seat, rest (see **area, rest**)

secondary radiation (see **radiation, secondary**)

second surgical stage (**subperiosteal**) The operation that is performed to insert an implant. (Oral Implant.)

secretary-receptionist The auxiliary whose chief responsibilities are to receive patients into the office, handle the correspondence and bookkeeping, order supplies, supervise housekeeping, and answer the telephone. (Pract. Man.)

secretomotor (sē′krĕ-tŏm′ō-tor) (**secretomotory**) Exciting or stimulating secretion; said of nerves. (Anesth.)

secretomotory (see **secretomotor**)

sectional impression An impression made in two or more parts. (M.F.P.)

sectioning, surgical Dividing a tooth to facilitate its removal. A variety of instruments, including osteotomes and power-driven burs, are used. (Oral Surg.)

sedation (sē-dā′shŭn) The production of a sedative effect; the act or process of calming. (Anesth.)

— The production of a calm, imperturbable state. (Oral Med.; Pharmacol.)

sedative (sĕd′ah-tĭv) (**amnesic, hypnotic**) A remedy that allays excitement and slows down the basal metabolic rate without impairing the cerebral cortex. (Anesth.)

— Productive of sedation. A drug that can produce sedation. (Oral Med.; Pharmacol.)

— Any one of the drugs that produces cortical depression of varying degrees. Their use in the psychic preparation of a patient is a good basic practice of therapeutics in dentistry. Many patients who frequently overreact to situations and show extreme anxiety are made amenable to suggestion and cooperation through the use of one of the drugs of this group. (Oral Physiol.)

seeds, radon (see **radon seeds**)

segment Any of the parts into which a body naturally separates or is divided, either actually or by an imaginary line. (Comp. Prosth.; Remov. Part. Prosth.)

selection Choosing among alternatives.

shade s. (**tooth color s.**) The determination of the color (hue, brilliance, saturation, and translucency) of the artificial tooth or set of teeth for a given patient. (Comp. Prosth.; Remov. Part. Prosth.)

tooth s. The selection of a tooth or teeth (shape, size, and color) to harmonize with the individual characteristics of a patient. (Comp. Prosth.; Fixed Part. Prosth.; Remov. Part. Prosth.)

tooth color s. (see **selection, shade**)

selective grinding (see **grinding, selective**)

selectivity, sensory The property of the specialized receptor end-organ by which it responds to one type of stimulus rather than another. All sensory stimuli are produced by changes in energy—mechanical, electrical, or chemical. It may be assumed that there is a great selectivity of the receptor end-organ because the forms of energy themselves are frequently multiple and change from one form to another. Thus the essential characteristic of a specialized receptor is that its threshold is much lower for one type of energy than for any other; e.g., a stimulus produces first a chemical reaction followed by a temperature change or a change from a solid to a gaseous state and thus stimulates different end-organs. (Oral Physiol.)

self-analysis Introspection of one's own behavior and actions in his total environment. (Pract. Man.)

self-curing resin (see **resin, autopolymerizing**)

self-tapping implant An implant that cuts its own path into bone. (Oral Implant.)

self-tapping screw A screw that cuts its own spirals into bone. (Oral Implant.)

sell In the context of the practice of dentistry, to convince a patient that he needs something whether he does or not. (Pract. Man.)

sella turcica (sĕl′ah tŭr′sĭ-kah) The center of the pituitary fossa of the sphenoid bone. (Orthodont.)

    floor of s. t. Lowermost point on the internal contour of the sella turcica. (Orthodont.)

Selter's disease (see **erythredema polyneuropathy**)

semicoma A mild coma from which the patient may be aroused. (Anesth.)

seminarcosis (see **sleep, twilight**)

semipermeable (sĕm″ē-per′mē-ah-bl) Permitting the passage of certain molecules and hindering that of others. (Anesth.)

senescence, dental (sĕ-nĕs′ĕns) A condition of the teeth and associated structures in which there is deterioration due to aging or premature aging processes. (Comp. Prosth.; Remov. Part. Prosth.)

sensation(s) (sĕn-sā′shŭn) An impression conveyed by an afferent nerve to the sensorium commune. (Anesth.)

    psychologic effects of s. Arousal, facilitation, and distortion of sensation by psychologic factors, the basis for which lies in the corticalization of the special senses. Thus, in the case of conversion hysteria, the general reorganization of cortical brain function produces complete unawareness of distortion of the special sense activities of vision, hearing, smell, taste, and pain, despite the anatomic intactness of the special sense system. This phenomenon explains the behavior of the disturbed patient whose color or dimension appreciation of a tooth, form, or position is bizarre and unesthetic but which, nonetheless, the patient demands. The bizarre request reflects the patient's conceptualization of esthetic values. (Oral Physiol.)

    referred s. A group of vaguely classified sensations that are a consequence of cortical experience. They are the sensory hallucinations, the paresthesias, and the phenomenon called phantom limb. Sensation and its localization do not depend solely on the stimulation of the sensorium for evocation. Any action or experience that arouses the cortical projection area of the brain will give a response of sensation. Consequently, if a projection region in the brain is aroused mechanically by a tumor, chemically by vascular changes, or by arousal of the residual nerve stumps anywhere along the nerve trunk, the patient will experience a sensation that corresponds not to the source of pain but to the region from which the nerve originally projected. Nonspecific and poorly localized pain in the alveolar ridges, which have poor vascular supply, may be evidence of this phantom limb phenomenon associated with neurotic behavior. (Oral Physiol.)

specialized s. Sensations that are perceived by the specialized end-organs associated with special senses, such as vision, hearing, and smell. These specialized end-organs are localized in narrow, sharply delineated organs. Although the distribution of the end-organs is wide, each end-organ is itself a highly specialized structure. There are also generalized sensory experiences that are perceived by the skin and mucous membrane. The sensations that the skin and mucous membrane of the mouth can perceive are those of touch (light touch, tactile discrimination, tactile localization, pressure, tickling, and itching), temperature (warmth and cold), and pain. Each of these finely discriminating sensory phenomena has its own specialized end-organ, with the exception of the pain sense. (Oral Physiol.)

    dissociation of s. s. The loss of the phenomena of touch, temperature, and pain, separately and in a sequence depending on the nature of the environment. Cold, anesthesia, and ischemia can each cause the senses to be lost in different sequences and to return in reverse order. (Oral Physiol.)

sense(s) A faculty by which the conditions or properties of things are perceived. Hunger, thirst, malaise, and pain are varieties of sense. (Anesth.)

special s. and learning The interaction of the special senses to produce growth and development of the emotional and intellectual capacities of a person. Learning to read and write and to develop other learned skills are the heritage of man, but relearning is necessary in each individual's lifetime. Motor acts associated with the oral structures, such as head posture, speech, and mastication, are learned experiences. Motor acts associated with swallowing and with respiration are present as reflexes at birth but have learned experiences superimposed on them. It can then be considered that the special senses alter, modify, and develop the co-ordinated muscular acts associated with the oral structures. (Oral Physiol.)

corticalization of special s. The projection of the stimuli from the organs of the special senses to the cortical areas of the cerebrum. This direct stimulation of the occipital projection area of the cerebral cortex produces a sensation of light even in the absence of an activation of the retinal receptor organs. Similarly, stimulation of other areas of the cerebral cortex will appropriately produce sensations of hearing, smell, and taste. This phenomenon implies that sensations are the consequence of the arousal of cortical projection areas and that experience and learning are affected by cortical connections with the special senses to a very significant degree; hence, patients who view, smell, taste, hear, and otherwise relate to clinical problems may have their sensations so modified by psychic phenomena that there will be gross distortions in the final perception of stimuli. (Oral Physiol.)

sensibility, deep Perception of pressure, tension, and pain from the deeper structures as contrasted with sensations derived from the superficial layers of the skin. (Anesth.)

sensitive Able to receive or to transmit a sensation; capable of feeling or responding to a sensation. (Anesth.)

sensitivity, tooth The state of responsiveness of teeth to external influences such as heat, sugar, and trauma. May be due to occlusal traumatism, especially if the anatomic relation of the apical foramen to the traumatized tissue is such that the circulation of the pulp is disturbed. (Oper. Dent.; Periodont.)

sensitization The process of rendering a cell sensitive to the action of a complement by subjecting it to the action of a specific amboceptor; anaphylaxis. (Anesth.)

sensorium Any sensory nerve center; more frequently, the whole sensory apparatus of the body. (Anesth.)

sensory Pertaining to or subserving sensation. (Anesth.)

separating medium (see **medium, separating**)

separating spring Spring placed between adjacent teeth to obtain separation. (Orthodont.)

separating wire (see **wire, separating**)

separator An instrument used to wedge teeth apart, out of normal contact by immediate separation; useful in the examination of proximal surfaces of teeth and in finishing proximal restorations. Must be used with care, and usually it should be stabilized against the teeth with modeling compound to prevent tissue damage. (Oper. Dent.)

Ferrier's s. One of a set of balanced, double-bowed adjustable separators designed by W. I. Ferrier. (Oper. Dent.)

noninterfering s. (see **separator, True's**)

True's s. (noninterfering s.) A single-bowed separator designed to give greater access to the surface being operated on; designed by Harry A. True. (Oper. Dent.)

sepsis, oral (sĕp'sĭs) A disease condition occurring within the mouth and/or adjacent areas that may affect the health and integrity of adjacent parts and/or the general health through the dissemination of toxins. (Periodont.)

septal space (see **space, septal**)

septicemia (sĕp″tĭ-sē′mē-ah) A condition in which pathogenic bacteria and bacterial toxins circulate in the blood. Manifestations include high temperature, leukocytosis, malaise, rapid pulse, and subsequent diffuse systemic degenerative disturbances. (Oral Med.; Oral Path.)

septum, interdental (interdental alveolar septum) The portion of the alveolar process extending between the roots of adjacent teeth. (Periodont.)

septum, nasal The thin, vertical bony septum separating the right and left nasal cavities. (Periodont.)

sequence Order of occurrence or performance. (Oper. Dent.)

sequestrum (sē-kwĕs′trŭm) A piece of dead bone that has become separated from vital bone. (Oral Path.)

— A piece of dead bone. Usually signifies necrotic bone that is being expelled from the body. (Oral Surg.)

serotonin (sē″rō-tō′nĭn) (**thrombocytin, thrombotonin**) A local vasoconstrictor (5-hydroxytryptamine) and general hypotensive agent produced by the enterochromaffin cells of the gastrointestinal mucosa. It is absorbed by platelets from the site of tissue damage, where it aids hemostasis locally by vasoconstriction and systemically by reducing blood pressure. (Oral Med.)

serozyme (ser′ō-zīm) (see **factor VII**)

serum (sē′rŭm) The fluid component of the blood containing all stable constituents except fibrinogen. When blood is allowed to clot and stand, a clear yellowish fluid, which is serum, separates. (Oral Med.)

s. accelerator globulin (see **accelerator, prothrombin conversion, I**)

s. protein determination, electrophoretic Separation of serum protein fractions (albumin, alpha globulins, beta globulin, and gamma globulin) based on their different isoelectric points and thus their mobility in an electric field. Electrophoretic patterns and concentrations are of value in evaluating the hyperglobulinemias. Electrophoretic evaluation of serum protein abnormalities is usually related to moving-boundary or paper-strip separation patterns. (Oral Med.)

s. prothrombin conversion accelerator (SPCA) (see **factor VII; thromboplastin, extrinsic**)

s. sickness Anaphylactoid or allergic reaction after injection of foreign serum; marked by urticarial rashes, edema, adenitis, arthralgia, high fever, and prostration. (Oral Diag.)

servant One who is employed to perform personal services (other than those that would be rendered in an independent calling) for his employer and who, in that service, remains entirely under the control of the employer. (D. Juris.)

loaned s. A person, the use of whose services has been granted by his employer to another person. (D. Juris.)

service(s) Performance of labor for the benefit of another. (D. Juris.)

denture s. Diagnosis and treatment of edentulous and partially edentulous patients, including the diagnosis of existing and potential oral pathosis, the planning of treatment for the preparation of the mouth for complete or partial dentures, the fabrication and adjustment of the prostheses, and the continuing observation of the changes in the oral conditions as the prostheses are in use. (Comp. Prosth.)

— Procedures that are involved in the diagnosis of oral conditions as well as the construction and maintenance of dental prosthetic appliances. (Remov. Part. Prosth.)

gratuitous s. A service that does not involve

a return, compensation, or consideration. (D. Juris.)

health s. Those services, including dentistry, which improve the general physical and mental well-being of the patient. (Pract. Man.)

set Term applied to a state of a plastic material after it has hardened or jelled by chemical action, cooling, or saponification. It is used in connection with impression materials, waxes, and gypsum materials. (Comp. Prosth.)

set-off (see **offset**)

setting expansion (see **expansion, setting**)

setting time (see **time, setting**)

setup The arrangement of teeth on a trial denture base. (Comp. Prosth.; Remov. Part. Prosth.)

— A procedure involving dissection of teeth from a plaster model and repositioning of the teeth in desired positions to aid in case analysis preliminary to constructing an appliance. (Orthodont.) (see also **arrangement, tooth**)

sex Classification of an individual as a male or female on the basis of anatomic, functional, hormonal, and chromosomal characteristics. (Oral Med.)

anatomic s. Classification of sex based on sexual differentiation of the primary gonads. (Oral Med.)

chromosomal s. (genotype) Chromosomal characteristics involving normally 44 somatic and 2 sex chromosomes, the latter designated as XX for the normal female and XY for the normal male. The presence of the Y chromosome is associated with a male phenotype and its absence with a phenotypic female. (Oral Med.)

s. chromosomes Chromosomes responsible for sex classification—XX for female, XY for male. (Oral Med.)

functional s. (phenotype) Designation of sex based on the state of maturation and potential for use of the external genitalia. (Oral Med.)

hormonal s. Contributory assignment of sex on the basis of adequate levels of estrogen and androgen for the development of typical phenotypic secondary sex characteristics. (Oral Med.)

legal s. That sex assigned at birth or legally by a court of law. (Oral Med.)

s. linkage (see **linkage, sex**)

nuclear s. Sex determination based on the presence or absence of the hyperchromatic nucleolar satellite in squamous cells from a buccal mucosa smear or of "drumsticks" in the polymorphonuclear neutrophil. Positives are normally seen in the female. (Oral Med.)

sharpening, instrument Establishing or restoring of a keen edge on a cutting instrument. (Oper. Dent.)

Sharpey's fibers (see **fiber, Sharpey's**)

shear (see **strength, shear; strength, ultimate**)

shearing cusps The upper buccal cusps, the lower lingual cusps, the upper canines, and the upper incisors. Each of these cusps help form the fossae that receive the stamp cusps. In the postcanine teeth, the triangular ridges of the shearing cusps are bold in arming the fossae with cutting ridges. (Gnathol.)

sheath, nucleated (see **neurilemma**)

sheath, primitive (see **neurilemma**)

sheath of Schwann (see **neurilemma**)

shedding (see **exfoliation**)

shelf, buccal The surface of the mandible from the residual alveolar ridge or alveolar ridge to the external oblique line in the region of the lower buccal vestibule. It is covered with cortical bone. (Comp. Prosth.)

shelf life The length of time a material may be stored without deterioration. The length of time it remains usable. (D. Mat.)

shellac base (see **base, shellac**)

shield, radiation A body of material used to prevent or reduce the passage of particles of radiation. A shield may be designated according to what it is intended to absorb (e.g., a gamma ray or a neutron shield) or according to the kind of protection it is intended to give (e.g., a background, biologic, or thermal shield). The shield of a nuclear reactor is a body of material surrounding the reactor to limit the escape of neutrons and radiation into the protected area. Shields may be required to protect personnel or to reduce radiation sufficiently to allow use of counting instruments for research or for locating contamination or airborne radioactivity. (Oral Radiol.)

shift, axis (see **axis shift**)

shift, chloride (see **phenomenon, Hamburger's**)

shift to right or left An arbitrary description of an increase in the number per unit volume of immature (shift to left) or mature (shift to right) forms of neutrophils, in the differential counting system of Schilling. (Oral Med.)

shingles (see **herpes zoster**)

shock A state of collapse of the body after injury or trauma. Shock may be either primary or secondary. The principal effects of shock are the slowing of the peripheral blood flow and a reduction in cardiac output. (Oral Physiol.)

— Circulatory insufficiency caused by a disparity between the circulating blood volume and the vascular capacity. (Oral. Surg.)

galvanic s. Pain produced as a result of galvanic currents caused by similar or dissimilar metallic restorations. (D. Mat.)

hemorrhagic s. An ineffectual circulating volume of blood due to loss of whole blood. (Oral Surg.)

insulin s. Coma due to too much insulin or an inadequate intake of food. Symptoms include wet or moist skin, hypersalivation or drooling, normal blood pressure, tremors, dilated pupils, normal or bounding pulse, and firm eyeballs. Sugar and acetoacetic acid may be present in bladder urine but will be absent in second specimen. The blood sugar will be low. (Oral Med.) (see also **coma, diabetic**)

neurogenic s. Shock caused by loss of nervous control of peripheral vessels, resulting in an increase in the vascular capacity. Onset is usually sudden but is quickly reversible if the cause is removed and treatment is instituted immediately. (Oral Surg.)

primary s. Shock that has a neurogenic basis in which pain and psychic factors affect the vascular system. Occurs immediately after an injury. (Oral Physiol.)

— Shock that is similar or identical to neurogenic shock. Often referred to as shock occurring immediately on receipt of injury. (Oral Surg.)

secondary s. Shock that occurs several hours after a traumatic or surgical wound. Characterized by a profound fall in blood pressure, pallor, coldness of the skin, cyanosis of the fingertips, a fall in body temperature and metabolic rate, rapid shallow breathing, a weak rapid pulse, and finally, apathy. (Oral Physiol.)

— Shock that occurs some time after the injury (6 to 24 hours later). Secondary shock is associated with changes in capillary permeability and subsequent loss of plasma into the tissue spaces. Changes in capillary permeability are probably related to histamine release associated with tissue injury. (Oral Surg.)

traumatic s. Any shock produced by trauma, whether psychic or physical. In general usage, this term refers to shock following physical trauma, with hemorrhage, peripheral blood vessel dilation, and/or changes in capillary permeability. (Oral Surg.)

shoeing cusps (see **restoration of cusps**)

short-cone technique (see **technique, short-cone**)

shoulder In extracoronal cavity preparations, the ledge formed by the meeting of the gingival wall and the axial wall at a right angle. (Fixed Part. Prosth.; Oper. Dent.)

    linguogingival s. The portion of a prepared cavity in the proximal surface of an anterior tooth that is formed by the angular junction of the gingival and lingual walls. Developed to facilitate the dense compaction of the gold in this area. (Oper. Dent.)

shrinkage Reduction or decrease in extent or quantity. (Oper. Dent.)

— Reduction in volume. (Remov. Part. Prosth.)

    casting s. Volume change (contraction) that occurs when the molten metal solidifies after being cast into the pattern mold. It is compensated for in three ways: by using the indicated water:powder ratio for the refractory investment to gain the maximum setting expansion of which that investment is capable; by exposing the investment to moisture as the refractory investment sets, causing some hydroscopic expansion; and by properly heating the mold to achieve thermal expansion. The total expansion must equal the contraction of the metal being cast. (Remov. Part. Prosth.)

    gingival s. (see **gingiva, shrinkage**)

shunt, arteriovenous (**arteriovenous aneurysm, arteriovenous fistula**) Abnormal communication between an artery and a vein; usually caused by trauma. (Oral Surg.)

shut The part of an anterior artificial tooth between the ridge lap and the shoulder. The pins for retaining the tooth in the base material are located in the shut. (Comp. Prosth.)

sialadenitis (sī″ăl-ăd″ĕ-nī′tĭs) Inflammation of the salivary gland, especially the accessory glands, due to trauma. (Oral Diag.)

sialoadenectomy (sī″ah-lō-ăd″nĕk′tō-mē) Excision of a salivary gland. (Oral Surg.)

sialoangiectasis (sī″ah-lō-ăn″jē-ĕk′tah-sĭs) (**ptyalectasis**) Dilation of the salivary ducts. (Oral Diag.)

— Operative dilation of the salivary ducts. (Oral Surg.)

sialodochitis (sī″ah-lō-dō-kī′tĭs) Inflammation of salivary gland ducts. (Oral Path.)

sialodochoplasty (sī″ah-lō-dō′kō-plăs″tē) A surgical procedure for the repair of a defect and/or restoration of a portion of a salivary gland duct. (Oral Surg.)

sialogogue (sī-ăl′ō-gog) A substance that increases the flow of saliva. (Anesth.; Oral Surg.)

sialograph (sī-ăl′ō-grăf) A radiograph made to determine the presence or absence of calcareous deposits in a salivary gland or its ducts. (Oral Radiol.)

sialography (sī″ah-log′rah-fē) Inspection of the salivary ducts and glands by x-ray film after injection of a radiopaque medium. (Oral Diag.)

— Production of a sialograph. (Oral Radiol.)

— Radiographic demonstration of the salivary ducts after injection of a radiopaque substance. (Oral Surg.)

sialolith (sī-ăl′ō-lĭth) A salivary calculus. (Oral Surg.) (see also **calculus, dental**)

sialolithiasis (sī″ah-lō-lĭ-thī′ah-sĭs) Presence of salivary gland or duct stones. (Oral Diag.)

— Formation of salivary calculi or the condition or infection caused by it. (Oral Path.)

sialolithotomy (sī″ah-lō-lĭ-thot′ō-mē) Removal of calculus from a salivary gland or duct. (Oral Surg.)

sialorrhea (sī″ah-lō-rē′ah) (**hypersalivation, ptyalism**) Excessive flow of saliva. It may be associated with acute inflammation of the mouth, mental retardation, neurologic disorders with lenticular involvement, mercurialism, pregnancy, ill-fitting dental appliances, dysautonomia, periodic diseases, cystic fibrosis of the pancreas, teething, alcoholism, and malnutrition. (Oral Diag.; Oral Med.)

    periodic s. Recurrent episodes of hypersalivation; of unknown cause but probably related to recurrent parotitis and other so-called periodic diseases. (Oral Med.)

sialoschesis (sī″ah-los′kĕ-sĭs) Suppression of salivary secretion (dry mouth). Usually this condition contraindicates the wearing of a dental prosthesis during sleep. (Oral Surg.; Remov. Part. Prosth.)

sialosemeiology (sī″ah-lō-sē″mī-ol′ō-jē) Analysis of the salivary secretion. The quantity and composition of saliva may be determined, although this procedure has not been used to any degree in oral diagnosis. (Oral Diag.)

sib (sĭb) Abbreviated form for sibling, meaning brother or sister. (Oral Med.)

sibilant (sĭb′ĭ-lănt) Accompanied by a hissing sound; especially a type of fricative speech sound. (Cleft Palate)

sickle (sĭk′l) (see **scaler, sickle**)

sicklemia (sĭk-lē′mē-ah) (see **anemia, sickle cell**)

side effect An effect not sought in the case under treatment. (Oral Med.; Pharmacol.)

sideropenic dysphagia (sĭd″er-ō-pe′nĭk dĭs-fā′jē-ah) (see **syndrome, Plummer-Vinson**)

side-shift Imprecise Anglo-Saxon–based term for

lateral thrust of the rotating condyle. The Latin-based term for side-shift is laterotrusion. (Gnathol.)

sigh (sī) An audible and prolonged inspiration, followed by a shortened expiration. (Anesth.)

sigmoid notch (sĭg'moid) (see **notch, mandibular**)

sign(s) (sīn) An indication of the existence of something; any objective evidence of a disease. (Anesth.)

Battle's s. The ecchymosis that appears near the mastoid process of the temporal bone; indicative of a fracture of the base of the skull. (Oral Surg.)

Bell's s. The turning up of the eyeball on the affected side when a patient with Bell's palsy attempts to close the eyelid. (Oral Diag.)

Hoover's s. A modification in the movement of the costal margins during respiration, caused by a flattening of the diaphragm; it is suggestive of empyema or other intrathoracic conditions causing a change in the contour of the diaphragm. (Anesth.)

Jackson's s. Greater movement of the paralyzed side of the chest than of the opposite side during quiet respiration, and less movement of the paralyzed side than of the other during forced respiration. (Anesth.)

Nikolsky's s. A diagnostic feature wherein apparently normal epithelium can be rubbed off with finger pressure. (Oral Path.)

s. and symptoms, diagnostic The objective and subjective features of disease that are carefully evaluated in order to establish a diagnosis. In periodontal disease, noteworthy features include changes in gingival color, form, position, and surface appearance; bleeding; pocket formation; presence of exudate; mobility; migration; occlusal alterations; radiographic changes in the alveolar process; and patient's symptoms (e.g., pain sensitivity and senses of taste and smell). (Periodont.)

Tinel's s. A paresthesia in the area served by a sensory nerve when the site of a lesion or injury to the nerve is percussed. Indicative of partial injury of a nerve or regeneration of an injured nerve. (Oral Surg.)

signa (sĭg'nah) (**signature**) The portion of a prescription that contains a statement of the directions for use. (Oral Med.; Pharmacol.)

signature (see **signa**)

silica (sĭl'ĭ-kah) (**quartz**) The purest of three major ingredients that make up dental porcelain. It imparts stiffness and hardness to the product and is the framework around which the kaolin and feldspar contract. (Fixed Part. Prosth.)

silicate cement (sĭl'ĭ-kāt) (see **cement, silicate**)

silicone (sĭl'ĭ-kōn) A compound of organic structural character in which all or some of the positions that could be occupied by carbon atoms are occupied by silicon. A plastic containing silicons. (Oral Med.; Pharmacol.)

silver amalgam (see **amalgam, silver**)

silver halide crystals (see **crystal, silver halide**)

silver nitrate, ammoniacal (ăm″ō-nī'ah-kal) (**ammoniated silver nitrate, Howe's silver nitrate**) An ammonium compound of silver nitrate, introduced by Percy R. Howe in 1917, that is more readily reduced to silver and silver proteinates than the usual silver nitrate; *formerly* used to disclose carious tooth structure and to immunize incipient carious lesions of the enamel. (Oper. Dent.)

silver nitrate, application The use of silver nitrate to reduce sensitiveness of areas on posterior teeth. Also, it is thought to be beneficial in deterring the development of dental caries in an area of enamel demineralization. (Remov. Part. Prosth.)

silver nitrate, Howe's (see **silver nitrate, ammoniacal**)

Simmonds' disease (see **disease, Simmonds'**)

sine curve The wave form of an alternating current characterized by a rise from zero to maximum positive potential, a descent back through zero to its maximum negative value, and then a rise back to zero. (Oral Radiol.)

single emulsion (**film**) (see **emulsion, single**)

sinus (sī'nŭs) A cavity, recess, or hollow space.

alveolar s. A passage connecting a pathologic cavity in the alveolus with the oral or nasal cavity and penetrating the mucous membrane. (Endodont.) (see. also **fistula, alveolar**)

s. balloon (see **balloon, sinus**)

carotid s. The dilated portion of the internal carotid artery. (Anesth.)

coronary s. The venous sinus in the groove between the left cardiac auricle and the left ventricle. (Anesth.)

maxillary s. (antrum of Highmore, maxillary antrum) The bony cavity in the body of the maxilla; it is superior to the alveolar process, lateral to the nasal cavity, and communicates with the middle meatus of the nose. (Oral Surg.)

— A large pyramidal cavity within the body of the maxilla. Its walls are thin and correspond to the orbital, nasal anterior, and infratemporal surfaces of the body of the maxilla. On dental radiographs, the floor of the sinus is often observed approximating the root apices of the teeth and is seen to extend from the cuspid or bicuspid region posteriorly to the molar or tuberosity region. (Periodont.)

paranasal s. Accessory sinuses of the nose. (Oral Surg.)

s. tract (see **tract, sinus**)

sinusitis Inflammation of the sinus. (Oral Diag.)

Siwe's disease (sē'vehz) (see **disease, Letterer-Siwe**)

Sjögren's syndrome (syĕh'grĕnz) (see **syndrome, Sjögren's**)

skeleton of partial denture (see **framework**)

skill Practical knowledge of an art, science, profession, or trade and the ability to apply it in practice in a proper manner. (D. Juris.)

— Technical ability of the dentist in performing professional services. (Pract. Man.)

reasonable s. That which is ordinarily possessed and exercised by persons of similar capacity engaged in the same employment or profession. (D. Juris.)

slander Oral defamation; the saying of false and malicious words about another, resulting in injury to the reputation of the other. (D. Juris.)

slant of occlusal plane The inclination measured by the angle it makes when extended to intersect with the axis-orbital plane. (Gnathol.)

sleep A period of rest for the body and mind, during which volition and consciousness are in partial or complete abeyance and the bodily functions partially suspended. (Anesth.)

twilight s. (seminarcosis) A state of amnesia and analgesia produced by an injection of scopolamine and morphine. (Anesth.)

slice In cavity preparation, a straight-line (plane) cut that removes a thin layer from an axial convexity. (Oper. Dent.)

slides Term that usually refers to the 2 × 2 inch transparencies from 35 mm film, used to help the patient visualize the esthetic effect of proposed treatment. (Pract. Man.)

slope, lower ridge The slope of the mandibular residual ridge in the second and third molar region as seen from the buccal side. (Comp. Prosth.)

— Any slope of the mandibular residual ridge as viewed from the buccal side. (Remov. Part. Prosth.)

slotted attachment (see **attachment, intracoronal**)

Sluder's neuralgia (see **neuralgia, Sluder's**)

smallpox (see **variola**)

smear, bacterial Bacteria taken from a lesion or area, spread on a slide, and stained for microscopic examination. (Oral Diag.)

sneeze An involuntary, sudden, violent expulsion of air through the mouth and nose; may be elicited during thiopental (Pentothal) anesthesia by corneal stimulation. (Anesth.)

Snyder's test (see **test, colorimetric caries susceptibility**)

soap A salt or mixture of salts, of aliphatic acids, such as palmitic, stearic, or oleic acid, with sodium or potassium used for cleaning purposes. (Oral Med.; Pharmacol.)

sob A short, convulsive inspiration, attended by contraction of the diaphragm and spasmodic closure of the glottis. (Anesth.)

socket An alveolus of the alveolar process in which the roots of a tooth are encased. It is lined by thin compact bone that is pierced by small openings through which blood vessels, lymphatics, and nerve fibers pass. (Periodont.)

dry s. (alveolalgia, infected s., localized alveolar osteitis) An osteitis or periostitis associated with infection and disintegration of the clot after tooth extraction. Because of its painful nature, it also is called alveolalgia. (Oral Diag.)

— The clinical appearance of a postextraction socket formed by necrotic bone and devoid of an organized clot. (Oral Path.)

— An infected socket. A tooth socket or alveolus in which clot formation has been interfered with and the bone is exposed to oral fluids. (Oral Surg.)

infected s. (see **socket, dry**)

sodium aluminum fluoride (see **cryolite**)

sodium fluoride (sō'dē-ŭm flor'īd) (NaF) A white, odorless powder used in 2% aqueous solution and applied topically to teeth as a caries-preventing agent; used as 33% NaF in kaolin and glycerin as a desensitizing agent for hypersensitive dentin. In drinking water, 1 part per million of NaF is used as a caries-prophylactic substance. (Periodont.)

sodium perborate (sō'dē-ŭm per-bor'āt) ($NaBO_2 \cdot H_2O_2 \cdot 3H_2O$) An oxygen-liberating antiseptic that has been used in the treatment of necrotizing ulcerative gingivitis and other forms of gingival inflammation. Prolonged and/or indiscriminate use has produced burns of the oral mucosa and hyperplasia of the filiform papillae of the tongue (black hairy tongue). (Periodont.)

sodium thiosulfate (sō'dē-ŭm thī"ō-sŭl'fāt) A powdered chemical, commonly called hypo, that is an ingredient of the fixing solution used in film processing. Its action is to clear the film of undeveloped silver halide crystals. (Oral Radiol.)

soft radiation (see **radiation, soft**)

soft tissue undercut (see **undercut, soft tissue**)

solarization (sō″lar-ĭ-zā′shŭn) A method of making an exact duplicate of a radiograph by exposing the original, with an unexposed film under it, to sunlight. Processing in light will first cause a reversal of the image to occur, but finally the same lights and shadows as those of the original film will be produced. This process may also be accomplished artificially by using the light from a radiographic view box, in which case the unexposed film is superimposed on the one to be duplicated. (Oral Radiol.)

solder, *n.* (sod′er) A fusible alloy of metals used to unite the edges or surfaces of two pieces of metal. (Comp. Prosth.; Orthodont.; Remov. Part. Prosth.)
— A relatively low-fusing alloy used to join metal parts. (D. Mat.)
—, *v.* To unite two pieces of metal by the proper alloy of the metals. (Comp. Prosth.; Orthodont.; Remov. Part. Prosth.)
— To join metals by use of an alloy of lower melting range than the metals being joined. (D. Mat.)

soldering flux (see **flux, soldering**)

soldering investment (see **investment, soldering; investment, refractory**)

solicitation The attempt to entice patients to obtain dental care by means not in keeping with the spirit of the Code of Ethics of the American Dental Association. (Pract. Man.)

solubility The quality or fact of being soluble; susceptible to being dissolved. (Anesth.)

solute The dissolved (usually the less abundant) constituent of a solution. (D. Mat.)

solution The process of dissolving. Also, a liquid consisting of a mixture of two or more substances that are molecularly dispersed through one another in a homogeneous manner; a loosening or separation. (Anesth.)
— A homogeneous mixture of different molecules, atoms, or ions whose composition may be varied within limits. (D. Mat.)
— In chemistry, a homogeneous dispersion of two or more compounds. In pharmacy, usually a nonalcoholic solution. Solutions containing alcohol are variously called elixirs, tinctures, spirits, essences, or hydroalcoholic solutions. (Oral Med.; Pharmacol.)

Carnoy's s. A sclerosing solution; mild; will not

cauterize normal oral mucosa if used judiciously. A mild hemostatic. (Oral Surg.)

chloramine s. A cleansing and irrigating solution used in pulp and root canal therapy and consisting of chloramine-T, 4 g; NaCl, 9 mg; and distilled H_2O, 100 ml. (Endodont.)

cleansing s. A solution especially suited to the removal of adherent food particles by immersion of the denture to avoid damaging the denture by brushing. (Remov. Part. Prosth.)

disclosing s. A topically applied substance used in aqueous solution to stain and reveal, to both the operator and the patient, the extent of calcareous and mucinous deposition on the teeth. An excellent disclosing solution is 4 minims of 1.9% basic fuchsin in 2 ounces of H_2O, as a rinse, although some question as to its carcinogenic properties has been raised. (Periodont.)

hardening s. An aqueous solution (often of 2% potassium sulfate) in which a hydrocolloid imperssion may be immersed to reduce or retard syneresis of the impression material. (Remov. Part. Prosth.)

parenteral s. A sterile solution or substance prepared for injection. (Anesth.)

pickling s. A solution of acid used for removing oxides and other impurities from dental castings; e.g., solutions of hydrochloric acid or sulfuric acid. (Comp. Prosth.; Oper. Dent.)

sclerosing s. An agent that will cause an intense inflammation, resulting in a fibrosis; used to treat subluxation of the temporomandibular joint, cauterize ulcers, arrest hemorrhage, treat hemangiomas, etc. (Oral Surg.)

solid s. An alloy all of whose constituents are mutually soluble in the solid state. (D. Mat.)

solvent The dissolving (usually the more abundant) constituent of a solution. (D. Mat.)
— A compound used for the removal of calculus from a removable partial denture; e.g., a dilute solution of acetic acid, or vinegar. (Remov. Part. Prosth.)

somatalgia (sō″mah-tăl′jē-ah) Bodily pain. (Anesth.)

somatic (sō-măt′ĭk) Pertaining to the body; especially pertaining to the framework of the body, as distinguished from viscera. (Anesth.)
— Derived from *soma,* meaning the body, as distinguished from the mind. The adjective pertains to the framework of the body, as distinguished from the viscera; hence the term

somatic nerves describes the nerves associated with the musculoskeletal function of the muscles of the body. (Oral Physiol.)

somatoprosthetics (sō″-mah-tō-prŏs-thĕt′ĭks) The art and science of prosthetically replacing external parts of the body that are missing or deformed. (M.F.P.)

somatotropin (sō″mah-tō-trō′pĭn) (see **hormone, growth**)

somnambulism Habitual walking in the sleep; a hypnotic state in which the subject has the full possession of his senses but no subsequent recollection. (Anesth.)

somnifacient (som″nĭ-fā′shĕnt) Causing sleep; hypnotic; a medicine that induces sleep. (Anesth.)

somniferous (som-nĭf′er-ŭs) Inducing or causing sleep. (Anesth.)

somnolence (som′nō-lĕns) Sleepiness; also unnatural drowsiness. (Anesth.)

somnolism A state of mesmeric or hypnotic trance. (Anesth.)

sonagram (sō′nah-grăm) The readily usable graph of the frequency bands (formants) produced by the sound spectrograph. (Cleft Palate)

sonagraph (sō′nah-grăf) A wave analyzer that produces a permanent visual record showing the distribution of energy in both frequency and time. (Cleft Palate)

sonant (sō′nănt) A speech sound that has in it a component of tone generated by laryngeal vibrations; e.g., "a-a-a" and "z-z-z." (Oral Physiol.)

soporific (sop′ō-rĭf′ĭk) A sleep-producing drug. (Anesth.)

sore, canker (aphthous ulcer, aphthous stomatitis) A shallow ulcer of the oral mucosa; characterized by a grayish-yellow base and erythematous halo; the result of local minor trauma or the rupture of vesicles produced by the herpes simplex virus. (Oral Med.)
—A vesicular lesion that rapidly ulcerates; often encountered on the oral mucous membrane. Generally singular, occasionally multiple; surrounded by a zone of erythema. Basic etiology unknown, but often precipitated by gastrointestinal disturbances, localized oral trauma, etc. (Periodont.)

sore, cold (see **sore, canker; herpes labialis**)

sore, denture (see **ulcer, decubitus**)

Sorrin's operation (see **operation, Sorrin's**)

source-collimator distance Distance from the focal spot to the diaphragm or collimator in an x-ray tube head. (Oral Radiol.)

source-film distance (SFD) Distance from the focal spot of an x-ray tube to the radiographic film. Also referred to as TFD (target-film distance). (Oral Radiol.)

source-object distance (SOD) Distance from focal spot to object of which a radiographic image is to be obtained. Also referred to as TOD (target-object distance). (Oral Radiol.)

space (spās) A delimited, three-dimensional region.

s. of Donders Space that lies above the dorsum of the tongue and below the hard and soft palates when the mandible is in the respiratory rest position. It can thus be considered the lumen of the digestive tract. When swallowing is to be effected, the lumen is obliterated and the bolus is passed backward. After the swallowing act is completed, the mandible and the tongue return to the respiratory rest position, which is the position of the mandible and its associated soft structures at the completion of the expiratory phase of the respiratory cycle. (Oral Physiol.)

free-way s. The interocclusal distance or separation between the occlusal surfaces of the teeth when the mandible is in its physiologic rest position. Interocclusal distance is the preferred term. (Periodont.) (see also **distance, interocclusal; clearance, interocclusal**)
—— The interocclusal space between mandibular and maxillary teeth when the mandible is in the physiologic rest position. (Periodont.)

interalveolar s. (see **distance, interarch**)

interocclusal rest s. (see **distance, interocclusal**)

interproximal s. The space between adjacent teeth in a dental arch. It is divided into the embrasure (occlusal to the contact point) and the septal space (gingival to the contact point). (Comp. Prosth.; Remov. Part. Prosth.) (see also **space, septal**)
—— The somewhat triangular-shaped space between approximating teeth; normally filled with gingival tissue (gingival papilla). (Oper. Dent.)

interradicular s. The area between the roots of a multirooted tooth; it is occupied by bony septum and the periodontal membrane. (Periodont.)

s. lattice (see **lattice, space**)

s. maintainer A fixed or removable appliance designed to preserve the space created by the premature loss of a tooth. (Oper. Dent.)

— An appliance that maintains a space. Also, an appliance that creates space by means of moving teeth apart while holding that space secured. (Orthodont.)

cast s. m. A space maintainer with one or two abutments for maintaining space for premolars and for guiding first permanent molars into their proper places in the dental arch. (Pedodont.)

orthodontic s. m. A removable or fixed appliance fabricated to maintain space in the arch for erupting permanent teeth. The appliance may be designed to regain space needed to accommodate the erupting tooth or teeth. (Periodont.)

removable s. m. A removable appliance, with or without artificial teeth, that is used for the maintenance of space when groups of primary teeth or permanent teeth are lost prematurely. (Pedodont.)

marrow s. Spaces in the spongiosa of bone; in the mandible and maxilla, the marrow spaces are occupied by fatty and/or hematogenic (red) marrow. When inflammation progresses into the marrow in these spaces, a change is noted in which the marrow becomes fibrous. The spaces enlarge in atrophy of disuse because of resorption of surrounding trabeculae, and the marrow remains fatty in nature. (Periodont.)

modification s. Term used to indicate an edentulous space additional to the area or areas that determine the primary classification of the partially edentulous condition. (Remov. Part. Prosth.)

s. obtainer An appliance used to increase the space between two teeth. (Orthodont.)

occupied s. The space that might be occupied by persons or radiation-sensitive materials and devices during the time that x-ray equipment is in operation or radiation is being emitted. (Oral Radiol.)

physiologic dead s. The air passages up to, but not including, the alveoli of the lungs; equal to about 150 cc. (Anesth.)

s. regainer A fixed or removable appliance capable of moving a displaced permanent tooth into its proper position in the dental arch. (Periodont.)

relief s. A slight elevation of a lingual bar type of major connector to allow for a minor degree of settling of a removable partial denture without impinging on the structures over which the bar passes. (Remov. Part. Prosth.)

retromylohyoid s. (rĕt″rō-mī″lō-hī′oid) The part of the alveololingual sulcus distal to the lingual tuberosity (the distal end of the mylohyoid ridge). (Comp. Prosth.)

septal s. The space, below the contact areas, between two approximating teeth in the same arch. (Remov. Part. Prosth.)

spasm (spăzm) A sudden involuntary contraction of a muscle or muscle group. It may cause a twitch or close a canal or passage, depending on its location. (Anesth.; Oral Diag.)

muscle s. Increased muscular tension and shortness that cannot be released voluntarily and that prevent lengthening of the muscles involved. Caused by pain stimuli to the lower motor neuron. (Comp. Prosth.; Remov. Part. Prosth.)

spasmolysant (spăz-mol′ĭ-zănt) Relieving or relaxing spasms; any agent that relieves spasm. (Anesth.)

spasmolytic (spăz″mō-lĭt′ĭk) Pertaining to a drug that reduces spasm in smooth or skeletal muscle. (Anesth.)

spastic (spăs′tĭk) Characterized by a more or less constant state of hypertonic contraction of a muscle or group of muscles. The condition is regarded as an abnormally heightened muscular tonus present even in states of inactivity. (Oral Physiol.)

spatula A flat-bladed instrument without sharp edges used for mixing certain dental materials, e.g., cement, plaster of paris, and impression pastes.

spatulate (spăt′ū-lāt) To manipulate or mix with a spatula. (Comp. Prosth.; Fixed Part. Prosth.; Remov. Part. Prosth.)

spatulation (spăt″ū-lā′shŭn) Manipulation of material with a spatula in order to mix it into a homogeneous mass. (Comp. Prosth.; Fixed Part. Prosth.; Oper. Dent.; Remov. Part. Prosth.)

spatulator (mechanical spatulator) A mechanical device that mixes ingredients to form a homogeneous mass. (Oper. Dent.)

mechanical s. (see **spatulator**)

SPCA Abbreviation for serum prothrombin conversion accelerator. (see **factor VII; thromboplastin, extrinsic**)

specialization The limiting of professional services to one isolated and distinct phase of dental practice. (Pract. Man.)

specific gravity (see **gravity, specific**)

spectrograph, sound (see **sonagraph**)

spectrum, antibacterial The range of antimicrobial activity of a drug. (Oral Med.; Pharmacol.)

spectrum, electromagnetic A family of radiant energies that travel in wave form, have neither mass nor charge, and travel at the speed of light. Radiations within the spectrum vary only in wavelength. X-ray photons and light rays are examples of electromagnetic radiation. (Oral Radiol.)

Spee, curve of (see **curve of Spee**)

speech Communication through conventional vocal and oral symbols. (Cleft Palate)

— A basic biologic function of the maxillofacial structures. The essential characteristic of the speech function is the production and organization of sound into symbols. The production of these sound symbols is a phenomenon of several highly integrated factors that are grouped into several components: respiration, phonation, resonance, articulation, and neurologic integration. The normal development of speech requires the normal growth and development of the maxillofacial structures and the pertinent neurologic apparatus. Conversely, lack of development or impairment or loss of the speech function is a symptom of a pathologic process. Thus any anomaly or pathology of the maxillofacial structures is generally reflected by evidence of some speech dysfunction. (Oral Physiol.)

s. aid (see **aid, speech**)

s. articulation (see **articulation, speech**)

delayed s. Failure of speech to develop at the expected age, usually due to slow maturation, hearing impairment, brain injury, mental retardation, or emotional disturbance. (Cleft Palate)

s. device A prosthesis that assists in the management of speech disorders associated with a congenital or acquired defect of the palate. (M.F.P.)

infantile s. A speech defect characterized by substitution of speech sounds similar to those used by the child who speaks normally in the early stages of speech development. (Cleft Palate)

s. phonation (see **phonation, speech**)

s. resonance (see **resonance, speech**)

retarded s. Slowness in speech development in which intelligibility is severely impaired; often preceded by late or delayed emergence of speech. (Cleft Palate)

visible s. Audible speech patterns that have been transformed by electronic apparatus into visual patterns that may be read by the deaf. (Cleft Palate)

speed Relative rapidity of motion; rate of motion. (Oper. Dent.)

film s. (see **film speed**)

high s. Relatively great rapidity of motion. In cavity preparations, rotary instruments are classified according to the number of revolutions per minute made by the cutting tool. Designation of each speed range presently varies with the author. In general, conventional speed is 10,000 to 60,000 rpm, high speed is 60,000 to 100,000 rpm, and ultrahigh speed is over 100,000 rpm. (Oper. Dent.)

s. of light A speed of 186,300 miles/sec. (Oral Radiol.)

s. of radiation (see **radiation, speed of**)

sphenoid bone (sfē′noid) (see **bone, sphenoid**)

spherocytosis, hereditary (sfēr″ō-sī-tō′sĭs) (see **jaundice, congenital hemolytic**)

spheroiding (sfē′roid-ĭng) Assuming the form of a sphere, globe, or ball. (Oper. Dent.) (see also **amalgam, spheroiding of**)

spicule, cemental (spĭk′ūl) (**cemental spike**) Calcification of a periodontal fiber adjacent to and continuous with the cemental covering of the root; a projection of cementum extending from the root surface into the periodontal membrane (usually along the path of the principal fibers). It represents calcification of the cemental fibers of the periodontal ligament and may not be true cementum. Hyperfunction is the etiologic agent for such spicules. (Periodont.)

spike, cemental (see **spicule, cemental**)

spillway A channel or passageway through which food escapes from the occlusal surfaces of the teeth during mastication. The occlusal, developmental, and supplemental grooves, as well as the incisal, occlusal, labial, buccal, and lingual embrasures, become spillways during function. (Oper. Dent.)

axial s. A groove that first crosses a cusp ridge or a marginal ridge and extends onto an axial (mesial or distal) surface of the tooth, just lingual to the contact area. It thus contributues to the self-cleansing ability of the tooth and to the stimulation of the investing tissues. In carving a restoration, an axial spillway should never extend into the contact area. (Oper. Dent.)

interdental s. A sluiceway formed by the interproximal contours of adjoining teeth. The spillways begin at the contact points and widen out toward buccal and lingual surfaces. The base of a spillway is formed by the interdental papilla with its vertical, linear depression (interdental grove). The architectural pattern of tooth contact, interproximal tooth contour, and shape of the interdental papilla assists in and permits the unimpeded flow of food away from the occlusal surfaces, over the gingival tissues, and toward the vestibular area. Spillways may also be present in the interproximal gingival tissues (the interdental grooves) or may be artificially created during therapy. (Periodont.)

occlusal s. A groove that crosses only a cusp ridge or a marginal ridge of the tooth; numerous on marginal ridges, thus increasing masticatory function. (Oper. Dent.)

spindle, muscle A fusiform body lying parallel to and between muscle fibers. It is composed of a conspicuously smaller modified muscle fiber that has its own motor end-plate to cause it to contract and its own special sensory end-organs (the flower spray ending and the anulospiral ending) that send information to the central nervous system regarding the state of contraction of the main muscle body. (Oral Physiol.)

spine, anterior nasal The small bony projection extending forward from the medial anterosuperior part of each maxilla. The tip of the anterior nasal spines may be seen on lateral radiographic head plates or cephalometric radiographs. (Orthodont.)

spine, posterior nasal The small, sharp, bony point projecting backward from the midline of the horizontal part of the palatine bone. (Orthodont.)

spinning, marginal (see **marginal spinning**)

spirit Any volatile or distilled liquid; also, a solution of a volatile material in alcohol. (Anesth.)

— A solution of a volatile drug or flavoring agent in alcohol. (Oral Med.; Pharmacol.)

spirograph (spī′rō-grăf) An instrument for registering the respiratory movements. (Anesth.)

spirography (spī-rŏg′rah-fē) The graphic measurement of breathing, including breathing movements and breathing capacity. (Anesth.)

spiroscope (spī′rō-skōp) An apparatus for respiration exercises by which the patient can see the amount of water displaced in a given time and thus gauge his respiratory capacity. (Anesth.)

splint(s) Metal, acrylic resin, or modeling compound fashioned to retain in position teeth that may have been replanted, are removable, or have fractured roots. (Endodont.)

— A rigid appliance for the fixation of dis-

placed or movable parts. (Oper. Dent.; Remov. Part. Prosth.)

— A support or brace used to fasten or to confine. (Oral Surg.)

— A device, appliance, or prosthesis designed to immobilize and stabilize the teeth and thus prevent them from being subjected to the effects of trauma from occlusal forces during mastication and during indulgence in clenching and grinding habits; e.g., acrylic resin bite-guard appliance, bite guard, provisional splint, or fixed splint. (Periodont.)

— A rigid support for the fixation of displaced or movable parts. (Oper. Dent.; Remov. Part. Prosth.)

— A device that maintains hard and/or soft tissue in a predetermined position. (M.F.P.)

abutment s. Adjacent tooth restorations that have been rigidly united at their proximal contact areas to form a single abutment with multiple roots. (Remov. Part. Prosth.)

acrylic resin bite-guard s. An acrylic resin appliance constructed for the purposes of immobilizing teeth, eliminating the effects of traumatic habit patterns on the teeth and periodontal structures, acting as a base for minor tooth movement, facilitating the establishment of centric relation and centric occlusion, etc. Basically it is designed so that it covers the occlusal and incisal surfaces of the dental arch for which it is constructed. (Periodont.)

bridge s. (see **splint, fixed partial denture**)

buccal s. A material (e.g., plaster) that can be placed on the buccal surfaces of assembled fixed partial denture units and onto which, after hardening, these components can be assembled and held in accurate relation. (Remov. Part. Prosth.)

cap s. Plastic or metallic fracture appliances that are designed to cover the crowns of the teeth; usually held in place by cementation. (Oral Surg.)

cast bar s. (Friedman s.) A provisional splint consisting of cast continuous clasps that follow the facial and lingual surfaces of the teeth at the height of contour. It is cemented onto the teeth to be splinted and simultaneously "wired closed" in order to bring the "clasps" into intimate contact with the teeth. May not be cemented in place to serve as a removable cast splint. (Periodont.)

continuous clasp s. A cast splint used for the provisional immobilization of teeth. (Periodont.)

copper band–acrylic s. A splint fabricated from copper bands and acrylic resin. (Periodont.)

crib s. An appliance used for temporary tooth stabilization; constructed of gold, acrylic resin, chrome-cobalt alloys, or combinations thereof. It consists of a continuous crib clasp covering the facial and lingual surfaces of the teeth to be splinted. (Periodont.)

cross arch bar s. A splint formed by a metal bar that unites one or more teeth of one side of the dental arch to one or more of the opposite side. Used to stabilize weakened teeth against lateral tilting forces. (Remov. Part. Prosth.) (see also **connector, cross arch bar splint**)

c. a. b. s., Bilson fixable-removable Type of cross arch bar splint. (Remov. Part. Prosth.)

fixed s. A fixed (nonremovable) restorative and replacement prosthesis utilized as a therapeutic aid in the treatment of periodontal disease. It serves to stabilize and immobilize the teeth, replace missing teeth, and, by the nature of its occlusal construction, to prevent the teeth and their attachment apparatus from being subjected to adverse occlusal forces. It must also possess axial, occlusal, proximal, and interproximal contours conducive to the maintenance of gingival health. (Periodont.)

fixed partial denture s. A fixed partial denture that is used to unite weakened teeth for the purpose of better resisting tilting stresses. A method frequently utilized to stabilize the second premolar when it stands alone, when the first premolar and molars are missing. (Fixed Part. Prosth.; Remov. Part. Prosth.)

Friedman s. (see **splint, cast bar**)

Gunning's s. A maxillomandibular splint used to support both the maxillae and mandible in mandibular and/or maxillofacial surgery. (Oral Surg.)

implant surgical s. (see **superstructure, temporary**)

inlay s. An inlay casting designed to give fixation or support to one or more approximating teeth. This may be accomplished by two inlays soldered together or a single casting made for prepared cavities in approximating teeth. (Oper. Dent.)

interdental s. An appliance, made of plastic or metallic materials, that is applied to the dentition of the labial and/or lingual as-

pects to provide points for applying mandibular and/or maxillofacial traction or fixation. (Oral Surg.)

labial s. An appliance of plastic, metal, or combinations of plastic and metal made to conform to the labial aspect of the dental arch. Used in the management of mandibular and maxillofacial injuries. (Oral Surg.)

lingual s. An appliance similar to a labial splint but conforming to the lingual aspect of the dental arch. (Oral Surg.)

occlusal s. A matrix similar to a buccal splint except that it is used on the occlusal surfaces for a similar assembly. (Remov. Part. Prosth.)

provisional s. A therapeutic appliance utilized to provide opportunities for healing, repair, and cure of periodontally involved teeth; it is further used to determine the prognosis of questionable teeth. It is semifixed in nature and consists of a series of connected full crowns of appropriate extent in order to stabilize the teeth during both functional and afunctional mandibular movements. It may be fabricated of gold and acrylic resin, acrylic resin alone, or combinations of copper bands and acrylic resin. (Periodont.)

Stader s. (see **appliance, fracture**)

splinting The ligating, tying, or joining of periodontally involved teeth to one another to stabilize and immobilize the teeth, thus preventing them from being adversely affected by occlusal forces. Splinting includes acrylic resin bite guards, orthodontic band splints, wire ligation, provisional splints, fixed prostheses, etc. Also serves to replace missing teeth. (Periodont.)

s. of abutments The joining of two or more teeth into a rigid unit by means of fixed restorations. (Comp. Prosth.; Oper. Dent.; Remov. Part. Prosth.)

cross arch s. The stabilizing of weakened teeth against tilting movements caused by laterally directed occlusal stress loads. This is accomplished by the use of a rigid connector that projects to the opposite side of the dental arch where attachment is made to one or more teeth, thus producing effective counterleverage. (Remov. Part. Prosth.)

Essig-type s. A method of stabilizing and repositioning injured teeth. Stainless steel fracture wire is passed labially and lingually around a segment of a dental arch, and the wire is held in position by individual ligatures around the contact areas of teeth. (Oral Surg.)

split cast mounting (see **mounting, split cast**)

split ring A casting ring made of three parts, designed to take advantage of the maximum expansion of the investment. (D. Mat.)

spongiosa (see **bone, cancellous**)

spoon An instrument with a round or ovoid-shaped working end; designed to be used in a scraping or scooping manner. (Oper. Dent.)

spot(s) A small circular area.

café-au-lait s. (kă-fā′ō-lā″) Brown-pigmented areas of the skin occurring particularly in neurofibromatosis. (Oral Diag.)

focal s. The specific area of the face of the anode or target that is bombarded by the focused electron stream when the x-ray tube is in action. It is usually an insert of tungsten. (Oral Radiol.)

effective f. s. (**prolonged focus**) The apparent size and shape of the focal spot when viewed from a position in the useful beam. With the use of a suitably inclined anode face, the area from which the useful beam stems is sharply concentrated, if seen from the perspective of the useful beam. (Oral Radiol.) (see also **line, focus**)

Fordyce's s. (**Fordyce's disease, ectopic sebaceous glands**) The chamois-colored, slightly raised spots on the oral mucosa or lips produced by sebaceous glands in those tissues. The term Fordyce's disease is sometimes erroneously applied to these spots, which are present in 70% to 80% of the population. (Oral Diag.)

Koplik's s. Oral lesions of measles (rubeola); usually occur on the buccal mucosa opposite the molar teeth as small white or bluish white spots surrounded by red zones. (Oral Diag.)

— Small bluish white spots surrounded by a red areola on the mucous membrane of the lips and buccal mucosa during the prodromal stage of measles. (Oral Path.)

pink s. (see **resorption, internal**)

sprain The stressing of a joint, with injury to its soft tissue supporting attachments. (Oral Surg.) (see also **strain**)

spray A liquid minutely divided, as by a jet of air or steam. (Anesth.)

spreader (see **condensor**)

spring An elastic wire attached to a denture or appliance. (Comp. Prosth.)

— A piece of metal having the physical charac-

teristic that, when bent, it returns to its original shape. (Orthodont.)

auxiliary s. (**finger s.**) A short piece of wire, attached to an orthodontic appliance at one end, that serves as a lever to apply force to a tooth or teeth. (Orthodont.)

coil s. A spiral winding of fine wire attached to an orthodontic appliance. (Orthodont.)

finger s. (see **spring, auxiliary**)

sprue (sprū) Wax, metal, or plastic used to form the aperture or apertures through which a material such as gold or resin may enter a mold to make a casting; also the material that later fills the sprue hole or holes. (Comp. Prosth.; Remov. Part. Prosth.)

— A hole that provides a pathway through the refractory investment in order to permit entry of the metal into the mold. (D. Mat.)

— In casting, the ingate through which melted metal passes into the heated mold. The waste piece of metal cast in the ingate. The pin or wax that attaches the pattern to the crucible former, or spruce base, and that creates the ingate through the investment when the pattern is invested. (Oper. Dent.)

s. base (see **sprue former; crucible former**)

s. former (**crucible former**) The base to which the sprue is attached while the wax pattern is being invested in a refractory investment in a casting flask. (Comp. Prosth.; Remov. Part. Prosth.)

— A cone-shaped base made of metal or plastic to which the sprue is attached. Forms a crucible in the investment material. (D. Mat.)

s. pin (see **pin, sprue**)

sputum (spū′tŭm) Matter ejected from the mouth; saliva mixed with mucus and other substances from the respiratory tract. (Anesth.)

stability The quality of a denture to be firm, steady, and constant in position when forces are applied. Refers especially to resistance against horizontal movement. (Comp. Prosth.)

— The characteristic of a removable denture which resists forces that tend to alter the relationship between the denture base and its supporting bony foundation. (Comp. Prosth.; Remov. Part. Prosth.)

dimensional s. The property of a material to retain its size and form. (Comp. Prosth.; Remov. Part. Prosth.)

emotional s. State of an individual that enables him to have appropriate feelings about common experiences and to act in a rational manner. (Oral Med.)

stabilization (stă″bĭ-lĭ-zā′shŭn) The seating or fixation of a fixed or removable denture so that it will not tilt or be displaced under pressure. (Comp. Prosth.)

— The control of induced stress loads and/or the development of measures to counteract these forces so effectively that the tilting of teeth or the movement of a prosthesis is minimized to a point within tissue tolerance limits. (Remov. Part. Prosth.)

stabilized baseplate (see **baseplate, stabilized**)

stabilizer An instrument used in an x-ray unit to render the milliamperage output of the tube constant. (Oral Radiol.)

stabilizing The process of fixing movable parts. Making firm and steady. The fixing of clamps, separators, or matrices to teeth by the application of tacky compound to the parts, then chilling the compound. In the case of clamps and separators, this serves the added purpose of distributing the force of operating over adjacent teeth as well as the one being operated on. (Oper. Dent.)

   s. circumferential clasp arm (see **clasp, circumferential, arm, stabilizing**)

stable Term applied to a substance that has no tendency to decompose spontaneously. As applied to chemical compounds, it denotes their ability to resist chemical alterations. (Anesth.)

   s. isotope (see **isotope**)

Stader splint (stā′der) (see **appliance, fracture**)

stage, surgical A period or distinct phase in the course of anesthesia. (Anesth.)

stain A discoloration accumulating on the surface of a denture or teeth. (Comp. Prosth.; Remov. Part. Prosth.)

   Gram s. A staining method for microorganisms that is used to place them into two broad groups: gram positive, which retain crystal violet stain, and gram negative, which decolorize but counterstain with a red dye. (Oral Diag.)

   methyl violet s. A dye used to color bacteria for microscopic examination. (Oral Diag.)

staining Modification of the color of the teeth or denture base to achieve a more lifelike appearance. (Comp. Prosth.; Remov. Part. Prosth.)

stainless steel (see **steel, stainless**)

stamp cusp A cusp made to work in a fossa. Basically, a stamp means a pestle used with a mortar. The maxillary lingual cusps are stamp cusps. In tooth-to-tooth occlusion, all lower buccal cusps may stamp into fossae. The lower lip teeth may also be regarded as flattened stamps. In tooth-to-two-tooth occlusion, the stamp cusps of the lower premolars may have their tips in embrasures and have only their shoulders in tiny fossae. (Gnathol.)

standard That which is established by authority, custom, or general acceptance as a model; criterion. (D. Juris.)

Staphylococcus albus (stăf″ĭ-lō-kok′ŭs ăl′bŭs) (**Staphylococcus pyogenes var. albus**) A species of spherical, gram-positive bacteria growing in grapelike clusters; of low pathogenicity, although occasional strains may be coagulase positive and produce hemolysis. Normally present as part of the oral flora and mucosa-lined cavities, such as the mouth and the nasal cavity. Can be isolated, along with *Staphylococcus aureus*, streptococci, pneumococci, fusiform bacilli, *Borrelia vincentii*, molds, yeasts, etc., from the gingival crevice by cultural examination. (Periodont.)

Staphylococcus aureus (stăf″ĭ-lō-kŏk′ŭs awr′ē-us) (**Staphylococcus pyogenes var. aureus**) A pathogenic variety of staphylococci that is capable of producing suppurative lesions; cultured colonies are golden-yellow. Produces hemolysis on blood agar, is coagulase positive, and may be resistant to commonly used antibiotics. Has been isolated along with other microorganisms (e.g., *Staphylococcus albus*) from the gingival crevice. (Periodont.)

Staphylococcus pyogenes var. albus (see **Staphylococcus albus**)

Staphylococcus pyogenes var. aureus (see **Staphylococcus aureus**)

stare decisis (stăr′ē dĭ-sī′sĭs) Latin phrase meaning to stand by decisions and not disturb settled matters; to follow rules or principles laid down in previous judicial decisions. (D. Juris.)

statement A printed form stating the balance of the account due the dentist. (Pract. Man.)

static electricity (see **film fault, static electricity**)

static relation (see **relation, static**)

stationary grid (see **grid, stationary**)

stationeries The various-sized sheets and envelopes on which the dentist has his letterhead printed. (Pract. Man.)

status (stā′tŭs) State or condition. (Anesth.)

   s. lymphaticus Enlargement of lymphoid tissue, particularly the thymus, in children. It may lead to sudden death in inhalation anesthesia. (Oral Diag.)

   s. thymicolymphaticus A constitutional disturbance of controversial existence thought to be responsible in some way for sudden and unexplained deaths from trivial causes such as the extraction of teeth. There is enlargement of the thymus and lymphoid tissue and underdevelopment of the adrenal glands, gonads, and cardiovascular system. (Oral Med.)

statute A law enacted and established by a legislative department of government. (D. Juris.)

s. of frauds A requirement that, for legal validity, contracts for conveying real property or contracts for the performance of personal services requiring a year or more to perform must be in writing. (D. Juris.)

s. of limitations A statute prescribing limitations to the right of action on certain causes of action that prescribes that no suit shall be maintained on them unless brought within a specified period after the right accrued. (D. Juris.)

wrongful death s. A statute that provides for the recovery of damages by one other than the party who received the fatal injuries. (D. Juris.)

steel crown (see **crown, steel**)

steel, stainless A steel that contains a minimum of 12% chromium and approximately 0.5% carbon. (D. Mat.)

Stellite (stĕl'ĭt) Any of various cobalt-chromium alloys. (D. Mat.)

— A very hard, noncorrosive alloy of cobalt, chromium, and sometimes tungsten used for special instruments, particularly surgical instruments. (Oper. Dent.)

stem, brain (see **brainstem**)

stenosis (stĕ-nō'sĭs) Narrowing or stricture of a duct, canal, or vessel. (Anesth.; Oral Surg.)

— A partial or complete stoppage of a passage by the narrowing of its lumen. (Oral Physiol.)

Stensen's duct (see **duct, Stensen's**)

stent A device used to hold a skin graft placed to maintain a body orifice, cavity, or space. An acrylic resin appliance used as a positioning guide or support. (Oral Surg.)

— An appliance that maintains tissue, e.g., a skin transplant, in a predetermined position. (M.F.P.)

step wedge (see **penetrometer**)

step-up transformer (see **transformer, step-up**)

stereoisomer (see **isomers**)

stereoscope An optical instrument for viewing photographs or radiographs; it produces binocular vision, or a blending of images, so that new perspectives can be seen with an appearance of depth. It operates on the same principle as the eyes; i.e., two views are registered on the retinas of the eyes, and the brain merges them into one. (Oral Radiol.)

stereoscopic radiograph (see **radiograph, stereoscopic**)

sterids (see **steroid**)

sterile Free from viable microorganisms. (Oral Surg.)

sterilization The act or process of rendering sterile; the process of freeing from germ life. (Anesth.)

— The process of freeing materials or areas of all microorganisms by means of heat or chemicals. (Oral Surg.)

sterilizer for root canal instruments A special device for heat sterilization of root canal instruments and dressings that depends on molten metal, glass beads, salt, or fine sand for the conduction of the heat. (Endodont.)

Sternberg-Reed cell (see **cell, Sternberg-Reed**)

steroid(s) (stĕr'oid) (**sterid**) A group name for compounds that resemble cholesterol chemically and that contain also a hydrogenated cyclopentanophenanthrene ring system. (Anesth.)

— Steroids having one or more carbonyl or carboxyl groups. Substances having a similar cyclic nucleus and resembling phenanthrene. Included are cholesterol, ergosterol, bile acids, vitamin D, sex hormones, adrenocortical hormones, and cardiac glycosides. (Oral Med.)

adrenocortical s. (**adrenal corticosteroid**) A hormone extracted from the adrenal cortex or a synthetic substance similar in chemical structure and biologic activity to such a hormone. (Anesth.)

— The biologically active steroids of the adrenal cortex, which include 11-dehydrocorticosterone (compound A), corticosterone (compound B), cortisone (compound E), 17α-hydroxycorticosterone (compound F, hydroxycortisone, or cortisol), and aldosterone. The effects of the corticosteroids include increased resorption of sodium and chloride by the renal tubules and metabolic effects on protein, carbohydrate, and fat. (Oral Med.)

— A steroid derived from the adrenal cortex. Also, a similarly acting substance prepared synthetically. (Oral Med.; Pharmacol.)

C-19 cortico-s. (**anabolic protein, N hormone**) Adrenocortical hormones similar in action to the male and female sex hormones. They cause nitrogen retention and, in excessive amounts, masculinization in the female. (Oral Med.)

C-21 cortico-s. (**glycogenic s., sugar hormone**) 21-Carbon adrenocortical hormones that are oxygenated at carbon 11 or at both carbon

11 and 17. They affect protein, carbohydrate, and fat metabolism; e.g., they elevate blood sugar, increase glyconeogenesis, decrease hepatic lipogenesis, mobilize depot fat, and increase protein metabolism. (Oral Med.)

glycogenic s. (see **steroid, C-21 cortico-**)

11-oxy-s. Term that refers collectively to the C-21 corticosteroids, all of which are oxygenated at carbon 11. (Oral Med.)

17 alpha-hydroxycortico-s. (**17-OHCS**) Term used for cortisol and other 21-carbon steroids possessing a dihydroxyacetone group at carbon 17. Serum and urinary determinations give a direct measurement of adrenocortical activity. (Oral Med.)

17-keto-s. (**17-KS**) Steroidal compounds with a ketone (carbonyl) group at carbon 17. Derived from cortisol and from adrenal and testicular androgen. Urinary neutral 17-ketosteroids represent the catabolic end products of the endocrine glands produced by the adrenal cortex and testes. Increased values occur in the adrenogenital syndromes, adrenocortical carcinoma, bilateral hyperplasia of the adrenal cortex, and Leydig's cell tumors. Normal adult values for a 24-hour urine sample are 10 to 20 mg for men and 5 to 15 mg for women. (Oral Med.)

sterols (stē'rolz) Steroids having one or more hydroxyl groups and no carbonyl or carboxyl groups; e.g., cholesterol. (Oral Med.)

stethospasm Spasm of the chest muscles. (Anesth.)

Stevens-Johnson syndrome (see **syndrome, Stevens-Johnson**)

Stillman's cleft (see **cleft, Stillman's**)

stimulant An agent that causes an increase in functional activity, usually of the central nervous system. (Anesth.)

psychomotor s. A drug that increases psychic activity. (Anesth.)

stimulation Increased functioning of protoplasm induced by some extracellular substance or agent. (Anesth.)

— The act of energizing or activating. Physiologically, this process readily may be carried beyond the point of benefiting an organ or structure and become an irritation. (Remov. Part. Prosth.)

stimulus A chemical, thermal, electrical, or mechanical influence that changes the normal environment of irritable tissue and creates an impulse. (Anesth.)

stippling An orange-peel appearance of the at-

tached gingiva believed to be due to the bundles of collagen fibers that enter the connective tissue papillae. (Periodont.)

— A roughening of the labial and buccal surfaces of denture bases to imitate the stippling of natural gingiva. (Comp. Prosth.)

basophilic s. (see **basophilia**)

gingival s. (see **gingiva, stippling**)

stipulation A material; an article in an agreement; an agreement in writing to do a certain thing. (D. Juris.)

Stokes' disease (see **disease, Adams-Stokes**)

stomatodynia (stō″mah-tō-dĭn′ē-ah) Sore mouth. (Oral Med.)

stomatitides (stō″mah-tĭ′tĭ-dēs) The oral lesions associated with various forms of stomatitis. (Oral Med.)

stomatitis (stō″mah-tĭ′tĭs) Inflammation of the oral cavity. This is used as a general term and for all practical purposes is synonymous with mucositis when applied to oral regions. Glossitis and gingivitis are more limiting terms, although essentially they are stomatitises. (Oral Diag.)

— Inflammation of the soft tissues of the mouth occurring as a result of mechanical, chemical, thermal, bacterial, viral, electrical, or radiation injury, reactions to allergens, or as secondary manifestation of systemic disease. (Oral Med.)

aphthous s. (**aphthae, canker sore**) Refers to recurrent ulcers of the mouth that appear to be the same clinically as herpetic ulcers and for that reason have been considered to be a manifestation of recurrent herpes simplex, although the herpesvirus has never been conclusively isolated from recurrent aphthae. (Oral Med.) (see also **gingivostomatitis, herpetic; stomatitis, herpetic; ulcer, aphthous**)

arsenical s. Oral manifestations of arsenical poisoning. The oral mucosa is dry, red, and painful. Ulceration, purpura, and mobility of teeth may also occur. (Oral Med.)

Atabrine s. A stomatitis considered by some to be associated with the use of the antimalarial and anthelmintic drug quinacrine hydrochloride (Atabrine) and characterized by oral changes simulating lichen planus. (Oral Med.)

bismuth s. A stomatitis resulting from systemic use of bismuth compounds over prolonged periods. Sulfides of bismuth are deposited in the gingival tissue, resulting in bluish black pigmentation known as a bismuth line. Oral manifestations of bismuth poisoning include gingivostomatitis like that of Vincent's infection, a blue-black line on the inner aspect of the gingival sulcus or pigmentation of the buccal mucosa, a sore tongue, metallic taste, and a burning sensation of the mouth. (Oral Med.)

— The deposition of bismuth sulfide in oral tissues due to a reaction of hydrogen sulfide, produced from degradation of oral food debris and necrotic tissue, on bismuth salts used for systemic medication. Bismuth stomatitis produces a bismuth line along the gingival margin. (Oral Path.)

catarrhal s. (see **gingivitis, catarrhal**)

epidemic s. (see **disease, foot-and-mouth**)

epizootic s. (see **disease, foot-and-mouth**)

gangrenous s. (**cancrum oris, noma**) Destruction of large masses of the oral tissues, particularly the cheek. It usually is found in weakened patients with very low resistance to infection due to lowered white blood cell count or other causes. In advanced states a large segment of the cheek may be lost, leaving the teeth visible through the defect. (Oral Diag.)

— Term used specifically for noma (cancrum oris) and collectively for several necrotizing stomatitides (e.g., noma, exanthematous necrosis, acatalasemia) and for involvement other than, or in addition to, the gingiva in necrotizing ulcerative gingivitis (Vincent's angina). (Oral Med.) (see also **noma**)

— A rapidly spreading gangrene occurring in the oral and facial tissues of debilitated patients. (Oral Path.)

gonococcal s. Inflammation of the oral mucosa caused by gonococci. (Oral Diag.)

herpetic s. Oral manifestations of primary herpes simplex infection. The term is also used by some for herpetiform ulcers considered to be oral manifestations of secondary or recurrent herpes simplex. (Oral Med.) (see also **ulcer, aphthous, recurrent**)

— Inflammation of the oral mucosa caused by herpesvirus. (Oral Diag.) (see also **gingivostomatitis, herpetic**)

acute h. s. (**acute herpetic gingivostomatitis**) The manifestations of clinically apparent primary herpes simplex characterized by regional lymphadenopathy, sore throat, and high temperature, followed by localized itching and burning, with the formation of small vesicles of an erythematous base that give way to plaques and then painful herpetic ulcers. The gingivae are swollen and erythematous and bleed

easily. Manifestations subside in 7 to 10 days, and recovery usually occurs within 2 weeks. (Oral Med.)

iodine s. (see **iodism**)

lead s. Oral manifestations of lead poisoning. Included are a bluish line along the free gingival margin, pigmentation of the mucosa in contact with the teeth, metallic taste, excessive salivation, and swelling of the salivary glands. (Oral Med.)

s. medicamentosa An allergic response of the oral mucosa to a systemically administered drug. Possible manifestations include asthma, skin rashes, urticaria, pruritus, leukopenia, lymphadenopathy, thrombocytopenic purpura, and oral lesions (erythema, ulcerative lesions, vesicles, bullae, and angioneurotic edema). (Oral Med.)

— Eruptive involvement of the oral mucosa resulting from an allergic reaction to some systemic medication such as antibiotics, arsenic, barbiturates, or salicylates. (Oral Path.)

— Stomatitis, varying from sensitive erythema to an ulcerative stomatitis and/or gingivitis, as a result of ingestion of certain drugs by an individual possessing a hypersensitivity or intolerance to them. Representative drugs include aspirin, iodine, iodoform, potassium iodide, phenobarbital, and amobarbital (Amytal). (Periodont.)

membranous s. Inflammation of the oral cavity, accompanied by the formation of a false membrane. (Oral Path.)

mercurial s. Oral manifestations of mercury poisoning consisting of hypersalivation, metallic taste, ulceration and necrosis of the gingivae with a tendency to spread posteriorly and to the buccal mucosa and palate, glossodynia, and periodontitis with loosening of the teeth in severe cases of chronic intoxication. (Oral Med.)

mycotic s. Infection of the oral mucosa by a fungus, most commonly *Candida albicans,* which produces moniliasis (thrush). (Oral Med.) (see also **moniliasis**)

s. nicotina (see **stomatitis, nicotinic**)

nicotinic s. (**s. nicotina**) An inflammation of the palate caused by irritation of tobacco smoke and characterized by raised small palatal lesions with red centers and white borders. The palatal mucosa usually has a generalized leukoplakia accompanying the smaller lesions. (Oral Diag.)

— Sialadenitis of minor salivary glands of the palate and inflammatory hyperplasia of the orifices of their ducts; related to smoking. (Oral Path.)

recurrent s. Recurrent manifestations of herpes simplex involving the lips and labial and buccal mucosa (fever blisters, cold sores). Considered by many to include also recurrent aphthae (canker sores). Episodes may result from fever, sunlight, menses, trauma, and gastrointestinal upset. Lesions begin as clear vesicles with an erythematous base that give way to ulcers and superficial crusts if the outer surfaces of the lip and skin are involved. (Oral Med.)

uremic s. Oral manifestations of uremia, consisting of varying degrees of erythema, exudation, ulceration, pseudomembrane formation, foul breath, and burning sensations. (Oral Med.) (see also **gingivitis, nephritic**)

s. venenata Inflammation of the oral mucosa caused by contact with a substance to which it is sensitive, e.g., a drug, food, or material. (Oral Diag.)

— Inflammation of the oral mucosa as the result of contact allergy. The most common causative agents are volatile oils, iodides, dentifrices, mouthwashes, denture powders, and topical anesthetics. Possible manifestations include erythema, angioneurotic edema, burning sensations, ulcerations, and vesicles. (Oral Med.; Oral Path.)

— Stomatitis that is similar to stomatitis medicamentosa but that results from direct application to the oral tissues of the drug or substance to which the individual is hypersensitive. (Periodont.)

stomatoglossitis (stō″mah-tō-glŏs-sī′tĭs) Inflammation involving oral mucous membranes and the tonuge. May be seen in nutritional disorders such as pellagra, beriberi, vitamin B complex deficiency, and infections. (Periodont.)

stomatognathic system (stō″mah-tō-năth′ĭk) (see **system, stomatognathic**)

stomatology (stō″măh-tol′ō-jē) The study of the structures, functions, and diseases of the mouth. (Comp. Prosth.; Fixed Part. Prosth.; Remov. Part. Prosth.)

— The study of the morphology, structure, function, and diseases of the contents and linings of the oral cavity. (Gnathol.)

stomion (stō′mē-ahn) The median point of the oral slit (orifice) when the mouth is closed. (Orthodont.)

stone An abrading instrument or tool. (Oper. Dent.)

Arkansas s. A fine-grained stone, novaculite,

used to make hones for the final sharpening of instruments. (Oper. Dent.)

— A stone, provided in suitable sizes, shapes, and abrasive consistencies, utilized to sharpen instruments. (Periodont.)

artificial s. (dental stone) A specially calcined gypsum derivative similar to plaster of paris; since its grains are nonporous, the product is stronger than plaster of paris. (Comp. Prosth.; Remov. Part. Prosth.)

carborundum s. A stone made of silicon carbide. (Oper. Dent.)

— An abrasive, handpiece-mounted rotary instrument of various sizes, shapes, and degrees of abrasiveness; used to contour the tooth structure in the various phases of selective grinding (occlusal adjustment). (Periodont.)

dental s. (Hydrocal) Alpha-hemihydrate of calcium sulfate. (D. Mat.)

  Class I Commonly referred to as Hydrocal. Harder and stronger than plaster of paris. (D. Mat.)

  Class II A dense, relatively hard stone of lower setting expansion than Class I stones; used for dies and working models. (D. Mat.)

— A gypsum product that, when combined with water in proper proportions, hardens in a plasterlike form. It is used for making casts and dies. (Oper. Dent.)

diamond s. Rotary instruments containing diamond chips as the abrasive. Available in various sizes, shapes, and abrasive consistency. Utilized for tooth reduction in operative dentistry and crown and bridge prosthesis, for tooth contouring in the occlusal adjustment procedure, for osseous and gingival contouring in periodontal surgery, etc. (Periodont.)

s. die (see **die, stone**)

lathe s. (lathe wheel) A grindstone mounted on a chuck and used on a lathe. (Oper. Dent.)

mounted point s. A small abrasive tooth of various shapes and sizes bonded or cemented onto a shaft or mandrel. (Oper. Dent.)

pulp s. (see **denticle**)

sharpening s. A hand stone, or a stone driven mechanically, that is used to sharpen instruments. (Oper. Dent.)

wheel s. A small grindstone of carborundum or corundum of various grits, mounted on a mandrel; of various thicknesses, ranging in diameter from ½ to 1 inch. (Oper. Dent.)

stop (see **rest**)

occlusal s. (see **rest, occlusal**)

stopping, temporary Gutta-percha mixed with zinc oxide, white wax, and coloring. Softens on heating and rehardens at room temperature. Used for temporary sealing of dressings in cavities. Lack of strength makes it ineffective in areas under occlusal stress. (Oper. Dent.)

storage Care of a prosthesis that is not being used. To avoid loss, accidental breakage, or desiccation of any resin part, a removable prosthesis should always be placed in an aqueous solution and in a place of safety. (Remov. Part. Prosth.)

Stout's method (see **wiring, continuous loop**)

straightening of teeth (see **orthodontics, corrective**)

strain Deformation induced by an external force. (D. Mat.)

— Deformation expressed as a pure number or ratio resulting from the application of a load. (Oper. Dent.)

— A traumatic stretching or compression of such tissues as the ligaments, capsule, or musculature associated with a joint. (Oral Surg.) (see also **sprain**)

s. hardening (see **hardening, strain**)

strangulation Choking or throttling. The arrest of respiration due to occlusion of the air passage or arrest of the circulation in a part due to compression. (Anesth.)

stray radiation (see **radiation leakage**)

strength Toughness; ability to withstand or apply force.

biting s. The force available for application against food or other material placed between the teeth. (Comp. Prosth.) (see also **force, masticatory**)

— The amount of force the muscles of mastication are capable of exerting. (Remov. Part. Prosth.) (see also **force, masticatory**)

compressive s. (crushing s.) Resistance to a pushing force. (D. Mat.)

— The amount of resistance of a material to fracture under compression. (Oper. Dent.) (see also **strength, ultimate**)

crushing s. (see **strength, compressive**)

dry s. Term generally used in conjunction with materials whose strengths vary markedly in the wet and dry states. The strength of gypsum products is usually reported in both wet and dry states. (D. Mat.)

edge s. Term indicative of the ability of fine margins to resist fracture or abrasion. There is no specific test for this property; it is a composite of ductility and shear, tensile, and other strength characteristics. (D. Mat.)

gel s. Usually, the ability of the material to withstand a load without rupture. (D. Mat.)

impact s. The ability of a material to withstand a striking force. (D. Mat.)

shear s. (shear) Resistance to a tangential force. (D. Mat.)

— Resistance to a twisting motion. (Oper. Dent.)

tensile s. Resistance to a pulling force. (D. Mat.)

— The amount of stress a material is able to withstand when being pulled lengthwise, before permanent deformation results. (Oper. Dent.)

— A measure of the resistance of a metal to permanent deformation by fracture. (Remov. Part. Prosth.)

ultimate s. (shear) The greatest stress that may be induced in a material or object before or during rupture; may be compressive, tensile or shear strength. (D. Mat.) (see also **strength, tensile**)

wet s. Term that refers to compressive strength while water in excess of that required for hydration of the hemihydrate is present in the specimen. Used in connection with gypsum products. (D. Mat.)

yield s. A definite proportionality obtained by drawing a line parallel to the proportional limit line. Yield strength is reported in terms of the degree of strain. (D. Mat.)

Streptococcus, alpha hemolytic (strĕp″tō-kok′ŭs, ăl′fah hē″mō-lĭt′ĭk) A spherical, gram-positive bacterium, occurring in chains of bacterial cells. Produces a zone of greenish discoloration around the colony in blood-agar medium. Part of an individual's normal oral flora; has been isolated from the gingival crevice. Capable of producing bacteremia and subsequent subacute bacterial endocarditis in patients with a history of rheumatic fever; thus prophylactic antibiotic therapy is necessary prior, during, and after periodontal, operative, and surgical therapy. (Periodont.)

Streptococcus viridans (strĕp″tō-kok′ŭs vĭ′rĭ-dănz) (see **Streptococcus, alpha hemolytic**)

streptothricosis (strĕp-tō-thrĭ-kō′sĭs) (see **actinomycosis**)

stress An external force that resists a load or force. (D. Mat.)

— A force induced by or resisting an external force; measured in terms of force per unit area. (Comp. Prosth.; Oper. Dent.)

— The force or energy directed against a tissue structure or against the function of tissue as the result of injury and trauma associated with fracture, burn, infection, surgical procedure, pharmacologic action, or anxiety states. The response to stress involves local metabolic function, the hormonal activity of the endocrine system regulated by the pituitary gland, and the autonomic and central nervous systems. The stress phenomenon is frequently associated with the general adaptation syndrome. (Oral Physiol.)

— Mutual force or action between contiguous surfaces of bodies caused by external force. (Remov. Part. Prosth.)

— Forcible pressure exceeding that produced in normal function. Stress exerted against the teeth and their attachment apparatus by occlusal forces may be within the adaptive capacities of the tissues, or the tissues may not be capable of compensation and adaptation, resulting in tissue destruction. (Periodont.)

— Adrenal dysfunction and associated bodily disturbances produced by physical and emotional disorders. (Periodont.) (see also **traumatism, occlusal**)

— In prosthetic dentistry, forcibly exerted pressure; e.g., the pressure of the upper teeth against the mandibular teeth or the pressure contact of a distorted removable partial denture on the supporting teeth or ridge structures. (Comp. Prosth.; Remov. Part. Prosth.)

axial s. Excessive force applied vertically to the teeth and their attachment apparatus. (Periodont.)

bone in s. Responses of bony structures to applied force. With application of excessive pressure stimuli to bone, adaptation may occur by the formation of thicker and more numerous trabeculae; or if tissue components cannot compensate for excessive stress, bone resorption will occur. (Periodont.)

buccolingual s. Excessive pressure exerted against teeth and their attachment apparatus from a buccal and/or lingual aspect. Lesions of the attachment apparatus associated with occlusal traumatism may occur. This stress usually (but not always) results in resorption of the thin crests of alveolar bone, with concurrent injury to the opposing apical bone and the other parts of the attachment apparatus and supporting bone. The attachment and supporting structures of the teeth are better able to withstand vertically applied forces than those applied horizontally. (Periodont.)

compressive s. The internal induced force that opposes shortening of the material in a direction parallel to the direction of the stress. (Comp. Prosth.; Remov. Part. Prosth.)

s. control (see **control, stress**)

shearing s. The internal induced force that opposes the sliding of one plane of the material on the adjacent plane in a direction parallel to stress. (Comp. Prosth.; Remov. Part. Prosth.)

tensile s. The internal induced force that opposes elongation of a material in a direction parallel to the direction of stress. (Comp. Prosth.; Remov. Part. Prosth.)

stress-bearing area (see **area, stress-bearing**)

stressbreaker (stress equalizer, stress divider) A device or system that is incorporated in a removable partial denture to relieve the abutment teeth of occlusal loads that may exceed their physiologic tolerance. (Remov. Part. Prosth.) (see also **connector, nonrigid**)

stress-breaking action of clasp (see **clasp, stress-breaking action of**)

stretch reflex (see **reflex, stretch**)

stretching, longitudinal The vertical elongations of gutta-percha that occur due to packing forces during the filling of large root canals. The material returns to the original form when force is released. (Endodont.)

stretching pliers (see **pliers, stretching**)

striations, muscle (strī-ā'shŭnz) The transverse alternating light and dark bands of skeletal muscles, which are due to differences in light absorption. The darker anisotropic band is very strongly birefringent, and the lighter isotropic band is relatively weakly birefringent. The difference between the bands is one of relative birefringence. Birefringence, or double refraction is a property of muscle fiber. There is a periodicity between the alternating light and dark bands. It is suggested that there are differences in chemical composition—that calcium, potassium, and magnesium are concentrated in the A band and that adenine derivatives and phosphogen are dominantly located in the I band. The muscle fibrils appear to run longitudinally through both bands. (Oral Physiol.)

stridor (strī'dor) A peculiar, harsh, vibrating sound produced during respiration. (Anesth.; Oral Diag.)

inspiratory s. The sound heard in inspiration through a spasmodically closed glottis. (Anesth.)

laryngeal s. Stridor due to laryngeal stenosis. (Anesth.)

strip A thin, narrow, comparatively long piece of material. (Oper. Dent.)

abrasive s. (linen s.) A ribbonlike piece of linen of varying lengths and widths on one side of which are bonded abrasive particles of selected grit; used for contouring and polishing proximal surfaces of restorations. (Oper. Dent.)

— A linen strip with abrasive texture supplied by silica, garnet, etc.; used to clean and polish proximal surfaces of the teeth. (Periodont.)

amalgam s. A linen strip with no abrasive; used to smooth proximal contours of newly placed amalgam restorations. (Oper. Dent.)

boxing s. A metal or wax strip used for making an enclosure to regulate the size and form of a cast. (Remov. Part. Prosth.)

Celluloid s. (see **strip, plastic**)

lightning s. (**separating s.**) A strip of steel with abrasive bonded on one side; used to open rough or improper contacts of proximal restorations or to begin the reduction of proximal excess of a foil restoration. (Oper. Dent.)

linen s. (see **strip, abrasive**)

plastic s. A clear plastic strip of Celluloid or acrylic resin that is used as a matrix when silicate cement or acrylic resin cement is inserted into proximal prepared cavities in anterior teeth. (Oper. Dent.)

polishing s. A strip with a very fine abrasive such as crocus powder. (Oper. Dent.)

separating s. (see **strip, lightning**)

stripping Removal of a very small amount of enamel from the mesial or distal surfaces of teeth to alleviate crowding. (Orthodont.)

— (**electrochemical milling**) The process of subjecting the surface of a gold casting, attached to an anode from a rectifier and transformer unit, to the dissolving action of a heated cyanide solution, the metal container for which is the cathode of the unit. A microscopic amount of the surface of the alloy is removed by the reverse electrolysis. The electrochemical milling is in contrast to electropolishing, wherein sharp edges are dissolved more rapidly than broader areas. (Oper. Dent.)

stroke A single, unbroken movement made by an instrument or the mandible.

circumferential s. One of the basic strokes utilized for root and gingival curettage; the blade of the periodontal curet is negotiated mesiodistally while it is in contact with either the root or the inner aspect of the soft tissue wall of the gingival or periodontal pocket. (Periodont.)

exploratory s. A phase of subgingival root scaling in which the curet is held in featherlike grasp to tactilely ascertain the amount and

extent of the accretions on the root surface; the ingress stroke into the pocket area. (Periodont.)

power s. The phase of the working stroke which is designed to split or dislodge calculus from the root surface. It is prefaced by the exploratory stroke and followed by the shaving stroke. (Periodont.)

shaving s. The phase of the working stroke of a periodontal curet that is designed to smooth or plane the root surface. It follows the power stroke, which is designed to dislodge calculus from the root surface. (Periodont.)

s. volume The volume of blood put out by the heart per heartbeat. Stroke volume is directly proportional to the volume of blood filling the heart during diastole. (Oral Physiol.)

stroma, colloidal (strō'mah) The concentration of colloidal proteins in the saliva. A theory of calculus formation (Prinz) postulates "that as saliva stagnates the colloidal proteins become concentrated at the surface and the protective colloidal action of proteins is lost." The calcium salts then precipitate and are carried down with the colloidal stroma. (Periodont.)

structure(s) The architectural arrangement of the component parts of a tissue, part, organ, or body. Also the individual components of the body. (Periodont.)

border s. (see **border structures**)

cored s. In metallurgy, a grain structure with composition gradients resulting from the progressive freezing of the components in different proportions. Nonmetals used in dentistry (e.g., zinc phosphate and silicate cements) are also cored structures in that they have a nucleus of undissolved powder particles surrounded by a matrix of reacted material. (D. Mat.)

denture-supporting s. The structures that make up the basal seat. The residual ridges that serve as the foundation or support for dentures. (Comp. Prosth.)

— The tissues, either teeth and/or residual ridges, that serve as the foundation or basal seat for removable partial dentures. (Comp. Prosth.; Remov. Part. Prosth.)

histologic s. The minute structure of organic tissues. (Oper. Dent.)

radiolucent s. (rā"dē-ō-lū'sĕnt) The structures or substances that permit the penetration of x radiation and are thus registered as relatively dark areas on the radiograph. (Periodont.)

radiopaque s. The structures that prevent the x rays from penetrating them because of their density, which causes them to appear as light areas on the radiograph. (Periodont.)

supporting s. The tissues that maintain or assist in maintaining the teeth in position in the alveolus; i.e., the gingivae, the cementum of the tooth, the periodontal membrane, and the alveolar and trabecular (supporting, cancellous, spongiosa) bone. (Periodont.)

functional form of s. s. Term that refers to the state of denture-supporting structures when they have been placed in such a position as to be able to begin resisting occlusal forces. (Remov. Part. Prosth.)

Stuart factor (see **factor X**)

study Pursuance of education; analysis.

s. cast (see **cast, diagnostic**)

graduate s. Postdoctoral educational efforts pursued for credit in institutions of higher learning. (Pract. Man.)

s. model (see **cast, diagnostic**)

postgraduate s. Postdoctoral educational endeavors that may or may not earn credits for advanced degrees. (Pract. Man.)

time s. The technique of random sampling used for analysis of the time spent for rendering each phase of each of the various professional services performed by the dentist. (Pract. Man.)

stupor The condition of being only partly conscious or sensible; also, a condition of insensibility. (Anesth.)

Sturge-Weber-Dimitri disease (see **disease, Sturge-Weber-Dimitri**)

stylet A wire inserted into a soft catheter or cannula to secure rigidity; a fine wire inserted into a hollow needle to maintain patency. (Anesth.)

stylus Ancient form of writing instrument. It is still used much as it was used when the Egyptians were figuring out geometry with a stylus and sand sprinkled on a polished stone. It has assumed importance in gnathology, since a well-pointed stylus can be slid on dust-covered glass with a minimum of friction, thereby making the jaw-writing data more accurate. (Gnathol.)

surgical indicator s. A small pointed instrument devised to mark the spot in the tissue where the intramucosal inserts will be placed. Styluses are seated in prepared depressions in the denture base and mark the mucosal tissue by puncturing it. (Oral Implant.)

s. tracer (see **tracer, needle point**)

s. tracing (see **tracing, needle point**)

styptic A hemostatic astringent. (Oral Med.; Pharmacol.)

sub- Prefix signifying under, beneath, deficient, near, almost. (Oper. Dent.)

subaxial Having the same relationship to axial that subpulpal has to pulpal. (Oper. Dent.)

subconscious Imperfect consciousness; the state in which mental processes take place without the mind's being distinctly conscious of its own activity. (Anesth.)

subgingival (sŭb-jĭn′jĭ-val) At a level apical to the gingival extent of the preparation or restoration. (Oper. Dent.)

subjacent tissue (sŭb-jā′sĕnt) (see **tissue, subjacent**)

sublabial adhesion (sŭb-lā′bē-al) (see **adhesion, sublabial**)

sublease A lease executed by the lessee of an estate to a third person, conveying the same estate for a shorter term than that for which the lessee holds it. (D. Juris.)

sublingual (sŭb-lĭng′gwal) Pertaining to the region of structures located beneath the tongue. (Comp. Prosth.; Remov. Part. Prosth.)

— Under the tongue. (Oral Surg.)

s. administration (see **administration, sublingual**)

s. crescent (see **crescent, sublingual**)

s. fold (see **fold, sublingual**)

subluxation (sŭb″lŭk-sā′shŭn) Incomplete dislocation of a joint. (Oral Diag.)

— Term applied loosely to the temporomandibular joint, indicating relaxation of the capsular ligaments and improper relationship of the joint components, resulting in cracking and popping of the joint during movement. (Oral Med.)

— An incomplete or partial dislocation. (Oral Surg.)

— Term used to characterize a mandibular joint of a patient whose condyle does not closely follow the contour of the eminence when he chews or when he is having his condyle movements projected on planes by jaw-writing devices. (Gnathol.)

submandibular Below the mandible. (Oral Surg.)

submarginal Pertaining to a deficiency of contour at the margin of a restoration or pattern. (Oper. Dent.)

submaxillary Situated beneath a maxilla. (Oral Surg.)

s. caruncle (see **caruncle, submaxillary**)

s. ganglion (see **ganglion, submaxillary**)

submental Situated below the chin. (Oral Surg.)

submucosa (sŭb″mū-kō′sah) The tissue layer beneath the oral mucosa. It contains connective tissues, vessels, and accessory salivary glands. (Oral Surg.)

submucous cleft (**occult cleft**) A congenital anomaly of the soft and/or hard palate, in which the midportion of the soft and/or hard palate lacks proper mesodermal development. Nonunion of bone and muscle tissues of the soft and hard palates and concealment by the superficial intact mucoperiosteum. (Cleft Palate)

subnasion (sŭb-nā′zē-ŏn) The point of the angle between the septum and the surface of the upper lip. It is sought at the point where a tangent applied to the septum meets the upper lip. (Orthodont.)

subnormality, mental (**mental retardation**) An individual, with or without brain damage, who is intellectually and socially inadequate in his society. (Pedodont.)

subocclusal connector (see **connector, subocclusal**)

subocclusal surface (see **surface, subocclusal**)

subpoena (sŭ-pē′nah) The process or writ issued by the court by which the attendance of a witness at a certain time and place is required in order that he may testify. It may also order him to bring with him any books, records, or other things under his control that he is bound by law to produce in evidence. (D. Juris.)

subpulpal (sŭb-pŭl′pal) In a prepared cavity, pertaining to a portion of the pulpal wall that is established pulpward from the level of the major pulpal wall; in a tooth from which the pulp has been removed, the base wall of the cavity extends to the floor of the pulp chamber and is then called the subpulpal wall. (Oper. Dent.)

subspinale (sŭb″spĭ-nā′lē) The deepest midline point on the premaxilla between the anterior nasal spine and the prosthion. (Orthodont.)

substitute One acting for or taking the place of another. (D. Juris.)

tinfoil s. Alginate material painted on gypsum molds to serve as a liner in preventing both the penetration of monomers into the surrounding investing medium and the leakage of water into acrylic resin. (D. Mat.)

substitution A standard or nonstandard speech sound used for another consonant speech sound; e.g., "w" for "l" (wady for lady). (Cleft Palate)

substructure A structure that is built to serve as a base or foundation for another structure. (Implantodont.)

implant s. (**implant denture s.**) A skeletal frame of inert material that fits on the bone under the mucoperiosteum. (Oral Implant.)
— The metal framework that is embedded beneath the soft tissues in contact with the bone for the purpose of supporting an implant superstructure. (Remov. Part. Prosth.)

i. s., abutment The portion of the implant that extends from the surface of the mucosa into the oral cavity for the retention of crowns, bridges, or superstructure bearing the teeth of the denture. (Oral Implant.)

i. s., auxiliary rest A small metal protrusion through the mucosa connected to the labial or buccal and lingual (peripheral) frame to furnish additional support for the superstructure between the abutments. (Oral Implant.)

i. s., interspaces Any one of the spaces between the primary and secondary struts that allows infiltration of tissue. (Oral Implant.)

i. s., neck (**implant post, i. s., post**) The constriction that connects the implant frame with the implant abutment. (Oral Implant.)

i. s., part The root section shaped in the form of a wire loop. This part of the substructure sinks into the alveolar socket or sockets after the extraction of one or two remaining anterior teeth. Newly formed bone tissue will grow through the loop and firmly affix the implant. (Oral Implant.)

i. s., peripheral frame The labial, buccal, lingual, and distal outline of the frame. (Oral Implant.)

i. s., post (see **substructure, implant, neck**)

i. s., primary struts The main traverse struts that connect the implant necks or posts with the peripheral frame. (Oral Implant.)

i. s., secondary struts The additional smaller transverse, diagonal, and longitudinal struts that are added when necessary to give additional strength and rigidity to the implant, to increase the area of bone support, and to afford additional intermeshing of the mucoperiosteal tissue. (Oral Implant.)

suction cup (see **cup, suction**)

suffocate Asphyxiate. (Anesth.)

suffocation Interference with the entrance of air into the lungs. (Anesth.)

suit Any proceeding in a court in which the plaintiff pursues the remedy that the law gives him for the redress of an injury or the recovery of a right. (D. Juris.)

sulcus (sŭl′kŭs) A furrow, trench, or groove, as on the surface of the brain or in folds of mucous membrane. A groove or depression on the surface of a tooth. A groove in a portion of the oral cavity. (Comp. Prosth.; Fixed Part. Prosth.; Remov. Part. Prosth.)

alveololingual s. (ăl-vē″ō-lō-lĭng′gwahl) The space existing between the alveolar or residual alveolar ridge and the tongue. It extends from the lingual frenum to the retromylohyoid curtain and is a part of the floor of the mouth. (Comp. Prosth.)

gingival s. (Preferred to gingival crevice.) The shallow groove between the gingiva and the surface of a tooth and extending around its circumference. (Oper. Dent.)

— The space between the free gingiva and the tooth, bordered on one side by the tooth surface and on the other side by the sulcular epithelium. Sulcular depths are subject to wide variations, the measurements ranging up to 6 mm under normal conditions. The shallower the sulcus, the more favorable is the maintenance of the health of the sulcus. Every sulcus may be regarded as within the norm regardless of its depth if there are no clinical or microscopic signs of a pathologic condition in the gingival tissues. (Periodont.)

implant g. s. A sulcus around the implant abutment post that resembles the sulcus around a healthy natural tooth. (Oral Implant.)

occlusal s. A groove or spillway on the occlusal surface of a tooth. (Remov. Part. Prosth.)

sulfa (sŭl′fah) (see **sulfonamide**)

sulfhemoglobinemia (sŭlf″hē-mō-glō′bĭ-nē′mē-ah) An abnormality of the heme moiety of the hemoglobin molecule due to inorganic sulfides (e.g., acetanilide). (Oral Med.)

sulfonamide (sŭl-fon′ah-mĭd) A derivative of sulfanilamide that is effective against microorganisms. (Oral Med.; Pharmacol.)

Sulkowitch's test (sŭl′kō-wĭch-ĕz) (see **test, Sulkowitch's**)

summation The phenomenon in which similar actions of more than one drug result in a total action that may be expressed as the arithmetic sum of the effects of the individual drugs. (Oral Med.; Pharmacol.)

summons A writ directed to the sheriff or other proper officer, requiring him to notify the person that an action has been begun against him in the court from which the writ issued and that he is required to appear on a certain day to answer the complaint. (D. Juris.)

superexcitation Excessive excitement. (Anesth.)

superplant A bayonet-shaped bar used as a subperiosteal implant whose purpose it is to serve as an abutment for a free end fixed prosthesis. (Oral Implant.)

supersaturation The addition to or presence of an ingredient in a solution in greater quantity than the solvent can permanently take up. (Periodont.)

superstructure A structure that is constructed on or over another structure. (Implantodont.)

s. casting In the subperiosteal implant, a surgical alloy bar designed with clasps, to telescope over the four abutments. To this casting is processed the final denture superstructure. (Oral Implant.)

implant s. (**implant denture s.**) A removable denture that fits snugly onto the protruding implant abutments. Sometimes called the implant denture. (Oral Implant.)

— The denture that is retained, supported, and stabilized by the implant denture substructure. (Remov. Part. Prosth.)

i. s. attaching material The denture resin by which the superstructure teeth are attached to the superstructure frame. (Oral Implant.)

i. s. attachment Any part of the superstructure that fits onto the implant abutments. May be a precision attachment coping, a conventional clasping, or a combination of precision attachment with clasps. (Oral Implant.)

i. s. connectors The rigid bars that unite the superstructure attachments into one strong element. (Oral Implant.)

i. s., denture (see **superstructure, implant**)

i. s. frame The metal skeleton of the superstructure, consisting of attachments and connnectors. (Oral Implant.)

i. s. teeth The artificial teeth of acrylic resin, metal, or porcelain that establish the occlusion of the superstructure with the opposing denture. (Oral Implant.)

temporary s. (**implant surgical splint**) An acrylic resin immediate appliance with six anterior teeth; has no metal clasps, precision coping, or frame; fitted loosely over the implant abutments immediately after the surgical insertion of the substructure. (Oral Implant.)

supervision The active administering and overseeing of all the functionings of the dental practice and the auxiliaries employed therein. (Pract. Man.)

support Resistance to vertical components of masticatory force in a direction toward the basal seat. (Comp. Prosth.)

ridge s. (see **area, supporting**)

supporting area (see **area, supporting**)

supporting bone (see **bone, cancellous**)

suprabony pocket (see **pocket, suprabony**)

suprabulge The portion of the crown of a tooth that converges toward the occlusal surface from the height of contour or survey line. (Remov. Part. Prosth.)

supraclusion (sū″prah-klū′zhŭn) Abnormally deep overlap of a dental arch or group of teeth over the opposing arch or group of teeth. A position occupied by a tooth that is too high in the line of occlusion. (Orthodont.)

supramentale (sū″prah-mĕn-tā′lē) The most posterior point in the concavity between the infradentale and the pogonion. (Orthodont.)

supraversion (sū″prah-ver′zhŭn) A condition in which teeth or other maxillary structures are situated above or below their normal vertical relationships. (Orthodont.)

surface(s) The outer portion of a mass or object.

basal s. (see **denture, basal surface of**)

buccal s. The side of a tooth or denture adjacent to the cheek. (Comp. Prosth.)

— Any surface adjacent to and facing the cheek. (Remov. Part. Prosth.)

foundation s. (see **denture, basal surface of**)

implant-bearing s. The area of bone that has been selected from the surgical bone impression to be in direct contact with the implant frame. (Oral Implant.)

impression s. (see **denture, basal surface of**)

occlusal s. The superior surface of a mandibular tooth or the inferior surface of a maxillary tooth. The working surface of the posterior teeth. The occluding surfaces of occlusion rims. (Comp. Prosth.) (see also **denture, occlusal surface of**)

— The anatomic surface of the posterior teeth that is limited mesially and distally by the marginal ridges and buccally and lingually by the buccal and lingual boundaries of the cusp eminences. (Periodont.)

balancing o. s. The surfaces of the teeth or denture bases that make contact to provide balancing contacts. (Comp. Prosth.)

working o. s. The surface or surfaces of the teeth on which mastication can occur. (Comp. Prosth.)

proximal s. The surface of a tooth or the portion of a cavity that is nearest to the adjacent tooth. The mesial or distal surface of a tooth. (Oper. Dent.; Periodont.)

smooth s. A surface of a tooth on which pits and fissures are not found normally. (Oper. Dent.)

subocclusal s. That portion of the occlusal surface of a tooth which is below the level of the occluding portion of the tooth. Its purpose is to assist in maintaining food in position on the occlusal surface of the lower teeth. (Comp. Prosth.)

surfactant (sŭr-făk′tănt) A surface-active agent. (Oral Med.; Pharmacol.)

surgeon One whose profession is to cure diseases or injuries by manual operation or by medication. (D. Juris.)

surgery, mucogingival Surgical procedures designed (1) to retain a functionally adequate zone of gingiva after surgical pocket elimination, (2) to create a functionally adequate zone of attached gingiva, (3) to alter the position of, or to eliminate, a frenum, or (4) to deepen the vestibule. (Periodont.)

adequate zone of attached gingiva in m. s. A portion of gingival tissue that will effectively dissipate muscular pull and remain healthy. (Periodont.)

apically repositioned flap in m. s. A surgically created flap of gingival tissue that is repositioned apically to maintain or create a functionally adequate zone of attached gingiva. In the surgical procedure, the existing attached and free gingiva is detached by employing a reverse bevel incision and apically repositioning the flap. (Periodont.)

full flap in m. s. A flap in which all the soft tissue elements are raised and repositioned, as opposed to the split-thickness flap. (Periodont.)

narrow zone of attached gingiva in m. s. (see **surgery, mucogingival, adequate zone of attached gingiva**)

oblique flap in m. s. An increased band of attached gingiva created by preparing a narrow papillary flap (to avoid donor site radicular recession), which is then rotated 90° and sutured into the prepared recipient site. (Periodont.)

pedicle flap in m. s. An increased band of attached gingiva created to repair a cleft by using proximal gingiva situated mesial and distal to the cleft, since gingiva in either location alone is not wide enough to cover the cleft if repositioned. The pedicles are repositioned laterally and sutured. (Also known as double papilla procedure.) (Periodont.)

surgery, osseous The therapeutic surgical measures employed and designed to (1) eliminate osseous deformities by means of ostectomy and or osteoplasty or (2) create a favorable environment by means of meticulous removal of the soft tissue contents of the infrabony osseous defect, for the formation of new bone, periodontal membrane, and cementum to fill in the area of bone resorption. (Periodont.)

access flap in o. s. A full- or split-thickness flap created for the purpose of gaining access to the alveolar bone when surgical remodeling is indicated. This procedure is the method of choice. (Periodont.)

crater in o. s. A troughlike two-walled osseous defect located interdentally at the place where the buccal and lingual walls are intact but the proximal walls are destroyed. (Periodont.)

crestal bone denudation in o. s. After periodontal flap surgery, the area where crestal bone is left exposed when the flap is repositioned. (Periodont.)

hemisepta in o. s. One-walled bony defect due to bone destruction that has left mesial or distal portions of the interdental septum standing alone. (Periodont.)

oral and vestibular defects in o. s. The result of reverse architecture caused by interdental bone resorption, with the result that the oral and vestibular bone margins over roots are left at a more coronal level than the interdental septa. (Periodont.)

periosteal retention in o. s. An infrequently used technique that involves excision of the gingiva or superficial tissues by one of a number of methods and leaves connective tissue covering the bone. (Periodont.)

presurgical preparation in o. s. A step immediately prior to surgery in which pocket depths are rechecked, an effort is made to visualize the alveolar topography, and any other necessary steps are taken to ensure a beneficial result. (Periodont.)

surgical centric registration The recording, after reflection of the overlying soft tissues, of the most retruded position the mandible can occupy from which lateral excursions may be made. This is done just prior to closure during the first surgical stage. (Oral Implant.)

surgical impression The registration of the exposed (host-site) mandibular bone. This is the purpose of the first surgical stage. From the cast made of this impression, the subperiosteal implant is fabricated. (Oral Implant.) (see also **implant, subperiosteal; stage, surgical**)

surgical occlusal rim A prosthodontic appliance used for recording the centric registration. (Oral Implant.) (see also **surgical centric registration**)

surgical preparation (see **preparation, surgical**)

surgical prosthesis (see **prosthesis, surgical**)

surgical template (see **template, surgical**)

surgical tray A prefabricated appliance constructed in advance of the first surgical stage and used for making an impression of the exposed mandibular bone. (Oral Implant.) (see also **stage, surgical**)

survey The study and examination of an area of consideration, of a diagnostic cast, or of a radiograph. (Oral Radiol.; Remov. Part. Prosth.)

s. line (see **line, survey**)

radiation s. Evaluation of the radiation hazards incidental to the production, use, or existence of radioactive materials or other sources of radiation under a specific set of conditions. It customarily includes a physical survey of the arrangement and use of equipment, as well as measurement of the dose rates of radiation under expected conditions of use. (Oral Radiol.)

radiographic s. The production of the minimum number of radiographic examinations necessary for a radiographic interpretation. (Oral Radiol.)

— An examination utilizing radiographs as a means of disclosing conditions that cannot be ascertained by direct or indirect vision. It should always precede any program of mouth rehabilitation. (Remov. Part. Prosth.)

roentgenographic s. (see **survey, radiographic**)

x-ray s. (see **survey, radiographic**)

surveying The procedure of studying the relative parallelism or lack of parallelism of the teeth and associated structures so as to select a path of placement for a restoration that will encounter the least tooth or tissue interference and that will provide adequate and balanced retention; locating guiding plane surfaces to direct placement and removal of the restoration, as well as to achieve the best appearance possible. (Remov. Part. Prosth.)

surveyor An instrument used to determine the relative parallelism of two or more surfaces of teeth or other portions of a cast of the dental arch. (Remov. Part. Prosth.)

Ney s. The paralleling instrument that was the first cast surveyor made available commercially. (Remov. Part. Prosth.)

susceptible The opposite of immune; having little resistance to disease. (Oper. Dent.)

suspension (sŭs-pĕn'shŭn) A mixture of two or more immiscible phases, such as a solid in a liquid or a liquid in a liquid. Suspensions differ from emulsions in that the former usually have to be shaken before each use. (Oral Med.; Pharmacol.)

Sutton's disease (see **periadenitis mucosa necrotica recurrens**)

suture, *n.* A surgical stitch or seam. Materials with which body structures are sewn, as after an operation or injury. (Oral Surg.)

  absorbable s. A suture that becomes dissolved in body fluids and disappears; e.g., catgut. (Oral Surg.)

  approximation s. A suture made to bring about apposition of the deeper tissues of an incision or laceration. (Oral Surg.)

  atraumatic s. A suture swaged into the end of a small eyeless needle. (Oral Surg.)

  button s. A suture passed through buttonlike disks on the skin to prevent the suture from cutting through the soft tissue. (Oral Surg.)

  chromic s. A chromatized sheepgut suture. (Oral Surg.)

  continuous s. A suture in which an uninterrupted length of suture material is used to close an incision or a laceration. (Oral Surg.)

  frontomalar s. Most lateral point of the suture between the frontal and malar bones. (Orthodont.)

  intermaxillary s. (median palatine s.) The line of fusion of the two maxillae, starting between the central incisors and extending posteriorly across the palate, "separating" it into two nearly equal parts. (Periodont.)

  interrupted s. Individual stitches, each tied separately. (Oral Implant.)

  mattress s. A continuous suture that is applied back and forth through the tissues in the same vertical plane but at a different depth or in the same horizontal plane but at the same depth. (Oral Implant.; Oral Surg.)

  median palatine s. (see **suture, intermaxillary**)

  nonabsorbable s. A suture that does not dissolve in body fluids; e.g., silk, tantalum, Nylon. (Oral Surg.)

  purse-string s. A horizontal mattress suture

employed generally about an implant cervix. (Oral Implant.)

  shoelace s. A continuous surgical suture for depression of the tongue and for retaining and holding the lingual flap out of the field of operation during the surgical impression. (Oral Implant.)

—*v.* To sew up a wound. (Oral Surg.)

swage (swāj) To shape metal by adapting or hammering it onto a die. Usually completed by forcing a counterdie into position on a die with the metal sheet interposed. (Comp. Prosth.; Fixed Part. Prosth.; Oper. Dent.; Remov. Part. Prosth.)

— To closely adapt a material to a given die or form. Platinum foil is swaged or closely adapted to a die in a Plasticine swager to form a matrix for a ceramic restoration; a wax pattern is pressed into close contact with the cavity form in a die by encompassing the wax and die in a Plasticine swager or by applying hydraulic pressure in a warm-water swager. (Oper. Dent.)

swager A laboratory instrument used for swaging. (Comp. Prosth.)

  wax s. An instrument used to swage wax to a die. (Oper. Dent.)

swaging A procedure analogous to bone grafting; also referred to as a contiguous autogenous transplant, which involves a greenstick fracturing of bone bordering an infrabony defect as well as displacement of the bone to eliminate the osseous defect. (Periodont.)

swallowing (see **deglutition**)

  s. threshold (see **threshold, swallowing**)

swear To take an oath; to become legally obligated by an oath properly administered. (D. Juris.)

sweat (swĕt) Perspiration. A clear liquid exuded or excreted from the sudoriferous glands. It possesses a characteristic odor, is slightly alkaline, is salty to the taste, and, when mixed with sebaceous secretion, is acid. Sweating is under the control of the sympathetic nervous system, although it can be stimulated by parasympathetic drugs. Thermoregulatory sweating is influenced by the blood temperature's affecting the nervous centers and by reflexes associated with heat receptors in the skin. (Oral Physiol.)

sweating, gustatory (see **syndrome, auriculotemporal**)

swelling, familial intraosseous (see **cherubism**)

Swift's disease (see **erythredema polyneuropathy**)

symbiotic relationship (sĭm"bī-ŏt'ĭk) In implantology, that relationship assumed by an implant and the natural teeth to which it has been splinted; the continuing existence of their relationship is based on their interdependence. (Oral Implant.)

symmetric Evenly balanced or uniformly developed. (Orthodont.)

sympathetic (sĭm″păh-thĕt′ĭk) The sympathetic nervous system. (Anesth.)

sympatholytic (sĭm″pah-thō-lĭt′ĭk) Pertaining to a drug that blocks the effects of stimulation of the sympathetic nervous system. (Anesth.) (see also **adrenolytic**)

sympathomimetic (sĭm″pah-thō-mĭ-mĕt′ĭk) Resembling the effect produced by stimulation of the sympathetic nervous system. (Anesth.) (see also **adrenergic**)

sympathy The art of projecting the feeling of sincere, kindly understanding to a patient. (Pract. Man.)

symptom(s) (sĭmp′tom) Any functional evidence or sign of a condition. (Oral Diag.; Oral Med.; Oral Path.)

    constitutional s. Symptoms related to the systemic effects of a disease; e.g., fever, malaise, anorexia, loss of weight. (Oral Med.)

    diagnostic signs and s. (see **signs and symptoms, diagnostic**)

synalgia (sĭ-năl′jē-ah) Pain felt in a distant part from an injury or stimulation of another part. (Anesth.)

synapse (sĭn′ăps) The region of contact between the processes of two adjacent neurons forming the place where a nervous impulse is transmitted from the axon of one neuron to the dendrites of another. It is called the synaptic junction. The mechanism of transmission is not clearly understood, although it is known to be associated with the chemical alterations of acetylcholine. It has been established, however, that impulses travel in one direction across the synaptic junction and that there is some chemical organization of the dendrite surface that boosts the electrical energy after transport across the synapse. (Oral Physiol.)

synarthrosis (sĭn″ar-thrō′sĭs) A joint formed by thin intervening layers of cartilage, by connective tissue, or by direct contact of bone to bone. It results in a rigid union, and there is little movement of the bones except during growth. Suture lines may be obliterated in adults with a synarthroidal joint when the bones joined together become fused as one bone. (Oral Physiol.)

syncope (sĭng′kō-pē) Swooning or fainting; temporary suspension of consciousness caused by cerebral anemia. (Anesth.)

— A loss of consciousness brought about by a decreased flow of blood to the brain. It may be due to vasovagal factors (e.g., prolonged standing), psychologic reactions to the sight of blood, syringes, etc., hypersensitive carotid sinus, postural hypotension, or cardiac disease. (Oral Med.)

— The sudden transient loss of consciousness of short duration. Frequently the events leading to syncope do not cumulatively cause loss of consciousness. In such instances, lightheadedness, a sinking sensation, numbness in the hands and feet, epigastric or precardial uneasiness, weakness, yawning, and nausea may be the only symptoms. There is facial pallor, the pupils are dilated, and respiration is slow. Fainting is sudden, and the body is limp and motionless. Recovery is achieved usually by placing the patient in a horizontal position. (Oral Physiol.)

— A peripheral cardiovascular collapse accompanied by a transient cerebral anemia causing unconsciousness. (Oral Surg.) (see also **shock**)

syndet (sĭn′dĕt) [*syn*thetic *det*ergent] Synthetic detergent. (Oral Med.; Pharmacol.) (see also **detergent, synthetic**)

syndrome (sĭn′drōm) A group of signs and symptoms that occur together and characterize a disease. Many syndromes are pertinent to oral surgery. (Oral Surg.)

    Adams-Stokes s. (see **disease, Adams-Stokes**)

    adaptation s. (see **disease, adaptation; syndrome, general adaptation**)

    adrenogenital s. Disorders of sexual development or function associated with abnormal adrenocortical function due to bilateral adrenal hyperplasia, carcinoma, or adenoma. Pseudohermaphroditism occurs congenitally, and masculinization occurs later in females. Precocious sexual development and occasionally feminization occur in males. (Oral Med.)

    Albright's s. A polyostotic form of fibrous dysplasia, usually associated with precocious puberty in females, endocrine disturbance influencing growth, and brown pigmentation of the skin. (Oral Diag.)

— A combination of a rare type of fibrous dysplasia, brown-pigmented areas of the skin, and occasionally the oral mucosa, and precocious sexual and somatic development in females. (Oral Med.)

— A symptom complex consisting of polyostotic fibrous dysplasia, skin pigmentation in the form of café-au-lait spots, endocrine dysfunction, and precocious puberty in females. (Oral Path.)

AHOP s. Adiposity, hyperthermia, oligomenorrhea, and parotitis appearing in females. Parotid gland enlargement begins at puberty and is followed by obesity, oligomenorrhea, and psychic disturbances. (Oral Med.)

Apert's s. (**acrocephalosyndactyly**) A congenital malformation consisting of pointed head and syndactyly of all four extremities. (Oral Diag.)

— Craniostenosis characterized by oxycephaly and syndactyly of the hands and feet. Facies manifestations include exophthalmos, high prominent forehead, small nose, and malformation of the mandible and mouth. (Oral Med.)

Ascher's s. Syndrome consisting of double lip, a redundance of the skin of the eyelids (blepharochalasis), and nontoxic thyroid enlargement. The sagging eyelids are obvious when the eyes are open and the double lip is seen when the patient smiles. (Oral Med.)

auriculotemporal c. (aw-rĭk″ū-lō-tĕm′pō-ral) (**Bogarad's s., Frey's s., Frey-Baillarger s., gustatory hyperhidrosis s., gustatory lacrimation, gustatory sweating s.**) The syndrome of lacrimation that accompanies eating. The patient usually notices that when he is eating, tears flow from the eye on the affected side. (Cleft Palate)

— Sweating and flushing in the preauricular and temporal areas when certain foods are eaten. May be related to parotid trauma or a complication of parotidectomy. (Oral Med.)

— Postsurgical sweating and flushing of the skin over a localized area occurring or associated with mastication. (Oral Surg.)

autoimmunization s. (see **disease, autoimmune**)

Behçet's s. (bā′sĕts) (**Behçet's disease**) A virus-induced disease characterized by oral aphthae, iridocyclitis, and genital ulcerations. (Oral Diag.)

— Recurrent iritis and aphthous ulcers of the mouth and genitalia. Other manifestations include arthralgia, hydrarthrosis, swelling of the salivary glands, cutaneous eruptions, and central nervous system disorders. (Oral Med.)

— A form of erythema multiforme in which oral, optical, and genital lesions are present. (Oral Path.)

Bloch-Sulzberger s. (**incontinentia pigmenti**) Syndrome in which there are pigmented skin lesions, defects of the eyes and central nervous system, skeletal anomalies, and hypoplasia of the teeth. (Oral Med.)

Bogarad s. (see **syndrome, auriculotemporal**)

Böök's s. Syndrome characterized by premature graying of the hair, hyperhidrosis, and premolar hypodontia. (Oral Med.)

Bourneville-Pringle s. (**epiloia**) Neurocutaneous complex consisting of adenoma sebaceum, mental deficiency, and epilepsy. (Oral Med.)

Caffey-Silverman s. (see **hyperostosis, infantile cortical**)

Christ-Siemens-Touraine s. (see **hypohidrotic ectodermal dysplasia**)

Costen's s. Various symptoms of discomfort, pain, or jaw pathosis claimed by Costen to be caused by lack of posterior occlusion, loss of vertical dimension, malocclusion, trismus, or muscle tremor. (Comp. Prosth.; Remov. Part. Prosth.)

cri-du-chat s. Clinical syndrome associated with the deletion of the short arm of a B chromosome. Manifestations include mental retardation, various congenital abnormalities, and an infant cry resembling the mewing of a cat. (Oral Med.)

crocodile tears s. A syndrome in which a spontaneous lacrimation occurs with the normal salivation of eating. It follows facial paralysis and seems to be due to straying of the regenerating nerve fibers, some of those destined for the salivary glands going to the lacrimal glands. (Oral Surg.)

Crouzon's s. (see **dysostosis, craniofacial**)

Cushing's s. (**Cushing's disease**) A symptom complex associated with an excess of adrenal steroids of all types due to hyperplasia of the adrenal cortex, malignant neoplasms, pituitary basophilia, or prolonged administration of ACTH. Manifestations include hypertension, buffalo obesity, diabetes mellitus, osteoporosis, purple striae of the skin in areas of tension, and disorders of glucose tolerance. (Oral Med.)

Down's s. (see **mongolism**)

Ehlers-Danlos s. A congenital or familial disorder characterized by fragility of the skin and blood vessels, hyperlaxity of the joints, hyperelasticity of the skin, subcutaneous pseudotumors, and a tendency to hemorrhage postoperatively. (Oral Med.)

Ekman's s. (see **osteogenesis imperfecta**)

Ellis–van Creveld s. (see **chondroectodermal dysplasia**)

Feer's s. (see **acrodynia**)

Frey-Baillarger s. (see **syndrome, auriculotemporal**)

Fröhlich's s. Adiposity and genital hypoplasia due to hypopituitarism or hypothalamohypophyseal dystrophy. (Oral Med.)

Gardner's s. Multiple osteomas, multiple polyposis of the large bowel, multiple epidermoid or sebaceous cysts, and multiple cutaneous fibromas. (Oral Med.)

— A hereditary condition manifested by multiple osteomas, epidermoid cysts, and dermoid tumors and polyposis of the bowel. (Oral Path.)

general adaptation s. (**adaptation s., GAS**) A three-stage physiologic response to physical or psychologic stress. The first stage is the *alarm* reaction, consisting of bodily changes typical of emotion. A second stage is *resistance to stress*, wherein an attempt is made to adapt to the physiologic changes. Certain hormones of the anterior pituitary gland and the adrenal cortex hypersecrete to increase resistance. Such resistance leads to diseases of adaptation, such as hypertension. Continual stress results in the third stage, *exhaustion*. (Oral Med.)

— The response of the body to stress. The response involves the entire organism, and all physiologic parts are closely related in terms of reaction. Stress may be caused by hemorrhage, wound, pain, radiation, nutritional deficiency, or psychic trauma. It may originate in the oral cavity and cause a general body reaction. Conversely, a nonspecific stress such as nutritional deficiency may cause a general body reaction, and the periodontium, for example, may also become a target organ. (Oral Physiol.)

Goldscheider's s. Dystrophic form of epidermolysis bullosa, leading to scars. The disturbance is inherited on an autosomal dominant or recessive basis. The form leading to retardation of mental and physical growth. (Oral Med.) (see also **syndrome, Weber-Cockayne**)

Greig's s. A condition manifested by ocular hypertelorism, often mental retardation, ectodermal and mesodermal abnormalities, and dental and oral anomalies. (Oral Med.)

Gunn's s. (**jaw-winking s.**) Movements of the upper eyelid in association with jaw movements. (Oral Surg.)

gustatory hyperhidrosis s. (see **syndrome, auriculotemporal**)

gustatory sweating s. (see **syndrome, auriculotemporal**)

Heerfordt's s. (see **fever, uveoparotid**)

Horner's s. A tetrad of symptoms due to paralysis of the cervical sympathetic trunk: (1) pupillary constriction; (2) ptosis of upper eyelid; (3) dilation of orbital blood vessels (redness of conjunctiva); and (4) blushing and anhidrosis of side of face. (Oral Physiol.)

Hunt's s. Herpetic inflammation of the geniculate ganglion, with herpes zoster of the soft palate, anterior tonsillar pillar, and auricular area. (Oral Med.; Oral Surg.) (see also **herpes zoster**)

Hurler's s. (**mucopolysaccharidosis I, gargoylism, dysostosis multiplex**) A heritable disorder of mucopolysaccharide metabolism in which excessive acid mucopolysaccharides—dermatan sulfate and heparitin sulfate—are made and stored in the tissues. Clinical manifestations include hypertelorism, open mouth with large-appearing tongue, thick eyelids and lips, anomalies of the teeth, and short, broad neck. The skeletal and facial deformities resemble the gargoyles of Gothic architecture. Mental retardation, corneal clouding, hepatosplenomegaly, deafness, and cardiac defects are present. (Oral Med.)

Hutchinson-Gilford s. (**progeria**) Syndrome of dwarfism, immaturity, and pseudosenility. Patient appears to be bald and elderly at an early age. There is hypoplasia of the mandible, and the face is small in relation to the neurocranium. (Oral Diag.; Oral Med.)

jaw-winking s. (**winking-jaw s.**) Congenital unilateral ptosis and elevation of the lid on opening of the jaw or moving of the mandible to the contralateral side. (Oral Med.)

Klinefelter's s. (**XXY s., chromatin-positive s., medullary gonadal dysgenesis**) Presence in men of an abnormal sex-chromosome constitution. Persons with XXY constitution show the clinical signs of sterility, aspermatogenesis, variable gynecomastia, and often mental retardation. About 50% of subjects with XXXXY variant have cleft palate. (Oral Med.)

Klippel-Feil s. Fusion of cervical vertebrae, short neck with limited head movement, and extension of the posterior hairline. (Oral Med.)

Lobstein's s. (see **osteogenesis imperfecta**)

Marfan's s. Tall, thin stature, long, tapered fingers and toes (arachnodactyly), dislocation of the lens of the eye (ectopia lentis), and aneurysm leading to rupture of the aorta. (Oral Med.)

Melkersson-Rosenthal s. Transient facial edema, especially swelling of the upper lip, facial paralysis, and lingua plicata. Plicated swelling of the mucosa of the tongue, palate, and buccal mucosa may not be present, or the paralysis may be incomplete. (Oral Med.)

Mikulicz' s. A condition characterized by swelling of the parotid, submandibular, sublingual, and lacrimal glands; associated with lymphosarcoma, leukemia, tuberculosis, sarcoidosis, or syphilis. (Oral Diag.)

— Enlargement of the salivary glands and lymph nodes due to a generalized disease such as lymphoma. (Oral Med.)

— Enlargement of the salivary glands due to leukemic infiltration, lymphosarcoma, or tuberculosis. (Oral Path.)

Möbius' s. Congenital facial diplegia consisting of facial paralysis as well as lingual and masticatory muscle paralysis, inability to abduct the eyes, and anomalies of the extremities. (Oral Med.)

myeloproliferative s. Extramedullary myelopoiesis in adults. It may follow contact with benzol compounds or polycythemia, or it may precede leukemia. (Oral Med.)

nephrotic s. (ně-frot'ĭk) Syndrome that includes proteinuria, hyperlipemia, hypoproteinemia, and edema. It occurs in a variety of conditions in which there is increased glomerular permeability and urinary loss of protein. (Oral Med.)

nonarticular pain s. One of several painful disorders that limit joint motion and that affect the periarticular structures: the tendons, tendon sheaths, bursae, connective tissue, and muscles. Patients commonly call this syndrome muscular aches and pains. The pains are chronic and nagging and may occur in acute exacerbations. The neck, shoulder, back, thighs, hands, and legs are common sites of irritation. The nonarticular disorders are associated with fibrositis, tenonitis, tenosynovitis, and periarticular muscle spasm. The precipitating agents are frequently obscure and may be associated with postural or personality disorders. When the acute symptoms of pain, stiffness, and restricted motion are reduced, the tissues resume their normal function. The common temporomandibular joint syndrome is thought to be caused by a postural occlusal

imbalance associated with the muscular tension induced by psychologic stress. The combination precipitates an acute muscle spasm in the muscles associated with the protection and movement of the joint. (Oral Physiol.)

paratrigeminal s. Trigeminal neuralgia, sensory loss, weakness and atrophy of the masticatory muscles, miosis, and ptosis of the upper eyelid on the affected side of the face due to a lesion of the semilunar ganglion and fibers of the carotid plexus. (Oral Med.)

Papillon-Lefevre s. Syndrome in which dental manifestations include loss of alveolar and supporting bone and premature exfoliation of primary teeth. Hyperkeratosis of the palmar surfaces of the hands and plantar surfaces of the feet is evident. Autosomal recessive mode of inheritance. (Pedodont.)

— Extensive periodontal disease (juvenile periodontosis) in young patients accompanied by keratotic lesions of the palmar and plantar surfaces. In some patients changes similar to hereditary ectodermal dysplasia are also present. (Oral Diag.)

— Syndrome consisting of hyperkeratosis of the palms and soles and severe periodontitis involving the primary and permanent dentitions. (Oral Med.)

Patau's s. (see **trisomy-D**)

Paterson-Kelly s. (see **syndrome, Plummer-Vinson**)

Peutz-Jegher s. Generalized multiple polyposis of the intestinal tract, consistently involving the jejunum, and associated with melanin spots of the lips, buccal mucosa, and fingers; autosomal dominant inheritance. (Oral Diag.; Oral Med.)

PHC s. (see **syndrome, Böök's**)

Pierre Robin s. (pē-air' ro'băn) A congenital defect, probably recessive (incomplete dominant), characterized by micrognathia, microglossia with retraction or prolapse, and cleft palate. (Oral Med.)

— Micrognathia of the newborn. Congenital retrognathism associated with cleft palate, glossoptosia, difficulty in swallowing, respiratory obstruction, and cyanosis. This congenital micrognathia will correct itself during the growth of the child if proper care is provided. (Oral Surg.)

Plummer-Vinson s. A group of symptoms seen in women past middle age; characterized by anemia, dysphagia, and atrophy of the oral mucosa, tongue, and upper gastrointestinal tract. (Oral Diag.)

— Syndrome consisting of dysphagia, atrophy of the oral mucosa, xerostomia, glossopyrosis, spoon-shaped fingernails, and hypochromic microcytic anemia. Hyperkeratotic lesions and mucosal changes predispose to the development of carcinoma. (Oral Med.)

— A symptom complex that includes fissures at the corners of the mouth, sore tongue, dysphagia, achlorhydria, and iron-deficiency anemia. Most comonly seen in females in the fourth and fifth decades of life and associated with a predisposition to carcinoma of the oral cavity and esophagus. (Oral Path.)

— A syndrome characterized by dysphagia, glossitis, hypochromic anemia, atrophic oral mucosa, and a marked propensity for the formation of oral carcinoma. (Oral Surg.)

Reiter's s. A syndrome that consists of arthritis (often of the rheumatoid type), conjunctivitis, nonspecific urethritis, and occasionally aphthous ulcers of the oral mucusa. (Oral Med.)

Rieger's s. Characteristics include hypodontia, conical crowns, enamel hypoplasia, dysgenesis of the iris and cornea, and myotonic dystrophy. (Oral Med.)

Riley-Day s. (familial dysautonomia) Disturbances of the autonomic and central nervous systems consisting of hypersalivation, defective lacrimation, excessive sweating, erythematous blotching after emotional upset, relative indifference to pain, and hyporeflexia. Normal growth and motor development are retarded. (Oral Med.)

Robin's s. (see **syndrome, Pierre Robin**)

Roger's s. Continuous excessive secretion of saliva as the result of cancer of the esophagus or other esophageal irritation. (Oral Surg.)

Rosenthal's s. (see **hemophilia C**)

rubella s. Enamel defects of the primary teeth attributed to prolonged effect of the rubella virus on ameloblasts during fetal life and in the postnatal period. (Oral Med.)

Scheuthauer-Marie-Sainton s. (see **cleidocranial dysostosis**)

sicca s. (see **syndrome, Sjögren's**)

Sjögren's s. (sicca s., xerodermosteosis) Acute recurrent swelling of the salivary glands associated with dry mouth, conjunctivitis sicca, and sometimes arthritis. (Oral Diag.)

— Condition related to deficient secretion of salivary, sweat, lacrimal, and mucous glands (xerostomia, keratoconjunctivitis, rhinitis, dysphagia), increased size of salivary glands, and polyarthritis. (Oral Med.)

— A syndrome characterized by dryness of all mucous membranes, swelling of the salivary glands, and polyarthritis. (Oral Path.)

Smyth's s. (see **hyperostosis, infantile cortical**)

Stevens-Johnson s. An acute inflammatory disease characterized by oral, ocular, and genital lesions with severe generalized symptoms. The oral lesions are irregularly shaped, painful ulcers. (Oral Diag.) (see also **erythema multiforme**)

— A symptom complex similar to erythema multiforme, with constitutional symptoms and vesicular, ulcerative, and bullous lesions of the oral mucosa, conjunctiva, genitalia, and skin. (Oral Med.)

— Clinical term that applies to a symptom complex consisting of oral lesions that may be vesicular or ulcerative and conjunctivitis with photophobia and cutaneous lesions that may be vesicular, bullous, or hemorrhagic. The etiology is unknown. (Oral Path.)

Sturge-Weber s. An encephalofacial angiomatosis characterized by cutaneous facial cerebral angiomatosis, ipsilateral gyriform calcifications of the brain, mental retardation, seizures (epilepsy), contralateral hemiplegia, and ocular involvement. Facial lesions (port-wine stain) may join intraoral angiomas on the buccal mucosa and gingiva. (Oral Med.)

Swift's s. (see **acrodynia**)

temporomandibular joint s. An acute muscle spasm in the muscles associated with the protection and movement of the joint. It is thought to be caused by a postural (occlusal) imbalance associated with the muscular tension induced by psychologic stress. The principal symptoms are pain in the region of the joint, limitation of mobility of the mandible, crepitus, clicking sounds in the joint, and frequently tinnitus. Thus, disability of the joint arises principally from the effect on the mobility of the mandible and its associated musculoskeletal structure. The etiology may be organic, functional, or both as a result of degenerative changes in the joint mechanism, the musculoskeletal system, or the nervous system. It may also result from hormonal dysfunction, surgical or traumatic impairment, dentoalveolar disease, agenesis, and/or disorganized dental occlusion. (Oral Physiol.)

thalassemia s. (**Cooley's anemia, Mediterranean anemia, hereditary leptocytosis**) Any of a group of closely related and genetically determined disorders in which there is a specific decrease in one of the polypeptide chains comprising hemoglobin. The defect results in hypochromic microcytic erythrocytes. There are alpha, beta, and delta variants as well as several subtypes based on biochemical techniques. (Oral Med.) (see also **thalassemia**)

Treacher Collins s. An incomplete mandibulofacial dysostosis in which there are congenital deformities of the eyelids, mandible, and malar bones, and malocclusion, cleft lip and palate, and nasal deformities. (Oral Med.)

Turner's s. (**XO s., gonadal dysgenesis, genital dwarfism**) Absence of one of the X chromosomes, with affected females being sterile and short of stature and having various congenital anomalies such as webbing of the neck, low-set ears, wide-set eyes, shieldlike chest, absence of breasts, and cubitus valgus. Common orofacial findings are hypoplastic mandible, high palatal vault, and dental anomalies. (Oral Med.)

Ullrich-Feichtiger s. Micrognathia, polydactyly, and genital malformations. (Oral Med.)

Urbach-Wiethe s. Hyalinosis of the skin and mucous membranes and hoarseness. The skin is infiltrated with yellowish waxy nodules and the oral tissues with similar plaques beginning before puberty and becoming increasingly severe. The teeth may be hypoplastic or may fail to develop. (Oral Med.)

vestibular disorder s. One of several syndromes involving the vestibule of the ear. The two most common syndromes of vestibular disorders are seasickness, which is due to the continuous movement of the endolymph in susceptible individuals (probably related to a disturbance in the reflex control of the eyeball movements), and Menière's syndrome, in which paroxysmal vertigo is the principal sign, but there are other associated vascular and metabolic disorders. When a patient suffers an acute attack of vertigo, he should be placed in a prone position with the position of the head varied from time to time. An appropriate hypnotic agent may be administered to the patient, and he should be sent home with a member of the family. (Oral Physiol.)

Waardenburg-Klein s. A syndrome consisting of congenital deafness, white forelock, increased distance between the inner canthi, the iris of the same eye or of the two eyes having different color (heterochromic irides), and prognathism. Inherited as an autosomal dominant disorder. (Oral Med.)

Weber-Cockayne s. Simple nonscarring form of epidermolysis bullosa; transmitted as an autosomal dominant trait. (Oral Med.) (see also **syndrome, Goldscheider's**)

Weech's s. (see **hypohidrotic ectodermal dysplasia**)

Witkop–von Sallman s. Hereditary benign intraepithelial dyskeratosis with gelatinous plaques on hyperemic bulbar conjunctiva and white folds and plaques involving the oral mucosa. (Oral Med.)

Zinsser-Engman-Cole s. Syndrome consisting of reticular atrophy of the skin, with pigmentation, dystrophic fingernails and toenails, and oral leukoplakia. Hyperhidrosis of the palms and soles is present, as well as acrocyanosis of the hands and feet. (Oral Med.)

syneresis (sĭ-nĕr'ĕ-sĭs) The exuding of water, as by a gel when stored. Associated with the hydrocolloid impression materials. (D. Mat.)

— A process by which a fluid exudate forms on the surface of a hydrocolloid gel, even when the gel is in water or in a humid atmosphere. It is accompanied by shrinkage of the gel. (Remov. Part. Prosth.)

synergism (sĭn'er-jĭzm) The ability of two drugs to increase the action of each other to an extent greater than the action of each when used alone. (Anesth.)

— Joint action of two drugs in such a manner that one supplements or enhances the action of the other to produce an effect greater than that which can be obtained with either one of the drugs in equivalent quantity, or to produce two or more effects that could not be obtained with any safe quantity of either drug, or both. (Oral Med.; Pharmacol.) (see also **potentiation**)

synthetic porcelain (see **cement, silicate**)

syphilid (sĭf'ĭ-lĭd) A cutaneous lesion of syphilis. (Oral Med.)

syphilis (sĭf'ĭ-lĭs) (**lues**) A contagious disease caused by *Treponema pallidum*. Oral lesions include the primary chancre, the secondary mucous patches and split papule, and the tertiary gumma. Congenital syphilis may lead to Hutchinson's incisors, mulberry molars, or rhagades. (Oral Diag.)

— A disease caused by the spirochete *Treponema pallidum* and manifested in three stages, producing a wide variety of cutaneous, osseous, vascular, mucosal, and nervous lesions. (Oral Med.)

— A contagious venereal disease due to *Treponema pallidum* and usually transmitted by direct contact. (Oral Path.) (see also **chancre; gumma; incisors, Hutchinson's; molar, mulberry; patch, mucous; Treponema pallidum**)

— A venereal disease due to the spirochetal microorganism *Treponema pallidum*. The primary lesion is the chancre. With spread of infection via the lymphatics to the skin and mucous membranes, a maculopapular rash will occur on dermal surfaces, with mucous patches present on mucosal surfaces. Tertiary stages involve gumma formation, with lesions occurring in bone, abdominal viscera, aorta, central nervous system, etc. Diagnosis is confirmed by serologic tests, dark-field examinations, etc. (Periodont.)

latent s. A stage of syphilis in which there are no clinical signs or symptoms of the disease. It is usually discovered by serologic tests. (Oral Med.)

Syrette (sǐ-rĕt′) Trade name for a small hypodermic syringe containing a dose of the drug to be administered. (Anesth.)

syringe (sǐ-rǐnj′; sǐr′ǐnj) An apparatus of metal, glass, or plastic material consisting of a nozzle, barrel, and plunger or rubber bulb; used to inject a liquid into a cavity or under the skin. (Anesth.)

air s. A device by which air may be applied to a given area. An instrument supplied as part of the dental unit, consisting of a hand grip, nozzle, pressure-regulating valve, and hose connected to the compressed air supply. It has a clamping device for the attachment of an air tip or a spray bottle. (Oper. Dent.)

hand a. s. An air syringe consisting of a metal tube bent at one end, terminating in a reduced diameter, and enlarged at the other end to engage a rubber bulb. The bulb is compressed by hand to supply a controlled spurt of air to a given area. The metal tip may be warmed so that the air will be correspondingly heated. Used to clear debris or moisture from a cavity, wax pattern, etc. (Oper. Dent.)

warm a. s. An air syringe equipped with an electric heating element to heat the room air to any desired temperature. (Oper. Dent.)

water s. A device, usually part of the dental unit, permitting controlled application of water to a given area. It has a flow control, pressure regulator, and heating element. (Oper. Dent.)

system A set or series of organs or parts that unite in a common function.

acid-base buffer s. The system by which a virtually constant pH of the blood and body fluids is maintained. The base and acid electrolytes associated with normal metabolism are continuously introduced into the bloodstream. Notwithstanding the marked amounts of base or acid or both introduced into the bloodstream during exercise, rest, hunger, or the ingestion of fluid and solid foods, the pH of the blood remains rather constant between the ranges of pH 7.3 and 7.5. There are four means by which this relatively narrow but constant pH is maintained: the buffer system of the blood, the tissue and cell fluids, and the mineral salts of the bone matrix; the excretion and retention of carbon dioxide by the lungs; the excretion of an acid or alkaline urine; and the formation or excretion of ammonia and/or organic compounds. (Oral Physiol.)

apothecaries′ s. A nondecimal system of weights and measures traditionally employed by druggists. (Oral Med.; Pharmacol.) (see also **system, avoirdupois**)

autonomic nervous s. The part of the nervous system that regulates the reflex control of bodily functions. It controls the functioning of glands, smooth muscle, and the heart. (Anesth.)

— An aggregation of peripheral nerves, ganglia, and plexuses situated outside the central nervous system. It provides the motor innervation for the viscera, glands, heart, blood vessels, and other smooth muscle structures of the body. The arrangement of the autonomic nerves is more complex and diffuse than the arrangement of the segmental spinal nerves with which they are intimately connected in both structure and function. The autonomic nerves are distributed widely over the body, but they are particularly concentrated in the regions of the head and neck and in the thoracic and abdominal cavities. (Oral Physiol.)

avoirdupois s. A commercial nondecimal system of weights and measures. (D. Mat.) (see also **system, apothecaries′**)

central nervous s. The brain and the spinal cord, including their nerves and end-organs; controls all voluntary acts. (Anesth.)

circulatory s., functions A conduction system

with a complex arrangement of vessels, or tubes, for the transport of metabolites to and from tissue cells. The metabolites are transported in solution in the blood fluid or in chemical union with blood cells. The circulatory system has several secondary but very important functions: to facilitate maintenance of fairly stable internal environment of the tissue cells; to be a reservoir for chemical buffers; to regulate body temperature; to provide bacteriostatic protection; to aid in repair of disease and injury; and to act as an accessory nervous system by the rapid circulation of endocrine secretions. (Oral Physiol.)

circulatory s., structures The heart and the blood vessels. There are three major groups of blood vessels: the arteries, the capillaries, and the veins. The arteries conduct the blood away from the heart; they vary in dimension and structure in accordance with their location and function. The capillaries are the reservoir for interchanges of blood fluid and metabolites between the vascular system and the tissue cells and also between the arterial and venous systems. The veins are the vessels that conduct the blood fluids back to the heart for recirculation. The heart, arteries, capillaries, and veins form a closed circulatory system in which the blood is continuously recirculated throughout life. (Oral Physiol.)

hematopoietic s. Term used to describe collectively the blood, bone marrow, lymph nodes, spleen, and reticuloendothelial cells. (Oral Med.)

masticatory s. The organs and structures primarily functioning in mastication: the jaws, the teeth and their supporting structures, the temporomandibular articulation, the mandibular musculature, the tongue, the lips, the cheeks, and the oral mucosa. (Comp. Prosth.; Orthodont.; Remov. Part. Prosth.)

metric s. A decimal system of weights and measures almost universally used in scientific and professional work, including the writing of perscriptions. The individual units are based on an international set of standards, notably the meter, the liter, and the kilogram. For details see the appendix. (Oral Med.; Pharmacol.)

musculoskeletal s. The system of body structures that provides the energy and movement necessary for the functions of life. The muscles, bones, and connective tissues

of the body are grouped together into one system, and they are intimately connected in their individual and combined functions; e.g., in order for muscle to accomplish its ultimate purpose of movement by contraction, bone, leverage, and connective tissue are required to transmit the force that the contraction generates. In the oral cavity and its related structures the musculoskeletal tissues fulfill the mechanical and structural requirements for movement of the mandible and for some related visceral functions such as respiration and digestion. (Oral Physiol.)

neurohormonal s. (nū″rō-hōr′mō-nal) The system by which the hormone secretions of the endocrine glands function, in part, as the regulator of both visceral and somatic function and have intimate anatomic and functional relationships with the nervous system by the union of the pituitary gland and the hypothalamus of the cerebrum. The pituitary gland has a pars nervosa, which is an extension of the anterior part of the hypothalamus, and a pars intermedia, which is an epithelial evagination of the secretory tissue from the stomodeum of the embryo. From its position in the cranial structures in the sella turcica, the pituitary gland regulates, by its union with the nervous system, the whole endocrine system with its many glands; these glands, in turn, partially regulate the viscera and the somatic muscle organs. (Oral Physiol.)

occlusal s. (occlusal scheme) The form or design and arrangement of the occlusal and incisal units of a dentition or of the teeth on a denture. (Comp. Prosth.; Remov. Part. Prosth.)

parasympathetic nervous s. One of the motor divisions of the autonomic nervous system. It is described as the craniosacral division and does not have the simplified structural apparatus of the strong sympathetic adrenal axis about which to function. The parasympathetic system inhibits the heart, contracts the pupils, and, in emotional states, produces a vagus-insulin axis of activity. The several parts function rather independently. The ocular division relates to the midbrain, and the bulbar division relates to the hindbrain. The bulbar division supplies the facial, glossopharyngeal, and vagus nerves. It also supplies the secretory and the vasodilator fibers of the salivary glands and the mucous membranes of the mouth and pharynx. In conditions of very loud noise or unusual anxiety states, the parasympathetic system will cause unaccounted-for spontaneous urination, excessive salivary and gastric juices, and either nausea or vomiting. (Oral Physiol.)

proaccelerin-accelerin s. (see **factor V**)

proconvertin-convertin s. (see **factor VII**)

stomatognathic s. The combination of all the structures involved in speech, and the reception, mastication, and deglutition of food. The system is composed of the teeth, jaws, muscles of mastication, and temporomandibular joints, and the nerves that control these structures. (Comp. Prosth.; Gnathol.; Periodont.; Remov. Part. Prosth.)

sympathetic nervous s. One of the two opposing motor systems in the autonomic nervous system that mediate the activity of the viscera. (The other is the parasympathetic system.) The sympathetic system is composed of 21 or 22 ganglia in chains on each side of the spinal cord. The fibers connect with the spinal cord through these ganglia. The actions of the sympathetic division of the autonomic nervous system are closely allied to the action of the medulla of the adrenal gland; thus a sympathetic-adrenal axis that functions as a unit to protect and regulate the body environment may be conceived. The sympathetic control is modified by the volitional somatic control of the patient. The volitional control, superimposed on the autonomic control, gives rise to great variations in motor patterns, as seen in the face in the presence of emotional changes, such as in the blushing of shame and the pallor of fear. (Oral Physiol.)

vascular s., closed tube The type of vascular system, as in humans, in which the blood circulates through the vessels (or tubes) and is not dissipated into the tissues. The closed vascular tube system offers resistance to the pumping action of the heart because the pressures are cumulative with each pumping action. The elastic walls in the arterial vessels, particularly in the aorta, absorb the additional energy and release its slowly, thus creating the possibility of mantaining a fairly steady and safe pressure head throughout the vascular system. The high-pressure point at the height of cardiac contraction is the systole, and the low point before the ventricular contraction is the diastole. (Oral Physiol.)

vascular s., open tube In some vertebrates, a vascular system with an open end that causes the blood fluid to dissipate into the tissues. This system starts with a maximum head pressure that diminishes until inertia in the blood is overcome. The blood is returned to the heart by muscle function, gravity, and diffusion. The blood pressure in this system fluctuates from a maximum at the heart to a minimum at the tissue cell. (Oral Physiol.)

venous s. A system of interconnected blood vessels that returns blood to the heart from the tissue and capillary bed through progressively larger vessels. The following affect the return of blood to the heart: thoracic pressure, associated with respiration; gravity, associated with body posture; the valves, the diameter of the lumen, and the muscle structure of the veins; muscle contraction of the somatic structures; the pressures in the arteriole system and the capillary bed; and the nervous and hormonal system controls that regulate cardiomuscular activity. The influences over the venous system circulation are collectively termed venopressor mechanisms. (Oral Physiol.)

systematically Done in a well-organized, carefully followed pattern of procedure. (Pract. Man.)

systole (sĭs'tō-lē) The period of contraction of the heart. The term specifically designates the contraction of the ventricles as distinguished from auricular contraction. It occurs synchronously with the first heart sound. The pressure from the systolic contractions is taken up and stored as potential energy by the elastic properties of the aorta and other great vessels of the arterial system. This storage of energy protects the smaller, more fragile vessels from undue pressure. The even flow and steady pressure of the blood are sustained by the controlled release of the potential energy stored in the arterial walls into kinetic energy for movement of the blood during the diastolic phase of heart function. The pressure recorded at the height of the ventricular contraction is the systolic pressure. In the adult, the normal blood pressure is 120/80 mm Hg (systolic/diastolic). It rises with advancing age to 135/89 at 60 years of age. (Oral Physiol.)

T

tabes dorsalis (tā′bēz dor-sā′lĭs) (**locomotor ataxia**) Degeneration of the dorsal tracts of the spinal cord, with loss of reflexes, incoordination, and other symptoms; caused by syphilis. (Oral Diag.)
— A form of neurosyphilis in which there is degeneration in the posterior roots of the spinal nerves and posterior column of the spinal cord. Manifestations include pains and paresthesias of the trunk, hands, and feet, abdominal pain crises, ataxia, Argyll Robertson pupil, atrophy of the optic nerve, and Charcot's joint. (Oral Med.; Oral Physiol.)

table, occlusal The occlusal surfaces of the bicuspids and molars; the basic collective topography including the form of the cusps, inclined planes, marginal ridges, and central fossae and grooves of the teeth. (Periodont.)
— Term referring to the total surface provided for occlusion by a complete or partial denture. In unworn teeth it is considerably narrower than the greatest buccolingual dimensions of the crown. Sometimes it is only about one half as great. (Comp. Prosth.; Fixed Part. Prosth.; Remov. Part. Prosth.)

tachycardia (tăk″ē-kar′dē-ah) Excessively rapid action of the heart; the pulse rate is usually above 100 beats/min. (Anesth.; Oral Surg.)

tachyphylaxis (tăk″ē-fĭ-lăk′sĭs) A decreasing response that follows consecutive injections at short intervals. (Anesth.)
— The rapid development of tolerance on administration of closely spaced successive doses of a drug or poison. (Oral Med.; Pharmacol.)

tachypnea (tăk-ĭp-nē′ah) Excessively rapid respiration. A respiratory neurosis marked by quick, shallow breathing. (Anesth.)

tailpiece (see **aid, speech, prosthetic, velar section**)

Takahara's disease (see **disease, Takahara's**)

take the bite Although objectionable in prosthetics, a term that is a more common and briefer descriptive term than others. In operative dentistry, it refers to the step in the making of an individual inlay wherein a registration is made, usually with inlay wax, of the occlusal relationships and the contact areas involved in the restoration. This interocclusal record (bite) becomes an integral part of the wax pattern of the cavity preparation. (Oper. Dent.) (see also **record, interocclusal**)

tang (see **connector, minor**)

tank, processing A receptacle used in the photographic or radiographic darkroom for the chemical solutions employed in the processing of films. (Oral Radiol.)

tantalum (tăn′tah-lŭm) A noncorrosive, malleable metal used for plates and devices to bridge bony defects, or as a wire mesh for sutures. (Oral Surg.)

tape, dental A ribbon of waxed nylon or silk used to aid the prophylaxis of interproximal spaces and the proximal surfaces of the teeth. The flattened, wide form of dental floss. (Oper. Dent.)

tapering A process of so shaping a clasp arm as to better distribute flexure throughout its length, thus reducing fatigue, strain-hardening, and resultant fracture. (Remov. Part. Prosth.)
t. arch (see **arch, tapering**)

target The small tungsten block, embedded in the face of the anode, that is bombarded by electrons from the cathode in an x-ray tube. (Oral Radiol.)

target-film distance (TFD) (see **distance, target-film; source-film distance**)

target-object distance (TOD) (see **source-object distance**)

tarnish Surface discoloration or loss of luster by metals. Under oral conditions, it is often due to hard and soft deposits. (D. Mat.)
— A chemical process by which a metal surface is discolored or its luster destroyed. (Oper. Dent.)

tartar (see **calculus, dental**)

taurodontism (taw″rō-don′tĭzm) A tooth in which the pulp chamber is elongated and extends deeply into the region of the roots. A similar condition is seen in the teeth of cud-chewing animals. (Pedodont.)
— Teeth with abnormally large pulp chambers and abnormal bifurcation development. (Oral Diag.)

tax A ratable portion of the proceeds or value of the property and labor of the citizen; any contribution imposed by government for the use and service of the state. (D. Juris.)

taxes The sum of monies collected by the various branches of a government. (Pract. Man.)

technic (tĕk′nĭk) (see **technique**)

technician A person skilled in the performance of technical procedures.

391

dental t. (see **technician, dental laboratory**)

dental laboratory t. (**dental t.**) A person trained and skilled in the laboratory phases of prosthodontics. (Remov. Part. Prosth.)

— One skilled in the art of executing the dentist's prescription for the mechanical fabrication of dental appliances. (Pract. Man.)

technique (těk-nēk′) A detailed method of procedure used in the preparation and construction of a prosthetic appliance. (Comp. Prosth.)

— A skillful and detailed method of executing procedures to accomplish a desired result. (Comp. Prosth.; Remov. Part. Prosth.)

— The method of performance or manipulation in any art; the terms technique and technic are used synonymously, but the word technique pertains more to the artistic skill involved. (Oper. Dent.)

— A certain prescribed procedure for obtaining a suitable radiogram. It includes the proper positioning of the patient and the selection of the correct physical factors such as tube angulation, milliampere-seconds, and kilovolt peak. (Oral Radiol.)

— A detailed method or procedure used in the preparation and construction of an orthodontic appliance. The skill in the execution of a procedure. (Orthodont.)

airbrasive t. (ār′brā-sĭv) A method of cutting tooth structure by means of finely divided aluminum oxide propelled by carbon dioxide gas at a high velocity. The cutting is controlled by the distance from the handpiece nozzle to the tooth and by the operator's direct vision (no tactile sense is involved). (Oper. Dent.)

bisection of the angle t. An intraoral radiographic technique whereby an angle formed by the mean plane of the tooth and the mean plane of the film is bisected and the central ray is directed through the tooth perpendicular to the bisection. This is the application of Cieszynski's rule of isometry. (Oral Radiol.) (see also **rule of isometry, Cieszynski's**)

calibrated angle t. An intraoral radiographic technique using a specified degree in vertical angulation from the horizontal plane. It is a variation of the bisection of the angle technique and assumed to be the correct angulation for the majority of patients. (Oral Radiol.)

chew-in t. (see **chew-in technique**)

double investing t. A method of investing wax patterns whereby the pattern is covered with a primary layer of investment; this core is then invested, before or after the primary investment has set, in an outer, thinner mix of the same or a different type of investing material. (Oper. Dent.)

Eames' t. In dental amalgam, a procedure utilizing mercury and alloy in approximately a 1:1 ratio, thus not having residual mercury in the plastic mix. (Oper. Dent.)

filling t. The method used to obliterate the space in the root of the tooth once occupied by the dental pulp. (Endodont.)

Fones' t. (see **method, Fones'**)

hydro-flow t. Synonym for a washed-field procedure; term originated by E. O. Thompson. The tooth being prepared is kept under a stream of water. (Oper. Dent.) (see also **dentistry, washed-field**)

impression t. A method and manner used in making a negative likeness. The series of operations or procedures used for making an impression. (Comp. Prosth.)

dual i. t. A technique by which the anatomic form of the teeth and immediately adjacent structures is recorded and by which the free-end denture foundation areas are registered in their functional form. (Remov. Part. Prosth.)

long cone t. The use of an extended cone distance, generally 14 inches or more, in oral radiography. It is generally used with, but not confined to, parallel film placement. (Oral Radiol.)

Nealon's t. A technique for the insertion of resin restorations whereby the monomer and polymer are applied with a brush. (D. Mat.)

— The procedure of incremental buildup of autopolymerizing resin in a prepared cavity. (Oper. Dent.)

open flap t. (see **open flap technique**)

parallel t. (**right-angle t.**) A technique in intraoral radiography in which the film is positioned parallel to the long axes of the teeth and the central ray is directed perpendicular to both the film and the teeth. (Oral Radiol.)

right-angle t. (see **technique, parallel**)

short cone t. The use of a short cone distance, usually 8 inches or less, that is supplied by the manufacturer as short cone. It is generally used with, but not confined to, the bisection of the angle technique. (Oral Radiol.)

telephone t. The friendly but businesslike conveying of ideas over the telephone. (Pract. Man.)

thermal expansion t. A casting procedure whereby compensation is made for metal shrinkage by thermal expansion of the refractory investment mold. (D. Mat.)

wax expansion t. A casting procedure whereby compensation is made for metal shrinkage by thermal expansion of the wax pattern prior to setting of the investment. (D. Mat.)

teeth (see **tooth**)

teething Eruption of primary teeth that is preceded by increased salivation. Young children may become restless during this period. Inflammation of the gingival tissues prior to complete emergence of the crown may cause a temporary painful condition. (Pedodont.)

Teflon A proprietary plastic material used in surgery as an implant. (Oral Surg.)

telangiectasia (tĕl-ăn″jē-ĕk-tā′zē-ah) Dilation of the capillaries and small arteries of a region. A hereditary form (hereditary hemorrhagic telangiectasia) may appear intraorally. (Oral Diag.)

— A disorder characterized by cutaneous and mucosal vascular macules, nodules, and arterial spiders that tend to bleed sporadically. (Oral Med.)

hereditary hemorrhagic t. (Rendu-Osler-Weber disease) Dilation of small vessels and capillaries, due to a genetic factor, with a tendency to bleed. The lesions may occur on the tongue as small, raised, red to bluish red elevations. (Oral Diag.)

teleradiography (tĕl″ĕ-rā″dē-ŏg′rah-fē) Radiography at a longer distance than is usually employed (6 feet). (Oral Radiol.)

telic (teleologic) Assigning purpose to functions as if they were provided by a creative planner. (Gnathol.)

temperature The degree of sensible heat or cold.

body t. The measurable temperature of the body (normal range of variation, 98° to 99° F orally and 99° to 100° F rectally, with much wider ranges for skin). (Oral Physiol.)

b. t. regulation Homeostasis of body temperature. Results from a balance of heat production (external heat plus heat from muscle contraction and other chemical processes) and heat loss (through lungs, sweating, surface radiation, and excretions). (Oral Physiol.)

casting t. The required degree of heat necessary to bring a metal to proper fluidity for introduction into a refractory mold. (Remov. Part. Prosth.)

recrystallization t. The temperature at which new equiaxial grains are formed during the annealing of cold-worked structures. (D. Mat.)

— The lowest temperature at which the distorted grain structure of a cold-worked metal is replaced by a new, strain-free grain structure during prolonged annealing. Time, purity of metal, and prior deformation are important factors. (Oper. Dent.)

tempering (hardening heat treatment) Hardening or toughening of steels by heating. Treatment of an alloy in such a manner that solid-solid transformation occurs. Precipitation of intermetallic substances occurs, increasing the proportional limit and hardness of the alloy. (D. Mat.)

— Bringing to a proper degree of hardness (metal) or viscosity (hydrocolloid). (Oper. Dent.)

gold t. The hardening of gold alloys by cold working or by heating and then cooling slowly. (Oper. Dent.)

hydrocolloid t. Storing of the material after liquefaction at a temperature that will increase the viscosity to the optimal manipulative degree of sol. (Oper. Dent.)

steel t. Counteracting of the hardening heat treatment to the extent needed for the particular tool or structure. It is heated to a predetermined temperature and then quenched in water or oil. (Oper. Dent.)

template (tĕm′plāt) A pattern or mold; a curved or flat plate used as an aid in setting teeth. (Comp. Prosth.; Remov. Part. Prosth.)

implant t. An early type of subperiosteal implant that was fabricated from a cast carved to simulate the host bone. Measurements made from radiographs taken with a template or wire mold resting on the soft tissues determined the carving of the cast. (Oral Implant.)

occlusal t. A stone or metal (electroformed) occlusal table made from a wax occlusal path registration of jaw movements and against which the opposing supplied teeth are occluded. (Remov. Part. Prosth.)

surgical t. A thin transparent resin base shaped to duplicate the form of the impression surface of an immediate denture and used as a guide for surgically shaping the alveolar process and its soft tissue covering to fit an immediate denture. (Comp. Prosth.; Remov. Part. Prosth.)

wax t. A wax recording of the occlusion of the teeth. (Periodont.)

temporal eminential angle The degree of slope between the axis-orbital plane and the discluding slope of the eminence. (Gnathol.)

temporary Pertaining to the interim restoration placed to protect a cavity preparation between appointments. (Oper. Dent.)

    t. base (see **baseplate**)

    t. prosthesis (see **prosthesis, temporary**)

    t. stopping (see **stopping, temporary**)

    t. superstructure A prosthodontic appliance (removable or fixed) which is used, often immediately postoperatively, as a transitional appliance either for cosmesis or splinting, or both. (Oral Implant.)

temporomandibular articulation (tĕm″pō-rō-măn″dĭb′ū-lar) (see **articulation, temporomandibular**)

temporomandibular extraoral radiographic examination (see **examination, radiographic, extraoral, temporomandibular**)

temporomandibular joint (see **articulation, temporomandibular**)

tenant One who has the temporary use and occupation of real property owned by another, the length and terms of his tenancy being usually fixed by a lease. (D. Juris.)

tender, legal The kind of coin or money that the law compels a creditor to accept in payment of his debt, when offered by the debtor in the right amount. (D. Juris.)

tensile strength (see **strength, tensile**)

tension (tĕn′shŭn) The state of being stretched, strained, or extended. (Comp. Prosth.; Fixed Part. Prosth.; Remov. Part. Prosth.)

    interfacial surface t. The tension or resistance to separation possessed by the film of liquid between two well-adapted surfaces; e.g., the thin film of saliva between the denture base and the tissues. (Comp. Prosth.; Remov. Part. Prosth.)

teratoma (tĕr″ah-tō′mah) A tumor arising from cells that retain their embryonic totipotentiality (ovary, embryonic rest, testis) and can differentiate into any of the three primary germ layers. (Oral Path.)

terminal hinge position (see **position, hinge, terminal**)

terminal jaw relation record (see **record, terminal jaw relation**)

terminology, technical The use of terms that are descriptive and meaningful to the dentist but that are not a part of the vocabulary of the patient. (Pract. Man.)

terra alba Gypsum added to plaster or stone to accelerate the setting reaction. (D. Mat.)

test(s) Any clinical or laboratory procedure designed to evaluate constituents or functions of the body. (Oral Med.)

    acetone t. (see **test, ketone bodies**)

    ACTH-stimulation t. (Thorn's t.) A test of adrenocortical reserve based on changes in the eosinophil count and urinary levels of 17-ketosteroids and 17-hydroxycorticoids as a result of intravenous infusion or intramuscular injection of ACTH. (Oral Med.)

    Addis' t. A renal concentration test that reflects the capacity of the tubule to perform osmotic work. The specific gravity of the urine is determined after fluids are withheld for 24 hours. The normal value for specific gravity should reach 1.025 or higher. (Oral Med.)

    allergy t., intradermal A test for allergy performed by injecting a preparation containing the suspected allergen into the dermis. (Oral Med.)

    amylase t. (ăm′ĭ-lās) Determination of serum amylase, which is useful in the diagnosis of acute pancreatitis and after operations in which the pancreas might have been injured. The Somogyi sarcogenic method is often used, and the results are given in Somogyi units, defined as the amount of amylase needed to digest 1.5 g of starch in 8 minutes at 37° C. The normal range is 60 to 200 units/100 ml. The serum amylase is also elevated in mumps and other diseases of the salivary glands. (Oral Med.)

    amyloid t. (ăm′ĭ-loid) Tests for amyloidosis based on disappearance of Congo red from serum or the metachromatic staining of a gingival biopsy specimen. (Oral Med.) (see also **test, Congo red**)

    antiviral antibody t. Antibody tests in viral diseases. Included are complement-fixation tests for poliomyelitis, psittacosis, and Coxsackie infections; hemagglutination-inhibition tests for mumps, influenza, and encephalitides; and neutralization tests. (Oral Med.)

    Aschheim-Zondek t. (ăsh′hīm-tson′dĕk) (see **test, pregnancy**)

    ascorbic acid t., intradermal A test for ascorbic acid deficiency based on the decoloration of an intradermal injection of a purple dye (2,6-dichlorphenol-indophenol). Normally with a wheal of 4 mm, using a dye concentration of N/300, decoloration occurs in 10 to 15 minutes. (Oral Med.)

    basophilic aggregation t. (bā″sō-fīl′ĭk) A test for lead poisoning based on increased stippling of erythrocytes. More than 2% stippled cells is seen in lead poisoning. (Oral Med.) (see also **test, lead**)

Bell's palsy t. Simple clinical tests such as motor function tests, in which the patient is asked to whistle, pucker the lips, smile, or wrinkle the forehead, and sensory function tests, in which the patient is asked to taste sweet with sugar, sour with citric acid, bitter with quinine, and salt with sodium chloride. (Oral Physiol.)

Benedict's t. A nonspecific test for glucose in the urine. Eight drops of urine are mixed with 5 ml of Benedict's qualitative sugar reagent in a test tube and placed in boiling water for 5 minutes. A color reaction of green to yellow, brown, orange, or red usually indicates glucose, although other reducing substances may cause a positive reaction. (Oral Med.)

bilirubin t. (bĭl″ĭ-roo′bĭn) Qualitative, presumptive, quantitative, or specific determinations for bilirubin in the urine and blood serum. Included are Gmelin's test and van den Bergh's test. (Oral Med.)

bleeding time t. Techniques for determining the time interval required for hemostasis to occur after a standardized wound has been made in the capillary bed. (Oral Med.) (see also **test, Duke's; test, Ivy's**)

Brinell hardness t. A means of determining surface hardness by measuring the amount of resistance to the indentation of a steel ball. Recorded as the Brinell hardness number (B.H.N.); the higher the number, the harder the material. Generally indicative of abrasion resistance. (D. Mat.)

— A laboratory test for determining the relative hardness of a metal. (Remov. Part. Prosth.)

Bromsulphalein (BSP) t. A test of liver function based on the removal of a known quantity of Bromsulphalein from the blood in a measured period of time. Normal values are less than 5% retention at the end of 45 minutes with an intravenous dose of 5 mg/ kg body weight. It is a useful test of hepatocellular disease and detoxifying ability but is not applicable in the presence of extrahepatic or intrahepatic obstructive jaundice. (Oral Med.)

Bunnell t. (see **test, Paul-Bunnell**)

capillary resistance t. (**Rumple-Leede-Hess t., Gothlin's t.**) A test of capillary fragility based on the number of petechiae that develop when a standardized intraluminal positive pressure is applied to the capillaries

either by a blood pressure cuff or a suction cup applied to the skin. (Oral Med.) (see also **test, tourniquet**)

— A test of the integrity of the capillary walls, in which a blood pressure cuff is applied to the arm with enough pressure to obstruct venous return but to permit arterial blood to pass; the number of petechiae thus produced are recorded. (Oral Surg.)

chemical t. A test employed especially for the diagnosis of deposits on the teeth; the disclosing solution shows up mucin plaques as well as materia alba. (Periodont.)

CO_2 capactiy t. (CO_2 combining power t.) A general measure of the alkalinity or acidity of the blood. Various normal adult ranges are given; e.g., 23 to 30 mEq/L of serum or 55 to 70 vol/100 ml of serum. A low value is found in diabetic acidosis, hyperventilation, certain kidney diseases, and severe diarrhea. A high value is found in excessive administration of ACTH or cortisone, intake of sodium bicarbonate, and persistent vomiting. (Oral Med.)

CO_2 combining power t. (see **test, CO_2 capacity**)

cold bends t. A mechanical test used for assessing ductility. (D. Mat.)

colorimetric caries susceptibility t. (**Snyder's t.**) A method of determining the concentration of acid-producing bacteria in the saliva by use of bromcresol green in a culture medium. The reliability of this and other salivary bacterial tests for dental caries susceptibility is questionable. (Oral Diag.)

Congo red t. A test of amyloid disease based on the more rapid disappearance of Congo red from the serum of affected patients than from that of normal individuals. Gingival biopsy and positive staining with methyl violet or crystal violet also indicate amyloidosis. (Oral Med.)

creatinine clearance t. (krē-ăt′ĭ-nĭn) A renal function test of exogenous creatinine clearance. It is a convenient clinical test of glomerular infiltration rate. It is calculated as the quotient of the product of urine creatinine (mg/L) and urine volume (L/24 hr) divided by the serum creatinine concentration (mg/L). The normal value for young healthy adults of average size (1.73 M^2 body surface area) is 115 to 155 L/24 hr (±15%). (Oral Med.)

dermal t. (see **test, skin**)

Dick's t. (**scarlet fever t.**) A skin test to determine susceptibility or immunity to scarlet fever. A positive test is indicated when an area of erythema and edema measuring more than 10 mm in diameter occurs 8 to 24 hours after an intradermal injection of a standardized erythrogenic toxin. (Oral Med.)

Duke's t. A test of bleeding time as indicated by the time that elapses before a puncture wound of the earlobe ceases to bleed. Normal range is 2 to 4½ minutes. (Oral Med.)

electric t. A test to determine whether a pulp is vital. (Periodont.)

false positive t. for reducing sugars False positive reactions in Benedict's test or similar tests because of nonfermentable substances such as glycuronates, aspirin, aminopyrine, morphine, para-aminobenzoic acid, and homogentisic acid and when uric acid, creatine, ascorbic acid, and penicillin are present in excessive amounts in the urine. (Oral Med.)

flow t. Used in the A.D.A. Specification for dental amalgam; measured as the percentage shortening of a cylinder of the material. (D. Mat.)

fluorescent treponemal antibody (FTA) t. Detection of specific treponemal antibody by an indirect technique using a fluorescent dye. (Oral Med.)

Foshay's t. A skin test for tularemia using the Foshay antigen. (Oral Med.)

Frei's t. (frīz) An intradermal skin test for lymphogranuloma venereum employing an antigen called Lygranum. It gives a specific dermal reaction in patients infected with lymphogranuloma venereum. A false positive test may occur with psittacosis. (Oral Med.)

Friedman's t. (frēd'mănz) (see **test, pregnancy**)

glucose paper t. A test in which paper is impregnated with glucose oxidase and other reagents (TesTape, Clinistix). When the paper is moistened with fresh urine, the presence of glucose will cause a change in color of the paper. (Oral Med.)

glucose tolerance t. (GTT) A test for abnormalities of carbohydrate tolerance by glucose loading and subsequent serial measurements of the concentration of glucose in the blood. Graphic representation of the concentration and the elapsed time make up the glucose tolerance curve. Abnormal curves occur in diabetes mellitus, thyrotoxicosis, Cushing's syndrome, acromegaly, and pheochromocytoma. (Oral Med.)

Göthlin's t. (see **test, capillary resistance**)

hardness t. (see **hardness, Mohs; test, Brinell hardness; test, Knoop hardness; test, Vickers hardness**)

Henderson's t. Test for acidosis. A normal person can hold his breath without preliminary deep inspiration for 30 seconds or more; the inability to hold it for more than 15 or 20 seconds in a person free from cardiorenal or pulmonary disease indicates the presence of acidosis. (Anesth.)

Hess' t. (see **test, capillary resistance**)

Hinton's t. A precipitation test for syphilis. (Oral Diag.)

histoplasmin t. A skin test to determine sensitization to *Histoplasma capsulatum*. A positive test indicates past or present infection (histoplasmosis). (Oral Med.)

infectious mononucleosis t. One of several tests for the diagnosis of infectious mononucleosis; e.g., Paul-Bunnell test. (Oral Med.)

inflammation and necrosis t. Tests of abnormalities in the blood associated with inflammatory and necrotizing processes. Most are nonspecific but are valuable when other possible sources of the reactants in the blood are excluded. Included are the erythrocyte sedimentation rate, latex fixation for rheumatoid arthritis, C-reactive protein for the exclusion of active rheumatic fever, and serum enzymes such as glutamic oxaloacetic transaminase for myocardial infarction. (Oral Med.)

intracutaneous t. (see **test, skin**)

intradermal t. (see **test, skin**)

Ivy's t. A test of bleeding time performed by making a wound 2 mm in length and depth with a Bard-Parker No. 11 blade just distal to the antecubital fossa. The blood is touched every 30 seconds with blotting filter paper. The normal range for the blood to cease staining the paper is ½ to 6½ minutes. (Oral Med.)

Janet's t. A test in which, with his eyes closed, the patient is instructed to say "yes" or "no" as he feels or does not feel the touch of the examiner's finger; in the case of functional anesthesia, he may say "no" when an anesthetized area is touched, but in the case of organic anesthesia, he will say nothing, being unaware that he is touched. (Anesth.)

Kahn's t. A precipitation test for the diagnosis of syphilis. (Oral Diag.; Periodont.) (see also **test, serologic**)

ketone bodies t. (acetone t., Rothera's t.)

Nitroprusside reaction tests for acetone and acetoacetic acid and the ferric chloride test for acetoacetic acid. Commercially prepared nitroprusside test tablets (Acetest) and powder (Acetone Test Denco) are available. (Oral Med.)

Kline's t. A flocculation test for syphilis based on the combination of the cardiolipin antigen with reagin to form grossly visible aggregates. (Oral Med.)

Knoop hardness t. A means of measuring surface hardness by resistance to the penetration of indenting tool made of diamond. Produces an indentation that has a diamond or rhombic shape. Especially preferred for testing hardness of tooth structure. (D. Mat.)

Küstner's t. (kĭst'nerz) (see **test, skin, indirect**)

laboratory t. Investigative procedures performed in the laboratory that are useful in the diagnosis of disease, including biopsy examination of tissue specimens, determination of type and characteristics of associated microorganisms, serology, blood and urine chemistry, hemogram (red cell count, hemoglobin content, white cell count, differential white cell count, etc.), metabolic studies (e.g., basal metabolic rate), etc. (Periodont.)

LE t. A test for lupus erythematosus based on the presence of a single (or multiple) homogenous basophilic inclusion in polymorphonuclear leukocytes. Such LE cells have also been found in cases of rheumatoid arthritis, allergic reactions to penicillin, hydrolazine toxicity, and "lupoid cirrhosis." (Oral Med.)

lead t. Any of several tests used to detect clinical lead poisoning or exposure to lead; e.g., coproporphyrinuria test, trace element analysis, urinary lead content test, and basophilic aggregation test. (Oral Med.)

Leede's t. (see **test, capillary resistance**)

liver function t. Tests to measure the severity of liver disease, to aid in the differential diagnosis of the various types of disease of the hepatobiliary system, and to follow the course of liver disease. Screening tests include urine bile, urine urobilinogen, Bromsulphalein (BSP) excretion, serum transaminases, thymol turbidity, cephalin-cholesterol flocculation, and van den Bergh's reaction (1 minute direct and total). (Oral Med.)

Mantoux t. (mahn-too') An intracutaneous tuberculin test using either old tuberculin (OT) or purified protein derivative (PPD). A positive reaction read 24 and 48 hours after injection shows erythema and edema greater than 5 mm in diameter and indicates past or present tuberculosis. (Oral Med.)

Mazzini's t. (mah-zē'nēz) A flocculation test for syphilis. (Oral Med.)

Meulengracht's t. (moi'lĕn-grăkts) (**icterus index**) A comparison of the yellow color of the serum with 1:10,000 solution of potassium dichromatic solution. Normal values are 4 to 6 units. Latent jaundice is indicated by values between 6 and 15 units, and clinical jaundice is usually noted when the values are above 15 units. This test is not frequently used now. (Oral Med.)

Mohs t. (see **hardness, Mohs**)

nontreponemal antigen t. Serologic tests for syphilis employing nontreponemal antigens. Such tests are not absolutely specific or sensitive for syphilis. Included are the Kline, Kahn, and Kolmer tests, and the VDRL slide test. (Oral Med.)

one-stage t. (see **time, prothrombin**)

pancreatic function t. Tests of enzyme levels in blood and urine (amylase, lipase), fecal fat content, trypsin activity, nitrogen content, alteration of digestive capacity, and alteration of pancreatic secretion via duodenal intubation. (Oral Med.)

patch t. (**percutaneous t.**) A test for allergy performed by placing the suspected allergen in direct contact with the skin or mucosa. (Oral Med.) (see also **test, skin**)

Paul-Bunnell t. A test for infectious mononucleosis based on increased agglutination of sheep red blood cells due to heterophil antibodies in the serum. Considered positive if dilution of serum of 1:80 or higher agglutinates the sheep cells. Elevated agglutinin titers are more likely to be found during the second or third week of the disease but the serum may not become positive until seven weeks have elapsed. (Oral Med.)

percussion t. A method of examination executed by striking the tissues of the area being examined with the fingers or an instrument, listening for resulting sounds, and observing the response of the patient. (Oper. Dent.)

percutaneous t. (per″kū-tā'nē-ŭs) (see **test, patch**)

phenolsulfonphthalein (PSP) t. (fē″nol-sŭl″fōn-thal'ēn) A renal test that roughly estimates glomerular function by measuring the rate of excretion of the dye after intravenous injection. Normally, after 15 minutes 25% or more of the dye should be excreted in the urine. (Oral Med.)

plasma ketone t. A test using nitroprusside for the detection of high levels of ketone bodies in the blood. The test is read 0 to 4+. A strongly positive reaction is seen in diabetic ketoacidosis. (Oral Med.)

Prausnitz-Küstner t. (prows'nĭts-kĭst'ner) (see **test, skin, indirect**)

pregnancy t. (Aschheim-Zondek t., Friedman's t.) Biologic or chemical tests to determine pregnancy; usually based on changes in the ovaries of an animal injected with the urine of a pregnant woman. Included are the Aschheim-Zondek test (using mice or rats) and the Friedman test (using virgin rabbits). Male frogs and female and male toads are also used. A saliva test has also been used. (Oral Med.)

prothrombin consumption t. (serum prothrombin time) A convenient screening test of the first stage of blood coagulation as determined by the quantity of prothrombin remaining after coagulation. The test reflects the formation of plasma thromboplastin, provided the one-stage prothrombin time of plasma is normal. Normally the prothrombin consumption of plasma is greater than 80% in 1 hour, and the serum prothrombin time is greater than 25 seconds. The time is reduced in a deficiency of plasma thromboplastin antecedent or component antihemophilic globulin, in a platelet factor deficiency secondary to thrombocytopenia, and in thrombasthenia. (Oral Med.) (see also **time, prothrombin**)

pulmonary function t. Tests used to evaluate respiratory function; e.g., tests of vital capacity, tidal volume, maximal breathing capacity, timed vital capacity, and arterial blood gases. (Oral Med.)

pulp t. A diagnostic test to determine clinical pulp vitality and/or abnormality. (Endodont.)

p. cavity t. The drilling into the coronal dentin with small burs without anesthesia to determine patient response. (Endodont.)

p. percussion t. Evaluation of periapical tissue response to striking the teeth. (Endodont.)

rapid reagin t. Serologic tests for syphilis that permit rapid and economical screening in the field. Included are the rapid plasma reagin (RPR) test and the unheated serum reagin (USR) test. (Oral Med.)

Reiter protein complement-fixation (RPCF) t. (rē'ter) Treponemal antigen test for syphilis using extracts from the nonpathogenic Reiter treponeme. (Oral Med.)

renal function t. Quantitative tests including inulin or mannitol clearance for the glomerular filtration rate (GFR), para-aminohippurate (PAH) clearance for renal plasma flow, and the maximum rate of tubular excretion of para-aminohippurate and the maximum rate of reabsorption of glucose for the measurement of excretory and reabsorptive functions of the renal tubules. Clinical renal tests are used to assess the extent of renal impairment. They include blood urea nitrogen (BUN), nonprotein nitrogen (NPN), urea clearance, endogenous creatinine clearance, filtration fraction, phenolsulfonphthalein (PSP), and concentration tests. (Oral Med.)

Rockwell t. An indentation test for hardness of a material. A static load is placed on a steel ball or diamond point, and the depth of the indentation is measured on the instrument. The depth of the indentation is remeasured after the load is increased. The hardness number is related to the type of point used and to the depth of the indentation. (Comp. Prosth.)

Rothera's t. (see **test, ketone bodies**)

routine t. A test or group of tests performed on most or all patients to detect relatively common disorders or to establish a base for further evaluation of a patient. (Oral Med.)

Rumple-Leede-Hess t. (see **test, capillary resistance**)

saline bleb t. Intradermal injection of isotonic saline solution, with observation of the disappearance time of the produced bleb. Time is considered to be shorter in patients with connective tissue disorders. (Oral Med.)

scarlet fever t. (see **test, Dick's**)

Schick t. A skin test to demonstrate the presence or absence of an immunity to diphtheria. (Oral Med.)

scratch t. (skin t.) A test for allergy performed by placing a preparation containing the allergen on the skin and scratching the skin. A positive reaction is indicated by the formation of a wheal and flare. (Oral Med.)

screening t. A group of tests especially chosen to detect specific abnormalities. (Oral Med.)

sedimentation t. A macroscopic test of the

blood used to detect severe infection. The blood cells are allowed to settle in the presence of an anticoagulant, and the time (sedimentation time) or quantity (sedimentation rate) of sedimentation is determined. The greater the time or rate, the more severe the infection. Pregnancy and menstruation affect the sedimentation. (Oral Diag.)

sensitivity t. In blood-grouping serology, the testing of the donor's and recipient's sera for possible Rh-Hr or other antibodies. In clinical microbiology the term refers to tests to determine the susceptibility of microorganisms to therapeutic agents, especially antibiotics. Also used loosely in reference to tests for hypersensitivity to allergens. (Oral Med.)

serologic t. (sĕ″rō-loj′ĭk) Tests of blood serum for the diagnosis of infectious diseases. Included are febrile agglutinations used in the diagnosis of fever of unknown origin; antistreptolysin-O (ASL-O) titer determination in the differential diagnosis of rheumatic fever; and flocculation (Kahn's, Kline's), complement-fixation (Wassermann), and *Treponema pallidum* immobilization tests for syphilis. (Oral Med.)

biologic false positive s. t. A positive serologic test for syphilis in the absence of syphilis. Such false positive tests may result from smallpox vaccination, malaria, measles, leprosy, and infectious mononucleosis as well as other diseases. (Oral Med.)

skin t. Tests to determine the sensitivity or susceptibility to infections by a specific agent, the presence of an allergy, or the presence of a nutritional deficiency. Included are the Mantoux, Schick, Dick, Frei, histoplasmin, and Foshay tests for infectious diseases (tests in which allergens are placed onto or into the skin) and the intradermal ascorbic acid, dermal, intradermal (intracutaneous), patch (percutaneous), scratch, and subcutaneous tests. (Oral Med.) (see also **test, skin, reactions**)

indirect s. t. (Prausnitz-Küstner t.) A valuable test for patients with atopic dermatitis. The patient's own serum is injected intracutaneously, and after 72 to 96 hours a suspected excitant is injected into the site of the previous serum injection. If a positive (immediate) reaction occurs in the sensitized site, a sensitizing antibody is considered to be present in the blood. (Oral Med.)

s. t. reactions An immediate-type (atopic, anaphylactoid) or delayed-type (bacterial, tuberculin) hypersensitivity reaction due to exposure to allergens or antigens. A positive reaction is manifested by a wheal or area of erythema and induration, occasionally accompanied by tissue necrosis and systemic manifestations. A positive test indicates past infection or active disease. A negative reaction may occur because of anergy or lateness of development of dermal sensitivity in some diseases. An immediate reaction occurs in about 15 minutes and is usually associated with an antigen other than from microorganisms. An immediate reaction occurs in trichinosis, echinococcosis, and toxoplasmosis. A delayed reaction of erythema and induration occurs within 24 to 48 hours and is seen in the tuberculin test, Foshay's test for tularemia, the histoplasmin test, and Frei's test for lymphogranuloma venereum. (Oral Med.)

tuberculin s. t. (tū-ber′kū-lin) Intradermal injection of old tuberculin (OT) or purified protein derivative (PPD) to determine a specific sensitivity or susceptibility to tuberculosis. (Oral Med.)

Snyder's t. (see **test, colorimetric caries susceptibility**)

subcutaneous t. (see **test, skin**)

Sulkowitch's t. A simple but roughly qualitative evaluation of calcium in the urine; 5 ml of Sulkowitch's reagent is added to 5 ml of a sample of filtered 24-hour urine. The degree of precipitate is noted as 0 or 1+ to 4+. If no precipitate is present, serum calcium is less than 7.5 mg/100 ml; a fine white cloud (1+) indicates a normal range (i.e., 9 to 11 mg/100 ml); a heavy milky precipitate (2+ or more) suggests hypercalcemia. The test is useful for excluding hyperparathyroidism and hypoparathyroidism. (Oral Med.)

syphilis t. Refers to any serologic test for syphilis based on the presence of a reagin, appearing during the second or third week of infection. Included are the Hinton, Kahn, Kline, Mazzini, Wassermann, and *Treponema pallidum* immobilization tests. (Oral Med.)

thermal t. The use of heat or cold as an aid in diagnosis; e.g., the use of heat or cold in testing the pulp. (Oral Diag.)

— Tests used to determine the health status

of pulps by applying heat and cold. (Periodont.)

— Tests to determine pulpal response to hot and cold stimuli. (Endodont.)

Thorn's t. (see **test, ACTH-stimulation**)

thromboplastin generation t. A test of the integrity of the first stage of blood coagulation and the nature of the defect. A patient's serum, plasma, or platelets are substituted in a system that is complete except for one of the factors to be tested for (antihemophilic factor, plasma thromboplastin antecedent, plasma thromboplastin component, or platelets), and the rate of thromboplastin generation is determined. (Oral Med.)

thyroid function t. Tests for thyroid function; e.g., radioactive iodine uptake, protein-bound iodine, basal metabolic rate, serum cholesterol, triiodothyronine suppression, and the thyroid-stimulating hormone tests. (Oral Med.)

tourniquet t. (toor'nĭ-kĕt) A test for capillary fragility based on counting petechiae in a given area of the arm after application of the rubber cuff of a sphygmomanometer for 15 minutes. (Oral Diag.)

—A test of capillary fragility performed by placing a blood presure cuff on the upper arm and inflating to 100 mm Hg for 10 minutes; 5 minutes after removal of the cuff, the number of petechiae in a circular area 2.5 cm in diameter and 4 to 5 cm below the antecubital fossa are counted. Normally there are 0 to 10 in women and children, with smaller numbers in males of the same age. Older persons have greater capillary fragility. The test is positive in hemorrhagic diseases involving vessel walls and platelet defects. (Oral Med.)

transaminase t. (trăns-ăm'ĭ-nās) Tests for serum glutamic oxaloacetic transaminase (SGOT) and serum glutamic pyruvic transaminase (SGPT). The normal value for serum glutamic oxaloacetic transaminase is 40 units or less; that for serum glutamic pyruvic transaminase, 35 units or less. The serum glutamic oxaloacetic transaminase value in myocardial infarction is 3 to 20 times the normal. (Oral Med.)

transillumination t. A test for a pulpless tooth in which the use of transmitted light shows a shadow of the root when the pulp is necrotic or has been replaced by a filling (not always reliable). (Endodont.)

treponemal antigen t. Tests for syphilis using *Treponema pallidum* or extracts from a treponeme as antigen. Included are *Treponema pallidum* immobilization (TPI), *Treponema pallidum* agglutination (TPA), fluorescent treponemal antibody (FTA), Reiter protein complement-fixation (RPCF), and *Treponema pallidum* complement-fixation (TPCF) tests. (Oral Med.)

Treponema pallidum immobilization (TPI) t. A test to confirm syphilis by demonstrating the immobilization of *T. pallidum* by specific antibodies in the serum of an infected individual. (Oral Med.)

t. for trigeminal nerve function Three simple clinical tests for trigeminal nerve function: *Sensation:* Apply the gentle touch wraps of cotton, pinpricks, or warm or cold objects to the areas supplied by the nerve and note responses. *Reflex:* Try the jaw jerk, eye, and sneeze reflexes. The jaw jerk is achieved by sharply tapping the lower incisor teeth with the back of a mirror handle while the mouth is partially open or by tapping the chin sharply with the hand. An appropriate response is for the mandible to elevate and the teeth to be brought into occlusal contact. *Motor function:* Test the patient's ability to chew and work against resistance. Ask the patient to clench his teeth and then observe contraction of the masseter and temporal muscles by visual examination and digital palpation. (Oral Physiol.)

tuberculin t. A test for past or present infection with tubercle bacilli. (Oral Med.) (see also **test, Mantoux**)

tularemia t. (see **test, Foshay's**)

Tzanck's t. A supplemental test for pemphigus based on the presence of degenerative changes in epithelial cells (Tzanck's cells) in the bullous lesions of pemphigus. Degenerative changes include swelling of the nuclei and hyperchromic staining. (Oral Med.)

urea clearance t. A clinical test of renal function determined by the clearance of urea from the plasma by the kidney each minute. The maximum clearance (urine flow of 2 ml/min or more) is calculated as the quotient of the product of the concentration of urea in the urine (mg/ml) and the urine flow (mg/ml) divided by the concentration of urea in the blood (mg/ml). Average normal value is 75 ml/min (75% to 125% of normal). (Oral Med.)

urine t., routine Routine examination of the

urine, including amount, appearance, pH, specific gravity, qualitative tests for sugar and protein, and microscopic examination of sediment. (Oral Med.)

van den Bergh's t. Tests for conjugated ("direct-reacting") 1-minute bilirubin, total serum bilirubin, and, by difference, unconjugated (indirect) bilirubin. An immediate direct reaction suggests obstructive jaundice, whereas an increased indirect value for bilirubin suggests hemolytic jaundice. The 1-minute direct-reacting bilirubin ranges from 0 to 0.25 mg/100 ml; the total bilirubin is normally less than 1 mg/100 ml. (Oral Med.)

VDRL (Venereal Disease Research Laboratory) t. A serologic nontreponemal antigen test for the detection of syphilitic reagin by means of a reaction between the reagin and a standard antigen. (Oral Med.)

Vickers hardness t. A penetration type of hardness test utilizing a square-based pyramid made of diamond. (D. Mat.)

viscosity of saliva t. A dental caries susceptibility test on freshly secreted saliva. An Oswald pipette is used in the determination of viscosity. (Oper. Dent.)

vitality t. The procedure using thermal, electrical, or mechanical stimuli to determine the response of the pulp in a tooth. This test is not infallible. (Endodont.)

—Measurement of the response of the dental pulp to various stimuli. (Pract. Man.)

Wassermann t. A complement-fixation test for syphilis. (Oral Diag.)

Zondek's t. (see **test, pregnancy**)

testimony Evidence of a witness, given orally under oath or affirmation. (D. Juris.)

tetany, hyperventilation (tĕt'ah-nē hĭ"per-vĕn"tĭ-lā'shŭn) The neuromuscular irritability and tonic carpopedal muscle spasm resulting from the alkalosis that may be caused by forced respiration over an extended length of time. (Oral Surg.)

tetracycline (tĕ"trah-sī'klēn) A type of antibiotic known to impart color to tooth enamel. (Pharmacol.)

Tg value Transition point of glass. In dentistry, the temperature at which resin becomes soft. (D. Mat.)

thalamus (thăl'ah-mŭs) An ovoid mass in the brain associated anatomically with the basal ganglion. It is the principal relay station in the forebrain for the sensory systems of the body. Sensory impulses from all over the body come to it for distribution to the conscious-

ness in the cerebral cortex and/or to the subcortical motor nuclei. It receives pain, temperature, tactile, and other exteroceptive and proprioceptive impulses. It also receives impulses from the special sense systems (auditory, visual, olfactory, and gustatory) and from the cerebrum and cerebellum. (Oral Physiol.)

thalassemia (thăl"ah-sē'mē-ah) (**hereditary leptocytosis, hereditary microcytosis**) A genetic disease characterized by anemia and bone changes (intraoral and extraoral). The peculiar bone patterns make it of oral interest. (Oral Diag.)

— A hereditary, chronic, hemolytic anemia with erythroblastosis. A complex of hereditary disorders characterized by microcytosis and increased red blood cell destruction and frequently associated with abnormal hemoglobins and increased normal trace hemoglobins. These disorders are prevalent in people of Mediterranean, African, and Asian ancestry. Disorders include Cooley's anemia, Cooley's trait, hemoglobin H disease, Hb S–thalassemia, Hb C–thalassemia, and Hb E–thalassemia. (Oral Med.)

— A chronic, hypochromic anemia with erythroblastosis; of familial origin, with numerous normoblasts in the blood. Lesions include mongoloid facies, splenomegaly, leukocytosis, osteoporosis, and hemolysis of the erythrocytes, seen in children of Mediterranean origin. Dental changes associated with overdevelopment of the maxillae and the malar bones produce malocclusion, open bite, and diastema. (Oral Med.; Periodont.)

— A microcytic, hypochromic, sex-linked anemia that when present homozygously creates the fatal thalassemia which is the major form of the condition. When present heterozygously, it is termed thalassemia minor, an anemia that carries an excellent prognosis. (Oral Path.)

t. major (Cooley's anemia, erythroblastic anemia, familial erythroblastic anemia, hereditary microcytosis, Mediterranean anemia, Mediterranean disease) The severe homozygous form of thalassemia characterized by a marked microcytic hypochromic anemia, atypical nucleated red blod cells, and skeletal changes (underdevelopment, mongoloid facies, anterior open bite). (Oral Med.)

t. minor (Cooley's trait) A heterozygous form of thalassemia that is a carried state with relatively mild manifestations. (Oral Med.)

theory (thē'ō-rē) An opinion or hypothesis not based on actual knowledge.

Prothero "cone" t. (see **retention**)

quantum t. The theory that in emission or absorption of energy by atoms or molecules, the process is not continuous but takes place by steps, each step being the emission or absorption of an amount of energy called a quantum. (Oral Radiol.)

somatotype t. The theory of W. H. Sheldon suggesting that body structure is correlated with certain temperaments and predisposes to mental disorders. (Oral Med.)

therapeutic index (thĕr"ah-pū'tĭk) (see **index, therapeutic**)

therapeutics The art and science of treatment of disease. (Oral Med.; Pharmacol.)

therapeutic vehicle A device used to transport and retain some agent for therapeutic purposes; e.g., a radium carrier. (M.F.P.)

therapy The treatment of disease.

antibiotic t. The treatment of disease states by the local or systemic administration of antibodies. (Periodont.)

indirect pulpal t. Application of a drug that heals the pulpal cells beneath a layer of sound or carious dentin, as in a moderately deep preparation for a restoration. (Pedodont.)

myofunctional t. (**myotherapeutic exercises**) Use of muscle exercises as an adjunct to mechanical correction of malocclusion. (Orthodont.)

periodontal t. Treatment of the periodontal lesion. Such therapy has two principal objectives: the eradication or arrest of the periodontal lesion with correction or cure of the deformity created by it, and the alteration in the mouth of the periodontal climate that was conducive or contributory to the periodontal breakdown. (Periodont.) (see also **aid in medicinal periodontal therapy**)

p. t., flap operation Surgical detachment of the gingivae, alveolar mucosa, and/or a portion of the palatal mucosa in order to secure greater access to granulating tissue and osseous defects. Its disadvantages are additional tissue injury and a tendency for improper gingival architecture to form postoperatively. (Periodont.)

p. t., maintenance phase The part of periodontal therapy that is necessary for the preservation of the results obtained during active therapy and for the prevention of further periodontal disease; an extension of active periodontal therapy, requiring the combined efforts of both the periodontist and the patient. (Periodont.)

p. t., osseous surgery The surgical procedures, properly and judiciously performed, employed to reshape the bone and secure physiologic architectural form and to eliminate the osseous defects associated with periodontal disease so that functional form of the bone and soft tissues may be obtained. (Periodont.)

pulp canal t. (see **endodontology**)

radiation t. (**radiotherapy**) Treatment of disease with any type of radiation. (Oral Radiol.)

replacement t. The administration, as a therapeutic agent, of an essential constituent in which the body is deficient; e.g., insulin in diabetes mellitus. (Oral Med.; Pharmacol.)

root canal t. (see **endodontology**)

speech t. The science that deals with the use of procedures, training, and remedies for the cure, alleviation, or prevention of speech disorders. (Cleft Palate)

thermal conductivity (see **conductivity, thermal**)

thermal expansion (see **expansion, thermal**)

thermionic emission The release of electrons when a material is heated; e.g., electron emission when the tungsten cathode filament of an x-ray tube is heated to incandescence by means of its low-voltage heating circuit. (Oral Radiol.)

thermocouple The joining of two dissimilar metals that reharden on cooling. The unequal thermal expansion of the two metals is used to indicate temperature changes. (Comp. Prosth.; Remov. Part. Prosth.)

thermoluminescence (ther"mō-lū"mĭ-nĕs'ĕns) The capability of certain crystalline compounds such as lithium fluoride to release stored energy as luminescent energy when heated. (Oral Radiol.)

thermoluminescent dosimetry (ther"mō-lū-mĭ-nĕs'ĕnt dō-sĭm'ĕ-trē) Determination of the amount of radiation to which a thermoluminescent material has been exposed. This is accomplished by heating the material in a specially designed instrument that relates the amount of luminescence emitted from the material to the amount of radiation exposure. (Oral Radiol.)

thermoplastic (ther'mō-plăs'tĭk) Term used in connection with resins. The property of becoming soft with the application of heat, rigid at normal temperature, and again soft with the reapplication of heat. A reversible physical phenomenon. (Comp. Prosth.; D. Mat.; Remov. Part. Prosth.)

thermosetting Having the property of becoming rigid or hardened with the application of heat. Not reversible. In dentistry, the term is used in connection with resins. (D. Mat.)

thermostat An automatic temperature control device. (D. Mat.)

thiamine (thī′ah-mĭn) (see **vitamin B₁**)

Thiersch's skin graft (tērsh′ēz) (see **graft, Thiersch's skin**)

thimble (see **coping**)

   t. ionization chamber (see **chamber, ionization, thimble**)

Thiokol (thī′ō-kol) Proprietary polysulfide polymer utilizing a mercaptan bond. The basic ingredient of rubber base impression materials. (D. Mat.) (see also **mercaptan**)

threat A menace; a statement of one's intention to harm or injure the person, property, or rights of another. (D. Juris.)

threshold The lowest limit of stimulus capable of producing an impression on the consciousness or of evoking a response in an irritable tissue. (Anesth.)

   t. dose (see **dose, threshold**)

   swallowing t. The moment the act of swallowing begins after the mastication of food. The critical moment of reflex action initiated by minimum stimulation prior to the act of deglutition. (Comp. Prosth.)

thrill A vibration felt on the chest wall over the heart. It is caused by eddy flow of the blood, which is produced by a structural defect in the heart. (Oral Med.)

— Palpable high-frequency vibration that may accompany cardiac murmurs or vascular disease. (Oral Diag.)

thrombasthenia (thrŏm″băs-thē′nē-ah) A hemorrhagic diathesis associated with qualitative abnormalities of the platelets. (Oral Med.)

thrombin (throm′bĭn) A proteolytic enzyme formed from prothrombin by the action of thromboplastin, Ca⁺⁺, and other factors. Thrombin forms fibrin from fibrinogen, speeds up the disruption of platelets, and activates factor V. (Oral Med.)

thrombocatalysin (thrŏm″bō-kă-tăl′ĭ-sĭn) (see **factor VIII**)

thrombocythemia (throm″bō-sī-thē′mē-ah) A continuing decrease in the number of blood platelets. (Oral Med.)

thrombocytin (throm″bō-sī′tĭn) (see **serotonin**)

thrombocytolysin (thrŏm″bō-sī-tol′ĭ-sĭn) (see **factor VIII**)

thrombocytosis (throm″bō-sī-tō′sĭs) Unusually large numbers of platelets in the circulating blood. It may occur after surgical procedures, parturition, and injury, or with thrombocythemia. (Oral Med.)

thrombogen (throm′bō-jĕn) Prothrombin. (see also **factor V**)

thrombogene (see **factor V**)

thrombokatilysin (thrŏm″bō-kă-tĭl′ĭ-sĭn) (see **factor VIII**)

thrombokinase (throm″bō-kī′nās) (see **factor III**)

thrombokinin (throm″bō-kĭn′ĭn) (see **factor III**)

thrombopenia, essential (throm″bō-pē′nē-ah) (see **purpura, thrombocytopenic**)

thromboplastic plasma component (TPC) (see **factor VIII**)

thromboplastin (throm″bō-plăs′tĭn) A substance necessary to coagulant activity of tissue extracts; also has been referred to as the direct activator of prothrombin and as a substance from plasma, platelets, and tissues that initiates thromboplastic activity in blood coagulation. (Oral Med.) (see also **factor III**)

   activated t. (see **thromboplastin, extrinsic**)

   cofactor of t. (see **factor V**)

   extrinsic t. (**prothrombinase, extrinsic prothrombin activator, proconvertin-convertin, cothromboplastin, activated t.**) A direct prothrombin activator formed by the interaction of brain extracts, factors V and VII, and Ca⁺⁺. (Oral Med.)

   incomplete t. Tissue thromboplastin. (Oral Med.)

   intrinsic t. (**plasma thromboplastin, intrinsic prothrombin activator**) A prothrombin activator formed from interaction of blood coagulation factors V, VIII, IX, and X and Ca⁺⁺ with a foreign surface. (Oral Med.)

   tissue t. A factor in tissue extracts responsible for coagulation of blood. (Oral Med.)

thromboplastinogen (throm″bō-plăs-tĭn′ō-jĕn) (see **factor VIII**)

thromboplastinogenase (throm″bō-plăs-tĭn′ō-jĕn-ās) (see **factor, platelet, 3**)

thrombosis (throm-bō′sĭs) Presence of a clot in a blood vessel. (Oral Diag.)

— Clogging of a blood vessel by a clot or deposit formed in situ; in contradistinction to an embolism, which is solid matter, such as a clot, a mass of vegetation, or the like, carried by the bloodstream to some point where the vessel's lumen narrows. (Oral Physiol.)

   cavernous sinus t. A blood clot in the cavernous

sinus occasionally arising from maxillary periapical infection. The prognosis is poor but not so grave as before antibiotic therapy. (Oral Diag.; Oral Surg.)

coronary t. Thrombosis of the coronary artery; also called heart attack and coronary occlusion. (Oral Med.)

thrombotonin (see **serotonin**)

thrombozyme (throm'bō-zīm) (see **factor II**)

thrombus (throm'bŭs) A blood clot in a vessel or in one of the chambers of the heart that remains at the point of its formation. (Oral Surg.)

thrush (**candidiasis, moniliasis**) A disease caused by *Candida albicans* and characterized by white patches that scrape off with some difficulty, leaving bleeding bases. This term usually is used for the intraoral disease, whereas moniliasis is the term applied to the condition in other areas of infection by the yeast, as well as to the oral cavity. (Oral Diag.)

— Infection of the oral mucous membrane by *Candida albicans*. Lesions are white, curdlike adherent patches that consist of pseudomycelium and desquamated epithelium. (Oral Med.) (see also **moniliasis**)

— *Candida albicans* infection characterized by white, curdlike raised patches with a diffuse erythematous background. (Periodont.) (see also **candidiasis; moniliasis**)

thyroid, lingual (thī'roid) Presence of thyroid tissue in the tongue, which is related to abnormal embryonic activity of the thyroglossal duct. (Oral Diag.)

thyroxine (thī-rok'sĭn) A secretion of the thyroid gland. Cretinism is a form of dwarfism and mental deficiency caused by a deficient secretion of thyroxine as a result of thyroid insufficiency. This deficiency causes a general retardation of skeletal development and growth. (Oral Physiol.)

tic An involuntary purposeless movement of muscle usually occurring under emotional stress. It is a survival in stereotyped form of a movement or muscle set once used voluntarily and purposefully. (Oral Physiol.)

— A spasmodic twitching or movement. (Oral Surg.)

t. douloureux Spontaneous trigeminal neuralgia associated with a "trigger zone" and causing spasmodic contraction of the facial muscles. (Oral Diag.; Oral Path.) (see also **neuralgia, trigeminal**)

tickling and itching Sensations thought to be caused by the total effects of light stimulation simultaneously to the touch and pain endings

of the skin and to the mucous membranes of the mouth and anus. (Oral Physiol.)

t.i.d. Abbreviation for *ter in die,* a Latin phrase meaning three times a day. (Oral Med.; Pharmacol.)

time A measure of duration.

clot retraction t. The time required for a given quantity of blood to separate in the tube in which it has been placed. For 3 ml of blood at room temperature, 1 hour is normal. It is very slow in thrombocytopenia. (Oral Diag.)

coagulation t. The time required for blood clotting to begin in a capillary tube, normally 2 to 8 minutes. A coagulation time three times normal is a definite danger sign. (Oral Diag.)

gel t. (**gelation t.**) The time required to pass from the sol (liquid) to the gel state. The interval of time is related to the sol temperature. (D. Mat.)

— The interval of time required for a colloidal solution to become a solid or semisolid jelly or gel. Usually refers to the working time of a hydrocolloid or alginate impression material. (Oper. Dent.)

gelation t. (see **time, gel**)

median lethal t. (LD_{50} **t., MLT**) The time required for 50% of a large group of animals or organisms to die after administration of a specified dose of radiation. (Oral Radiol.)

prothrombin t. (**one-stage test**) A gross but useful screening test of the completeness of the second and third stages of blood coagulation. Normal prothrombin time by the Quick method is 12 to 15 seconds. The time will be affected by deficiencies of factor V or factor VII as well as of prothrombin. (Oral Med.) (see also **test, prothrombin consumption**)

serum prothrombin t. (see **test, prothrombin consumption**)

setting t. The length of time for a mixed preparation of materials to reach a state of hardness, measured from the start of the mixing. The end point for dental materials is usually determined by a penetration test. (Oper. Dent.)

timer A radiographic timer similar to either a watt-hour meter or a clocklike timing device. Its function is to act both as an automatic exposure timer and as a switch to control the current to the high-tension transformer and filament transformer. The face of the timer is calibrated in seconds and fractions of seconds.

A device controls the total time that the current passes through the x-ray tube and thus the time during which the x rays are emitted. The timer activates a switch or contractor that closes and opens the low-voltage circuit of the high voltage. (Oral Radiol.)

electronic t. An electronic vacuum tube device, with no moving parts, that covers a time range of 1/20 to 10 seconds. It automatically sets itself, is more accurate than mechanical timers, and meets all the needs of modern high-speed dental techniques. (Oral Radiol.)

foot t. A timer with an attachment that permits the timing device to be activated by foot pressure. This is the preferred type of timer. (Oral Radiol.)

hand t. An attachment to or part of a timer that requires thumb or finger pressure to activate the timing device. (Oral Radiol.)

mechanical t. A timer using a spring mechanism for determination of length of exposure. Accuracy of timing is not assumed in exposure of less than 1 second with a mechanical timer. (Oral Radiol.)

tinfoil (see **foil, tin**)

   t. substitute (see **substitute, tinfoil**)

tin octoate (ŏk′tō-āt) Substance used to accomplish vulcanization of silicone rubber impression materials. It is not a true catalyst since it becomes part of the final polymer. (D. Mat.)

tincture (tĭngk′tūr) An alcoholic, hydroalcoholic, or ethereal solution of a drug. (Oral Med.; Pharmacol.)

Tinel's sign (tĭn-ĕlz′) (see **sign, Tinel's**)

tinnitus (tĭ-nī′tŭs) Noises or unpleasant sounds in the ears, such as ringing, buzzing, roaring, or clicking; is usually high pitched and heard by many persons with auditory impairment. Clicking tinnitus may be heard by others. (Oral Physiol.)

tinted denture base (see **base, denture, tinted**)

tipping of cusps (see **restoration of cusps**)

tissue(s) An aggregation of similarly specialized cells united in the performance of a particular function. (Comp. Prosth.)

— The various cellular combinations that make up the body. (Remov. Part. Prosth.)

Antoni type A t. An aggregation of what are believed to be Schwann's cells arranged to form distorted oblong spheroid masses. The nuclei of the cells of each mass are in the same place, and when tissue so arranged is cut, the nuclei may appear in rows (palisades) or as circles or parts of circles

(Verocay bodies). Such tissue is seen in the neurilemoma. (Oral Path.) (see also **body, Verocay; neurilemoma**)

Antoni type B t. Tissue composed of a mixture of cells arising from the fibroblasts of the nerve sheath and the cells of the sheath of Schwann, loosely arranged and often showing microcysts. The tissue is a component of a neurilemoma and composes a neurofibroma. (Oral Path.)

t.-borne partial denture (see **denture, partial, tissue-borne**)

compression of t. (see **tissue displaceability**)

connective t. The binding and supportive tissue of the body; derived from the mesoderm; depending on its location and function, it is composed of fibroblasts, primitive mesenchymal cells, collagen fibers, and elastic fibers, with associated blood and lymphatic vessels, nerve fibers, etc. (Periodont.)

critical t. Tissue that either reacts most unfavorably to radiation or, by its nature, attracts and absorbs specific radiochemicals. (Oral Radiol.)

t. displaceability The quality of oral tissues that permits them to be placed in, or to assume, other than their relaxed position. (Comp. Prosth.; Fixed Part. Prosth.; Remov. Part. Prosth.)

t. displacement Change in the form or position of tissues as a result of pressure. (Comp. Prosth.; Fixed Part. Prosth.)

flabby t. (see **tissue, hyperplastic**)

hyperplastic t. (**flabby t.**) Excessively movable tissue about the mandible or maxillae due to an increase in the number of normal cells. (Comp. Prosth.; Fixed Part. Prosth.; Remov. Part. Prosth.)

interdental t. The gingivae, the cementum of the teeth, the free gingival and transseptal fibers of the periodontal membrane (ligament), and the alveolar and supporting bone. (Periodont.)

t. molding (see **border molding**)

peripheral t. (see **border structures**)

t. placement Establishment of yielding structures in that position where they are capable of initiating denture support or border seal without injury. (Comp. Prosth.; Remov. Part. Prosth.)

redundant t. (see **epulis fissuratum**)

subjacent t. (sub-jā′sĕnt) The structures that underlie or are in border contact with a denture base; they may or may not have a supporting relationship to the overlying base. (Comp. Prosth.; Remov. Part. Prosth.)

titer (tī′tĕr) The standard amount by volume of a material required to produce a desired reaction with another material. (Comp. Prosth.; Pharmacol.)

title Evidence of the right of a person to the possession of property. (D. Juris.)

titration (tī-trā′shŭn) Incremental increase in drug dosage to that level which provides the optimal therapeutic effect. (Oral Med.)

toilet of cavity (see **cavity, toilet**)

tolerance The ability to endure the influence of a drug or poison, particularly acquired by continued use of the substance. (Anesth.)

— A state in which more than the usual quantity of drug is required to elicit a standard response. (Oral Med.; Pharmacol.) (see also **resistance**)

    acquired t. Tolerance that develops with successive doses of a drug. If it develops within in a short span of time, such as 24 hours, it is called tachyphylaxis. Slowly acquired tolerance is sometimes called mithridatism. (Oral Med.; Pharmacol.)

    carbohydrate t. The ability of the body to utilize carbohydrates. A decrease in tolerance is seen in diabetes mellitus, liver damage, and some infections and in the presence of hyperactivity of the adrenal cortex or pituitary gland. (Oral Med.) (see also **test, glucose tolerance**)

    cross t. Tolerance to a number of drugs of similar mode of action or chemical structure. (Oral Med.; Pharmacol.)

    individual t. Tolerance characteristic of an individual. (Oral Med.; Pharmacol.)

    pseudo-t. A state of apparent tolerance because the drug does not reach its usual receptor sites. (Oral Med.; Pharmacol.)

    species t. Tolerance characteristic of a species of animal. (Oral Med.; Pharmacol.)

    tissue t. The ability of structures to endure environmental change without ill effect. (Remov. Part. Prosth.)

tomogram (see **examination, radiographic, extraoral body section**)

tongue The muscular organ which is the main articulatory element in the production of speech and accounts for the clarity and fluidity of speech. The muscle fiber and bundle arrangement of the tongue provide for the extremely rapid change in position and morphology required for speech and mastication. There are two groups of tongue muscles, the intrinsic and the extrinsic, which are united into one organ. Each group, however, has

separate structural and functional characteristics. (Oral Physiol.)

    amyloid t. (amyloid macroglossia) Enlargement of the tongue due to amyloidosis. (Oral Med.)

    antibiotic t. A glossitis caused by sensitivity to an antibiotic, by vitamin B complex deficiency associated with antibiotic therapy, or by thrush associated with antibiotic therapy. (Oral Diag.)

    bald t. (see **glossitis, atrophic**)

        Sandwith's b. t. A condition in which the tongue is very smooth due to a loss of fusiform papillae and is fiery red and enlarged due to severe inflammation; seen in pellagra. (Oral Path.)

    beefy t. Erythematous and/or atrophic glossitis. (Oral Diag.) (see also **glossitis, atrophic; glossitis, Moeller's**)

    — A severe form of Sandwith's bald tongue in which red, irregular ulcerations are seen on the dorsal surface. (Oral Path.) (see also **tongue, bald, Sandwith's**)

    bifid t. (cleft t.) A tongue divided by a midline cleft. (Oral Diag.)

    cleft t. (see **tongue, bifid**)

    coated t. A tongue with a white to brown film that is readily removed by scraping. The film consists of desquamated cells, food debris, and microorganisms. Reduced function, as in general illness or laryngitis, is a primary cause. (Oral Diag.)

    — Nonspecific term used to describe the condition of the tongue due to whitish or otherwise discolored accumulations of food debris, bacterial plaques, and hyperplastic filiform papillae. (Oral Med.)

    cobblestone t. Hyperplasia and hyperemia of fungiform and filiform papillae of the tongue in riboflavin deficiency. Formerly used to describe syphilitic glossitis with leukoplakia. (Oral Med.)

    fissured t. (furrowed t.) A tongue traversed by clefts that may be arranged like the veins of a leaf or that may be such as to give the tongue a "pavement block" appearance. It is seen in 5% of all dental patients but in 13% of those past 50 years of age. (Oral Diag.)

    flat t. Paralysis of the transverse lingual muscles such that the borders of the tongue cannot be rolled; due to congenital syphilis. (Oral Med.)

    t. function The role of the tongue in mastication and deglutition, and as an important accessory organ for speech, a sensory organ for taste, etc. During mastication of some foods, the tongue has a direct crushing action, pressing the food against the hard palate. The tongue aids in forming a compact bolus of food and in placing the bolus on the occlusal platform for tooth action. The tongue also serves as a mechanism of cleansing of the lingual surfaces of the teeth and stimulates the lingual gingival tissues. (Periodont.)

furrowed t. (see **tongue, fissured**)

geographic t. (benign migratory glossitis, glossitis areata exfoliativa, glossitis migrans, wandering rash) An inflammation of the tongue characterized by anular patterns with red centers and white borders. The dorsum and borders of the tongue may be involved, with loss of papillae in the central red zones. The pattern changes slowly from time to time—hence the term migratory. The cause is not known. (Oral Diag.)

— A condition characterized by a chronic, circumscribed, more or less circinate desquamation of the superficial epithelium of the dorsum of the tongue. The spots of desquamation migrate continuously, usually passing from the region near the vallate papillae toward the tip of the tongue. (Periodont.)

— A tongue with denuded areas surrounded by areas of normal or hyperkeratotic epithelium which by contrast appear white. The areas that are denuded frequently change position. (Oral Path.)

hairy t. Hyperplasia of the filiform papillae of the tongue associated with use of sodium perborate, smoking, use of antibiotics, and oral moniliasis. (Periodont.)

black h. t. (lingua nigra) A black appearance of the dorsal surface of the tongue; caused by elongated filiform papillae and an accumulation of dark pigments. (Oral Diag.)

— Presence of a brown, black, or green furlike covering on the dorsum of the tongue due to hypertrophy of the filiform papillae and excess deposition of keratin. The coloration is due to the impaction of food debris. (Oral Path.)

white h. t. (lingua alba, lingua villosa alba) Hairy tongue characterized by elongation of the filiform papillae but without the dark staining seen in lingua nigra (black hairy tongue). (see also **tongue, hairy, black**) (Oral Diag.)

lobulated t. A congenital defect with a sec-

ondary lobe of the tongue arising from its surface. (Oral Diag.)

magenta t. (mah-jĕn′tah) The reddish purple tongue of riboflavin deficiency. (Oral Med.)

t. room (see **tongue space**)

smooth t. (see **glossitis, atrophic**)

t. space The space available for functioning of the tongue. (Remov. Part. Prosth.)

strawberry t. The red, inflamed tongue with prominent fungiform papillae characteristic of scarlet fever. (Oral Diag.)

— Changes in the tongue in scarlet fever, consisting of changes in the epithelium and accentuation of the filiform and fungiform papillae. (Oral Med.)

t. thrust Pressing of the tongue against or between the maxillary and mandibular teeth as a habit pattern. (Orthodont.)

t. thrusting The interposition of the tongue between the opposing occlusal surfaces during the act of swallowing. Although it is frequently associated with children and adolescents, it is also prevalent among adults and the aging population. In some instances it appears during adolescence, when there are marked changes in the growth and development of the dental occlusion and the facial skeleton. It also appears in adults in whom there is modification in the occlusion and musculoskeletal architecture of the face. The presence of tongue thrusting may or may not be considered pathologic. There are times when it may be considered physiologically normal; e.g., when the infant swallows. The tongue is used to brace the mandible against the maxillae in order to elevate the structures of the floor of the mouth. (Oral Physiol.)

tonofibril (tōn-ō-fi′bril) A fibril emanating from epithelial cells. Recent electron microscopy has shown such fibrils to be irregular formations of the cell membrane. (Periodont.)

tonofibrils A light-microscope structure made up of fibers that appear to course from epithelial cell to epithelial cell across the intercellular bridges. (Periodont.)

tonsillitis (ton″sĭ-li′tĭs) Inflammation of the tonsils. (Oral Diag.)

lingual t. A form of tonsillitis at the posterior part of the base of the tongue in the lymphoid masses (lingual tonsils) located there. (Oral Diag.)

tonus, muscle (tō′nŭs) The steady reflex contraction that resides in the muscles concerned in maintaining erect posture. Tonus has its basis in the positional interactions of the muscle and its accompanying nerve structure; e.g., a muscle holds the body (mandible) in a given position, and the awareness of this position is constantly being relayed by the sensory approaches to the cortex. Any change in position or contractility of the muscle that affects its tonus is immediately relayed by the sensory apparatus for readjustment. (Oral Physiol.)

facial m. t. The tone of the facial musculature, which is a major factor in providing the esthetic values of the human face. The configurations of the face, which are maintained by good muscle tonus, are the modiolus, the philtrum, the nasolabial sulcus, and the mentolabial sulcus. These functional contours are present when the nerve tissue is intact. They are altered by the loss of teeth or impaired nerve function. Their presence is an indication of the good state of health of the nerve and possibly of the dental arch. (Oral Physiol.)

tooth, teeth Organs of mastication. (Comp. Prosth.; Remov. Part. Prosth.)

— One of the hard bodies or processes usually protruding from and attached to the alveolar process of the maxillae and the mandible; designed for the mastication of food. (Oper. Dent.)

abutment t. A tooth or teeth selected to support a bridge on the basis of the total surface areas of a healthy attachment apparatus. (Periodont.)

accessory t. (ăk-sĕs'ō-rē) Supernumerary teeth that do not resemble normal teeth in size, shape, or location. (Oral Diag.; Oral Path.) (see also **distomolar; mesiodens; paramolar; tooth, supernumerary**)

acrylic resin t. (ah-krĭl'ĭk) A tooth made of acrylic resin. (Comp. Prosth.)

anatomic t. (ăn"ah-tom'ĭk) An artificial tooth that closely resembles the anatomic form of a natural unabraded tooth. An artificial tooth that has notable triangular (pyramidal) eminences on the masticating surfaces, which are designed to occlude primarily in the sulci and fossae of the teeth of the opposing denture or dentition. (Comp. Prosth.; Remov. Part. Prosth.)

ankylosed t. (ăng'kĭ-lōsd) A primary tooth, with or without a permanent successor, that fails to erupt into occlusion with its opponent as a result of a union of the alveolar bone and dentin of the root structure. Tooth has the appearance of being "submerged." The occurrence is noted to have a familial tendency and is probably a nonsex-linked trait. (Pedodont.)

anterior t. One of the incisor or canine teeth. (Orthodont.)

artificial t. A tooth fabricated for use as a substitute for a natural tooth in a prosthesis; usually made of porcelain or plastics. (Comp. Prosth.; D. Mat.; Remov. Part. Prosth.)

canine t. The four cuspids; the third tooth located distal to the midline in any one of the four quadrants of the dentition. (Periodont.)

conical t. (**peg-shaped t.**) Failure of morphologic development of the tooth germ found in ectodermal dysplasia and other disorders and occasionally found in normal children. (Pedodont.)

cross-bite t. Posterior teeth designed to permit the modified buccal cusps of the upper teeth to be positioned in the central fossae of the lower teeth. (Comp. Prosth.; Remov. Part. Prosth.)

t. curvatures, faulty Improper or imperfect form of the crown or root, especially those crowns or roots that do not provide adequate protection to the gingival tissue. (Periodont.)

cuspless t. Teeth designed without cuspal prominences on the masticatory surfaces. (Comp. Prosth.; Remov. Part. Prosth.)

deciduous t. (see **deciduous; tooth, primary**)

devital t. (see **tooth, pulpless**)

drifting t. Slow physiologic movement of a tooth into an adjacent edentulous space. (Orthodont.)

—— The migration of teeth from their normal positions in the dental arches as a result of such factors as loss of proximal support, loss of functional antagonists, occlusal traumatic tooth relationships, inflammatory and retrograde changes in the attachment apparatus and oral habits. (Periodont.)

embedded t. An unerupted tooth, usually one completely covered with bone; also spelled imbedded. (Oral Surg.) (see also **tooth, impacted**)

evulsed t. (**avulsed t.**) A tooth that has been abnormally luxated from its alveolar support commonly as a sequela to trauma. (Oral Surg.)

t. form (see **form, tooth**)

fulcrum of t. The axis of movement of a tooth when lateral forces are applied to the tooth. The fulcrum is considered to be at the middle third of the portion of root embedded in the alveolus and thus moves apically as the bone resorbs in periodontal disease. (Periodont.)

fused t. Two teeth united during development by the union of their tooth germs. The teeth may be joined by the enamel of their crowns, by their root dentin, or by both. (Oral Diag.)

— Developmental anomaly in which two tooth buds are united early in development to form a single large crown. Two root canals are usually present. (Oral Path.)

— The fusion of two adjacent tooth germs. (Pedodont.)

geminated t. (jĕm′ĭ-nā-tĕd) Teeth with bifid crowns and confluent root canals resulting from the division of the enamel organ during the developmental period. (Pedodont.)

grinding of t. The afunctional movements of the mandible, with the teeth in contact, occurring in bruxism. Also, the selective modification of tooth form and contour in the occlusal adjustment operation in order to eliminate occlusal interferences and establish tooth contours conducive to the health of the periodontium. (Periodont.) (see also **bruxism**)

    g. of t., buccolingual diameter A phase of selective grinding (occlusal adjustment) in which the buccolingual dimension of a tooth is narrowed. The purposes are to bring forces applied to the tooth closer to its center and the center of rotation within its root and to unlock the teeth during the functional and nonfunctional movements of the mandible. (Periodont.)

hereditary brown t. (see **hypoplasia, enamel, hereditary**)

hutchinsonian t. Teeth with defective clinical crowns as a result of congenital syphilis. (Comp. Prosth.; Oral Diag.)

hypoplasia of t. (hī″pō-plā′zē-ah) A reduction in the amount of enamel formed, resulting in irregular pits and grooves of the enamel. (Pedodont.)

— Defective or incomplete development and formation of the teeth or portions thereof; e.g., amelogenesis imperfecta and dentinogenesis imperfecta. (Periodont.)

impacted t. A condition in which the unerupted or partially erupted tooth is positioned against another tooth, bone, or soft tissue so that complete eruption is unlikely. An impacted third molar tooth may be further described according to its position: buccoangular, distoangular, vertical, etc. An impacted maxillary cuspid tooth may also be further described according to its position: palatal (maxillary cuspid), lingual (mandibular cuspid), labial, vertical, etc. (Oral Surg.)

implant superstructure t. (see **superstructure, implant, teeth**)

inclination of t. The angle of slope of teeth from the vertical planes of reference. Thus a tooth may be mesially, distally, lingually, buccally, or labially inclined. (Periodont.)

loosening of t. Mobility of teeth associated with alterations of the attachment apparatus, such as that occurring with periodontitis, periodontosis, periapical inflammation, etc. Sequelae include resorption of alveolar and supporting bone; a degenerative and heterogeneous appearance of periodontal fibers, especially of the alveolar group; etc. (Periodont.)

loss of t. The separation of a tooth from its investing and supporting structures as a result of (1) normal exfoliation attending loss of deciduous dentition, (2) exfoliation as a sequela to excessive bone resorption and periapical migration of the epithelial attachment in periodontal disease, and (3) instrumentation for extraction necessitated by pathologic involvement of the dental pulp, the periodontium, the periapical tissues, etc. (Periodont.)

mesial movement of t. Migration of teeth toward the midline, occurring as a phenomenon associated with the action of the anterior component of force. Mesial migration of teeth occurs with the wear of their proximal surfaces due to the buccolingual movements of the teeth. (Periodont.)

metal insert t. An artificial tooth, usually of acrylic resin, containing an inserted ribbon of metal, or a cutting blade, in its occlusal surface, with one edge of the blade exposed; sometimes used in removable dentures. (Comp. Prosth.; Remov. Part. Prosth.)

migration of t. The movement of teeth into altered positions in relationship to the basal bone of the alveolar process and to adjoining and opposing teeth as a result of loss of approximating or opposing teeth, occlusal interferences, habits, inflammatory and dystrophic disease of the attaching and supporting structures of the teeth, etc. (Periodont.)

— The drifting, separating, tipping, etc. that occurs after a void has been created in the dental arch by the loss of one or more teeth. (Remov. Part. Prosth.)

missing t. The absence of teeth from the dentition because of congenital factors, exfoliation, extraction, etc. (Periodont.)

t. mobility The movability of a tooth resulting from loss of all or a portion of its attachment and supportive apparatus. Seen in periodontitis, occlusal traumatism, and periodontosis. (Periodont.)

t. morphology The science of the anatomic topography of the teeth. (Oper. Dent.)

t. movement (see **movement, tooth**)

natal t. Primary teeth found in the oral cavity at birth. (Pedodont.)

neonatal t. A primary tooth that erupts into the oral cavity during the neonatal period (from birth to 30 days). (Pedodont.)

nonanatomic t. Artificial teeth so designed that the occlusal surfaces are not copies from natural forms, but rather are given forms which, in the opinion of the designer, seem more nearly to fulfill the requirements of mastication, tissue tolerance, etc. (Comp. Prosth.; Remov. Part. Prosth.)

peg-shaped t. (see **tooth, conical**)

permanent t. (see **dentition, permanent**)

pink t. (see **resorption, internal**)

plastic t. Artificial teeth constructed of synthetic resins. (Comp. Prosth.; Remov. Part. Prosth.)

polishing of t. The removal of film, plaque, soft deposits, etc. from the teeth by appropriate hand- and/or engine-driven instrumentation. Abrasive cups, wheels, or disks are often used in conjunction with abrasive pastes such as pumice and water. (Periodont.)

t. position (see **position, tooth**)

posterior t. The maxillary and mandibular premolars and molars of the permanent dentition, or the bicuspids and molars of prostheses. (Comp. Prosth.; Periodont.; Remov. Part. Prosth.)

primary t. Term used by some in preference to deciduous teeth; however, it has not received the approval of preference by the American Dental Association. (Oper. Dent.) (see also **deciduous**)

— The College Committee Report of Dentistry for Children, in 1942, as a result of a survey of the terminology employed to name the teeth of the first dentition, recommended the use of primary teeth as the term preferred to deciduous, first, milk, temporary, baby, or foundation teeth. The term "primary" was suggested as a word "which may be acceptable to the dental profession, significant in its meaning, with no connotation of impermanence, and readily understood by nonprofessional people." (Pedodont.)

pulpless t. A tooth from which the dental pulp has been removed or is missing. (Remov. Part. Prosth.)

replaced t. (see **tooth, supplied**)

rotated t. An altered position of the tooth in relation to the adjacent and opposing teeth and to its basal alveolar process; in such an altered position the tooth has been turned on its long axis and is in a state of torsiversion. The result is an altered contact with adjacent teeth that produces a possible locus for food impaction between the teeth, with consequent gingival damage. (Periodont.)

t. selection (see **selection, tooth**)

sensitivity of t. A painful pulpal response to external stimuli such as heat, cold, and sweet substances. The most common clinical finding is a hyperesthetic state of the root surface due to loss of a portion of the cemental covering, with exposure of the dentin. (Periodont.)

drugs for s. of t. The medicaments used to treat hypersensitivity of the teeth; they should cause relatively little pain when applied; should be easily applied, rapid in action, and permanently effective; and should not discolor the teeth or unduly irritate the pulp. Substances used include 33% sodium fluoride in kaolin and glycerin, a 25% aqueous solution of strontium chloride, hot medicinal olive oil, 0.9% solution of sodium silicofluoride, etc. (Periodont.)

separation of t. The action of moving a tooth mesially or distally out of contact with its neighboring tooth. (Oper. Dent.)

immediate s. of t. Separation of teeth accomplished rapidly by the wedging action of an appliance. (Oper. Dent.)

slow s. of t. Separation of teeth accomplished over a long period of time, usually by the wedging action of a material such as gutta-percha, orthodontic wire, thread, or fibers. (Oper. Dent.)

set of t. Term that usually refers to a full complement of maxillary and/or mandibular artificial teeth, as they are carded by the manufacturer. (Comp. Prosth.)

setting up of t. The arranging of teeth on a trial denture base; includes proper relation with occluding teeth. (Comp. Prosth.; Remov. Part. Prosth.)

shell t. A form of dentinal dysplasia characterized by large pulp chambers, meager coronal dentin, and, usually, no roots. (Oral Diag.)

supernumerary t. Extra erupted or unerupted teeth that resemble teeth of normal shape. (Oral Path.; (Pedodont.)

supplied t. (replaced t.) Artificial replacements for natural teeth. (Comp. Prosth.; Remov. Part. Prosth.)

supportive mechanism of t. The anatomic structures that function to maintain or to aid in maintaining the teeth in position in their alveoli: the gingivae, cementum of the tooth, periodontal membrane, and alveolar and supporting bone. (Periodont.) (see also **structures, supporting**)

suspension of t. Most likely, the connective tissue fiber apparatus of the periodontal membrane, arranged with a predominance of oblique fibers with a fluid displacement mechanism. The attachment apparatus serves to transmit masticatory forces to the supporting structures of the tooth. The intermediate plexus plays a role in transmission and dissipation of force in that a shock-absorption quality of a loose connection operates, whereas the fluid component of the periodontal membrane (ligament) serves as a hydraulic system for eliminating excessive stress. (Periodont.)

tube t. Artificial teeth constructed with a vertical, cylindric aperture extending from the center of the base up into the body of the tooth into which a pin or cast post for the attachment of the tooth to a denture base may be placed. (Comp. Prosth.; Remov. Part. Prosth.)

Turner's t. A permanent tooth showing hypoplasia due to injury or inflammation of the precedent deciduous tooth. (Oral Diag.)

vital staining of t. The staining of enamel and dentin of primary and permanent teeth during development with vital stains; e.g., with bile pigment in Rh incompatibility or with tetracyclines. (Pedodont.)

zero degree t. Prosthetic teeth having no cusp angles in relation to the horizontal plane; cuspless teeth. (Comp. Prosth.; Remov. Part. Prosth.)

tooth-borne Term used to describe a prosthesis or a part of a prosthesis that depends entirely on the abutment teeth for support. (Fixed Part. Prosth.; Remov. Part. Prosth.)

t.-b. base The denture base restoring an edentulous area that has abutment teeth at each end for support. The tissue that it covers is not used for support of the base. (Fixed Part. Prosth.; Remov. Part. Prosth.)

toothbrushing The use of a brush of varying design to brush the teeth and gingivae for cleanliness and to massage for oral hygiene. (Periodont.)

faulty t. The improper performance of toothbrushing, resulting in defective cleansing, inadequate stimulation of the gingival tissues, or destructive effects on the teeth and marginal gingivae due to overzealous brushing. (Periodont.)

toothpick A wood sliver used to cleanse the interdental space. (Periodont.)

balsa wood t. A triangular wedge of balsa wood used to cleanse teeth interproximally and to stimulate the interdental gingival tissues. (Periodont.)

topesthesia (top″ĕs-thē′zē-ah) Ability through tactile sense to determine any part that is touched. (Anesth.)

topographic intraoral radiographic examination (see **examination, radiographic, intraoral, true occlusal topographic**)

toponarcosis (tŏp-ō-nar-kō′sĭs) Local insensibility or anesthesia. (Anesth.)

torque (tork) A rotary force applied to a denture base. (Comp. Prosth.)

— Force applied to a tooth to produce rotation of a tooth on a mesiodistal or buccolingual (labiolingual) axis. (Orthodont.)

— A force that produces or tends to produce rotation in a body. Such force applied to a tooth tends to cause rotation around its long axis. (Remov. Part. Prosth.)

t. wire An auxiliary wire used to torque the roots of the anterior teeth. (Orthodont.)

torsion In dentistry, the twisting of a tooth on its long axis. (Orthodont.; Remov. Part. Prosth.)

clasp t. The twisting of the retentive clasp arm on its long axis. It has been suggested that a retentive clasp be formed so that it traverses a vertical distance before encircling the abutment in order to increase the torsion component of the clasp opening as compared to the flexure that it underwent. (Remov. Part. Prosth.)

torsiversion An axially rotated tooth position. (Orthodont.)

tort A legal wrong perpetrated on a person or his property independent of contract. (D. Juris.)

torus A bulging projection of bone. (Comp. Prosth.; Remov. Part. Prosth.)

t. mandibularis A bony enlargement (hyperostosis) appearing unilaterally or bilaterally on the lingual aspect of the mandible in the cuspid-premolar region of about 7% of the population. (Oral Diag.)

— Exostosis occurring on the lingual surface of the mandible in the region of the cuspid and first bicuspid. (Comp. Prosth.; Oral Path.; Remov. Part. Prosth.)

t. palatinus A bony enlargement (hyperostosis) occuring in the midline of the hard palate in about 20% of the population. (Oral Diag.)

—An osseous protuberance, or exostosis, on the hard palate near the intermaxillary (median palatine) suture. (Comp. Prosth.; Oral Path.; Remov. Part. Prosth.)

total body radiation (see **radiation, total body**)

total filtration (see **filtration, total**)

touch, light Tactile sense, the principal organs of which are Meissner's corpuscles, which are large in size and oval in shape. Each capsule receives several nerve fibers that shed their myelin sheath and coil into a spiral complex network. Associated with Meissner's corpuscles in the perception of light touch are both Merkel's disks and a basketlike arrangement of nerve fibers around the hair follicles. (Oral Physiol.)

toxic Poisonous; produced by a poison. (D. Juris.; Oral Med.)

toxicity (tok-sĭs′ĭ-tē) The quality of being toxic; the kind and amount of poison produced by a microorganism. (Anesth.)

— The ability of a drug or other chemically active substance to produce harm, especially to cause permanent injury or death. Usually distinguished from allergenic properties. Also various quantitative measures of harmful or lethal dosage, e.g., LD_{50} values. (Oral Med.; Pharmacol.)

acute t. A condition produced after short-term use of a toxic agent. (Oral Med.; Pharmacol.) (see also **dose, lethal, median; dose, lethal, minimum**)

chronic t. A condition produced after long-term use of a toxic agent. (Oral Med.; Pharmacol.)

toxicologist (tok″sĭ-kol′ō-jĭst) One versed in toxicology. (Anesth.)

toxicology The science of the nature and effects of poisons, their detection, and the treatment of their effects. (Anesth.)

toxoplasmosis (tok″sō-plăz-mō′sĭs) A disease caused by protozoa in the bloodstream and body tissues. (Oral Diag.)

TPC (thromboplastic plasma component) (see **factor VIII**)

TPI (see **test, Treponema pallidum immobilization**)

tracer A mechanical device used to trace a pattern of mandibular movements. A mechanical device with a marking point is attached to one jaw, and a graph plate is attached to the other jaw. It is used to indicate or record the direction and extent of movements of the mandible or to indicate the relative position of the mandible to the maxillae. (Comp. Prosth.; Fixed Part. Prosth.; Oral Radiol; Remov. Part. Prosth.)

— A foreign substance mixed with or attached to a given substance to enable the distribution or location of the latter to be determined subsequently. A radioactive tracer is a physical or chemical tracer having radioactivity as its distinctive property. (Oral Radiol.)

Gothic arch t. (see **tracer, needle point**)

needle point t. A mechanical device consisting of a weighted or a spring-loaded needle that is attached to one jaw and a coated plate that is attached to the other jaw. Movement of the mandible causes a tracing to be formed on the horizontally placed plate. When the needle point is in the apex of the tracing, the mandible is said to be in the horizontal position of centric relation. (Comp. Prosth.)

sea gull t. (see **tracer, needle point**)

trachea (trā′kē-ah) The windpipe; a cartilaginous and membranous tube extending from the lower end of the larynx to its division into two bronchi. (Anesth.)

tracheal tugging (trā′kē-ăl) The downward tugging movement of the larynx. (Anesth.)

tracheo- (trā′kē-ō) Combining form denoting connection with or relation to the trachea. (Anesth.)

tracheobronchial (trā″kē-ō-brŏng′kē-al) Pertaining to the trachea and a bronchus or bronchi. (Anesth.)

tracheobronchoscopy (trā″kē-ō-brong-kōs′kō-pē) Inspection of the interior of the trachea and bronchus. (Anesth.)

tracheolaryngeal (trā″kē-ō-lah-rĭn′jē-al) Pertaining to the trachea and larynx. (Anesth.)

tracheolaryngotomy (trā″kē-ō-lar″ĭng-got′ō-mē) Incision into the larynx and the trachea; tracheotomy and laryngotomy. (Anesth.)

tracheoscopy (trā″kē-os′kō-pē) Inspection of the interior of the trachea by means of a laryngoscopic mirror and reflected light or through a bronchoscope. (Anesth.)

tracheostenosis (trā″kē-ō-stĕ-nō′sĭs) Abnormal constriction or narrowing of the trachea. (Anesth.)

tracheostomy (trā″kē-os′tō-mē) The formation of an opening into the trachea and the suturing of the edges of the opening to an opening in the skin of the neck. (Anesth.)

— Surgical formation of an opening into the trachea, usually through the tracheal rings below the cricoid cartilage, to give the patient an airway. (Oral Surg.)

tracheotome (trā′kē-ō-tōm″) A cutting instrument used in tracheotomy; a tracheotomy knife. (Anesth.)

— An instrument for use in creating an airway through the skin into the trachea below the cricoid cartilage. (Oral Surg.)

tracheotomist (trā″kē-ot′ō-mĭst) One skilled in performing tracheotomies. (Anesth.)

tracheotomize (trā″kē-ot′ō-mīz) To perform a tracheotomy on a living animal. (Anesth.)

tracheotomy (trā″kē-ot′ō-mē) The operation of cutting into the trachea to give the patient an airway. (Oral Surg.)

tracing A line or lines or a pattern scribed by a pointed instrument or stylus on a tracing plate or tracing paper.

arrow point t. (see **tracing, needle point**)

cephalometric t. A line drawing of pertinent features of a cephalometric radiograph made on a piece of transparent paper placed over the radiograph. (Comp. Prosth.; Fixed Part. Prosth.; Orthodont.; Remov. Part. Prosth.)

extraoral t. A tracing of mandibular movements made outside the oral cavity. (Comp. Prosth.; Fixed Part. Prosth.; Remov. Part. Prosth.)

Gothic arch t. (see **tracing, needle point**)

intraoral t. A tracing of mandibular movements made within the oral cavity. (Comp. Prosth.; Fixed Part. Prosth.; Remov. Part. Prosth.)

needle point t. (arrow point t., Gothic arch t., sea gull t., stylus t.) A tracing made by a mechanical device consisting of a weighted or spring-loaded stylus that is attached to one jaw and contacts a coated plate attached to the other jaw. Movement of the mandible causes a tracing to be formed on the horizontally placed coated plate. When the stylus point is in the apex of the tracing, the mandible is said to be in the horizontal position of centric relation. The shape of the tracing depends on the relative location of the marking point and the tracing table. The various tracing shapes have been called Gothic arch, arrow point, and sea gull tracings. The apex of a properly made tracing is considered to indicate the most retruded unstrained relation of the man-

dible to the maxillae, i.e., the centric relation. The tracings are made by a stylus (or needle point) by the movement of the mandible. Unless otherwise designated, stylus tracings are made by lateral movements registered on a horizontal plate. (Comp. Prosth.; Fixed Part. Prosth.; Remov. Part. Prosth.)

sea gull t. (see **tracing, needle point**)

stylus t. (see **tracing, needle point**)

tracings, pantographic Mandibular tracings, made on maxillary held planes, that record movements made by the mandible about its axes as they are moved in the "cams" of the joints. (Gnathol.)

tract, sinus A communication between a pathologic space and an anatomic body cavity or between a pathologic space and the skin. A sinus tract may . or may not be lined with epithelium. (Oral Surg.)

traction The act of drawing (pulling).

external t. A fracture reduction appliance principally used in the management of midfacial fractures. Points of fixation are located in the oral cavity and over the cranial area, with elastic or rigid connectors between the cranial and oral points of fixation. (Oral Surg.)

intermaxillary t. (see **traction, maxillomandibular**)

internal t. A pulling force created by using one of the cranial bones, above the point of fracture, for anchorage. (Oral Surg.)

maxillomandibular t. (intermaxillary traction) The technique for reducing fractures of the maxillae or mandible into functional relations with the opposing dental arch through the use of elastic or wire ligatures and interdental wiring and/or splints. (Oral Surg.)

tragion (trā′jē-on) The notch just above the tragus of the ear. It lies 1 to 2 mm. below the spina helicis, which may be easily palpated. (Orthodont.)

tragus (trā′gŭs) A prominence in front of the opening of the external ear. (Oral Surg.)

trait, Cooley's (see **thalassemia minor**)

trait, sickle cell A form of sickle cell disease in which patients are asymptomatic but their erythrocytes can be caused to assume a sickle shape under certain conditions. The trait is present when one parent has the gene (heterozygous condition) for sickle cell disease. (Oral Med.) (see also **disease, sickle cell**)

tranquilizer (trăn′kwĭ-lī″zer) Layman's term for

a calming agent that reduces anxiety and tension without depressing mental or motor functions; a psychosedative. (Anesth.)

— One of a poorly defined group of drugs designed to produce a calm and relaxed state without interfering with physical responsiveness or mental clarity. (Oral Med.; Pharmacol.)

transaminase (trăns-ăm′ĭ-nās) One of several enzymes involved in conversion of NH_3, formed in metabolic processes, to urea or its transfer to an amino acid. Characteristic high values are seen in myocardial infarction and viral hepatitis. (Oral Med.)

transfer, linear energy (**LET**) Linear energy transfer per unit length. This term is comparable to specific ionization except that specific ionization ordinarily implies the number of ion pairs per unit length of track in air, whereas linear energy transfer refers to the transfer of energy in tissues. This transfer of energy includes the energy required to produce ions and the energy imparted to other atoms and molecules that are not ionized but become "excited." (Oral Radiol.)

transformer An electrical device that increases or reduces the voltage of an alternating current by mutual induction between primary and secondary coils or windings. (Oral Radiol.)

auto-t. (see **autotransformer**)

Coolidge filament t. A step-down transformer that reduces the line voltage of 110 volts to one of 12 volts, which in turn heats the tungsten filament of the Coolidge tube for the production of electrons. (Oral Radiol.)

step-down t. A transformer in which the secondary voltage is less than the primary voltage. (Oral Radiol.)

step-up t. A transformer in which the secondary voltage is greater than the primary voltage. (Oral Radiol.)

transillumination (trăns′ĭ-lū″mĭ-nā′shŭn) A test in which the use of transmitted light may disclose a discoloration of the coronal aspect, indicating dentinal tubular hemorrhage as a result of trauma and/or pulpal necrosis, or a fracture. (Endodont.)

— Examination of an organ, cavity, or tissue (e.g., a tooth or gingival tissue) by transmitted light. A valuable aid in detecting carious lesions, disclosing carious or demineralized dentin during cavity preparation, checking the finish or gingival margins of restorations, and revealing cement, debris, or calculus subgingivally. (Oper. Dent.)

— Examination of tissues by means of a light placed so that the region under study is between the light source and the observer. (Oral Diag.; Periodont.)

transition point (see **Tg value**)

transitional denture (see **denture, transitional**)

translation Movement of a rigid body in which all parts move in the same direction at the same speed. (Comp. Prosth.)

translatory movement (see **movement, translatory**)

transosteal implant jig An instrument designed to guide a bone drill from inferior border through alveolar ridge to create a path for the seating of a transosteal implant. (Oral Implant.)

transpirable Capable of passing in a gaseous state through the respiratory epithelium or skin. (Anesth.)

transplant, *n.* Implantation of living or nonliving tissue or bone into another part of the body; it then serves as a scaffold in the healing process and is progressively resorbed and replaced by newly formed bone. (Periodont.)

—, *v.* To remove and plant in another place, as from one body or part of a body to another. (M.F.P.)

— To move a tooth or tissue from one site to another, often but not always autogenously. (Oral Implant.)

transplantation, tooth The transfer of a tooth from one alveolus to another. (Oral Surg.)

autogenous t. t. Transplantation of a tooth from one position to another in the same individual. (Implantodont.)

homogenous t. t. Transplantation of a tooth from one human to another. (Implantodont.)

transseptal fiber (see **fiber, transseptal**)

transtrusion, magnitude of The amplitude of condylar transtrusion, which varies among persons as determined clinically by measuring it in the jaw tracings at the levels of the tragi from a few millimeters to 7 mm. The side shifts of many condyles equal the fore shifts. The transtrusion increases the capacity of the person to manage larger boluses by lengthening the lateral stroke of the lower cusps. This evidence is recordable in the horizontal and frontal craniofacial space planes. (Gnathol.)

transudate (trăn′sū-dāt) Any substance that has passed through a membrane. Usually a fluid not associated with inflammation. Noninflammatory edema such as is encountered in heart failure and renal disease. It is low in proteins and colloids and has a specific gravity usually below 1.012. (Oral Path.)

transversion Eruption of a tooth in the wrong position. (Orthodont.)

trauma (traw′mah) A hurt; a wound; an injury damage; impairment; external violence producing bodily injury or degeneration. An actual alteration of tissues produced by dental disharmony. (Comp. Prosth.; Oper. Dent.)

— In medical jurisprudence, a wound; an injury to the body caused by external force. (D. Juris.)

— A hurt; a wound; an injury; damage or impairment; generally caused by external violence. (Oral Path.; Remov. Part. Prosth.)

   occlusal t. Abnormal occlusal relationships of the teeth, causing injury to the periodontium. (Oral Diag.)

      injury in o. t. The damaging effects of occlusal trauma, which are of a dystrophic nature and affect the tooth and its attachment apparatus. In pure occlusal traumatism the integumenal gingivae are not affected. Lesions include wear facets on the tooth, root resorption, cemental tears, thrombosis of blood vessels of the periodontal membrane, necrosis and hyalinization of the periodontal membrane on the pressure side, resorption of alveolar and supporting bone, etc. Clinically, tooth mobility and migration may be evident; radiographically, evidence is the widening of the periodontal membrane space and fraying or fuzziness of the lamina dura, formation of infrabony resorptive defects, etc. Pocket formation is not a sequela to occlusal traumatism. (Periodont.)

      pocket in o. t. (see **pocket in occlusal trauma**)

traumatic (traw-măt′ĭk) Of, or pertaining to, or caused by an injury. (Comp. Prosth.; Fixed Part. Prosth.; Remov. Part. Prosth.)

   t. occlusion (see **occlusion, traumatic**)

   t. shock (see **shock, traumatic**)

traumatism (traw′mah-tĭzm) A form of periodontal disease caused by excessive occlusal trauma. (Oral Diag.)

   t. by food Impingement of the gingival margin by coarse foodstuff; caused by improper contour of the tooth or faulty position of the tooth. (Periodont.)

   occlusal t. Lesions of the attachment apparatus; caused by force placed on the tooth in excess of that which the supporting structures can withstand. (Periodont.)

      primary o. t. The force, or forces, that are caused by mandibular movement and re-sultant tooth percussion and that are capable of producing pathologic changes in the periodontium. (Periodont.)

      secondary o. t. Destruction of the attachment apparatus by factors other than those of occlusion (e.g., periodontitis). In secondary occlusal traumatism, even the forces of mastication become pathologic in nature. (Periodont.)

   periodontal t. The application of stress to the structures comprising the attachment apparatus, which exceeds the adaptive capacities of the tissues, with resultant tissue destruction. (Periodont.)

traumatogenic (traw″mah-tō-jĕn′ĭk) Capable of producing a wound or injury. (Comp. Prosth.; Fixed Part. Prosth.; Remov. Part. Prosth.)

   t. occlusion (see **occlusion, traumatogenic**)

tray A receptacle or device that holds or carries.

   acrylic resin t. A tray made of acrylic resin. (Comp. Prosth.)

   impression t. A receptacle or device that is used to carry the impression material to the mouth, to confine the material in apposition to the surfaces to be recorded, and to control the impression material while it sets to form the impression. (Comp. Prosth.; Remov. Part. Prosth.)

   — A receptacle into which a suitable material is placed to make an impression. A device that is used to carry, confine, and control an impression material for making an impression. (Oper. Dent.)

Treacher Collins syndrome (see **syndrome, Treacher Collins**)

treatment The mode or course pursued for remedial ends. (Oper. Dent.)

— Services received by the patient and provided by the dentist. (Pract. Man.)

   heat t. Subjecting a metal to a given controlled heat, followed by controlled sudden or gradual cooling to develop the desired qualities of the metal to the maximum degree. (Oper. Dent.)

— A process of giving a metal predetermined physical properties by controlled temperature changes. (Remov. Part. Prosth.)

   hardening h. t. (see **tempering**)

   homogenizing h. t. (see **anneal**)

   softening h. t. (see **anneal**)

   indirect pulp capping t. Application of a drug or material to a layer of carious or sound dentin in the deepest part of the carious lesion. The treatment material is placed as an aid in promoting repair of the pulp and deposition of secondary dentin. (Pedodont.)

partial denture t. (see **denture, partial, treatment**)

t. prescription The formal outline of the projected treatment of a patient; e.g., the blueprint from which the dentist projects his treatment. (Oral Diag.)

rest t. (sedative t.) Use of a drug sealed into a root canal to relieve pain or discomfort; not used primarily for its antiseptic value. (Endodont.)

root canal t. The techniques and pharmaceuticals used in removing pulp tissue, sterilizing the root canal, and preparing the root canal for filling. (Endodont.)

sedative t. (see **treatment, rest**)

tremolo (trĕm'ō-lō") An irregular and exaggerated speech pattern. It may be the symptom of an emotional disturbance or of various diseases affecting the nervous control of the organs of respiration and phonation. (Oral Physiol.)

trench mouth (see **gingivitis, necrotizing ulcerative**)

Trendelenburg position (trĕn-dĕl'ĕn-bĕrg) (see **position, Trendelenburg**)

trepanation (trephination) The act of surgically cutting a round hole. (Oral Implant.)

trephine (trĕ-fīn') A circle-cutting surgical instrument designed to remove a circumscribed portion of tissue. It permits the insertion of the heads of the intramucosal inserts into the tissue. (Oral Implant.)

Treponema (trĕp"ō-nē'mah) A genus of schizomycetes composed of parasitic and pathogenic spiral microorganisms. (Oral Path.)

T. pallidum The spirochete that causes syphilis in man. (Oral Path.; Periodont.)

T. vincenti A spirochete associated with necrotizing ulcerative gingivitis. (Periodont.)

triad, Hutchinson (trī'ăd) Interstitial keratitis, deafness, and hutchinsonian teeth due to congenital syphilis. (Oral Med.)

trial An examination before a competent tribunal of the facts or law in issue in a cause of action for the purpose of determining the issue. (D. Juris.)

t. base (see **baseplate**)

triangle A three-cornered area.

Bolton t. A triangle formed by drawing a line from the nasion to the sella turcica and from there to the Bolton point. (Orthodont.)

Bonwill's t. An equilateral triangle with 4-inch sides bounded by lines from the con-

tact points of the lower central incisors (or the median line of the residual ridge of the mandible) to the condyle on either side and from one condyle to the other. It is the basis for Bonwill's theory of occlusion. (Comp. Prosth.; Fixed Part. Prosth.; Remov. Part. Prosth.)

Lesser's t. A surgical landmark for locating the lingual artery; the triangle is located above the hyoid bone and is formed by the posterior belly of the digastric muscle and the posterior edge of the mylohyoid muscle below and the hypoglossal nerve above. The floor of the triangle is the hyoglossus muscle, and directly below the hyoglossus muscle is the lingual artery. (Oral Surg.)

trichoepithelioma (trĭk"ō-ĕp"ĭ-thē"lē-ō'mah) (see **epithelioma adenoides cysticum**)

tridymite (trĭd'ĭ-mīt) A physical form of silica used in combination with cristobalite to limit thermal expansion. (D. Mat.)

trifurcation Division into three parts or branches, as the three roots of a maxillary first molar. (Oper. Dent.)

trimmer, gingival margin (margin trimmer) A binangled, double-paired, chisel-shaped, single-beveled, double-planed, lateral cutting instrument. The blade is curved left or right like a spoon excavator; the cutting edge is straight and not perpendicular to the axis of the blade. The pair with the end of the cutting edge farthest from the shaft forming an acute angle is termed distal and is used to bevel a distal gingival margin or accentuate a mesial axiogingival angle; the pair with the acute angle of the cutting edge closest to the shaft is called mesial and is used to bevel a mesial gingival margin or accentuate a distal axiogingival angle. When one of these trimmers is used, all four must be used. (Oper. Dent.)

trimmer, margin (see **trimmer, gingival margin**)

trimming, tissue (see **border molding**)

tripoding (trī'pŏd-ĭng) The marking of a cast at three points in the same plane as a means of repositioning the cast in that plane during subsequent procedures. (Remov. Part. Prosth.)

tripodism A widely used principle to gain instant stability on uneven terrains in all landings. It is referred to as a three-point landing. Watch-makers use tripodism to keep delicate mechanisms well balanced. Stamp cusps in well-organized occlusion have only three-point contacts with their fossa brims (none with their tips). (Gnathol.)

trismus (trĭz'mŭs) Spasms of the muscles of mastication, resulting in inability to open the mouth; often symptomatic of pericoronitis. (Oral Diag.; Periodont.)

trisomy (trī'sō-mē) An additional chromosome in the normal complement, so that in each nucleus a chromosome is represented three times rather than twice. (Oral Med.) (see also **mongolism**)

trisomy-D (**trisomy 13-15, Patau's syndrome**) Clinical syndrome associated with an autosomal abnormality in which the extra chromosome occurs in the 13-15 group. Numerous anatomic defects are present, including hemangiomas, hernia, arrhinencephaly, eye anomalies, cleft lip and palate, and characteristic changes in the footprint and palm print. (Oral Med.)

trituration (trĭt"ū-rā'shŭn) The process of mixing together silver alloy fillings with mercury to produce amalgam. (Oper. Dent.)

  hand t. The mixing of ingredients by hand in a mortar and pestle. (Oper. Dent.)

  mechanical t. The mixing of constituents in a mechanical device or amalgamator. (Oper. Dent.)

troche (trō'kē) (see **lozenge**)

Trousseau's twitching (see **twitching, Trousseau's**)

True's separator (see **separator, True's**)

truss arm (see **connector, minor**)

try-in A preliminary placement of trial dentures (complete or removable partial), a partial denture casting, or a finished restoration to evaluate fit, appearance, maxillomandibular relations, etc. (Comp. Prosth.; Remov. Part. Prosth.)

tryptase (trĭp'tās) (see **plasmin**)

TSH (see **hormone, thyrotropic**)

tube A hollow cylindrical structure. (Anesth.)

  buccal t. A section of tubing attached to the buccal side of a molar band in a horizontal position, serving as an attachment for the labial arch wire, which slides into the tube. (Orthodont.)

  Coolidge t. An x-ray tube in which the gas pressure is purposely made so low that it plays no role in the operation of the tube, the operation depending on the emission of electrons by the heated filament of the cathode. (Oral Radiol.) (see also **x-ray tube, Coolidge**)

  Crookes' t. A vacuum-discharge tube used by Sir William Crookes in early experimental work with cathode rays. The tube usually contained a Maltese cross at the antecathode end that would cast a shadow on the wall of

a darkened room, providing the existence of a stream of cathode rays. (Oral Radiol.) (see also **x-ray tube, Crookes'**)

  discharge t. Any vacuum tube in which a high-voltage electric current is discharged; e.g., an x-ray tube. (Oral Radiol.)

  gas t. An early x-ray tube in which the available electrons were produced by the disruption of the residual gases within the tube. It utilized a bianode and a regulator in addition to the anode and cathode. (Oral Radiol.) (see also **x-ray tube, gas**)

  horizontal t. A metal tube attachment that is placed in a horizontal position on the buccal surface of each anchor molar tooth to allow for the insertion of the labial arch wire. (Orthodont.)

  intubation t. A tube for insertion into the larynx through the mouth. (Anesth.)

  line focus t. An x-ray tube in which the target face is about 20 inches from the cathode face. The focal spot is rectangular, with the length approximately three times the width. The acute angle provides an effective focal spot area approximately square and a fraction of the actual area. (Oral Radiol.)

  protective t. housing An x-ray tube enclosure that provides radiation protection. (Oral Radiol.)

    p. t. h., diagnostic A tube housing that reduces the leakage radiation to, at most, 0.10 r/hr at a distance of 1 mm from the tube target when the tube is operating at its maximum continuous rated voltage. (Oral Radiol.)

    p. t. h., therapeutic A tube housing that reduces the leakage radiation to, at most, 1 r/hr at a distance of 1 meter from the tube target when the tube is operating at its maximum continuous rated current for the maximum rated voltage. (Oral Radiol.)

  right-angle t. An x-ray tube in which the target is at right angles to the cathode. (Oral Radiol.)

  t. tooth (see **tooth, tube**)

  vertical t. An attachment that is usually placed on the lingual surface of the anchor band to allow for the insertion of the lingual wire. (Orthodont.)

  x-ray t. (see **x-ray tube**)

tubercle, genial (tū'ber-kl, jē'nē-al) (**geniohyoid tubercle**) A small rounded elevation on the lingual surface of the mandible on either side of the midline near the inferior border of the body of the mandible, serving as a point of insertion for the geniohyoid muscles. (Comp. Prosth.; Oral Physiol.)

superior g. t. The small spines on the lingual surface of the mandible that serve as the attachment for the genioglossus muscles. On resorbed mandibles, these tubercles may be at or above the crest of the residual ridge. (Comp. Prosth.)

tubercle, geniohyoid (tū'ber-kl, jē"nē-ō-hī'oid) (see **tubercle, genial**)

tuberculosis An infectious disease caused by *Mycobacterium tuberculosis* and characterized by the formation of tubercles in the tissues. (Oral Path.)

tuberosity, maxillary The most distal aspect of the maxillary alveolar process. Appears as normal bone, with its posterior border curving upward and distally. (Periodont.)

tuberosity reduction Surgical excision of excessive fibrous or bony tissue in the area of the maxillary tuberosity prior to the construction of prosthetic appliances. (Oral Surg.)

tumor(s) A swelling. Through usage the term is now used synonymously with neoplasm. (Oral Path.) (see also **neoplasm**)

Brooke's t. (see **epithelioma adenoides cysticum**)

brown t. A central giant cell tumor of the bone; associated with parathyroidism. (Oral Diag.)

carotid body t. A tumor formed about the carotid artery. (Oral Diag.)

collision t. A rare condition in which two neoplasms, both growing in the same general area, collide with the tumor elements and become intermingled. (Oral Path.)

Ewing's t. (**endothelioma, Ewing's sarcoma**) A malignant connective tissue neoplasm believed to arise from young reticular cells of the bone marrow. It occurs chiefly in young people and may involve the mandible as well as other bones. (Oral Diag.)

— A rare malignant tumor of disputed histogenetic origin in bone. It is characterized by a presenting symptom of pain, a radiographic appearance called onionskinning, and a histologic picture consisting of solid sheets of small round cells that appear on the many small blood vessels present. (Oral Path.)

giant cell t. A benign neoplasm of bone, producing resorption and characterized by giant cells. (Oral Diag.)

hormonal t. Localized enlargements of the gingivae that have the appearance of neoplasms and are associated with hormonal imbalance during pregnancy. (Oral Diag.)

mixed t. One of a group of neoplasms of the salivary glands whose histologic appearance suggests both epithelial and connective tissue origin, although they presently are considered of epithelial origin only. There are benign and malignant types. (Oral Diag.)

— Any tumor arising from cells derived from more than one germ layer. (Oral Path.)

basaloid m. t. (see **carcinoma, adenocystic**)

mucoepidermoid t. A tumor of the salivary glands composed of mucous cells, epidermoid cells, and clear cells. Benign and malignant forms are recognized. (Oral Path.)

odontogenic t. (ō-don"tō-jěn'ĭk) A neoplasm produced from tooth-forming tissues; e.g., odontogenic fibroma, odontogenic myxoma, ameloblastoma. (Oral Diag.) (see also **calcifying epithelial odontogenic tumor**)

— Any tumor arising from the dental lamina or its derivatives, the dental papilla, or the dental sac. (Oral Path.)

pregnancy t. A localized tumorlike enlargement of the gingivae during pregnancy due to hormonal imbalance. It is not a true neoplasm. (Oral Diag.)

— A pyogenic granuloma arising in the gingivae about the third month of pregnancy. (Oral Path.) (see also **granuloma, pyogenic**)

— A gingival enlargement seen during pregnancy, the microscopic examination of which reveals the features of a pyogenic granuloma. (Periodont.)

turban t. (see **carcinoma, basal cell**)

Warthin's t. (see **cystadenoma, papillary, lymphomatosum**)

turbulence Casting term used to denote irregular flow of the metal into the mold. May result in porosity. (D. Mat.)

Turner's tooth (see **tooth, Turner's**)

twilight sleep (see **sleep, twilight**)

twins Two siblings produced in the same pregnancy and developed from one egg (identical, monozygotic) or from two eggs fertilized at the same time (fraternal, dizygotic). (Oral Med.)

twin-wire (see **appliance, twin-wire**)

twist drill A spiral bone bur. (Oral Implant.)

twitch A short, sudden pull or jerk. (Anesth.)

twitching An irregular spasm of a minor extent. (Anesth.)

Trousseau's t. A twitching of the face which the patient can exhibit at will and which occurs obsessively to relieve tension. (Oral Diag.)

type A hepatitis (see **hepatitis, infectious**)

type B hepatitis (see **hepatitis, homologous serum**)

typewriter ribbon as a marking medium Typewriter ribbon is more desirable than carbon paper when setting teeth because the porcelain tooth that is being adjusted will not perforate the ribbon and abrade the surface of the stone template record of jaw movement. (Remov. Part. Prosth.)

typical implant connective tissue The tendon-like condensed elongated avascular tissue formed in direct contact with implant infrastructure metal underlaid by normal collagenous fibrous connective tissue. (Oral Implant.)

typodont (tĭ'pō-dont) An artificial model containing artificial or natural teeth used for teaching technique exercises. (Oper. Dent.)

Tzank cell (tsănk) (see **cell, Tzank**)

Tzank's test (see **test, Tzank's**)

U

ulalgia (ū-lăl′jē-ah) Pain in the gums. (Anesth.)

ulcer A loss of covering epithelium from a surface that leaves the underlying tissue exposed to irritation by bacteria and other factors. (Oral Diag.)

— Localized loss of epithelium of the skin or mucous membranes. (Oral Med.)

— A loss of substance on a cutaneous or mucous surface, causing gradual disintegration and necrosis of the tissues. (Oral Path.)

— A wound or break with loss of the covering epithelium on the surface of the skin or mucous membrane; results from necrosis. (Periodont.)

  aphthous u., recurrent (ăf′thŭs) (**RAU, canker sore, recurrent aphthae**) Periodic episodes of aphthous lesions ranging from one week to several months. Trauma, menses, immunologic factors, upper respiratory infections, herpes simplex and other exciting causes have been suggested. The single or multiple discrete or confluent ulcers have a well-defined marginal erythema and central area of necrosis with sloughing. The herpetic appearance suggests a common mechanism with herpes simplex, but no known infectious agents have been demonstrated. (Oral Med.)

  autochthonous u. (ăw-tok′thō-nŭs) (see **chancre**)

  decubitus u. (dē-kū′bĭ-tŭs) (**traumatic u.**) A bedsore. Loosely used to refer to a traumatic ulcer of the oral mucosa. (Oral Med.)

  — An ulcer that develops as a result of physical irritation or injury. (Oral Path.)

  diabetic u. (dī″ah-bĕt′ĭk) An ulcer, usually of the lower extremities, associated with diabetes mellitus. (Oral Med.)

  herpetic u. (her-pĕt′ĭk) An ulcer that is secondary to the vesicle of herpes simplex. A shallow ulcer with an irregular, erythematous border and a yellow-gray base. (Oral Med.)

  Mikulicz' u. (mĭk′ū-lĭch) (see **periadenitis mucosa necrotica recurrens**)

  peptic u. (pĕp′tĭk) An ulcer of the stomach or duodenum; probably due in large part to an increased secretion of hydrochloric acid. Nervous, emotional, and endocrine factors have been implicated. (Oral Med.)

  pterygoid u. (tĕr′ĭ-goid) (see **aphtha, Bednar's**)

  rodent u. (see **carcinoma, basal cell**)

  traumatic u. (see **ulcer, decubitus**)

ulceration The process of forming an ulcer or of becoming ulcerous. (Periodont.)

ultimate strength (see **strength, ultimate**)

ultra (ul′trah) Beyond; in addition; in excess of (D. Juris.)

  damages, u. Damages beyond those paid in court. (D. Juris.)

ultrasonic handpiece (see **handpiece, ultrasonic**)

ultrasonics (ŭl″trah-son′ĭks) Instruments that function by the physical principle of magnetostriction and serve to aid in calculus removal, especially large and hard deposits. (Periodont.)

unconscious Insensible; not receiving any sensory impression and not having any subjective experiences. (Anesth.)

undercut The portions of a tooth that lies between its height of contour and the gingivae, only if that portion is of less circumference than the height of contour. The contour of a cross section of a residual ridge of dental arch that would prevent the placement of a denture or other prostheses. (Comp. Prosth.; Fixed Part. Prosth.; Oper. Dent.; Remov. Part. Prosth.)

— The contour of flasking stone that interlocks in such a way as to prevent the separation of parts. (Comp. Prosth.; Fixed Part. Prosth.; Oper. Dent.; Remov. Part. Prosth.)

— The portion of a prepared cavity that creates a mechanical lock or area of retention; may be desirable in a cavity to be filled with gold foil or amalgam but undesirable in a cavity prepared for a restoration to be cemented. (Oper. Dent.)

  u. gauge (see **gauge, undercut**)

  retentive u. An area of the abutment surface suitable for the location of a retentive clasp terminal which, to escape the undercut, would be forced to flex and thus generate retention. (Remov. Part. Prosth.)

  soft tissue u. An undercut in a residual ridge or soft tissue covering of a dental arch that would prevent or influence the placement of a removable denture. (Remov. Part. Prosth.)

unusable u. The area of an abutment tooth or soft tissue across which a unit of the removable parietal denture must pass without interference and hence must be blocked out (filled with wax or clay) before the master cast is duplicated. A surveyor can be used to produce a surface that is parallel to the proposed path of a placement and removal. (Remov. Part. Prosth.)

undermine To surgically separate the skin or mucosa from its underlying stroma so that it can be stretched or moved to cover a defect or wound. (Oral Implant.)

unerupted Not having perforated the oral mucosa. In dentistry, used with reference to a normal developing tooth, an embedded tooth, or an impacted tooth. (Oral Surg.)

unification The act of uniting or the condition of being united; e.g., the result of joining the components of a removable partial denture by connectors. (Remov. Part. Prosth.)

unilateral One-sided. (Orthodont.)

unit One of the components of a whole. (Remov. Part. Prosth.)

Ångström u. (ăng'strom) (Å, A.U.) The unit of measure of wavelengths; one one-hundred millionth of a centimeter. (Oral Radiol.)

dental u. An article of equipment in which are assembled numerous items used in dental operations, such as a dental engine, cuspidor, or operatory light, bracket, working table, saliva ejector, water supply, electric outlets, compressed air, and miscellaneous instruments. (Oper. Dent.)

— Basically, the tooth, the attachment apparatus, and the gingival unit—all of which are necessary for proper masticatory activity. (Periodont.)

dentoperiodontal u. Term referring to the tooth and periodontium together. (Periodont.)

gingival u. The tough collagenous and epithelial covering of the neck of the tooth and the underlying attachment apparatus. (Periodont.)

partial denture u. The individual parts of the partial denture, each constributing some particular function. (Remov. Part. Prosth.)

x-ray u. A device designed to produce x rays. (Oral Radiol.)

x.u. calibration The determination of the kilovoltage peak (KVP) value of each autotransformer tap at various milliamperages, checking these values by means of a sphere gap or a prereading voltmeter. (Oral Radiol.)

unmedullated (ŭn-mĕd'ŭ-lāt'ĕd) Not possessing a medulla or medullary substance. (Anesth.)

unpolarized Not polarized. (Anesth.)

unsharpness, geometric (see **geometric unsharpness**)

unstable Capable of undergoing spontaneous change. A nuclide in an unstable state is called radioactive. An atom in an unstable state is called excited. (Oral Radiol.)

upright arm (see **connector, minor**)

uprighting spring An auxiliary wire used to torque roots mesially or distally. (Orthodont.)

uremia (ū-rē'mē-ah) Presence of urea or its components in the circulating blood. (Oral Diag.)

— A clinical syndrome indicating renal failure, with symptoms due to altered body chemistry, excretory defects, and associated effects of extrarenal, vascular, cardiac, or cerebral disease when present. Manifestations include weakness, headache, confusion, vomiting, and coma, and in terminal chronic renal disease, purpura and epistaxis may be present. (Oral Med.) (see also **stomatitis, uremic**)

urticaria (ur"tĭ-kā'rē-ah) (**hives**) Smooth, elevated, blanched areas on the skin surrounded by a zone of redness; results from allergy, trauma, exercise, or emotion. (Oral Med.)

— A vascular reaction pattern of the skin marked by the transient appearance of smooth, slightly elevated patches that are either more red or more pale than the surrounding skin and attended by severe itching. (Oral Path.)

giant u. (see **edema, angioneurotic**)

USAN Council The United States Adopted Names Council, which is responsible for the selection of appropriate nonproprietary names for drugs used in the United States. (Oral Med.; Pharmacol.)

useful beam (see **beam, useful**)

U.S.P. *The Pharmacopeia of the United States.*

ut dict. Abbreviation for *ut dictum*, a Latin phrase meaning as directed. (Oral Med.; Pharmacol.)

uveoparotitis (ū"vē-ō-păr"ō-tī'tĭs) (see **fever, uveoparotid**)

uvula, bifid (ū'vū-lah) A congenital cleft resulting in a split uvula. (Oral Surg.)

❧ V ❧

Vacudent A proprietary suction apparatus designed to remove strongly but gently any fluids and debris from an operating field. (Oper. Dent.)

vacuum (see **oral evacuator**)

vacuum mixing (see **mixing, vacuum**)

vacuumizing A method of handling a material (e.g., plaster of paris) in a partial vacuum in order to reduce its air content. (Remov. Part. Prosth.)

vagomimetic (vā″gō-mī-mĕt′ĭk) Pertaining to a drug with actions similar to those produced by stimulation of the vagus nerve. (Anesth.)

values, normal laboratory Generally, statistically and biologically significant qualitative and/or quantitative measurements of cellular and clinical components of the body. The values derived from such measurements are based on averages of a survey of presumably healthy persons. The concept of individual normal values is based on an acceptable response (comparable with known evidence of health or disease) of the individual to a known alteration of cellular and/or chemical components or systems. (Oral Med.)

values, phonetic (fō-nĕt′ĭk) The character or quality of vocal sounds. (Comp. Prosth.; Remov. Part. Prosth.)

valve A membranous structure or fold that prevents reflux of the contents of a canal or passage. (Anesth.)

exhalation v. A valve that permits escape of exhaled gases into the atmosphere and prevents them from being rebreathed. (Anesth.)

van den Bergh's test (see **test, van den Bergh's**)

vapor Steam, gas, or exhalation. (Anesth.)

Vaquez' disease (vah-kāz′) (see **erythremia**)

varicella (văr″ĭ-sĕl′ah) (**chickenpox**) An acute communicable disease, usually found in children, caused by the herpesvirus and marked by the eruption of macular vesicles. (Oral Diag.; Oral Path.)

— A contagious viral disease having an incubation period of 2 or 3 weeks. Manifestations include coryza, fever, malaise, and headache, followed in 2 or 3 days by crops of pustules and vesicles that last for 1 to 3 days. (Oral Med.)

variola (**smallpox**) (vah-rī′ō-lah) An acute, viral contagious disease transmitted by the respiratory route and direct contact. The incubation period is 1 or 2 weeks. Manifestations include headache, chills, and temperature up to 106° F, followed by macules on the third and fourth day, which then become papules, and then constitutional symptoms abate. On the sixth day the papules become vesicles and then pustules, with desquamation occurring in about 2 weeks. (Oral Diag.; Oral Med.)

varnish (**cavity liner**) A clear solution of resinous material or natural gum, such as copal or rosin dissolved in acetone, ether, or chloroform, that is capable of hardening without losing its transparency. Used in cavity preparations to seal cut dentinal tubules, *to reduce microleakage,* and to insulate the pulp against shock from thermal changes. (Oper. Dent.)

cavity v. A cavity liner prepared from a solution of gums, rosins, or resins in organic solvents. Used as a protective agent under certain restorative materials. (D. Mat.)

vasoconstrictor (**vasopressor**) An agent that causes a rise in blood pressure by constricting the blood vessels. In local areas, it causes constriction of the arterioles and capillaries. (Anesth.)

vasodepressor An agent that depresses circulation and causes vasomotor depression. (Anesth.)

vasodilator An agent that causes dilation of the blood vessels. Also, a drug that relaxes the smooth muscle walls of the blood vessels and increases their diameter. (Anesth.)

vasomotor (văs″ō-mō′tor) Pertaining to any agent or nerve that causes expansion or contraction of the walls of blood vessels. (Anesth.)

vasopressin (see **hormone, antidiuretic**)

vasopressor (see **vasocontrictor**)

vault A cavity or specially prepared area within the bone for placement of the implant magnet. (Oral Implant.)

vehicle An excipient substance that lends form or substance to a drug. (Anesth.)

— A pharmaceutic ingredient, usually a liquid, employed as a medium for dissolving or dispersing the active drug in a mass suitable for its administration. (Anesth.; Oral Med.; Pharmacol.)

Veillonella alcalescens (vā″yon-ĕl′ah ăl-kah-lĕs′ĕnz) An organism of the genus *Veillonella.* A schizomycete that has been found in the flora of the periodontal pocket and, by association, has been implicated in the origin and perpetuation of periodontitis in human beings. (Periodont.)

veins The blood vessels that conduct the blood from the capillary bed back to the heart. They range in increasing size from the venules, to small veins, to large veins. The lumens of the veins are generally much larger than the comparable arterial vessels, and their walls are thinner. This difference is due to the marked reduction in the muscle and connective tissue components. The three divisions—the tunica intima, the tunica media, and the tunica adventitia—exist, but they are not so prominent. The venules are small veins that are of special clinical interest to dentists. (Oral Physiol.)

velopharyngeal adequacy (vel″ō-fah-rĭn′jē-ăl) (see **adequacy, velopharyngeal**)

velopharyngeal closure (see **closure, velopharyngeal**)

velopharyngeal inadequacy (see **inadequacy, velopharyngeal**)

veneer In the construction of crowns or pontics, a layer of tooth-colored material, usually porcelain or acrylic resin, attached to the surface by direct fusion, cementation, or mechanical retention. (Fixed Part. Prosth.)

venipuncture (ven″ĭ-pŭng′tūr) Surgical or therapeutic puncture of a vein. (Anesth.)

ventilation The constant supplying of oxygen through the lungs. (Anesth.)

  air v. The process of supplying alveoli with air or oxygen. (Anesth.)

  respiratory v. The process of getting air into and out of the lungs. The air enters the mouth and nose and must go through the conduction system (the pharynx, the larynx, the trachea, and the bronchial tree) into the lungs. This ventilating process involves many other structures as well, including the abdomen, the thorax, and the maxillofacial tissues. The latter structures make two significant contributions to the respiratory process: they provide the portal of entry and egress for the air to and from the lungs, and they alter the physical properties of the inspired air for the protection of the very sensitive lung tissues. (Oral Physiol.)

venue (ven′ū) The neighborhood, place, or county in which an injury is declared to have occurred or fact is declared to have happened; also designates the county in which an action or prosecution is presented for trial. (D. Juris.)

venule (ven′ūl) The smallest of the venous blood vessels. Consists of an endothelial tube enclosed in a variable amount of elastic and col-

lagenous tissue. Smooth muscle is introduced in the media as the caliber of the vessel increases. The muscle fibers are distributed sparsely in the smaller vessels and coalesce into circumferential bands in the larger vessels. (Oral Physiol.)

verbal By word of mouth; oral, as a verbal agreement. (D. Juris.)

verdict The formal decision or finding of a jury on the matters or questions duly submitted to them at the trial. (D. Juris.)

vernier (ver′nē-er) (see **gauge, Boley**)

Verocay body (see **body, Verocay**)

verruca (vĕ-roo′kah) A wartlike lesion. (Oral Diag.)

  v. carcinoma A squamous cell carcinoma, usually intraoral, that is exophytic and has a papillary appearance. (Oral Path.)

  v. leukoplakia (lū-kō-plā′kē-ah) Leukoplakia that is exophytic and clinically appears to be papillary in form. (Oral Path.) (see also **leukoplakia**)

  v. senilis (sĕ-nĭl′ĭs) (see **keratosis, seborrheic**)

  v. vulgaris (**wart**) A common wart of the skin or mucosa. (Oral Diag.)

  — A benign epithelial tumor that is elevated and papillomatous and covered with keratin. Histologically, marked hyperkeratosis, parakeratosis, and acanthosis are seen. Rete pegs are elongated, and the lateral ones turn toward the center of the base of the lesion. (Oral Path.)

vertical Perpendicular; in an up and down direction.

  v. angulation (see **angulation, vertical**)

  v. dimension (see **dimension, vertical**)

  v. fulcrum line (see **line, fulcrum, vertical**)

  v. lug (see **connector, minor**)

  v. opening (see **dimension, vertical**)

  v. overlap (see **overlap, vertical**)

  v. relation (see **relation, vertical**)

vertigo (ver′tĭ-gō) A sensation described as dizziness. (Anesth.)

— A sensation of the room revolving about the patient or the patient revolving in space. It is a form of dizziness, but the terms are not synonymous. (Oral Diag.)

vesicant (ves′ĭ-kănt) A chemically active substance that can produce blistering on direct contact with the skin or mucous membrane. (Oral Med.; Pharmacol.)

vesicle (ves′ĭ-kl) A small blisterlike elevation of the skin or mucous membrane due to an intraepithelial collection of fluid. It is a primary type of lesion and may be seen in herpes simplex, recurrent herpes, recurrent aphthae, stomatitis medicamentosa, stomatitis venenata, erythema multiforme, Reiter's syndrome, Behçet's syndrome, Stevens-Johnson syndrome, herpangina, varicella, and many others. (Oral Diag.; Oral Med.)

— A circumscribed, elevated lesion of the skin containing fluid and having a diameter up to 5 mm. (Oral Path.)

vessels, blood, visualization of Any one of various methods by which the blood vessels are seen by the examiner. Direct visualization of blood vessels is possible only to a limited extent. The blood vessels in the retina can be directly visualized; the capillary loops in the fingernail can be seen by microscopy, and the blood vessels in the oral mucosa and gingivae can be visualized by infrared photography. More recently, radiopaque substances can be visualized by radiography and cineradiography. The methods can reveal the actual blood column, its width, variation in contour, and tortuosity. Arteriograms and venograms are useful in revealing spasms, obstructions, congenital defects, and collateral circulation of the deeper tissues. (Oral Physiol.)

vestibule of oral cavity The part of the oral cavity that lies between the teeth and gingivae or between the residual ridges and the lips and cheeks. (Comp. Prosth.; Fixed Part. Prosth.; Remov. Part. Prosth.)

— The part of the oral cavity lateral to the teeth and medial to the labial and buccal tissues. (Oral Surg.)

buccal v. The space between the alveolar or residual ridge and the cheek, distal to the buccal frenum. (Comp. Prosth.; Fixed Part. Prosth.; Remov. Part. Prosth.)

lower b. v. The space between the mandibular residual alveolar ridge and the cheek; bounded anteriorly by the lower buccal frenum and posteriorly by the distobuccal end of the retromolar pad. (Comp. Prosth.)

upper b. v. The space between the maxillary residual alveolar ridge and the cheek, bounded anteriorly by the upper buccal frenum and posteriorly by the hamular notch. (Comp. Prosth.)

labial v. The space between the alveolar or residual ridge and the lips anterior to the buccal frenum. (Comp. Prosth.; Fixed Part. Prosth.; Remov. Part. Prosth.)

vestibuloplasty (věs-tĭb′ū-lō-plăs″tē) Any of a series of surgical procedures designed to restore alveolar ridge height by lowering muscles at-

taching to the buccal, labial, and lingual aspects of the jaws. (Oral Surg.)

viable (vī′ah-bl) Capable of life; able to live. (D. Juris.)

vibrating line (see **line, vibrating**)

Vicat needle (vē-kah′) (see **needle, Vicat**)

Vickers hardness number (see **number, Vickers hardness**)

Vickers hardness test (see **test, Vickers hardness**)

Vincent's angina (see **angina, Vincent's**)

Vincent's bacillus (see **Fusobacterium fusiforme**)

Vincent's gingivitis (see **gingivitis, necrotizing ulcerative**)

Vincent's infection (see **gingivitis, necrotizing ulcerative**)

Vincent's organism (see **organism, Vincent's**)

vinegar as a solvent A warm dilute solution of household vinegar; used, as a substitute for acetic acid, to dissolve accumulated dental calculus from a removable dental prosthesis. (Remov. Part. Prosth.)

Vinethene (vĭn′ě-thēn) Proprietary name for vinyl ether. (Anesth.)

violence Severe physical force; the assault of a person with great force. (D. Juris.)

violation Injury; encroachment; breach of right, obligation, or law. (D. Juris.)

violet, gentian (vī′ō-lět, jěn′shŭn) A rosaniline dye, useful as a protective covering and an antiseptic in the treatment of minor lesions of the oral mucosa. It is an effective fungicide and is therefore of value in the treatment of moniliasis. (Periodont.)

violet stain (see **stain, methyl violet**)

vinyl resin (vī′nĭl) (see **resin, vinyl**)

virus Latin word meaning poison. One of a heterogeneous group of widely differing agents that infect animals, plants, insects, bacteria, and fungi. Viruses are intracellular parasites. (Periodont.)

v., herpes simplex (see **herpes simplex**)

vision Sight; the faculty of seeing.

field of v. The portion of space that the fixed eye can see. When a patient has a modified or restricted field of vision due to either optical or neurologic dysfunction, the dentist should approach the patient so that the latter observes the dentist's movements and actions before instruments or hands touch the face or mouth of the patient. This permits the patient to adjust more readily to a treatment procedure. This adjustment is required especially in anxious, neurotic, or chronically ill children. (Oral Physiol.)

function of v. The performance of the eye, based on specific sensitivity to light. In many animals, such sensitivity is concentrated in special cells or cell clusters frequently called eyespots. From this primitive eyespot, there is evolutionary progress to an organized photoreceptive structure, the eye, with a lens for concentrating light on sensitive cells contained in a closed chamber. Many such light-sensitive organs in lower phyla are merely receptors for light in bulk; with better organization, the sensory cells are arranged to receive patterns, and true vision, as in man, results. (Oral Physiol.)

pattern v. Pattern vision in man depends on two processes: the capacity for accommodation to view near and distant objects and the coordination of the visual fields of the two eyes to give binocular, or stereoscopic, vision. The purpose of accommodation is to obtain definition of objects at varied distances. (Oral Path.)

stereoscopic v. Vision in which the visual fields of the two eyes are unified. Sensations from a common object received by the two eyes are superimposed, and as a result of the slight differences in the fields and the superimposition of the fields, the effects of depth and shape of the object are attained. This phenomenon of stereoscopic vision is accomplished in the central nervous system after incomplete decussation of the fibers of the optic nerves. The visual area of each brain hemisphere thus builds up a half picture of the total visual field. By further interconnections between hemispheres, the two halves of the picture are welded together as a double exposure to emerge in the consciousness as a single stereoscopic view. Stereoscopic vision is characteristic of mammalian life. (Oral Physiol.)

visual acuity (see **acuity, visual**)

visual disorders (see **disorders, visual**)

vital Necessary to or pertaining to life. (Anesth.)

v. capacity (see **capacity, vital**)

vitalometer (vī″tăl-om′ĕ-ter) An electric-powered instrument for delivering and measuring an electrical stimulus to a tooth. (Endodont.) (see **pulp tester**)

vitalometry (vī″tăl-ŏm′ĕ-trē) The use of high-frequency pulp-testing equipment to establish the vital condition of the pulp of a tooth. (Remov. Part. Prosth.)

vitamin A protein substance essential to the metabolic processes and intimately associated with enzyme function. Vitamins differ essentially from enzymes in that they are not produced by the human body. They must ulti-

mately come from plant sources and thus must be ingested in the diet. (Oral Physiol.)

v. A Two closely related forms of a fat-soluble alcohol found in man and in saltwater fish (A_1) and freshwater fish (A_2). Vitamin A is essential for the integrity of epithelial cells and the regeneration of visual purple. It is also concerned with the development of bone and teeth. A deficiency results in hyperkeratinization of nonsecretory protective epithelium, deranged secretory function of the mucous membrane, dark dysadaptation (night blindness), and possibly, enamel hypoplasia. (Oral Med.)

v. B complex Collectively, the various B vitamins: thiamine, riboflavin, nicotinic acid, pyridoxine, biotin, para-aminobenzoic acid, folic acid, pantothenic acid, cyanocobalamin, and others that are unknown. (Oral Med.)

v. B$_c$ (folic acid, pteroylglutamic acid, vitamin M) A vitamin whose most important activity is the synthesis of compounds that are utilized for the formation of nucleoproteins. A deficiency of nucleoproteins leads to megaloblastic arrest of normal red blood cell maturation in the bone marrow. A deficiency of vitamin B$_c$ results in a macrocytic anemia without nervous system involvement. Vitamin B$_c$ is effective in the treatment of the megaloblastic anemias of pregnancy and infancy, nutritional macrocytic anemia, the sprue syndrome, and the anemic syndrome due to the folic acid antagonist aminopterin. (Oral Med.; Pharmacol.)

v. B$_1$ (thiamine) A vitamin that is necessary for normal carbohydrate metabolism. It is found in whole-grain cereals, pork, eggs, yeast, green leafy vegetables, legumes, and other foods. A deficiency impairs carbohydrate metabolism in the pyruvate state. The clinical result of a deficiency results in beriberi. (Oral Med.)

v. B$_2$ (lactoflavin, riboflavin, vitamin G) A vitamin that plays an intimate role in cellular reactions because it forms a part of the prosthetic group of several enzymes. Small amounts are synthesized in the intestinal tract. A deficiency results in ariboflavinosis. It is found in green leafy vegetables, whole grains, eggs, liver, milk, legumes, and other foods. (Oral Med.)

— A heat-stable member of the B complex group of vitamins; $C_{17}H_{20}N_4O_6$. Deficiency of vitamin B$_2$ along with other B complex vitamins, may result in angular stomatitis, glossitis, gingival ulcerations, etc. (Oral Med.; Periodont.)

v. B₆ (pyridoxine) A vitamin that functions as the coenzyme for several enzyme systems for normal amino acid metabolism. A deficiency may result in convulsive seizures in infants. Used prophylactically in tuberculosis patients on prolonged isoniazid therapy. Sources are liver, meats, whole-grain cereals, and a number of vegetables. (Oral Med.)

v. B₁₂ (antipernicious factor, cyanocobalamin, erythrocyte-maturing factor [EMF], extrinsic factor) A vitamin essential for the maturation of erythrocytes. A deficiency is due primarily to a lack of the intrinsic factor. It is important in the treatment of pernicious anemia. (Oral Med.)

v. Bₓ (vitamin H, second meaning) Para-aminobenzoic acid.

v. C (ascorbic acid) A vitamin that plays an important role in the metabolism of amino acids because it is necessary for the hydroxylation of proline in collagen synthesis and probably for polysaccharide synthesis. It is essential for the normal elaboration of fibrous tissues, mucoprotein matrices in teeth, cartilage, and bone, and for the integrity of capillary walls. It is found in citrus fruits, tomatoes, potatoes, cantaloupes, and minimally cooked vegetables. A frank deficiency leads to scurvy. (Oral Med.)

— A water-soluble vitamin found in citrus fruits, tomatoes, cabbage, and other fresh fruits and vegetables; necessary for the formation of collagen and tissue ground substance and for the maintenance of the integrity of the walls of blood vessels. (Periodont.)

v. D One of several sterol compounds capable of preventing or curing rickets. Of primary importance are D₂ (ergocalciferol) and D₃ (cholecalciferol), which is formed in the skin on exposure to sunlight and is also found in fish-liver oils. Vitamin D increases the absorption of dietary calcium, maintains proper calcium and phosphorus levels in the blood, and favors mineral metabolism of the teeth and bones. A primary deficiency results from inadequate exposure to sunlight and deficient dietary intake. Secondary deficiencies occur from abnormalities of intestinal resorption. Manifestations of a deficiency include rickets and enamel hypoplasia in infants and children and osteomalacia in adults. (Oral Med.)

v. E (alpha-tocopherol) A vitamin that is an essential dietary factor for a number of animals; however, there is no conclusive evidence that vitamin E is essential in man or is of value in sterility, multiple sclerosis, or heart disease. It is available in most diets. (Oral Med.)

v. G (see **vitamin B₂**)

v. H (biotin) One of the B complex vitamins found in organ meats (e.g., liver, heart, and kidney), egg yolk, cauliflower, chocolate, and mushrooms. Since it is also furnished through synthesis by intestinal bacteria, no human deficiency disease has been established. (Oral Diag.; Oral Med.)

— (see **vitamin Bₓ**)

v. K One of many naphthoquinone compounds with vitamin K activity. Vitamin K₁ is found chiefly in leafy vegetables; K₂ is synthesized by human intestinal bacteria; and K₃ (menadione, N.F.) is a synthetic compound. Vitamin K is essential for the synthesis of prothrombin by the liver. A dietary deficiency of vitamin K is rare, however. The vitmain has been used in conjunction with extensive oral antibiotic therapy, hemorrhagic disease of the newborn, hemorrhage of obstructive jaundice, and sprue, and during anticoagulant therapy. Prothrombin, Stuart factor, Christmas factor, and serum prothrombin conversion accelerator require vitamin K for their synthesis. (Oral Med.)

v. M (see **vitamin B₆**)

v. P.-P. (see **acid, nicotinic**)

vitiate (vĭsh′ē-āt) To weaken; to make void or voidable. (D. Juris.)

vitiligo (vĭt-ĭ-lī′gō) A skin condition characterized by spotty areas of depigmentation. (Oral Diag.)

vitrification (vĭ″trĭ-fĭ-kā′shŭn) The act, instance, art, or process of converting dental porcelain (frit) to a glassy substance; the process of becoming vitreous by heat and fusion. (Fixed Part. Prosth.)

vocal cords (see **cords, vocal**)

voice Sound produced primarily by the vibration of the vocal bands. (Cleft Palate)

void Ineffectual; having no legal or binding effect. (D. Juris.)

volatile (vol′ah-tĭl) Having a tendency to evaporate rapidly. (Anesth.)

v. oil (see **oil, essential**)

volt The unit of electromotive force. It is the unit that is used to measure the tendency of a charge to move from one place to another. The unit of electrical pressure or electromotive force; the force necessary to cause 1 ampere of current to flow against 1 ohm of resistance. (Oral Radiol.)

electron v. The kinetic energy gained by an electron in falling through a potential difference of 1 volt. It is equivalent to 1.6×10^{-12} ergs. Kev and mev refer to one thousand and one million electron-volts, respectively. (Oral Radiol.)

voltage The potential of electromotive force of an electric charge, measured in volts. (Oral Radiol.)

volume Measure of the quantity of a substance, such as air. (Anesth.)

expiratory reserve v. (**reserve air, supplemental air, supplemental v.**) The maximum volume that can be expired from the resting expiratory level. (Anesth.)

v. index of blood (see **blood, volume index of**)

inspiratory reserve v. (**complemental air**) The maximum volume that can be inspired from the end of tidal inspiration. (Anesth.)

packed-cell v. (see **hematocrit**)

residual v. (**residual air**) The volume of air in the lungs at the end of maximal expiration. (Anesth.)

stroke v. (see **stroke volume**)

supplemental v. (see **volume, expiratory reserve**)

tidal v. (**tidal air**) The volume of gas inspired or expired during each respiratory cycle. (Anesth.)

von Recklinghausen's disease of bone (von rĕk'lĭng-how"zĕnz) (see **hyperparathyroidism; osteitis fibrosa cystica, generalized**)

von Recklinghausen's disease of skin (see **neurofibromatosis**)

voucher A receipt or release that may serve as notice of payment of a debt or may prove the accuracy of accounts. (D. Juris.)

vowel A conventional vocal sound in the production of which the speech organs offer little obstruction to the airstream and form a series of resonators above the level of the larynx. (Cleft Palate)

vs. Abbreviation for versus (against); commonly used in legal proceedings, particularly in designating the title of cases. (D. Juris.)

vulcanite (vŭl'kah-nīt") An obsolete denture-base material that may be used for making impression trays. (Comp. Prosth.)

— A combination of caoutchouc and sulfur that hardens in the presence of suitable wet heat and pressure. (Comp. Prosth.; Remov. Part. Prosth.)

— A hard rubber formerly used for denture bases. (D. Mat.)

vulcanization The process of treating crude rubber to improve strength, hardness, etc. Usually consists of heating the rubber with sulfur in the presence of moisture, the sulfur uniting with the rubber to produce saturated double bonds. (D. Mat.)

vulcanize To produce flexible or hard rubber, as desired, by subjecting caoutchouc, in the presence of sulfur, to heat and high steam pressure in a vulcanizer. (Comp. Prosth.; Remov. Part. Prosth.)

W

wages The compensation agreed on by an employer to be paid to an employee hired to do work for him. (D. Juris.)

waiver (wā′ver) Repudiation, abandonment, or surrender of a claim, right, or privilege. (D. Juris.)

wall The outside layer of material surrounding an object or space; a paries.

  cavity w. One of the enclosing sides of a prepared cavity. It takes the name of the surface of the tooth adjoining the surface involved and toward which it is placed. Parts of a surrounding or peripheral wall are the cavosurface angle, the enamel wall, the dentinoenamel junction, and the dentin wall. (Oper. Dent.)

  gingival c. w. The peripheral wall that most closely approximates the apical end of the tooth. (Oper. Dent.)

  peripheral c. w. (see **wall, cavity, surrounding**)

  surrounding c. w. (peripheral c. w.) One of the external, bounding side walls of a cavity; one side forms a part of the cavosurface angle of the preparation. (Oper. Dent.)

  enamel w. The portion of the wall of a prepared cavity that consists of enamel. (Oper. Dent.)

  finish of e. w. The planing of the enamel in finishing a cavity preparation; includes the treatment of the cavosurface angle. (Oper. Dent.)

  incisal w. The wall of a prepared cavity in an anterior tooth that is closest to or in direct relation to the incisal edge of the tooth. (Oper. Dent.)

wandering Mobility of the teeth, a major symptom in periodontal disease; also seen is migration of the teeth, resulting in loss of proximal contact and movement from the arch form. (Periodont.)

  pathologic w. Migration or movement of a tooth or teeth from their normal positions in the dental arch as a result of destructive changes in the principal fiber apparatus of their periodontal membranes, such as those seen in occlusal traumatism, periodontosis, advanced periodontitis, etc. (Periodont.)

Wanscher's mask (vahn′sherz) (see **mask, Wanscher's**)

ward An infant (minor) placed by authority of law under the care of a guardian; the person over whom or over whose property a guardian is appointed by a court. (D. Juris.)

warp Torsional change of shape or outline, such as that which may occur in swaging sheet metal, in denture material, or in other materials exposed to varying temperatures. (Comp. Prosth.; Fixed Part. Prosth.; Remov. Part. Prosth.)

wart (see **verruca vulgaris**)

Warthin's tumor (see **cystadenoma, papillary, lymphomatosum**)

wash, Karo syrup A mixture of Karo syrup in warm water (1 tbs.: ½ glass [4 oz.] warm water) used as a protective soothing rinse in the treatment of inflammatory lesions of the oral mucous membrane. (Periodont.)

Wassermann test (see **test, Wassermann**)

water The transport agent for food and metabolites; regulates temperature and participates in chemical reactions. It is under the very precise control of the central and autonomic nervous systems, which determine the need for water, locate the water, and, with the aid of the hormonal mechanisms, direct the transport and usage of water. (Oral Physiol.)

  w. depletion Loss of water from the tissues before salt is lost, resulting in cellular dehydration while the extracellular fluid level is maintained. The water loss results from lack of water intake, dysphagia, excessive sweating, diabetes insipidus, and diuresis. The symptoms are thirst, dry skin, dry mucous membranes, scanty, highly concentrated urine, high hematocrit concentration, high blood count, and high non-protein nitrogen. Ultimately, death may result from a rise in osmotic pressure in the tissue cells. (Oral Physiol.)

  w. need The amount of water needed to maintain normal metabolism. Water is not stored in the body beyond its physiologic need. The daily obligatory expenditure of water is 1000 ml/day. In addition, the kidney requires 1000 ml to excrete the solids it concentrates. Thus, patients who suffer acute trauma or disease processes require at least 2000 ml of water daily. (Oral Physiol.)

  w. syringe (see **syringe, water**)

water:powder ratio (see **ratio, water:powder**)

Waters extraoral radiographic examination (see **examination, radiographic, extraoral, Waters**)

Waters view (see **examination, radiographic, extraoral, Waters**)

wave, electromagnetic Energy manifested by movements in an advancing series of alternate elevations and depressions. (Oral Radiol.)

wavelength The distance between the peaks of waves in any wave form, such as light, x rays, and other electromotive forms. In electromagnetic radiation, the wavelength is equal to the velocity of light divided by the frequency of the wave. (Oral Radiol.)

  effective w. The wavelength that would produce the same penetration as an average of the various wavelengths in a heterogeneous bundle of x rays. (Oral Radiol.)

wax One of several esters of fatty acids with higher alcohols, usually monohydric alcohols. Dental waxes are combinations of various types of waxes compounded to provide the desired physical properties. (D. Mat.)

— An ester derived from an aliphatic acid and a high molecular weight monobasic alcohol. (Oral Med.; Pharmacol.)

  baseplate w. A hard pink wax used for making occlusion rims and baseplates for occlusion rims. (Comp. Prosth.)

  — A sheet of wax used as a template for the examination of the occlusion. (Periodont.)

  bone w. A plastic mixture that may contain antiseptic and hemostatic drugs, designed for temporary application to freshly cut bone to prevent hemorrhage and infection. (Oral Med.; Pharmacol.)

  boxing w. A soft wax used for boxing impressions. (Comp. Prosth.)

  w. burnout (see **burnout, inlay; wax elimination**)

  carnauba w. (kar-now'bah) A hard, high-melting wax used for the control of the melting range of dental waxes. (D. Mat.)

  casting w. A composition containing various waxes with controlled properties of thermal expansion and contraction; used in making patterns to determine the shape of metal castings. (Comp. Prosth.; Fixed Part. Prosth.; Remov. Part. Prosth.)

  w. elimination (**w. burnout**) The procedure of removing the wax from a wax pattern invested in a mold preparatory to the introduction of another material into the resulting cavity. May be done by dry heat alone or by irrigation with boiling water followed by use of dry heat. (Comp. Prosth.; Oper. Dent.; Remov. Part. Prosth.)

  w. expansion A method of expanding the wax patterns to compensate for the shrinkage of gold during the casting process. (Comp. Prosth.; Fixed Part. Prosth.; Remov. Part. Prosth.)

  fluid w. A series of waxes, each having different physical properties, used for making a correctable impression of the foundation structures that are to support a free-end partial denture (or complete denture) base. The term indicates that the wax is applied in fluid form as required. (Comp. Prosth.; Remov. Part. Prosth.)

  inlay w. Wax used in making patterns for dental restorations. Composed of a variety of waxes. Usually listed as soft, medium, or hard, depending on the melting range and carving characteristics. (D. Mat.)

  w. out (see **blockout**)

  w. pattern (see **pattern, wax**)

  w. template (see **template, wax**)

waxing (waxing up) The contouring of a wax pattern or the wax base of a trial denture into the desired form. (Comp. Prosth.; Fixed Part. Prosth.; Remov. Part. Prosth.)

  functional determinant w. The occlusion determinately derived is functional because the laboratory processing entails constant consultation of all the factors of occlusion that have been put into the articulator setting. (Gnathol.)

wear A loss of substance or a diminishing through use, friction, etc.

  compensatory w. Term sometimes used to designate the mechanical action of the files or reamers in modifying curves in root canals in order to obtain a direct approach to the apex. (Endodont.)

  interproximal w. A loss of tooth substance in contact areas through functional wear and friction, resulting in broadening and flattening of the contacts and a decrease of the mesiodistal dimension of the teeth and of the dentition as a whole. (Oper. Dent.)

  occlusal w. Attritional loss of substance on opposing occlusal units or surfaces. (Comp. Prosth.; Remov. Part. Prosth.) (see also **abrasion**)

  — The morphology of the occlusal surface of a tooth, modified so as to partly or totally eradicate the contour established by the marginal ridges, grooves, and inclined planes. Normal anatomic convexities assume flattened characteristics. (Periodont.)

  abnormal o. w. Wear that exceeds the physiologic wear patterns associated with the attritional effects of food substances; the excessive wear of the teeth occurring as a result of continued afunctional gyrations of the mandible. (Periodont.)

w. pattern (see **pattern, wear**)

physiologic w. Attrition or abrasion of tooth substance occurring as a result of the abrasive consistency of the normal diet, the slight buccolingual movement of the teeth possible in the masticatory process, etc. It does not include the wear produced by habits, occlusal prematurities, etc. (Periodont.)

Weber's disease (see **telangiectasia, hereditary hemorrhagic**)

Weber-Dimitri disease (see **disease, Sturge-Weber-Dimitri**)

Wedelstaedt chisel (věd′el-staht) (see **chisel, Wedelstaedt**)

wedge, step (see **penetrometer**)

wedging Packing or fixing tightly by driving in a wedge or wedges. (Oper. Dent.)

w. effect (see **effect, wedging**)

weekly permissible dose (see **dose, weekly permissible**)

weight The downward pressure due to gravity that is diminished by the centrifugal force caused by the earth's rotation. (Remov. Part. Prosth.)

    maxillary extension base, w. An important factor in the construction of a partial denture, due to the effect of gravity as a dislodging force. (Remov. Part. Prosth.)

    molecular w. (mō-lĕk′ū-lar) The sum of atomic weights of all the atoms in a molecule. (Anesth.)

    rubber dam w. A piece of metal, varying in shape and weight, attached to a clip that is hung on the bottom of a placed rubber dam to increase the tension. (Endodont.)

    — A weight with a component clip that is attached to a lower border of a rubber dam to keep the field of operation clear. (Oper. Dent.)

Weil's disease (vīlz) (see **disease, Weil's**)

welding A process used to join metals. (D. Mat.)

    arc and gas w. (see **welding, fusion**)

    cold w. Property of welding at room temperature, when clean surfaces are pressed into contact. Exhibited to the highest degree by gold in the form of foil or crystals. (Oper. Dent.)

    fusion w. (arc and gas w.) A process in which parts are melted and fused together. (D. Mat.)

pressure w. (resistance w., spot w.) A welding process in which the parts are not melted, although heat is usually required. Recrystallization across the interface occurs. Gold foil is welded by pressure without temperature elevation. (D. Mat.)

w. property The characteristic of certain materials, especially metals, to unite together firmly when subjected to heat and/or pressure in a suitable environment. (Oper. Dent.)

resistance w. (see **welding, pressure**)

spot w. (see **welding, pressure**)

Werlhof's disease (verl′hofs) (see **purpura, thrombocytopenic**)

wet strength (see **strength, wet**)

wetting agent (see **agent, wetting**)

Wharton's duct (see **duct, Wharton's**)

wheal (whēl) Edematous elevation of the skin or mucosa. (Anesth.) (see also **urticaria**)

wheel, Burlew (see **Burlew wheel**)

wheel, lathe (see **stone, lathe**)

wheel stone (see **stone, wheel**)

wheeze A whistling sound made in breathing that is caused by a foreign body in the trachea or bronchus. (Anesth.)

wife A woman united to a man in lawful wedlock; a married woman whose husband is alive and from whom she is not divorced; a spouse. (D. Juris.)

willfully Intentionally; purposefully. (D. Juris.)

Williams' probe (see **probe, Williams'**)

Wilson curve (see **curve of Wilson**)

window, beryllium (see **beryllium window**)

winking, jaw (see **syndrome, Gunn's**)

wire A circular, flexible metal structure.

    alignment w. An arch-shaped wire adjusted to lie across the buccal and labial, or the lingual, surfaces of the teeth. It is attached to molar bands and serves to control the movement of the teeth into desired positions. (Orthodont.)

    arch w. An alignment wire used in orthodontics as a source of force to direct teeth to move in desired directions. According to the shape of its cross section, the wire may be described as ribbon, rectangular, round, etc. (Orthodont.)

    — A wire, usually steel or gold, adapted so as to conform to facial or lingual aspects of the teeth; provides tooth stabilization and/or is used as a basis for orthodontic tooth movement. (Periodont.)

diagnostic w. (see **wire, measuring**)

Kirschner w. A surgical steel wire of heavy gauge with pointed ends; used in the reduction and fixation of bone fragments by being passed through the cancellous portion of the bone and spanning the fracture site. (Oral Surg.)

ligature w. A soft, thin wire used to tie an arch wire to the band attachments. (Orthodont.)

measuring w. (diagnostic w.) A wire or other, similar metal placed in a root canal; made for the purpose of determining the length of the canal. A radiogram is used to make the determination. (Endodont.)

orthodontic w. Stainless steel and wrought gold wire of various dimensions used in orthodontic treatment. (D. Mat.)

Risdon w. (rĭz′don) A wire arch bar tied in the midline. (Oral Surg.)

separating w. Wires threaded interproximally between two adjacent teeth and tightened by twisting the ends together so as to wedge the teeth slightly apart. Used preparatory to adapting bands to teeth having tight contacts with adjacent teeth. (Orthodont.)

wrought w. A wire formed by drawing a cast structure through a die. Used in dentistry for partial denture clasps and orthodontic appliances. (D. Mat.)
— A form of metal resulting from the swaging, rolling, and drawing of a metal ingot into a desired shape and size. (Remov. Part. Prosth.)

wiring An arrangement of a wire or wires.

circumferential w. To maintain mandibular and maxillofacial surgical appliances, the placement of a wire around a bone contiguous to the oral cavity, with the ends exiting in the oral cavity; e.g., circumferential mandibular wiring and circumzygomatic wiring. (Oral Surg.)

continuous loop w. (multiple loop w.) A technique for wiring the teeth for the reduction and fixation of fractures. (Developed by Colonel R. A. Stout, Dental Corps, U. S. Army, and commonly referred to as Stout's method.) (Oral Surg.)

craniofacial suspension w. A method of wiring using areas of bones not contiguous with the oral cavity for the support of fractured jaw segments; e.g., piriform aperture; zygomatic arch; zygomatic process of the frontal bone. (Oral Surg.)

Ivy loop w. A method utilizing a wire around two adjacent teeth, providing a loop useful for fixation of a fracture. (Oral Surg.)

multiple loop w. (see **wiring, continuous loop**)

perialveolar w. (pĕr″ē-ăl-vē′ō-lar) A method of wiring a splint to the maxilla by passing a wire through the bone from the buccal plate to the palate. (Oral Surg.)

piriform aperture w. A method of wiring using that area of the nasal bones for the stabilizing of fractures of the jaws. (Oral Surg.)

witness One who has knowledge of an event; a person whose declaration under oath is received as evidence for any purpose. (D. Juris.)

hostile w. A witness who manifests so much hostility or prejudice under examination (in chief, or direct) that the party who has called him, or his representative, is allowed to cross-examine the witness, i.e., to treat him as though he had been called by the opposite party. (D. Juris.)

w. marks The small hemispheric depressions that may be prepared in the bone surface in lieu of abutment grooves as a guide for seating the abutment posts of the implant. (Oral Implant.)

Wolf's law (see **law, Wolf's**)

work hardening (see **hardening, work**)

work sheet The office form used for a complete planning program for the completion of dental servies. (Pract. Man.)

work simplification The application of the principles of the scientific method to increase the ability to produce without sacrificing quality. (Pract. Man.)

working contact (see **contact, working**)

working occlusal surfaces (see **surface, occlusal, working**)

working occlusion (see **occlusion, working**)

working side The lateral segment of a denture or dentition toward which the mandible is moved. (Comp. Prosth.; Fixed Part. Prosth.; Remov. Part. Prosth.)
— The side of the mouth on which the bolus is being formed. In good mouths first one side and then the other is used to form the bolus. The condyle on that side is called the working side condyle or the rotating condyle. The teeth on that side are called the working teeth. As soon as the side to do the chewing is chosen, its condyle moves upward, backward, and usually outward, and the other condyle is pulled downward, forward, and inward. The motions on the food side turn the bolus over and cock the jaw to bite or crush the bolus in an upward and sagittal direction, which becomes more vertical as the stamp cusps near their fossae in the successive strokes. (Gnathol.)

workload The working activity of an x-ray unit measured in milliampere minutes per week. (Oral Radiol.)

Workmen's Compensation Board of Industrial Commission An administrative body that receives claims for injuries and refers them to certain physicians or dentists for treatment, if indicated, with the express or implied assurance to the claimant that the expense will be defrayed by the employed under the Workmen's Compensation Law. The determination of the Industrial Commission is subject to an appeal to court. The federal agency for these matters is the Bureau of Employees Compensation. (D. Juris.)

wound Any injury that affects either the hard or the soft parts of the body, including bruises, fractures, and contusions. (D. Juris.)

incised w. In medical jurisprudence, a cut or incision on a human body; a wound made by a cutting instrument. (D. Juris.)

writ of execution A writ to implement the judgment or decree of a court; e.g., a contract or a deed. (D. Juris.)

writing Any written or printed paper or document; e.g., a contract or a deed. (D. Juris.)

wrong An injury; a tort; a violation of right or of law; an injustice; a violation of right resulting in damage to another. (D. Juris.)

wrought clasp (wraht) (see **clasp, wrought**)

wrought metal (see **metal, wrought**)

wrought wire (see **wire, wrought**)

X

xanthogranuloma (zăn″thō-grăn″ū-lō′mah) A benign lesion of infancy, usually solitary and composed of lipid-laden histiocytes with varying numbers of Touton giant cells. In the oral cavity the lesion occurs most often on the tongue and regresses spontaneously. (Oral Path.)

xanthoma (zăn-thō′mah) Small yellow nodules, composed of lipid-laden macrophages, which generally occur in subcutaneous tissue. (Oral Path.)

   x. palpebrarum (zăn-thō′mah păl-pĕ-brā′rŭm) (**xanthelasma palpebrarum**) Small yellowish plaques on the eyelids due to accumulation of lipids in reticuloendothelial cells. They are a frequent occurrence in diabetics. (Oral Diag.)

xanthomatosis (zăn″thō-mah-tō′sĭs) A disease characterized by the accumulation of excess lipids. (Oral Diag.) (see also **histiocytosis X**)

X-bite (**cross-bite**) A malrelation of teeth in which the buccal cusps of the mandibular bicuspids and/or molars occlude buccal to the buccal cusps of the maxillary posterior teeth, and/or the maxillary anterior teeth occlude lingual to the mandibular anterior teeth. (Orthodont.)

xerodermosteosis (zē″rō-dĕrm-os″tē-ō′sĭs) (see **syndrome, Sjögren's**)

xerophthalmia (zē″rof-thăl′mē-ah) Dryness of the conjunctiva caused by functional or organic disorders of the lacrimal apparatus. It may be found in vitamin A deficiency or Sjögren's syndrome and may follow chronic conjunctivitis. (Oral Med.)

xerostomia (zē″rō-stō′mē-ah) Dryness of the mouth due to functional or organic disturbances of the salivary glands and lack of the normal secretion. (Oral Diag.; Oral Med.; Oral Surg.) (see also **hyposalivation**)

— Lack of saliva and resultant overgrowth of oral organisms, and frequently a drying of the soft tissues and rampant caries. (Periodont.)

X-linkage (see **linkage, sex**)

x ray Roentgen ray; called x ray by its discoverer because of its enigmatic character. (D. Juris.)

— A type of electromagnetic radiation characterized by wavelengths between approximately 1000 Å and 10⁻⁴ Å, corresponding to photon energies of about 20 ev to 125 mev. They are invisible, penetrative especially at higher photon energies, and travel with the same speed as visible light. They are usually produced by bombarding a target of high atomic number with fast electrons in a high vacuum; they are also emitted as a product of some radioactive disintegrations (specifically originating from the extranuclear part of the atom). X rays were first discovered by Wilhelm C. Roentgen in 1895; hence the term "roentgen rays," often applied to mechanically generated x rays. Roentgen called them x rays after the mathematic symbol "x" for an unknown. (Oral Radiol.)

monochromatic x r. An x ray that has a single wavelength or an extremely narrow band of wavelengths. (Oral Radiol.)

x-ray beam The spatial distribution of radiation emerging from an x-ray generator or source. (Oral Radiol.)

   x. b., central ray The straight line passing through the center of the source and the center of the final beam-limiting diaphragm. (Oral Radiol.)

   x. b., edges The lines joining the center of the anterior face of the source to the diaphragm edges farthest from the source. (Oral Radiol.)

   x. b., field size The geometric projection, on a plane perpendicular to the central ray, of the distal end of the limiting diaphragm as seen from the center of the front surface of the source. The field is thus the same shape as the aperture of the collimator, and it can be defined at any distance from the source. (Oral Radiol.)

   x. b., principal plane A plane that contains the central ray and, in the case of rectangular section beams, is parallel to one side of the rectangle. (Oral Radiol.)

x-ray film, diagnostic A radiograph showing a wire, cone, or instrument in a root canal. The length of the pulp canal is usually determined from this type of radiogram. (Endodont.)

— A film that is sensitive to roentgen rays.

When exposed, it provides evidence of diagnostic value. (Pract. Man.)

x-ray film, full-mouth (see **survey, radiographic**)

x-ray mount (see **mount, x-ray**)

x-ray tube An electronic tube in which x rays can be generated. (Oral Radiol.)

   Coolidge x. t. A vacuum tube in which x rays are generated when the target (integral with the anode) is bombarded by electrons that are emitted from a heated filament (on the cathode) and accelerated toward the anode across a high potential difference. Modern x-ray tubes are of this type. (Oral Radiol.) (see also **tube, Coolidge**)

   Crookes' x. t. A vacuum discharge tube used by Sir William Crookes in early experimental work with cathode rays. Wilhelm C. Roentgen first discovered that in addition to the production of cathode rays, x rays were emitted during the operation of these tubes. (Oral Radiol.) (see also **tube, Crookes'**)

   gas x. t. An early type of x-ray tube in which electrons were derived from residual gases within the tube. (Oral Radiol.) (see also **tube, gas**)

x-ray unit (see **unit, x-ray**)

xylene (zī'lēn) (**xylol**; $C_6H_4(CH_3)_2$; **dimethylbenzene**) A colorless, flammable fluid used as a solvent and clarifying agent in the preparation of tissue sections for microscopic study. (Oral Med.)

xylol (zī'lol) (see **xylene**)

Y

Y axis (see **axis, Y**)

Yankauer's mask (yăn′kow-erz) (see **mask, Yankauer's**)

yaws (frambesia) A disease that is usually non-venereal although its lesions are similar to those of syphilis. The causative agent is *Treponema pertenue*. (Oral Path.)

yield point (see **point, yield**)

yield strength (see **strength, yield**)

yokes Metal clamps with adjustable screws that secure the cylinders to the apparatus or reducing valves. They are equipped with nipples that fit snugly into the inlet socket or part of the cylinder valve. (Anesth.)

Young's modulus (see **elasticity, modulus of**)

Young's rule (see **rule, Young's**)

Z

Z A symbol for atomic number. (Oral Radiol.)

zinc oxide and eugenol (zǐngk ok'sīd ū'jĕ-nol)
Two substances that react chemically to form a relatively hard mass. When modified by certain additives, the material is used for impression pastes, root canal fillings, surgical dressings, temporary filling materials, and cementing media. (D. Mat.; Oral Med.; Pharmacol.)

— A combination used in paste form for making impressions of the basal surface of the oral cavity, which supports the denture base of complete or removable partial dentures. (Comp. Prosth.; Remov. Part. Prosth.)

zinc oxide–eugenol cement (zǐngk ŏk'sīd ū'jĕ-nol) (see **cement, dental, zinc oxide–eugenol**)

zinc phosphate cement (zǐngk fos'fāt) (see **cement, zinc phosphate**)

Zinsser-Engman-Cole syndrome (see **syndrome, Zinsser-Engman-Cole**)

ZnOE Zinc oxide and eugenol. (D. Mat.; Oral Med.; Pharmacol.)

zone A region or area with certain characteristics.

    incubation z. An area or place that provides a favorable environment for the multiplication of microorganisms and is thus conducive to the initiation or perpetuation of a pathologic process; e.g., a gingival flap on a partly erupted third molar may form an area of incubation by providing a cul-de-sac between the tissues and the tooth. (Periodont.)

    neutral z. The potential space between the lips and cheeks on one side and the tongue on the other. Natural or artificial teeth in this zone are subject to equal and opposite forces from the surrounding musculature. (Comp. Prosth.; Remov. Part. Prosth.)

Z-plasty A surgical procedure utilizing the transposition of tissue flaps to ensure the release of contractures, as in ankyloglossia. (Oral Surg.)

zygomaxillare (zī″gō-măks'ĭl-ăr-ē) (see **ridge, key**)

436

APPENDIX*

WEIGHT (MASS)

Troy weight

Grains* (gr)	Pennyweights (dwt)	Ounces (oz t)	Pound (lb t)	SI† equivalent
1	0.041667	0.0020833	—	64.7989 mg
24	1	0.05	0.0041667	1.55517 g
480	20	1	0.083333	31.10348 g
5760	240	12	1	373.2418 g

(1 carat = 3.168 gr = 205.6 mg)

Apothecaries' weight

Grains* (gr)	Scruples (Ə or s ap)	Drams (ʒ or dr ap)	Ounces (℥ or oz ap)	Pound (lb ap)	SI equivalent
1	0.05	0.016667	0.0020833	—	64.7989 mg
20	1	0.33333	0.041667	0.003472	1.295978 g
60	3	1	0.125	0.0104167	3.88794 g
480	24	8	1	0.083333	31.10348 g
5760	288	96	12	1	373.2418 g

Avoirdupois

Grains* (gr)	Drams (dr av)	Ounces (oz av)	Pound (lb av)	SI equivalent
1	0.03657	—	—	64.7989 mg
27.34375	1	0.0625	—	1.771845 g
437.5	16	1	0.0625	28.3495 g
7000	256	16	1	453.5924 g

*Note that the grain has the same mass (0.064798918 g) in each system. Precious metals and their alloys are weighed in troy units, whereas the ordinary items of commerce are weighed in avoirdupois units, when SI units are not used.

†The International System of Units.

---

*Prepared by Duncan McConnell, Ph.D.

LIQUID MEASURE (CAPACITY)

United States system					
Gills (gi)	Pints (pt)	Quarts (qt)	Gallons (gal)	Cubic inches (in³)	SI equivalent*
1	0.25	0.125	0.03125	7.21875	118.292 ml
4	1	0.5	0.125	28.875	0.473167 l
8	2	1	0.25	57.749	0.946333 l
32	8	4	1	231	3.78533 l

(1 gill = 4 ʒ)

Apothecaries' fluid measure				
Minims (min or ♏)	Fluid drams (ʒ or fl dr)	Fluid ounces (℥ or fl oz)	Pints (pt)	SI equivalent*
1	0.016667	0.0020833	—	0.06161 ml
60	1	0.125	—	3.69661 ml
480	8	1	0.0625	29.5729 ml
7680	128	16	1	0.473167 l

1 drop = 1 ♏; 1 teaspoon = 3 ʒ; 1 tablespoon = ½ ℥)

*The International System of Units (SI) does not provide for the use of "liter" for accurate measurements. As used here, 1 liter is the capacity equivalent to a volume of 1000.027 cm³, which is the volume occupied by 1 kg of water at 4° C and 760 mm pressure.

LENGTH

United States system					
Inch (in)	Feet (ft)	Yards (yd)	Rods (rd)	Miles (mi)	SI equivalent
1	0.08333	—	—	—	2.5400 cm
12	1	0.3333	—	—	0.3048 m
36	3	1	0.181818	—	0.9144 m
198	16.5	5.5	1	0.003195	5.0292 m
63,360	5280	1760	320	1	1.60935 km

TEMPERATURE (THERMOMETER SCALES)

	Celsius (C)	Fahrenheit (F)	Kelvin (K)
Freezing point (water)	0°	32°	273°
Boiling point (water)	100°	212°	373°
Body temperature	37°	98.6°	310°
Room temperature	21°	70°	294°

To convert °F to °C: subtract 32°, multiply by 5, and divide by 9.
To convert °C to °F: multiply by 9, divide by 5, and add 32.
To convert to °K: add 273° to Celsius temperature.

INTERNATIONAL SYSTEM (SI)

Of primary interest are the units of mass, length, area, and volume: the kilogram (kg), meter (m), square meter (m²), and cubic meter (m³). (The liter [l] is now defined as 1 dm³ = 10^{-3} m³, and the metric ton [t] at 10^3 kg.) The following prefixes are used to designate some of the principal multiples and decimal fractions:

0.001 m	0.001	0.01	0.1	1	10	100	1000	1000 k
micro	milli	centi	deci	—	deka	hecto	kilo	mega
μ	m	c	d		dk	h	k	M
$\times 10^{-6}$	$\times 10^{-3}$	$\times 10^{-2}$	-10^{-1}	10^0	$\times 10^1$	$\times 10^2$	$\times 10^3$	$\times 10^6$

Certain additional units may be used for length:

1 micrometer (formerly 1 micron) (μm) = 0.001 mm or 1×10^{-6} m
1 nanometer (formerly 1 millimicron) (nm) = 0.001 μm or 1×10^{-9} m
1 angstrom (Å) = 0.1 nm or 1×10^{-8} cm
1 myriameter = 10,000 m

Certain additional units may be used for weight:

1 metric carat = 200 mg = 3.0864712 gr
1 quintal (metric) = 100 kg
1 myriagram = 10,000 g = 10 kg

Useful approximations in terms of common objects or dimensions:

1 centimeter = approx. 0.4 in
Approximately 25 mm = 1 in
1 meter = approx. 39⅓ in
1 kilometer = approx. 0.62 mile
1 United States 5-cent coin weighs approx. 5 g
1 pint of water weighs approx. 475 g or slightly more than 1 lb
1 ounce (avoirdupois) = approx. 28 ⅓ g
1 liter = approx. 34 fl oz or slightly more than 1 qt

MISCELLANEOUS INFORMATION

Specific gravity

Specific gravity is the weight of an object (in grams) in air divided by the weight of an equal volume of water (of density 1). The weight of the equivalent volume of water is equal to the loss of weight when the object is suspended in water (i.e., its displacement). To correct for the departure of the density of water from unity (4° C) the result is divided by 0.998 at 21° C, for example.

Specific gravity (density) values for common materials (at 20° C):

Aluminum	2.70	24K Gold	19.33
Balsa	0.11-0.14	Lead	11.35
Beeswax	0.96-0.97	Mercury	13.55
Bone	1.7-2.0	Platinum	21.37
Brass, bronze	8.45-8.70	Porcelain	2.3-2.5
Copper	8.9	Rubber	0.9-1.1
Dental plastics	1.1-1.3	Silver	10.50
Dental stone	2.3	Steel	7.8
Ebony	1.11-1.33	Wood's metal	10.56
Glass	2.4-5.9	Woods (most)	0.40-0.93

(To convert specific gravity to density expressed in pounds per cubic foot multiply by 62.43.)

Hardness

In addition to the several methods for measuring penetration, resistance to scratching can be expressed in terms of the arbitrary standards of Mohs: 10 diamond, 9 corundum, 8 topaz, 7 quartz, 6 orthoclase, 5 apatite, 4 fluorite, 3 calcite, 2 gypsum, 1 talc. The hardness of crystalline materials will vary with direction; e.g., a diamond will grind (abrade by scratching) another diamond only in certain directions. Hardness of metals is usually expressed in terms of a penetration test, whereas the hardness of brittle materials may be expressed in terms of the Mohs scale of numbers.

Strength

The ultimate tensile strength of metals may be above 320,000 lb/in² for steel or as low as 20,000 lb/in² for gold. In general, metals have moderately high compressive strengths also, but some of them are ductile even at room temperatures (mercury, of course, is a liquid). Inorganic, nonmetallic substances may have high compressive strengths, but their tensile strengths are comparatively low and may be merely 10% of the compressive strength. Plastic materials of the kind used for dentures may have tensile strengths between 4000 and 12,000 lb/in², with compressive strengths slightly higher. (To convert kg/cm² to lb/in² multiply by 14.223.)

Yield strength is more important for most purposes than is the ultimate strength because significant permanent deformation may result when this value has been exceeded. Repeated stresses which approach the yield strength may cause failure through fatigue.

Alloys

Fineness of silver is expressed in parts per thousand by weight, with "sterling" being 925. The amount of gold in an alloy is frequently similarly expressed as "fineness," but an earlier designation still persists. Gold is 24K (carat) when pure, whereas 22K gold contains about 92% by weight, the remainder being silver and copper. Dental gold alloys frequently contain platinum and/or palladium in order to increase the modulus of elasticity, hardness, and melting range as these alloys progress from group I to group III. However, the physical properties of any alloy depend on its previous mechanical and thermal history as well as its composition.

Stainless steels, used extensively in orthodontics, are generally of the 18-8 type, containing approximately 18% chromium and 8% nickel, which impart corrosion resistance. The physical properties, however, depend on the formation of carbides; thus the mechanical and thermal treatment is extremely important with respect to proper utilization of these alloys.

Cobalt-chromium alloys, which may also contain various amounts of nickel, molybdenum, tungsten, and/or manganese, are used for castings. Such "stellites" have excellent corrosion resistance, but the techniques required for fabrication of appliances are more complex than those for gold alloys.

Solder compositions vary widely depending on the intended uses, and solders intended for use on gold alloys are distinctly different from those intended for stainless steels, where electric welding is frequently employed advantageously.

Further information on alloys for use in dentistry can be found in the latest editions of *Skinner's Science of Dental Materials,* by Ralph W. Phillips, and *Restorative Dental Materials,* edited by F. A. Peyton and R. G. Craig, as well as *Guide to Dental Materials and Devices,* published by the American Dental Association.

COMMON NAMES OF CHEMICALS

Common names	Chemical names	Formulas
Acetic ether	Ethyl acetate	$CH_3CO_2C_2H_5$
Alum	Potassium aluminum sulfate	$K_2AL_2(SO_4) \cdot 24H_2O$
Alumina	Aluminum oxide	Al_2O_3
Aniline	Phenyl amine	$C_6H_5NH_2$
Apatite	Calcium phosphate (mineral)	$Ca_{10}(PO_4)_6(F,OH,Cl)_2$
Aqua fortis	Nitric acid	HNO_3
Aqua regia	Mixture of acids	$HNO_3 + 3HCl$
Aspirin	Acetyl salicylic acid	$C_6H_4(CO_2H)(OCOCH_3)$
Baking soda	Sodium bicarbonate	$NaHCO_3$
Bentonite	Impure montmorillonite	(An aluminum silicate mineral)
Benzine	Petroleum distillate	—
Benzol	Benzene	C_6H_6
Bleaching powder	Calcium chlorohypochlorite	$CaOCl_2$
Blue stone } Blue vitriol }	Copper sulfate	$CuSO_4 \cdot 5H_2O$
Bone ash	Impure calcium phosphate	—
Bone mineral	Carbonate hydroxyapatite	—
Boracic acid	Boric acid	H_3BO_3
Borax	Sodium tetraborate	$Na_2B_4O_7 \cdot 10H_2O$
Brimstone	Sulfur	S
Carbolic acid	Phenol	C_6H_5OH
Carborundum	Silicon carbide	SiC
Caustic	Hydroxide of a metal	—
Chalk	Calcium carbonate (natural)	$CaCO_3$
Clove oil	Eugenol (predominately)	$CH_2 \cdot CHCH_2C_6H_3(OCH_3)OH$
Corundum	Aluminum oxide	Al_2O_3
Dental plaster } Dental stone }	Calcium sulfate hemihydrate	$CaSO_4 \cdot \frac{1}{2}H_2O$
Emery powder	Impure aluminum oxide	Al_2O_3
Epsom salt	Magnesium sulfate	$MgSO_4 \cdot 7H_2O$
Feldspar	Aluminum silicate mineral	—
Fluorspar	Fluorite (calcium fluoride)	CaF_2
Fusel oil	Mixed amyl alcohols	$C_5H_{11}OH$
Gypsum	Natural calcium sulfate	$CaSO_4 \cdot 2H_2O$
Hydrocal	(Trade name)	$CaSO_4 \cdot \frac{1}{2}H_2O$
Hypo	Sodium thiosulfate	$Na_2S_2O_3 \cdot 5H_2O$
Kaolin	Kaolinite (mineral)	Hydrated aluminum silicate
Kieselguhr	Siliceous earth	SiO_2
Lanolin	Cholesterol	$C_{27}H_{46}O$
Lime	Calcium oxide	CaO
Limestone	Impure calcium carbonate	$CaCO_3$
Litharge	Lead monoxide	PbO
Lysol	(Trade name)	Solution containing cresol
Marble	Crystallized limestone	$CaCO_3$
Milk of lime	Solution of calcium hydroxide	$Ca(OH)_2$
Molybdenite	Molybdenum sulfide (mineral)	MoS_2
Muriatic acid	Hydrochloric acid	HCl
Naphtha (petroleum)	Petroleum distillate	—
Naphtha (solvent)	Coal tar distillate	—
Niter	Potassium nitrate	KNO_3
Oil of vitriol	Sulfuric acid	H_2SO_4
Plaster of paris	Calcium sulfate hemihydrate	$CaSO_4 \cdot \frac{1}{2}H_2O$

COMMON NAMES OF CHEMICALS—cont'd

Common names	Chemical names	Formulas
Plumbago	Graphite (mineral)	C
Pumice powder	Crushed volcanic glass	—
Putty	Mixture of whiting and oil	—
Putty powder	Impure stannic oxide	SnO_2
Quartz	Silicon dioxide (natural)	SiO_2
Rochelle salt	Potassium sodium tartrate	$KNaC_4H_4O_6 \cdot 4H_2O$
Rock salt	Sodium chloride	$NaCl$
Rouge	Ferric oxide (hematite)	Fe_2O_3
Silica	Silicon dioxide	SiO_2
Soda (washing)	Sodium carbonate	Na_2CO_3
Sugar of lead	Lead acetate	$Pb(C_2H_3O_2)_2 \cdot 3H_2O$
Talc	Hydrated magnesium silicate (mineral)	—
Toluol	Toluene	$C_6H_5CH_3$
Washing soda	Sodium carbonate	Na_2CO_3
Water glass	Solution of sodium silicate	—
Whiting	Calcium carbonate	$CaCO_3$
Wood alcohol	Methanol	CH_3OH
Wood's metal	Alloy of 50Bi, 25Pb, 12.5Sn, 12.5 Cd	
Zinc white	Zinc oxide	ZnO